THE ADRENAL GLAND

CURRENT ENDOCRINOLOGY: BASIC AND CLINICAL ASPECTS
Louis V. Avioli, *Series Editor-in-Chief*

TITLES IN **CURRENT ENDOCRINOLOGY**

ENDOCRINE CONTROL OF GROWTH
William H. Daughaday, *Editor-in-Chief*

GLUCAGON
Roger H. Unger and Lelio Orci, *Editors-in-Chief*

PROLACTIN
Robert B. Jaffe, *Editor-in-Chief*

ENDOCRINE ASPECTS OF AGING
Stanley G. Korenman, *Editor-in-Chief*

PROSTAGLANDINS
James B. Lee, *Editor-in-chief*

CLINICAL REPRODUCTIVE NEUROENDOCRINOLOGY
Judith L. Vaitukaitis, *Editor-in-Chief*

THE PINEAL GLAND
Richard Relkin, *Editor-in-Chief*

THE ADRENAL GLAND
Patrick J. Mulrow, *Editor-in-Chief*

THE ADRENAL GLAND

Edited by

Patrick J. Mulrow, M.D.
Professor and Chairman
Department of Internal Medicine
Medical College of Ohio
Toledo, Ohio

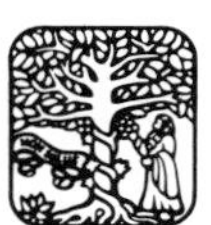

ELSEVIER
New York • Amsterdam • Oxford

Elsevier Science Publishing Co., Inc.
52 Vanderbilt Avenue, New York, New York 10017

Sole distributors outside the United States and Canada:

Elsevier Science Publishers B.V.
P.O. Box 211, 1000 AE Amsterdam. The Netherlands

Library of Congress Cataloging in Publication Data

Main entry under title:

The Adrenal gland.

(Current endocrinology)
Includes bibliographies and index.
1. Adrenal gland—Diseases. 2. Adrenal gland.
3. Adrenocortical hormones—Physiological effect.
I. Mulrow, Patrick J. (Patrick Joseph), 1926–
II. Series. [DNLM: 1. Adrenal Gland Diseases.
2. Adrenal Glands. WK 700 A2421]
RC659.A37 1985 616.4′5 85-20448
ISBN 0-444-00862-4

Current printing (last digit):
10 9 8 7 6 5 4 3 2 1

Manufactured in the United States of America

CONTENTS

Foreword xi
Preface xiii
Contributors xv

ADRENAL MEDULLA 1
Jerome A. Levin, Ph.D.

Introduction 1
Synthesis of Catecholamines 2
Transport of Tyrosine into Adrenal Medullary Cells 4
Tyrosine Hydroxylase 5
Aromatic-L-amino Acid Decarboxylase 6
Dopamine-β-Hydroxylase 6
Phenylethanolamine-N-methyl Transferase 8
Regulation of Catecholamine Synthesis 10
Storage of Catecholamines in the Adrenal Medulla 13
Chromaffin Granule Membrane 13
Chromaffin Granule Matrix 16
Catecholamine Storage Complex 21
Release of Catecholamines 23
References 32

SELECTED MORPHOLOGICAL ASPECTS OF HUMAN SUPRARENAL GLANDS 45
Richard A. Yeasting, Ph.D.

Introduction 45
Gross Anatomy 46

Microscopic Anatomy 49
Anatomic–Physiologic Correlations 56
Developmental Anatomy 59
References 62

ADRENAL STEROID BIOSYNTHESIS AND METABOLISM 65
John P. Rapp, D.V.M., Ph.D.
Biosynthesis of Adrenal Steroids 65
Electron Transport and Steroid Hydroxylation in Adrenal Cortical Mitochondria 66
Cholesterol Side Chain Cleavage 68
Conversions from Pregnenolone 69
21-Hydroxylation 71
11β- and 18-Hydroxylase System 72
Formation of Aldosterone 73
Formation of Androgens and Estrogens 74
Metabolism of Adrenal Steroids 74
Metabolism of Cortisol 75
Metabolism of Aldosterone 77
References 78

METABOLIC AND PHARMACOLOGIC ACTIONS OF GLUCOCORTICOIDS 85
Richard P. McPartland, Ph.D.
Introduction 85
Effects of Adrenocorticoid Deficiency 86
Effects of Glucocorticoids on Glucose Metabolism 87
Effects of Glucocorticoids on Glucose Uptake 89
Actions of Glucocorticoids on Lipid Mobilization and Glucose Metabolism in Adipose Tissue 90
Effects of Glucocorticoids on Protein Metabolism 93
Biochemical Changes in Target Tissues 94
Lymphoid Tissues 94
Glucocorticoid Effects on the Liver 97
Glucocorticoid Effects on Muscle 100
Glucocorticoid Effects on the Lung 100
Glucocorticoid Effects on Vascular Tissues 101
Glucocorticoid Effects on the Heart 102
Glucocorticoids as Antiinflammatory Agents and Immunosuppressive Agents 103
Glucocorticoid Effects on the Pituitary 105
Glucocorticoid Effects on Bone 107
Conclusions 108
References 108

CONTROL MECHANISMS IN THE PITUITARY–ADRENAL SYSTEM 117
Murray Saffran, Ph.D.
Introduction 117
Neural Events 118
Neurohormones 119
ACTH 123
Adrenal ACTH Receptor 125
Adrenocortical Membrane 128
Phospholipids 129
Prostaglandins 132
Calcium Ions 132

Cyclic Nucleotides 134
"Labile Protein" 136
Which Reaction in Steroid Biosynthesis Is Stimulated? 139
Ascorbic Acid 142
Feedback Control 143
Summary 145
References 145

CONTROL OF ADRENAL SECRETION OF MINERALOCORTICOIDS 153
S.Y. Tan, M.D.
The Renin-Angiotensin System 153
Potassium 158
ACTH 159
Other Factors 160
Sodium 160
Central Nervous System 160
Miscellaneous 161
References 162

RECEPTORS FOR HORMONES OF THE ADRENAL CORTEX 169
Judith Saffran, Ph.D.
Introduction 169
Distribution of Glucocorticoid Receptors in Various Tissues 170
Mineralocorticoid Receptors 175
Properties of Glucocorticoid Receptors 176
Activation or Transformation of Glucocorticoid Receptors 178
Nuclear Binding 181
Multiple Receptor Forms 183
Membrane Receptors 184
Regulation of Receptor Concentrations in Vivo 185
Correlation of Physiologic Activity with Receptors 187
Ontogeny of Receptors 187
Structure-Activity Relationships 189
Receptors and Disease States 190
Summary 190
References 191

EFFECT OF ADRENAL HORMONES ON WATER AND ELECTROLYTE METABOLISM 201
Paul H. Brand, Ph.D., and James T. Higgins, Jr., M.D.
Introduction 201
Cellular Action of Mineralocorticoid Hormones 202
Aldosterone Binding and Cell Response 202
Physiologic Role of the Aldosterone-Induced Proteins 207
Aldosterone Effect on Energy Generation 211
Adrenocorticoid Action at the Organ Level 214
Na^+ and K^+ Transport in the Urinary Tract 214
Renal H^+ Secretion 219
Glucocorticoids and Glomerular Filtration Rate 224
Adrenocorticoids and Water Balance 224
Adrenocorticoids and the Colon 227
Clinical Disorders of Water and Electrolyte Metabolism Caused by Adrenocorticoid Hormone Abnormalities 230

Adrenocortical Hormone Insufficiency 230
Adrenocortical Hormone Excess 233
Summary and Conclusions 237
References 238

DISEASES OF THE ADRENAL CORTEX 247
Roberto Franco-Saenz, M.D.
Cushing's Syndrome 247
Definition and Historical Perspective 247
Classification and Pathogenesis 248
Clinical Manifestations 257
Diagnosis 261
Screening Tests 261
Diagnostic Tests 264
Differential Diagnosis of Cushing's Syndrome 265
Other Tests 268
Treatment 274
Course and Prognosis 279
Complications of Therapy 280
Virilizing Tumors of the Adrenal 281
Suppression and Stimulation Test 282
Feminizing Tumors of the Adrenal 283
Hypofunction of the Adrenal Cortex 284
Definition and Historical Perspective 284
Classification 284
Primary Adrenocortical Insufficiency, or Addison's Disease 285
Clinical Manifestations and Pathophysiology 292
Laboratory Findings 294
Diagnosis of Addison's Disease 295
Test Used for the Differential Diagnosis of Adrenal Insufficiency 297
Therapy 298
Course and Prognosis 300
Secondary Adrenocortical Insufficiency 300
Acute Adrenocortical Insufficiency 302
References 302

DISEASES OF HYPER- AND HYPOMINERALOCORTICOID PRODUCTION 325
S.Y. Tan, M.D.
Hypermineralocorticoidism 325
Primary Aldosteronism: Incidence and Clinical Manifestations 325
Diagnosis 327
Forms of Primary Aldosteronism 328
Differential Diagnosis 330
Treatment of Primary Aldosteronism 333
Low Renin Hypertension: A Mineralocorticoid Excess Syndrome? 334
Secondary Aldosteronism 336
Aldosterone During the Menstrual Cycle and in Pregnancy 336
Secondary Aldosteronism with Edema 340
Secondary Aldosteronism without Edema 344
Hypomineralocorticoidism 346
Adrenal Insufficiency 346
Selective Hypoaldosteronism 346
Congenital Adrenal Hyperplasia 349
Pseudohypoaldosteronism 350
References 350

CONGENITAL ADRENAL HYPERPLASIA 363
Paul V. DeLamater, M.D.
History 363
Genetics 364
Clinical Presentation and Diagnosis 365
21-Hydroxylase Deficiency, Simple Virilized 365
21-Hydroxylase Deficiency, Salt-Wasting, and Virilizing 367
11-β-Hydroxylase Deficiency 369
3-β-Hydroxysteroid Dehydrogenase Deficiency 370
17-α-Hydroxylase Deficiency 370
Cholesterol Desmolase Deficiency 371
18-Hydroxylase Deficiency 371
18-Dehydrogenase Deficiency 372
Dexamethasone-Suppressible Hyperaldosteronism 372
Acquired 21-Hydroxylase Deficiency, Partial 11- and 21-Hydroxylase Deficiency 373
Treatment 373
Hormonal Treatment 373
Surgical Treatment 375
Psychological Treatment 376
References 376

PHEOCHROMOCYTOMA 383
David Juan, M.D.
Introduction 383
History 384
Incidence 384
Etiology 385
Pathology 386
Embryology and Apudomas 386
Location, Weight, and Size 387
Gross, Histological, and Ultrastructural Features 387
Clinical Manifestations 390
Signs and Symptoms 390
Catecholamine Cardiomyopathy and Electrocardiographic Change 394
Pheochromocytoma in Pregnancy 395
Pheochromocytoma in Children 396
Pheochromocytoma of the Bladder 397
Familial Pheochromocytoma and MEN Syndromes 398
Malignant Pheochromocytoma 400
Neuroectodermal Dysplasias and Other Associated Diseases 402
Drug-Induced Hypertensive Crises 403
Diagnosis 404
Plasma Catecholamines 407
Provocative Tests: Physical and Chemical 409
Other Laboratory Abnormalities 411
Preoperative Localization: Noninvasive vs. Invasive Procedures 411
Treatment: Medical and Surgical 414
Surgery of Pheochromocytoma 417
Summary 420
References 422

Index 433

FOREWORD

Although endocrinology textbooks satisfy a fundamental educational need and are routinely used as reference standards, an information gap often exists between the current state of the art and the published contents. Refinements in laboratory methods and assay techniques, the ever increasing awareness of metabolic and endocrine correlates that were once unapparent, and the dramatic discoveries in molecular biology and genetics make it extremely difficult to present an up-to-date volume at time of publication. The endocrinology textbook may effectively serve the academic community only for 3–5 years.

Despite the constant change in the state of the art, new discoveries defining relationships between endocrinology and molecular biology, physiology, genetics, biochemistry, biophysics, and immunology do not proceed at comparable rates.In fact, certain areas of endocrinology have been dormant for years.

In an attempt to offer timely reviews, a number of well-established authorities were offered the challenge of editing small editions that characterize the state of the art in *specific* areas of endocrinology. This format relieves the editor (or editors) from the nearly impossible task of producing a "current textbook" of endocrinology and facilitates the process of rapid and timely revision. Moreover, a specific endocrine discipline review can be revised if and when necessary without revising an entire textbook.

Endocrine Control of Growth, edited by W. Daughaday, was the first review in this series, *Current Endocrinology: Basic and Clinical Aspects.* This has been followed by individual texts on *Glucagon, Prostaglandins, Prolactin, Clinical Reproductive Neuroendocrinology, Endocrine Aspects of Aging,* and *The Pineal Gland.* The series presents those current aspects of endocrinology of interest to the basic scientist, clinician, house officer, trainee, and medical student alike. These initial volumes will be followed by others on *Thyroid, Posterior Pituitary, Biochemical Action of Steroid Hormones, Disorders of the Parathyroid Gland,* and *Gastrointestinal Hormones.* We are confident that this complete series and its revised editions, when appropriate, will serve the academic community well.

Louis V. Avioli, M.D.

PREFACE

In 1855, Addison attributed a life-maintaining role to the adrenal cortex but nearly 70 years elapsed before this concept was generally accepted. It was not until the early 1930s that systematic investigation of the role of the adrenal cortex in both glucose and salt and water metabolism began in earnest. The isolation and chemical characterization of the many adrenal steroids and of ACTH formed the basis for major discoveries in the biochemical, physiological, and clinical functions of the adrenal cortex. Practically every tisue in the body is affected by the action of these hormones and numerous diseases are associated with malfunction of the adrenal cortex. The main thrust of today's research is to understand the molecular basis by which steroids alter gene function. With advances in this field, the clinician-scientist will surely recognize new diseases.

The adrenal gland is composed of more than the adrenal cortex. In it center lies the adrenal medulla, the body's "stress" gland. The two major products of the adrenal medulla, norepinephrine and epinephrine, have been the subject of numerous investigations for many decades. Although the medulla is not necessary to maintain life, it makes important contributions to glucose metabolism and blood pressure control, especially under conditions of stress. The adrenal medulla is famous to clinicians for one of its tumors: pheochromocytoma.

As you will see, the adrenal gland is a marvelous endocrine organ. It is really several separate, yet interrelated endocrine systems. The zona glomerulosa has a control mechanism and function separate from the zona fasciculata, and the zona reticularis may well have a control mechanism and function different from the zona fasciculata, the major source of glucocorticoid secretion. The adrenal cortex is wrapped around the medulla, a catecholamine-secreting organ. We still are not sure why these two glands are so closely related anatomically.

This book on the adrenal gland attempts to describe the basic biochemical and physioloigical aspects of the gland and then apply these concepts to the understanding of the diseases of the adrenal gland. The book may serve to broaden the horizons of the scientist investigating a limited area and serve as a resource for the student and clinician who wishes a detailed description of diseases related to the adrenal gland and a knowledge of the basic mechanisms involved in the disease process.

Patrick J. Mulrow, M.D.

CONTRIBUTORS

PAUL H. BRAND, Ph.D.
Department of Physiology, Medical College of Ohio, Toledo, Ohio

PAUL V. DeLAMATER, M.D.
Associate Professor, Department of Pediatrics, Medical College of Ohio, Toledo, Ohio; Mercy Hospital, Toledo, Ohio

ROBERTO FRANCO-SAENZ, M.D.
Professor of Medicine, Chief, Division of Endocrinology and Metabolism, Medical College of Ohio, Toledo, Ohio

JAMES T. HIGGINS, JR., M.D.
Department of Medicine, Medical College of Ohio, Toledo, Ohio

DAVID JUAN, M.D.
Clinical Pharmacy Center, Department of Medicine, Northwestern University Medical School, Chicago, Illinois, formerly Department of Medicine, Medical College of Ohio, Toledo, Ohio

JEROME A. LEVIN, Ph.D.
Department of Pharmacology, Medical College of Ohio, Toledo, Ohio

RICHARD R. McPARTLAND, Ph.D.
Program Director, Bacterial Disease Diagnostics, Wampole Laboratories, Half Acre Road, Cranbury, New Jersey, formerly Department of Medicine, Medical College of Ohio, Toledo, Ohio

JOHN P. RAPP, D.V.M., Ph.D.
Professor, Departments of Medicine and Pathology, Medical College of Ohio, Toledo, Ohio

JUDITH SAFFRAN, Ph.D
Departments of Biochemistry and Pathology, Medical College of Ohio, Toledo, Ohio

MURRAY SAFFRAN, Ph.D.
Department of Biochemistry, Medical College of Ohio, Toledo, Ohio

S.Y. TAN, M.D.
Associate Professor, Department of Medicine, University of Hawaii, John A. Burns School of Medicine, Honolulu, Hawaii, formerly Department of Medicine, Medical College of Ohio, Toledo, Ohio

RICHARD A. YEASTING, Ph.D.
Associate Professor of Anatomy, Department of Anatomy, Medical College of Ohio, Toledo, Ohio

JEROME A. LEVIN, Ph.D.

ADRENAL MEDULLA

INTRODUCTION

The central core of the adrenal gland, the adrenal medulla, is an endocrine gland separate from the adrenal cortex. The two portions of the adrenal gland differ in many important ways—their anatomical arrangement, the chemical nature of the hormones they secrete, the effects of these hormones, the fact that the adrenal medulla is innervated, etc. However, there are a few important similarities and interrelationships that exist between the adrenal cortex and medulla. First, it appears that the adrenal medulla receives a portal circulation from the cortex (47), although this has recently been disputed (48). Second, glucocorticoids released from the adrenal cortex can influence the synthesis of catecholamines, which are the hormones of the adrenal medulla. The presence of a portal circulation, therefore, takes on great significance by providing a mechanism for the exposure of the adrenal medulla to very high concentrations of adrenal cortical hormones. Last, both the glucocorticoids and the catecholamines (epinephrine and norepinephrine) are important for adaptation of the organism to stressful perturbations of homeostasis.

This chapter will focus primarily on the synthesis, storage, and release

From the Department of Pharmacology, Medical College of Ohio, Toledo, Ohio.

of catecholamines from the adrenal medulla. The effects produced by catecholamines and the mechanisms of their inactivation will not be considered here since these processes occur outside of the adrenal medulla. The reader is referred to other sources for a consideration of these latter topics (15,47,86,139,165,196,212,228).

SYNTHESIS OF CATECHOLAMINES

The currently accepted scheme of the synthesis of catecholamines was suggested by Blaschko in 1939 (26). This metabolic pathway is illustrated in Figure 1 and summarized diagrammatically in Figure 2. Although tyrosine can be formed from phenylalanine, tyrosine will be treated as the beginning of the pathway because tyrosine is a normal dietary constituent

FIGURE 1. Metabolic pathway for the synthesis of catecholamines.

HO-C_6H_4-CH_2-CH(COOH)-NH_2
Tyrosine

↓ Tyrosine Hydroxylase

(HO)$_2$-C_6H_3-CH_2-CH(COOH)-NH_2
3,4-Dihydroxy phenyl alanine (DOPA)

↓ L-Aromatic amino acid decarboxylase

(HO)$_2$-C_6H_3-CH_2-CH_2-NH_2
3,4-Dihydroxy phenyl ethylamine (Dopamine)

↓ Dopamine β-hydroxylase

(HO)$_2$-C_6H_3-CH(OH)-CH_2-NH_2
Norepinephrine

↓ Phenethanolamine N-methyl transferase

(HO)$_2$-C_6H_3-CH(OH)-CH_2-NH-CH_3
Epinephrine

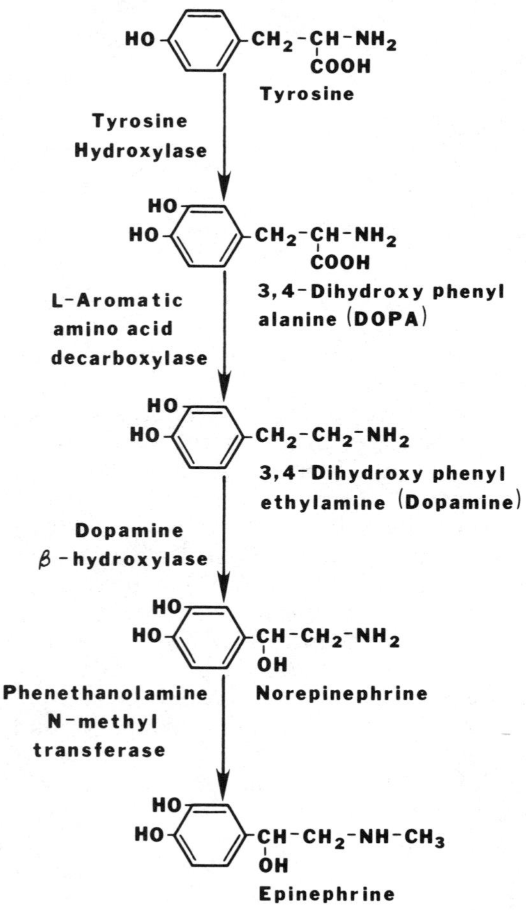

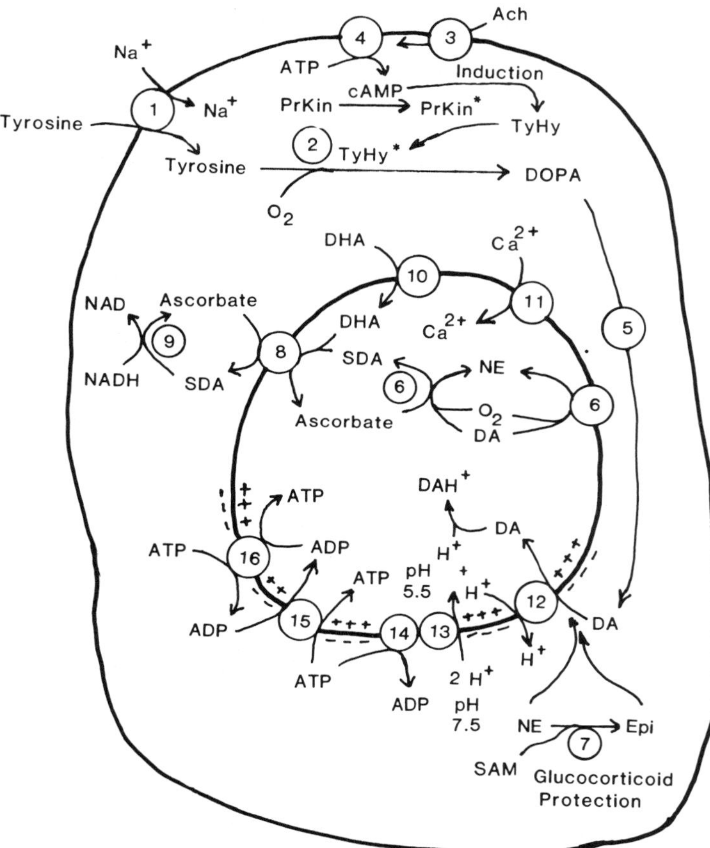

FIGURE 2. Diagram of the synthesis and accumulation of catecholamines in the adrenal medulla. Diagram of a single chromaffin cell containing a single large chromaffin granule (other cellular constituents were omitted; chromaffin cells actually contain numerous small granules). The upper portion of the diagram illustrates synthesis and the lower portion illustrates accumulation of catecholamines. Numbered items represent unique proteins: *1*—neutral amino acid transporter; *2*—tyrosine hydroxylase plus tetrahydrobiopterin; *3*—nicotinic cholinergic receptor; *4*—adenylate cyclase; *5*—aromatic amino acid decarboxylase plus pyridoxal phosphate; *6*—dopamine β-hydroxylase; *7*-phenethanolamine N-methyl transferase; *8*—cytochrome b-561; *9*—semidehydroascorbate reductase; *10*—dehydroascorbate entry (probably by a passive mechanism); *11*—calcium transporter; *12*—catecholamine transporter; *13*—proton transporter; *14*—magnesium adenosine triphosphatase; *15*—nucleotide transporter; *16*—phosphoryl group transferring enzyme.

Abbreviations used in the diagram are as follows: ACH—acetylcholine, ADP—adenosine diphosphate; ATP—adenosine triphosphate, cAMP—cyclic adenosine-3′,5′-monophosphate; DA—dopamine; DOPA—dihydroxyphenylalanine; Epi—epinephrine; NAD—nicotinamide adenine dinucleotide; NADH—reduced NAD; NE—norepinephrine; Pr Kin—protein kinase; * indicates activated form; SAM—S-adenosylmethionine; and TyHy— tyrosine hydroxylase; * indicates activated form.

and most of the control of catecholamine synthesis occurs at the conversion of tyrosine to dihydroxyphenylalanine (see below). A more detailed discussion of the synthesis of catecholamines can be found elsewhere in the literature (108,142,207).

Transport of Tyrosine into Adrenal Medullary Cells

The first step in the synthesis of catecholamines is not a metabolic transformation, but rather the uptake of the precursor, tyrosine, into the adrenal medullary cells (#1 in Figure 2). Although there do not appear to be reports in the literature dealing with the uptake of tyrosine by the adrenal medulla, there are studies of the uptake of tyrosine by neuronal tissue. These studies indicate that the transport of tyrosine into nerve tissue is a carrier-mediated facilitated diffusion which most resembles the L-system (leucine-preferring) for neutral amino acids described by Christensen (40). This transport system is not energy-dependent; it is sensitive to sulfhydryl reagents and is inhibited by some structural analogs of tyrosine; it is independent of chloride concentration, and is slightly inhibited by a decrease in the extracellular sodium or potassium concentration (10,33,115,182). Archer et al. (10) studied the uptake of tyrosine (and phenylalanine) in three clones of neuroblastoma which differed in the neurotransmitters that they synthesized: one synthesized primarily catecholamines, the second synthesized primarily serotonin, and the third synthesized large amounts of acetylcholine (ACH). They found that the uptake of tyrosine was similar in all three clones with respect to kinetics and the effects of metabolic inhibitors and sodium deprivation.

Bruinvels (32,33) demonstrated an interesting effect of sodium on the uptake of tyrosine by rat brain synaptosomes. When the concentration of sodium in the incubation medium was reduced to 25%−50% of control, there was a modest decrease in the uptake of tyrosine by the synaptosomes. However, in a sodium-free medium, the accumulation of tyrosine was increased. In contrast, the accumulation of norepinephrine (NE) was markedly suppressed in a sodium-deficient or sodium-free medium as reported by other investigators (233). Bruinvels (32,33) suggested that the increase in tyrosine uptake in the absence of sodium could lead to an increase in catecholamine synthesis in response to increased nerve discharge. An increase in nerve activity would be expected to decrease the concentration of sodium in the extracellular fluid immediately adjacent to the nerve terminal due to the influx of sodium associated with the nerve-action potential. It is questionable, however, whether the concentration of sodium, even in this superficial layer of extracellular fluid, would decrease to an essentially sodium-free state during nerve activity. It has also been suggested that tyrosine uptake is controlled by cyclic nucleotides since tyrosine accumulation in neuroblastoma was increased by analogs of cyclic AMP (cAMP) (232).

Etiologically, it does not seem reasonable to control catecholamine synthesis at the level of tyrosine uptake, since control at this level would nonselectively affect all of the metabolic pathways in which tyrosine participates. For example, in the whole vas deferens (229) and in neuroblastoma cultures (232), considerably more of the accumulated tyrosine is incorporated into protein than is converted to catecholamines. In tissues such as the vas deferens, this may be due to the large mass of non-neuronal tissue (e.g., smooth muscle) which would synthesize protein but not catecholamines. Therefore, experiments were performed to measure the incorporation of ^{3}H-tyrosine into protein and catecholamines in the isolated adventitia of the rabbit aorta. The isolated adventitia contains the adrenergic nerve terminals of the aorta but very few non-neuronal elements (128). The incorporation of ^{3}H-tyrosine into protein and catecholamines was measured by standard techniques (229). We found that only 0.3% of the total tyrosine taken up by the adventitia was converted to catecholamines, whereas 5% of the tyrosine accumulated (almost 17 times more) was incorporated into protein. The remainder was present as free tyrosine. Therefore changes in tyrosine uptake would probably affect the synthesis of proteins as well as catecholamines.

Tyrosine Hydroxylase

Tyrosine hydroxylase (tyrosine-3-monooxygenase, EC 1.14.13.a) catalyzes the following reaction (199):

$$\text{L-tyrosine} + \text{tetrahydrobiopterin} + 0_2 \longrightarrow$$
$$\text{3,4-dihydroxyphenylalanine (DOPA)} + \text{quinoid dihydrobiopterin} + H_20.$$

Tyrosine hydroxylase (# 2 in Fig. 2) is the rate-limiting enzyme in catecholamine synthesis (129). Since this reaction represents the first committed step in the synthesis of catecholamines, it is logical that most of the control of catecholamine synthesis is exercised here (see below). As indicated above, tyrosine hydroxylase requires a reduced pterin cofactor. Many properties of the enzyme are influenced by the nature of the cofactor used in the assay. In general, the affinity of the enzyme for both substrates and inhibitors is higher with tetrahydrobiopterin than with synthetic cofactors (105). Tyrosine hydroxylase is an iron-containing enzyme. The iron is quite tightly bound to the enzyme and cannot be removed by iron chelators (95).

There has been considerable controversy over whether tyrosine hydroxylase is a soluble or particulate enzyme. The distribution of tyrosine hydroxylase between the soluble and particulate fractions is influenced by the nature of the buffer used to homogenize the tissue (119,152). Particulate tyrosine hydroxylase can be solubilized by treatment with trypsin to yield an enzyme with a molecular weight of 34,000 (199). Some of the enzyme in tissue homogenates also exists in this low molecular-weight form. The significance of higher molecular weight aggregates and particulate forms of the enzyme is questionable, since tyrosine hydroxylase interacts with polyanions (95,104,146) and the chromaffin granule membrane contains large numbers of anionic groups (19,138, 235). Moreover, high molecular-weight aggregates of tyrosine hydroxylase contain large amounts of nucleic acids and low molecular-weight forms of the enzyme do not form aggregates when reexposed to the same conditions used to isolate the enzyme from the tissue (220). All of this evidence tends to support the concept that tyrosine hydroxylase is normally a soluble enzyme.

Neither tyramine, m-tyrosine, nor D-p-tyrosine are substrates for tyrosine hydroxylase (154). However, phenylalanine is hydroxylated especially when tetrahydrobiopterin serves as the cofactor (199). There are at least three classes of tyrosine hydroxylase inhibitors: 1) substituted tyrosine analogs such as alpha-methyltyrosine and halogenated tyrosine derivatives; 2) iron chelators such as alpha-dipyridyl and o-phenanthroline; and 3) catechol compounds, such as the catecholamines, 4-isopropyltropolone, and 3,4-dihydroxyphenylacetamide, which compete with the pterin cofactor (142).

Aromatic-L-amino Acid Decarboxylase

This enzyme (EC 4.1.1.26) catalyzes the decarboxylation of dihydroxyphenylalanine (DOPA) to dopamine and was originally called DOPA decarboxylase. However, this same enzyme also catalyzes the decarboxylation of tryptophan, 5-hydroxy-tryptophan, m- and p-tyrosine, histidine, and alpha-methyldopa (55,142). Therefore, aromatic-L-amino acid decarboxylase (AAAD) (#5 in Figure 2) is a more accurate name and reflects the substrate specificity of this enzyme.

The enzyme AAAD is soluble, with a molecular weight of about 110,000. It appears to be composed of three subunits of different molecular weights. Pyridoxal phosphate is the cofactor for AAAD and 1 mole of pyridoxal phosphate is tightly bound to each mole of enzyme as a Schiff base (55,142).

Many inhibitors of AAAD have been developed. Initially, it was hoped that these drugs would be useful therapeutically as inhibitors of catecholamine synthesis. However, AAAD is so widespread throughout the body and present at such a high level of activity compared to tyrosine hydroxylase, that it is not practical to inhibit catecholamine synthesis by inhibiting AAAD. Many of the inhibitors of AAAD are simple analogs of DOPA, such as alpha-methyldopa, which is actually a competitive substrate for the enzyme. Other classes of AAAD inhibitors include: hydrazine acids, hydrazines, and benzyloxyamines (55,142,206). Diarman et al. (56) isolated and partially characterized a specific endogenous inhibitor of AAAD from the rat submaxillary gland. The significance of this inhibitor is unknown.

Dopamine-β-Hydroxylase

The third step in the synthesis of catecholamines is the beta-hydroxylation of dopamine (DA) to form norepinephrine (NE) (#6 in Figure 2). This reaction is catalyzed by dopamine-β-hydroxylase (3,4-dihydroxyphenylalanine, ascorbate: oxygen oxidoreductase [β-hydroxylating] EC 1.14.17.1). Dopamine-β-hydroxylase is a glycoprotein that contains

N-acetylglucosamine, mannose, and fucose. The native enzyme has a molecular weight of 290,000 and is composed of four subunits. It appears that there are two different polypeptide chains with a molecular weight of about 78,000 each. Two of these monomers are joined by a disulfide linkage to form a dimer, two of which interact in a noncovalent manner to form a tetramer. The enzyme also contains about 4 mol of copper/mol of enzyme tetramer (80,131,162,223).

Like tyrosine hydroxylase, dopamine-β-hydroxylase is a mixed-function oxidase. In this reaction, dopamine-β-hydroxylase is first reduced with electrons donated by intragranular ascorbate. The reduction appears to be due to a decrease in the valence state of the enzyme-bound copper (73,74,202). The reduced enzyme then reacts with molecular oxygen and DA to yield NE, water, and regenerated enzyme (82). Originally it was thought that each molecule of ascorbate provided two electrons to the enzyme and was converted to dehydroascorbate (82). More recent evidence suggests that each molecule of ascorbate contributes only one electron to the enzyme so that the product of this reaction is the ascorbate-radical, semidehydroascorbate (60,61,201).

In order for NE synthesis to continue, the ascorbate must be regenerated. Diliberto et al. suggest that semidehydroascorbate is converted back to ascorbate by semidehydroascorbate reductase (60,61) (#9 in Figure 2). However, this enzyme is localized on the outer membrane of mitochondria and does not appear to be associated with chromaffin granules (61). The authors maintain that semidehydroascorbate could diffuse out of the chromaffin granule and be reduced to ascorbate at mitochondria. However, this would deplete the chromaffin granule of even more reducing equivalents since ascorbate itself can not enter the granule—it is only accumulated as dehydroascorbate (213, see below). Recently, Njus et al. (158) demonstrated that reducing equivalents could be transferred into the chromaffin granule by electron transport by cytochrome b-561 in the granule membrane (#8 in Figure 2). This would serve to regenerate intragranular ascorbate from cytosolic ascorbate so that NE synthesis could continue. Semidehydroascorbate in the cytoplasm would then be converted back to ascorbate by semidehydroascorbate reductase. Thus, this mitochondrial enzyme serves to maintain intragranular ascorbate in the reduced form, but only through the intermediate action of cytochrome b-561 as an electron transporter.

The substrates of dopamine-β-hydroxylase are phenylethylamines. Addition of a phenolic hydroxyl in the meta- or para-position (or both) increases the affinity of the substrate (54). There are endogenous inhibitors of dopamine-β-hydroxylase in most tissues which act by chelating copper (41). Disulfiram also inhibits dopamine-β-hydroxylase by copper chelation (153). Phenylethylamine analogs (e.g., the picolinic acid derivatives such as fusaric acid) also inhibit dopamine-β-hydroxylase, but their action does not involve copper chelation (155).

Dopamine-β-hydroxylase activity is found in the catecholamine storage granules of the adrenal medulla and adrenergic nerves (120,235). Approximately half of the enzyme is bound to the vesicular membrane and the remainder is in the soluble contents of the vesicle. These two forms of the enzyme are virtually identical enzymatically and immunologically (142,235). However, the membrane-bound dopamine-β-hydroxylase appears to have a hydrophobic "tail" that anchors it to the membrane (25). Membrane-bound dopamine-β-hydroxylase is oriented to the inside of the vesicle (99,112) and the activity of the enzyme is influenced by the state of the membrane (11). Therefore, the substrates for dopamine-β-hydroxylase must be taken up into the storage vesicle to gain access to the enzyme and the rate at which any potential substrate is β-hydroxylated by whole vesicles or intact tissue will be influenced by the rate of its uptake by the transport system.

Phenylethanolamine-N-methyl Transferase

The last step in the synthesis of epinephrine (Epi) is the N-methylation of NE which is catalyzed by phenylethanolamine-N-methyl transferase (PNMT; EC 2.1.1.28). The methyl group which is transferred to NE is the "activated" methyl group of S-adenosyl methionine (SAM) which ultimately comes from methionine (109) (#7 in Figure 2). The enzyme has a molecular weight of about 38,000 but dimeric and tetrameric aggregates have been observed. The enzyme PNMT contains 8.5 mol of sulfhydryl groups per mol of enzyme and inactivation of only two of these sulfhydryl groups will cause almost a complete loss of enzyme activity. PNMT has a relatively large content of acidic amino acids (especially glutamic acid) and contains a small amount of hexosamine. It has been reported that there are two charge isozymes of PNMT in the bovine adrenal medulla. PNMT does not require any cofactors, not even magnesium, which is required by other methyl transferases. The kinetics of PNMT are somewhat complicated but suggest a random binding of the substrates with the kinetic preference for S-adenosyl methionine to be the first substrate bound (44,100).

The substrate specificity of PNMT is quite prominent for phenylethanolamines rather than phenylethylamines. Secondary amines (such as Epi) can be N-methylated but to a much lesser extent than the corresponding primary amines (such as NE) (14). On the basis of the substrate specificity of PNMT (and other information), it has been suggested that the final steps in the synthesis of Epi are the β-hydroxylation of DA to form NE followed by the N-methylation of NE to form Epi. The reverse sequence of steps would be the N-methylation of DA to form epinine (N-methyldopamine) followed by the β-hydroxylation of epinine to form Epi. This latter sequence was ruled out because DA (a phenethylamine) was shown not to be a substrate for PNMT (14). However, in view of the accepted localization of the enzymes involved, it is difficult to understand the operation of the generally accepted pathway: DA to NE to Epi. As noted above, dopamine-β-hydroxylase is a particulate enzyme associated with the catecholamine storage vesicles, whereas PNMT has generally been considered to be a soluble enzyme. In this case, DA must be taken up into the storage vesicles to be converted to NE which then must pass out into the cytosol again to be N-methylated to Epi. The Epi would then be taken back into the vesicles where it is stored. Based on our current understanding (which may be erroneous), this seems very inefficient. Moreover, in view of the relatively stable storage complex for catecholamines which exists in these vesicles (see below), it seems unlikely that NE could diffuse out of the granule at a sufficient rate for the synthesis of Epi.

For these reasons, Laduron (118) investigated further the possibility that epinine may be the intermediate in the formation of Epi from DA. He found that DA is, in fact, a substrate for PNMT but that its affinity for the enzyme is much less (500-fold) than the affinity of NE for PNMT. Nonetheless, he suggested that epinine might still be the intermediate for Epi formation if PNMT had much better access to DA than to NE. This would appear to be the case since most of the DA and PNMT are localized in the cytosol, whereas most of the NE is localized in the storage vesicles. However, Schumann and Brodde (193) were unable to detect any epinine in the rat adrenal medulla even under conditions designed to maximize its formation (cold exposure and administration of DOPA to increase catecholamine synthesis plus administration of a monoamine oxidase and a dopamine-β-hydroxylase inhibitor to decrease the breakdown of any epinine which might be formed). The lack of epinine formation is readily understood since the fate of DA is primarily dependent on its concentration in the cytosol and on the kinetic constants of the various pathways competing for it. Since the K_m of the vesicle transport system for DA is much lower (204) than the K_m of PNMT for DA (118), most of the DA will be taken up into the storage vesicle when the concentration in the cytosol is low. The fact that DA is taken up by storage vesicles is supported by the fact that DA can be released from the rat adrenal gland along with NE and Epi (205).

As noted above, PNMT is generally considered to be a soluble enzyme (14,100). Van Orden et al. (219) used an immunocytochemical technique to study the localization of PNMT. They found that virtually all of the PNMT in the rat adrenal medulla was associated with the catecholamine storage vesicles. They suggested that the binding of PNMT to the storage vesicles might be readily reversible so that it is readily solubilized during tissue homogenization. It might appear that this observation clarifies the problem of the multiple translocations required for synthesis of Epi if PNMT were a soluble enzyme. However, Van Orden et al. (219) noted that most of the PNMT appeared to be localized on the periphery of the storage vesicles (on the cytosol face). If this indicates that PNMT is located on the outside of the vesicle membrane then the problem is unresolved since dopamine-β-hydroxylase is located on the inside of the storage granule. Dopamine would still have to be transported into the vesicle to be converted to NE and then the NE would have to pass out of the vesicle to gain access to the PNMT. Further investigations will be required to clarify our understanding of this final step in catecholamine synthesis.

In contrast to the other enzymes discussed above, PNMT is found almost exclusively in the adrenal medulla (83,142). However, immunohistochemical studies indicate that only a portion of the cells in the adrenal medulla contain PNMT (75). This is consistent with the earlier observation that certain cells in the adrenal medulla contain primarily Epi whereas other cells contain primarily NE (48). Presumably, Epi would only be synthesized and stored in the cells which contain PNMT.

Regulation of Catecholamine Synthesis

There are many factors that influence the rate of catecholamine synthesis in the adrenal medulla and in adrenergic nerve terminals (142,227). Physiologically, the most important mechanism is the increase in synthesis which occurs with an increase in the rate of release of catecholamines due to neurogenic activation of the adrenal medulla. The capacity of the adrenal medulla to increase its synthesis of catecholamines in response to stimulation of the splanchic nerve has been recognized for over 25 years (36).

It was generally accepted that this stimulation of catecholamine synthesis resulted from a decrease in the feedback inhibition of tyrosine hydroxylase by catecholamines. As noted above, tyrosine hydroxylase is the rate-limiting enzyme in the synthesis of catecholamines, and, since it catalyzes the first committed step in the synthesis of catecholamines, it is most reasonable that regulation of catecholamine synthesis should occur here. In fact, the increase in catecholamine synthesis accompanying sympathetic nerve stimulation results, at least in part, from an increase in tyrosine hydroxylation (194). Nagatsu et al. (154) showed that catecholamines inhibit tyrosine hydroxylase in vitro and suggested that the enzyme was controlled by feedback inhibition. Taken together, these observations lead to the hypothesis that nerve stimulation increases the release of catecholamines from the nerve terminal and that the resulting decrease in the intraneuronal concentration of catecholamines decreases the feedback inhibition of tyrosine hydroxylase and therefore increases the rate of catecholamine synthesis. Although this is an attractive hypothesis and some data are consistent with the idea that catecholamines produce a feedback inhibition of tyrosine hydroxylase in situ, one very important discrepancy is that tyrosine hydroxylase is a soluble enzyme whereas most, if not all, of the catecholamines are bound in the storage granules. Free catecholamines in the cytoplasm are rapidly inactivated by monamine oxidase. Moreover, the catecholamines released by nerve stimulation come directly from the storage granules (see below). Therefore, it is difficult to understand how the activity of soluble tyrosine hydroxylase can be regulated by the level of catecholamines which are localized in a different compartment.

The first evidence that the increase of tyrosine hydroxylase activity produced by nerve stimulation does not result from a decrease in feedback inhibition by NE comes from the studies of Weiner et al. (43,230). They performed a detailed study of the kinetics of inhibition of catecholamine synthesis produced by catecholamines and the stimulation of catecholamine synthesis produced by sympathetic nerve stimulation.

They found that these two processes were operating by different mechanisms. It now appears that there are at least two mechanisms by which nerve stimulation increases the activity of tyrosine hydroxylase in the adrenal medulla. First, acute stimulation of the adrenal medulla produces a rapid onset activation of tyrosine hydroxylase which appears to result from phosphorylation of the enzyme. Second, more prolonged stimulation of the adrenal medulla causes an induction of the synthesis of tyrosine hydroxylase resulting in an increase in the quantity of enzyme in the tissue (see top portion of Figure 2).

Several investigators have demonstrated an increase in tyrosine hydroxylase activity when the enzyme is exposed to protein phosphorylating conditions. Incubation of tyrosine hydroxylase in the presence of cyclic AMP (cAMP), protein kinase, ATP, and magnesium increases the affinity of the enzyme for its cofactor and decreases the affinity for catecholamines as inhibitors of tyrosine hydroxylase without changing the affinity for tyrosine (5,95,133,145). This same process appears to be initiated in vitro by stress-induced stimulation of the adrenal medulla, which causes a shift of tyrosine hydroxylase from a less active to a more active form (137). Initial attempts to demonstrate the phosphorylation of tyrosine hydroxylase under these conditions were unsuccessful. This led to the suggestion that an activator of tyrosine hydroxylase was phosphorylated and thereby "turned on" under these conditions (132). More recently however, direct phosphorylation of tyrosine hydroxylase by cAMP-dependent protein kinase accompanied by an increase in enzyme activity has been demonstrated (126,127,239,240).

Phospholipids, such as phosphatidylserine, and polyanionic substances, such as heparin and ATP, have also been shown to increase tyrosine hydroxylase activity by increasing its affinity for the pterin cofactor (95,104,146). Activation of tyrosine hydroxylase by phosphatidylserine is not additive with the activation produced by protein phosphorylating conditions (132). This supports the suggestion by Lovenberg et al. (133) that the activation produced by anionic substances and the activation produced by phosphorylation (which introduces an anionic group into the enzyme) act through a common mechanism. They suggested that an appropriately placed anionic group may be necessary for high-affinity binding of the cofactor.

Other mechanisms have also been suggested to play a role in the acute activation of tyrosine hydroxylase. Polyanionic substances activate tyrosine hydroxylase by an electrostatic effect resulting in an increase in the affinity of the enzyme for its cofactor. Katz et al. (104) suggested that tyrosine hydroxylase may exist in two forms that differ in charge density and activity; and that the more active form of the enzyme has at least local areas of higher positive-charge density. Polyanionic substances would bind to this form of the enzyme and stabilize the enzyme in this more active form. They noted that some membranes are polyanionic and that binding of tyrosine hydroxylase to these membranes could activate the enzyme. It has also been reported that tyrosine hydroxylase is activated by calcium. This observation lead to the hypothesis that the influx of calcium that accompanies activation of the cell and is essential for catecholamine release (see below) is also responsible in some manner for activation of tyrosine hydroxylase and the increase in catecholamine synthesis (144,186). However, other investigators have been unable to demonstrate that calcium activates tyrosine hydroxylase (104,231).

As noted above, more prolonged stimulation of the adrenal medulla causes an increase in the synthesis of tyrosine hydroxylase. Much of our current understanding of the process involved in the induction of tyrosine hydroxylase, as well as a review of this process (85), comes from Costa's laboratory. The induction of tyrosine hydroxylase requires a more prolonged stimulation of the adrenal medulla (at least 60−90 minutes) than is required for activation of the enzyme. The increase in the amount of tyrosine hydroxylase is due to an increase in tyrosine hydroxylase synthesis rather than a decrease in the breakdown of the enzyme. The steps involved in this process have been identified, but the manner by which some of them occur is still unknown. Activation of nicotinic receptors on the plasma membrane of adrenomedullary cells increases the activity of adenylate cyclase and thereby increases the synthesis and tissue levels of cAMP (#3, #4, in Figure 2). This increase in cAMP level is self-limiting and its duration is never more than 90 minutes regardless of the duration of the initial stimulus. The tissue levels of cAMP return to normal as a result of the cellular release of a protein which, in combination with calcium, activates the high K_m form of cyclic nucleotide phosphodiesterase, thereby increasing the rate of cAMP breakdown. The increase in the tissue level of cAMP, although it is transient, activates protein kinase in the cytosol by causing a dissociation of the free, active catalytic subunit from its complex with the regulatory subunit. The adrenal medulla, along with many other tissues, contains two types of cAMP-dependent protein kinase, which have been designated PK_1 and PK_2. The free catalytic subunit of PK_1 is taken up into the cell nucleus thereby increasing nuclear protein phosphorylation. It is presumed that the protein kinase phosphorylates a chromosomal regulatory protein which is in turn responsible for the observed increase in mRNA synthesis and the subsequent increase in the synthesis of tyrosine hydroxylase.

Procedures which increase sympathetic discharge (143) or administration of nerve growth factor (164) have been shown to increase the activity of dopamine-β-hydroxylase in sympathetically innervated tissues and in the adrenal medulla without affecting the tissue level of enzymes which are not involved in catecholamine synthesis. Gagnon et al. (78) demonstrated that this is due to induction of the synthesis of new dopamine-β-hydroxylase molecules. Waymire et al. (224) showed that an analog of cAMP increased the levels of tyrosine hydroxylase and dopamine-β-hydroxylase. The lag time for this response was consistent with an increased synthesis of mRNA as an intermediate step. Thus it appears that the process described above for induction of tyrosine hydroxylase also causes a simultaneous induction of dopamine-β-hydroxylase.

The final step in the synthesis of catecholamines, the N-methylation of NE to form Epi, is also under control. The activity of PNMT in the adrenal medulla is markedly increased by glucocorticoids. In contrast to the increase in the activity of tyrosine hydroxylase and dopamine-β-hydroxylase, this increase in PNMT activity results from a decrease in the rate of PNMT proteolysis rather than an increase in the rate of PNMT synthesis. Glucocorticoids appear to increase the tissue level of a substance which stabilizes PNMT against degradation. This stabilizing factor appears to be SAM, the methyl donor of PNMT (23). The stabilizing effect of SAM on PNMT is considerably enhanced by its substrate NE (136). Since glucocorticoids do not increase the synthesis of PNMT, they would not be expected to induce synthesis of PNMT in NE-storing cells, thereby converting these cells into Epi-synthesizing cells. This conclusion is supported by the observations of Hersey and Distefano (90). Epinephrine has been reported to decrease PNMT activity in the adrenal medulla by decreasing the tissue level of the enzyme (35). The mechanism of this effect of Epi is unclear.

STORAGE OF CATECHOLAMINES IN THE ADRENAL MEDULLA

Thirty years ago, two laboratories reported simultaneously that the catecholamines of the adrenal medulla are stored in a particulate subcellular fraction (27,93). The following outline will be used in reviewing the knowledge about these storage vesicles or chromaffin granules: 1) characterization of the vesicular membrane; 2) soluble contents of the vesicle and the mechanisms of accumulation of the vesicular contents; and 3) the nature of the storage complex. Detailed reviews on the composition and biogenesis of these storage vesicles have been published elsewhere (235,236).

Chromaffin Granule Membrane

Under the electron microscope, the limiting membrane of the chromaffin granule appears as a standard bilaminar-unit membrane. This membrane is composed of lipids and proteins. There appear to be a large number of different proteins associated with the chromaffin-granule membrane. Aunis et al. (12) found 37 different proteins with a molecular weight over 27,000. Abbs and Phillips (1) identified 40–60 different proteins in the chromaffin-granule membrane. Most of these proteins are exposed to the cytosol. Among the proteins, at least nine enzymes have been identified: magnesium-ATPase (18); cytochrome b-561 (18,72,200); NADH:oxidoreductase (72); phosphatidyl inositol kinase (151); tyrosine hydroxylase (215); the regulatory subunit of type II cAMP-dependent protein kinase (215); a Ca^{+2}–calmodulin-dependent protein kinase (215); a phosphoryl-group transferring enzyme (208); and, as discussed above, about half of the granular dopamine-β-hydroxylase is bound to the vesicular membrane. The ATPase generates a proton (pH) gradient which provides the energy for catecholamine uptake by the granule (see below). It has been suggested that phosphatidyl inositol kinase is involved in the release of catecholamine from the storage granule (125). Dopamine-β-hydroxylase constitutes about 25% of the total membrane proteins (237). Its function has been discussed at length. It is unclear at the present time whether the membrane bound and/or the soluble form of dopamine-β-hydroxylase is responsible for conversion of DA to NE. The functional role of the NADH: oxidoreductase in the granular membrane has not been identified. The two protein kinases in the granule membrane phosphorylate membrane proteins and there are also some proteins which are phosphorylated by a cAMP, Ca^{+2}–calmodulin-independent mechanism (113,215). Among the seven membrane proteins that were phosphorylated, only two have been identified: the type II cAMP-dependent protein kinase phosphorylates itself, and the membrane-bound tyrosine hydroxylase. The significance of this membrane-bound tyrosine hydroxylase is uncertain. Konings and DePotter (113) showed that inhibition of phosphorylation of proteins in the chromaffin-granule membrane was associated with inhibition of catecholamine release from granules. In these experiments the catecholamine release was induced by adding chromaffin-cell-plasma membrane fragments to the chromaffin granules. Therefore, the authors suggested that phosphorylation of proteins in the chromaffin-granule membrane may be involved in exocytosis.

Chromomembrin B is another protein which constitutes a major fraction of the proteins of the chromaffin-granule membrane (235,238). Until recently, the function of this protein was unknown. Now Apps et al. have shown that it is identical with cytochrome b-561 and that it has an apparent molecular weight of about 22,000 (7) (#8 in Figure 2). This protein appears to be a transmembrane protein (1) and it has been implicated in the transfer of electrons across the granule membrane (158). This electron transport is essential to maintain ascorbic acid in its reduced form for oxidation of DA to NE (see above). Huber et al. (99) reported that there are five glycoproteins in the vesicular membrane one of which they identified as dopamine-β-hydroxylase. Abbs and Phillips (1) identified 13 different glycoproteins. Although both groups indicate that the carbohydrate portion of these proteins faces the inside of the granule, other investigators report that the carbohydrate portion of some membrane glycoproteins is oriented to the outstide (140).

Recently it has become clear that some contractile proteins are associated with the chromaffin-granule membrane. Both immunocytochemical staining of intact cells and direct analysis of chromaffin-granule membrane proteins by gel electrophoresis have shown that these membranes contain both actin and alpha-actinin (12,16,124). Actin also appears to be attached to the chromaffin-cell-plasma membrane and localized in the cytoplasm as microfilaments (12,124). Thus, actin may be involved in maintaining cell structure and in the growth of the cell in culture as well as playing an important role in catecholamine release. Alpha-actinin may serve as the anchoring site on the chromaffin granule for attachment of actin microfilaments (12,16,124).

The major lipids of the vesicular membrane are cholesterol and phospholipids and the ratio of cholesterol:phospholipds is relatively high compared to other membranes (average about 0.6) (235). The most striking feature of the lipids of these granules is the relatively high lysolecithin content. Since lysolecithin induces fusion of cell membranes (4), it has been suggested that lysolecithin plays an important role in fusion of the vesicular membrane to the plasma membrane which is a necessary step in the release of catecholamines (see below). However, as noted below, the phospholipids of the granule membrane are not readily accessible from the cytoplasmic face (34). More specifically, only 10% of the lysolecithin is oriented to the outside of the membrane (163). Finally, Creutz (52) recently showed that certain cis-unsaturated fatty acids cause fusion of previously aggregated chromaffin granules. However, lysolecithin did not promote fusion of chromaffin granules in this system. Thus, it does not seem that lysolecithin plays an important role in membrane fusion for exocytosis. These membranes also contain appreciable amounts of sphingomyelin, phosphatidyl choline and phosphatidyl ethanolamine and smaller amounts of phosphatidyl inositol, phosphatidyl serine, and gangliosides (68,180,235). Buckland et al. (34) found that only half (fraction varies for the specific phospholipids) of these phospholipids are accessible to phospholipases or to a phospholipid-specific reagent. This was the case for both intact granules and their ghosts. In other types of membranes, virtually all of the phospholipids can be hydrolyzed after the cell or organelle is ruptured. It is unclear how the phospholipids of the chromaffin-granule membrane are protected or shielded from these enzymes.

The lipid and protein composition of the chromaffin-granule membrane has been compared with the composition of the membrane of the endoplasmic reticulum (97) and Golgi apparatus (216). In view of the marked differences observed, the authors concluded that chromaffin-granule membranes are not formed simply by bulk flow of membranes from either of these structures without some specific process of differentiation which could account for the differences observed. There are also marked differences in the lipid and protein composition of chromaffin-granule membranes and plasma membranes of adrenal medullary cells (243). Thus, although the chromaffin-granule membrane fuses with the plasma membrane during release of catecholamine (see below), the plasma membrane is not composed of the remains of chromaffin granules after catecholamine release. Instead, the chromaffin-granule membranes are recovered, probably for reuse.

The permeability characteristics of the storage-granule membrane have been investigated (101,148,167). The granules behave as very good osmometers in hypertonic solutions but undergo lysis in hypotonic solutions. The water space of the granule is 0.6 at 300 mOsm. The granule membrane is impermeable to sodium, potassium, and hydrogen ions and the divalent cations calcium and magnesium. The permeability to nonelectrolytes is dependent on the molecular size and temperature. Above 20°C the granule membrane is permeable to hexoses and therefore appears to possess hydrophilic pores with a radius of 4.2 Å. Below 15°C, the membrane is impermeable to the larger (5–6 carbon) nonelectrolytes. The internal pH of the granules is maintained at about 5.5 even at an external pH of 7.4 (101). This pH gradient appears to be essential for uptake of catecholamines by the granule and may also increase the stability of stored catecholamines (which are more stable in an acid environment) and increases the activity of dopamine-β-hydroxylase which has an acidic pH optimum.

Chromaffin Granule Matrix

The soluble contents of the storage granules are obtained by lysis of the granules (hypotonic or freeze–thaw) and centrifugation of the membranes. The soluble contents include: proteins, catecholamines, nucleotides, calcium, ascorbic acid, and possibly some phospholipids. There are two specific soluble proteins which have been identified and characterized. First, soluble dopamine-β-hydroxylase constitutes about 5% of the soluble proteins (98) and has already been described. The remainder of the soluble proteins are called chromogranins and one of these proteins, chromogranin A, accounts for about 50% of the soluble proteins. Chromogranin A has been purified and characterized. It is an acidic protein with a molecular weight of about 78,000 and the configuration of a random-coil polypeptide. There are conflicting reports as to whether it is a glycoprotein or not (235). It appears that chromogranin A can serve as a substrate for protein carboxymethylase, but the significance of carboxymethylation of chromogranin A is uncertain (30). Chromogranin A serves to stabilize the catecholamine storage complex (see below). The mechanism by which these proteins are incorporated into the storage granules is uncertain but it has been shown that soluble dopamine-β-hydroxylase and chromogranin A are incorporated into the granules at different rates although they are synthesized simultaneously (122).

The other major soluble components of the storage granules are the catecholamines and nucleotides. The major catecholamine is Epi, but NE accounts for about 25% of the catecholamines. The primary nucleotide in the chromaffin granule is ATP but there are also significant amounts of ADP, AMP, UTP, and GTP (218,235). Many investigators have noted that the molar ratio of catecholamines to ATP in the storage granules is approximately 4:1 (235). Since the catecholamines have a single positive charge and ATP has four negative charges at physiologic pH, it has been suggested that an ionic interaction between the catecholamine and ATP is involved in the formation of the storage complex (see below). It should be noted that some investigators report that the molar ratio of catecholamines to ATP is in the range of 8:1 up to 12:1 (211, 218). If this is the case, the catecholamines cannot be stored entirely in a simple ionic complex with ATP. Terland et al. (211) reported the isolation of a relatively pure fraction of NE storage granules from the adrenal medulla. Their analyses indicate that these granules have a higher content of catecholamine and ATP than the total population of granules but that the ratio of catecholamines to ATP was lower in the NE granules than in the total population of granules.

The uptake of catecholamine by chromaffin granules was described shortly after the discovery of the granules, and this uptake was shown to be markedly enhanced by ATP and magnesium (107). As noted above, the vesicular membrane contains a magnesium ATPase (18,92,110) (#14 in Figure 2). Inhibitors of this ATPase will inhibit ATP–magnesium-stimulated uptake of catecholamines (96,191,214). However, there is not a direct correlation between catecholamine uptake and ATPase activity under all conditions. For example, very low concentrations of reserpine will block catecholamine uptake without affecting ATPase activity, and uncouplers of oxidative phosphorylation will inhibit catecholamine uptake but stimulate ATPase activity in chromaffin granules (20,96,214). Therefore, the ATPase must not be directly responsible for catecholamine uptake, but rather it appears that the energy from ATP hydrolysis is stored in some other form which can then be used for catecholamine uptake.

Several recent studies have clarified this issue. Many of these studies have been reviewed by Njus and Radda (159) and Njus et al. (160). It now appears that the ATPase in the vesicular membrane is coupled to a proton (H^+) pump which generates an appreciable H^+ electrochemical gradient. This gradient serves as the energy source for catecholamine uptake. The chromaffin granule ATPase is similar in many ways to the mitochondrial F_1 ATPase, similar in structure and in the effects of many inhibitors. However, the two enzymes are definitely different. They can be differentiated immunologically and on the basis of some selective inhibitors (8,9,42). This chromaffin granule ATPase has a K_m for ATP (69 μM) which is well below the cytosolic concentration of ATP. The pH optimum of the enzyme is 7.4 (22) which means that it should function well since it is oriented to the cytoplasm (6) where the pH is about 7.4, in contrast to the interior of the granule where the pH is much more acidic. The internal pH of the chromaffin granule is about 5.5–6.0, thus there is about a 30- to 100-fold concentration gradient for hydrogen ion across the vesicular membrane (20,39,161,175). This large gradient is possible because the membrane has a low permeability to H^+ and the intragranular buffering capacity is high (101). In the absence of exogenous ATP, the membrane potential of the chromaffin granule is negative inside. Addition of exogenous ATP and magnesium in the presence of an anion that the membrane is permeable to (a permeant anion, e.g., chloride) will cause a further decrease in internal pH due to a relatively large accumulation of hydrogen ion with the accompanying anion. In the absence of a permeant anion the membrane potential reverses and becomes about 30–80 mV inside positive due to the uptake of hydrogen ion without an accompanying anion (22,39,96,161,169). Thus, there is a large electrochemical gradient (up to 200 mV) for hydrogen ion across the vesicular membrane (22).

The ATPase is distinct from the proton pump (#13 in Figure 2) as indicated by differential purification of the two activities in reconstitution experiments (81) and by the differential effects of some drugs (9). For example, the proton channel appears to be preferentially blocked and labeled by dicyclohexyl carbodiimide (9). Although the ATPase and the proton channel are separate entities, they appear to be tightly coupled. The ATPase is stimulated by a decrease in either the pH gradient or the transmembrane potential (22). In addition, the tight coupling can be demonstrated in reverse. Adenosine triphosphate can be synthesized by an artificially imposed proton electrochemical gradient in chromaffin-granule ghosts (185) or artificially reconstituted chromaffin membranes (81). It has been estimated that there are approximately 20 molecules of ATPase per granule and about 240 proton channels per granule (8). The stoichiometry of the proton pumping is such that two protons are pumped into the granule for each ATP that is hydrolyzed (22).

It appears that both the pH gradient (hydrogen-ion-concentration gradient, inside acid) and the membrane potential (inside positive in the presence of ATP–magnesium and absence of a permeant anion) can supply energy for catecholamine uptake (22,111). Schuldiner et al. (191) suggested that only the pH gradient could supply this energy and that the membrane potential did not contribute to ATP-stimulated uptake of catecholamines. However, their experiments were performed in the presence of a permeant anion which would collapse the membrane potential.

At least three roles have been suggested for the hydrogen ion electrochemical gradient of the chromaffin granules. First, if the vesicular membrane is only permeable to the unprotonated form of the catecholamine, the catecholamine will concentrate in the more acidic interior due to ion trapping, i.e., the concentration of the uncharged form of the amine is the same on both sides of the membrane but there will be a higher concentration of hydrogen ions inside (20,39,191). An artificially imposed pH gradient (inside acid) will cause catecholamine accumulation in liposomes (156) and will drive carrier-mediated transport of biogenic amines in chromaffin granule membrane vesicles (164,191). However, this passive accumulation based on ion trapping due to a pH gradient cannot nearly account for the magnitude of the ATP-stimulated catecholamine accumulation (111). Second, the large electrochemical gradient for H^+ can serve as the energy source for carrier-mediated accumulation of catecholamines. This is generally accepted as the mechanism for catecholamine accumulation by the chromaffin granules (see below). Third, it was suggested that the more acid pH inside the storage granule may help to prevent oxidation of the stored catecholamine since catecholamines are more stable in an acid environment (20).

Thus, the magnesium ATPase of the chromaffin granule generates the electrochemical gradient necessary for catecholamine accumulation. However the ATPase does not serve as the carrier as well. Transport of catecholamines is effected by a different molecular species (#12 in Figure 2) since various drugs will selectively interfere with the generation of the gradient or the accumulation of catecholamines (9). For example, reserpine is a competitive inhibitor of catecholamine accumulation (102) but it does inhibit the ATPase or uncouple the granule membrane (20). There was some confusion regarding the action of reserpine because it appeared to be a competitive inhibitor of catecholamine accumulation in isolated granules, but it was irreversible in its actions. It now appears that the irreversibility is just due to the high lipophilicity of this drug (103).

Classically, the adrenal medulla is relatively insensitive to the actions of reserpine in vivo. This may be because of the high lipid solubility of reserpine and the relatively low blood flow to the adrenal medulla. Recently, Gabizon et al. developed a photoaffinity label for the catecholamine transporter (77). This compound is a competitive, reversible inhibitor of the catecholamine transporter in the dark. When exposed to light, it binds irreversibly and selectively to the transporter. Using this compound, they were able to determine that the molecular weight of the transporter is 45,000 and that it represents about 3% of the proteins in the granule membrane.

The stoichiometry of the coupling between catecholamine influx and H^+ efflux has been examined by determining the accumulation of catecholamines under various conditions of pH gradient and transmembrane potential. These studies indicate that catecholamine accumulation is electrogenic. The number of protons leaving the granule exceeds by one the charge which enters the granule with the catecholamine. For example, if the catecholamine is transported in as a cation then two H^+ is transported out in exchange for one molecule of catecholamine. If the catecholamine is transported in as a neutral species then one H^+ is transported out in exchange. In this latter case an additional H^+ would be used to form the cation form of the catecholamine which predominates at the intragranular pH so that two H^+ are consumed all together (22,111). Although the neutral form of the catecholamines is a very minor species at physiologic pH, this is probably the species which is transported by the carrier. Studies of the pH-dependency of catecholamine binding to the carrier indicate that the neutral form of the catecholamines has the highest affinity for the carrier (187). The overall stoichiometry of ATP-dependent catecholamine accumulation is: one ATP hydrolyzed = two protons pumped in = one catecholamine accumulated. All three components of this accumulation process, the ATPase, the proton pump, and the catecholamine transporter, are now subject to analysis since they have been solubilized and reconstituted back to a functional system (81,134).

The ATP present in chromaffin granules is partially synthesized in mitochondria and then transported into the chromaffin granules (166). At least two mechanisms have been described by which this transport might occur. First, there appears to be a carrier-mediated transport system in the vesicular membrane for uptake of the nucleotides (#15 in Figure 2). This transport of ATP is specifically and competitively blocked by atractyloside, whereas reserpine specifically blocks catecholamine uptake. Therefore, separate carriers are involved in the transport of catecholamines and nucleotides. Both transport processes are inhibited by ATPase inhibitors and uncouplers of oxidative phosphorylation so that both types of transport utilize the electrochemical proton gradient generated by the ATPase as the source of energy to drive the transport (2). As noted above, both the chemical portion of the gradient and the electrical portion of the pH gradient can drive the transport of catecholamines. However, only the electrical portion of this gradient provides energy for the transport of nucleotides. Thus abolition of the pH gradient by incubating the granules with nigericin plus K^+ or with NH_4^+ does not decrease nucleotide uptake (2). However, when the membrane potential is short-circuited by incubating the granules with lipid permeable anions such as Cl^- or SCN^-, nucleotide accumulation is markedly reduced (225). The affinity of this nucleotide transporter for ATP is fairly low (K_m about 1 mM) but still higher than the affinity for ATP in the presence of Mg^{+2} (K_m about 3 mM). Thus it appears that ATP is the species which is transported rather than an ATP-Mg^{+2} complex (225). The specificity of the nucleotide transporter is also quite low. Not only does this carrier transport other nucleotides such as GTP and UTP (225), it also handles other divalent strongly negative-charged groups. Thus the same transport system accumulates phosphate, sulfate, and phosphoenol pyruvate. These compounds block accumulation of ATP and of each other. The accumulation of these compounds by chromaffin vesicles is inhibited by atractyloside and permeant anions suggesting that they use the same carrier as ATP and the same driving force (226). Since this carrier can transport inorganic phosphate, the inorganic phosphate found in chromaffin granules may be taken up from the cytosol rather than resulting from breakdown of the ATP.

Another possible mechanism for transport of ATP from mitochondria to the chromaffin granules was suggested by Carmichael and Smith (37,38) as a result of their electron-microscope study of adrenal medullary cells. These investigators identified tubular channels which could serve as a direct connection between mitochondria and chromaffin granules. They suggested that these channels could permit the movement of nucleotides from the mitochondria to the chromaffin granules circumventing the need for the nucleotide to diffuse through the cytoplasm. However, if these channels function as suggested, they should allow large concentrations of catecholamines to diffuse into the mitochondria. This does not occur.

The chromaffin granules also appear to be capable of synthesizing ATP from ADP. A large proportion of the ADP accumulated by these granules is converted to ATP within the granule (2). This conversion appears to take place by transfer of the terminal phosphoryl group from ATP outside the granule to ADP within the granule (208,209). The reaction is catalyzed by a phosphoryl group transferring enzyme in the vesicular membrane (#16 in Figure 2). This enzyme can be differentiated from the ATPase in the membrane. Taugner and Wunderlich (208) suggested that this reaction may facilitate the accumulation of ATP within the granule. Since the membrane is more permeable to ADP than ATP (2), the major portion of the ATP molecule may be accumulated as the diphosphonucleotide which is then phosphorylated within the granule by the phosphoryl group transferring enzyme. Thus the ATP would be transported into the granule in two separate pieces (ADP and a high energy phosphate group) by two different mechanisms.

Not all of the ^{32}P accumulated by chromaffin granules from ^{32}P-ATP appears as ATP within the granular matrix. Some of the ^{32}P is incorporated into membrane lipids and some appears to be ATP, which is firmly bound to the granular membrane (209). It is uncertain whether the phosphorylation of membrane lipids utilizes ATP from inside or outside the granule. However, if this or any other reaction hydrolyzes intragranular ATP, the phosphoryl-group-transferring enzyme described above may serve as a mechanism for regeneration of intragranular ATP from the intragranular ADP and extragranular ATP. This would eliminate the need for the granule to take up a whole molecule of ATP.

The chromaffin granules also contain a very high concentration of calcium (15 mM) compared to the concentration in cytoplasm (10^{-4}M) (58). Along with mitochondria, the chromaffin granules represent the major site of calcium localization in the adrenal medullary cell (181). The uptake of calcium by chromaffin granules was studied by Kostron et al. (114). They demonstrated that calcium uptake in chromaffin granules is carrier-mediated (#11 in Figure 2) by showing that the uptake is markedly temperature dependent, exhibits saturation kinetics and is inhibited by strontium ion. Once accumulated by the chromaffin granule, the calcium is firmly bound within the granule. The uptake of calcium into chromaffin granules was readily distinguished from calcium uptake by mitochondria since the uptake by chromaffin granules is not blocked by azide or dinitrophenol and is not stimulated by ATP plus magnesium.

One other soluble constituent of chromaffin granules has been identified. Terland and Flatmark (210) reported that these organelles contain ascorbic acid in a concentration of 13 mM and suggested that the ascorbic acid might serve as an electron donor in the oxidation of DA to NE. Tirrell and Westhead (213) reported that ascorbic acid was accumulated by chromaffin granules only after oxidation to dehydroascorbate (#10 in Figure 2). The uptake of dehydroascorbate did not appear to be carrier-mediated. The rate of accumulation of ascorbic acid was quite slow compared to the rate of uptake of catecholamines, calcium and ATP. In order to serve in the oxidation of dopamine to NE, the dehydroascorbate first has to be reduced back to ascorbic acid. As noted above, cytochrome b-561 appears to transport electrons into the chromaffin granules to maintain ascorbic acid in the reduced state (158). Since ascorbic acid can only cross the chromaffin-granule membrane as dehydroascorbate, and since there is an efficient electron transport system in the membrane to convert intragranular dehydroascorbate to ascorbate, these two processes will serve to maintain ascorbic acid in the storage granule.

Newly accumulated ascorbic acid is released along with catecholamines by isolated chromaffin cells (59). Although there are many similarities between the release of catecholamines and the release of ascorbic acid, there are significant differences in the effects of some drugs and the temporal relationships. This led the authors to suggest that ascorbic acid was being released from a different compartment than the catecholamines, possibly from the cisternae of the endoplasmic reticulum.

Catecholamine Storage Complex

As noted above, catecholamines and ATP exist in a 4:1 molar ratio in the storage granules and thus at physiological pH there is a balance of ionic charges between these two substances. These facts led to the assumption that these two constituents form some sort of storage complex in the chromaffin granule (28). The concentration of catecholamines (0.55 M) and nucleotides (0.18 M) is such that the storage vesicles could not be osmotically stable unless some interaction takes place that decreases the osmotic activity of these substances in solution. Pletscher et al. (171) have used several techniques to show that such complexes do exist in vitro. The apparent average molecular weight (as determined by analytical ultracentrifugation) of catecholamines and ATP in an aqueous solution increases markedly with increasing concentration reaching a maximum value when the molar ratio of NE to ATP is 4:1. Addition of small amounts of calcium or magnesium to this solution increased the molecular weight even more; therefore, under optimum conditions the apparent molecular weight of the complex NE, ATP, and calcium is greater than 10,000. Finally, addition of chromogranins to this mixture leads to the formation of a single peak with an even higher molecular weight, whereas albumin did not form a complex with these small molecules. Thus, all four components appear to interact in a more or less specific manner to form a complex which allows high concentrations of catecholamine to be stored at a reduced osmotic pressure. Moreover, the catecholamines appear to interact with ATP in the intact chromaffin granules (171).

More recently several laboratories have used nuclear magnetic resonance spectroscopy to examine the nature of the storage complex in vivo. These studies indicate that a similar interaction occurs between the catecholamine, ATP, chromogranin, and divalent metal ions in the chromaffin granules in vivo. The results of these studies indicate that ATP serves as a central component of the complex to cross link the other components. Thus at the acidic pH found within the granules, catecholamines do not chelate divalent metals; instead, the catecholamines interact with ATP, which in turn chelates the metal ions (84). However, within this complex the catecholamine is influenced by the presence of metal ions. The interaction between ATP and the catecholamine appears to involve both an ionic bond and the weaker forces associated with vertical stacking of their aromatic rings. Moreover, ATP appears to crosslink catecholamine and chromogranin, and within this complex the catecholamine and protein also interact (57,197,198). The evidence indicates that this complex is relatively weak so that a considerable portion of the catecholamine may be in free solution and there is a rapid equilibrium between the catecholamine in free solution and the catecholamine in the complex (57). Little if any of the catecholamines or ATP are firmly bound in the storage granules. Finally, about half of the soluble protein within the storage granule (probably proteins other than chromogranin) appears to be involved in high molecular weight soluble complexes. The role of these protein complexes is uncertain (195).

Some of the catecholamines may be stored loosely bound to anionic groups on the granule membrane. These membranes can bind a considerable amount of catecholamine at a pH of 7.4, but the binding capacity decreases with decreasing pH. Relatively little catecholamine is bound by these membranes at a pH of 5.5, which is the normal intragranular pH

(217). Therefore the extent of this binding depends on whether it occurs on the inner or outer surface of the membrane which will have a profound effect on the pH at this binding site.

RELEASE OF CATECHOLAMINES

The release of catecholamines is obviously the *raison d'etre* of the adrenal medulla. This process is diagramatically summarized in Figure 3. Catecholamine release starts with stimulation of the medullary cells. The best recognized example of this is stimulation of the adrenal medulla by acetylcholine released from the splanchic nerves innervating the medulla. The activated cell responds with a series of seven steps terminating in catecholamine release. Douglas and Rubin (63) referred to this process as "stimulus–secretion coupling." This process is dependent on calcium just as excitation–contraction coupling is. It is now generally accepted that catecholamine release occurs by exocytosis (62,221,238). This process is, figuratively, phagocytosis in reverse. Briefly, exocytosis begins with fusion of the membrane of the storage granule to the inside of the plasma membrane. Then the membrane opens at the point of fusion so that the inside of the granule is continuous with the outside of the cell. The entire soluble contents of the granule can then diffuse into the extracellular space, but none of the membrane bound components are released. Finally the membrane reseals and the empty storage granule is retrieved to be refilled and used again (221,236). Several lines of evidence indicate that the release of catecholamines occurs in an all-or-none fashion both in vivo by exocytosis and in vitro from isolated granules (69,70,149,203,238).

There are many substances which can stimulate the release of catecholamines from the adrenal medulla. In addition to acetylcholine and other cholinergic agonists, the adrenal medulla is also stimulated by angiotensin, serotonin, histamine, bradykinin, increased potassium, barium, and β_2-adrenergic agonists (63,65,87,174). However this discussion will focus on stimulation of the adrenal medulla by acetylcholine. The cholinergic receptors are primarily nicotinic in most species (item C in Figure 3). However, many investigators have suggested that muscarinic receptors are also present (67,71,94,130,189,241). This suggestion is based on the fact that atropine can inhibit the effects of cholinergic agonists. These observations must be interpreted with caution, since Wilson and Kirshner (234) reported that atropine interferes with the specific binding of α-bungarotoxin (a specific nicotinic ligand) to cholinergic receptors in the adrenal medulla. However, there do appear to be muscarinic receptors in the adrenal medulla of the rat and chick (106,121). In the bovine adrenal medulla the nicotinic receptors are located on the plasma membrane and the density of the receptors is somewhat less than in brain or skeletal muscle (234).

The first studies on the electrophysiology of the adrenal medulla concluded that these cells were electrically inexcitable. The cells were reported to have a low membrane-resting potential and although they

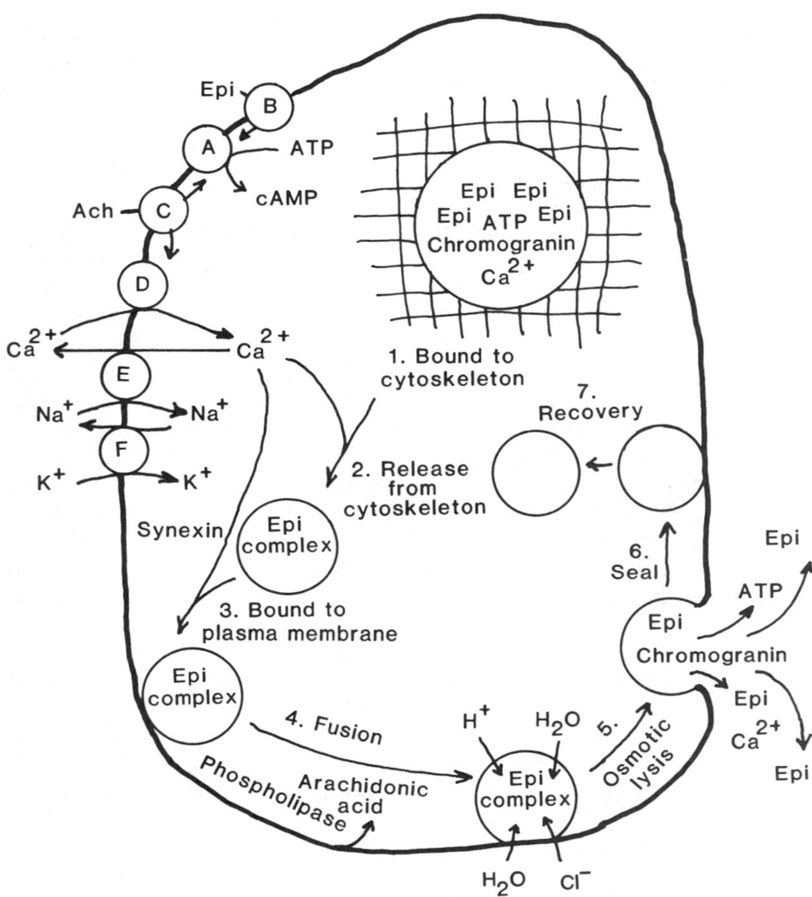

FIGURE 3. Diagram of the storage and release of catecholamines. This diagram of a single chromaffin cell shows a granule with the major components of the storage complex in the upper right. Starting from that point, the seven steps involved in exocytosis are diagrammed. The components of the plasma membrane represent: A—adenylate cyclase; B—β_2-adrenergic receptor; C—nicotinic cholinergic receptor; D—calcium channel; E—sodium–calcium exchanger; F—Na^+, K^+-activated ATPase. Abbreviations used in this diagram are as follows: Ach—acetylcholine; ATP—adenosine triphosphate; cAMP—cyclic adenosine-3′,5′-monophosphate; Epi—epinephrine.

could be depolarized by acetylcholine, they did not generate all-or-none action potentials (66,67). More recent studies have indicated that these negative results were probably due to injury of the cells. Adrenal medullary cells from the rat, gerbil and human can have a resting membrane potential as high as -50 mV (24,31). The resting membrane potential increases considerably in a sodium-free medium indicating that the resting membrane is more permeable to sodium than many other excitable membranes but the membrane resistance and capacitance are similar to other excitable cells. As long as the resting membrane potential is high enough, these cells generate all-or-none action potentials spontaneously and in response to acetylcholine, increased potassium or current pulses. The action potential results primarily from an increase in sodium conductance but there is also a small inward calcium current (item D in Figure 3).

Thus, calcium enters the cell during the action potential. Efflux of calcium from adrenal medullary cells occurs, at least in part, by a sodium–calcium exchange mechanism (item E in Figure 3). There is also a calcium–calcium exchange mechanism in the plasma membrane of adrenal medullary cells. The significance of this latter process is uncertain (3,184). The influx of calcium is essential for the release of catecholamines in response to acetylcholine and other cholinergic agonists, increased potassium, biogenic amines, and polypeptides (63,174), but is not essential for the release of catecholamines elicited by β-adrenergic agonists (29). The necessity for calcium ion in the release of catecholamines caused by tyramine appears to be species dependent (221).

Influx of calcium alone is sufficient to initiate catecholamine release from adrenal medullary cells. This has been demonstrated by the reintroduction of calcium after exposure of the adrenal medulla to a calcium-free medium (63), by the use of calcium ionophores to facilitate calcium uptake (94) and methoxyverapamil to block calcium uptake (170). The fact that calcium influx is a stimulus for catecholamine release was also demonstrated by using calcium-loaded liposomes to facilitate calcium entry (88) and in isolated adrenal medullary cells rendered permeable to calcium by high-voltage electric discharge (17). As with many other calcium-dependent processes, the release of catecholamines from the adrenal medulla is inhibited by an increase in magnesium ion (17,64). It has been suggested that the inhibitory effect of magnesium occurs at an intracellular site rather than by inhibition of calcium influx (3).

Thus, acetylcholine-induced stimulation of the adrenal medulla leads to an influx of sodium and calcium. Calcium has several possible roles in the exocytotic release of catecholamines, which will be examined later. First let us consider some of the other biochemical or biophysical actions of acetylcholine that may be important for the release of catecholamines. One of the most interesting phenomena was reported by Schneeweiss et al. (188). They measured the fluidity of chromaffin-cell-plasma membranes from the depolarization of a lipid-soluble fluorescent probe. They found that acetylcholine, nicotine, and potassium increase the fluidity of these membranes. The action of potassium was selectively antagonized by calcium addition, whereas hexamethonium blocked the effect of nicotine. The investigators suggested that the increased fluidity of the membrane lipids resulted from membrane depolarization and the consequent alteration in the ionic environment. They also suggested that an increase in cell-membrane fluidity may be essential for fusion of the storage-granule membrane with the cell membrane leading to exocytosis. Recently, Rimle et al. (183) studied the same phenomena using a different technique, electron spin resonance. They did *not* find any effect of acetylcholine on membrane fluidity using two different nitroxide spin labels. They suggested that the effects observed by Schneeweiss et al. (188) may be due to artifacts created by the fluorescent probe that they used. Further studies may be required to clarify this issue.

As noted above, Costa et al. demonstrated that stimulation of the adrenal medulla by acetylcholine also causes an increase in adrenal medullary cAMP which they suggested is involved in the regulation of tyrosine hydroxylase activity (85). Others have suggested a role for cAMP in the release of catecholamines from the adrenal medulla (173). However, Gutman and Boonyaviroj (29,87) have presented evidence that acetylcholine itself does not increase cAMP in the adrenal medulla. Rather, catecholamines released by the acetylcholine activate β_2-receptors (item B in Figure 3) on the plasma membrane of adrenal medullary cells which results in activation of adenylate cyclase, an increase in tissue cAMP levels and a further release of catecholamines. Acetylcholine itself does not activate adenylate cyclase in adrenal medullary cell membranes but β-adrenergic agonists do (29). One function of this arrangement might be to ensure activation of all adrenal medullary cells by catecholamines released from a few activated cells without the need for all cells to be innervated. One very disturbing aspect of this hypothesis is that stimulation of these β-receptors causes the release of more catecholamines, which would further activate the β-receptors creating a positive-feedback loop. In the absence of any other control mechanisms, an initial stimulation of the adrenal medulla should result in the release of more and more catecholamines. This obviously does not occur.

This apparent dilemma may be resolved by the observation of Nikodijevic et al. (157). They reported that there is an adenylate cyclase activity associated with the membranes of the catecholamine storage vesicles. In contrast to the adenylate cyclase of the plasma membrane, this adenylate cyclase is inhibited by β-adrenergic agonists such as Epi and isoproterenol. This observation may clarify the problem just described, i.e., the possibility of a positive-feedback loop in the release of catecholamines from the adrenal medulla. As noted above, during the release of catecholamines the vesicular membrane fuses with the plasma membrane and the inside of the granule becomes continuous with the outside of the cell. Thus the vesicular membrane is temporarily incorporated into the plasma membrane. This would result in the incorporation into the plasma membrane of some adenylate cyclase which is inhibited by catecholamines in addition to the already present adenylate cyclase which is stimulated by catecholamines. This could put a brake on the positive feedback mechanism and make the release of catecholamines self-limiting.

The mechanism by which calcium causes catecholamine release is uncertain, although several possibilities have been suggested. In 1966, Banks (19) suggested that calcium could neutralize the negative charge, which was present on the outside surface of the chromaffin granule and on the inside of the plasma membrane (due to the membrane potential), and thereby facilitate fusion of these membranes. This conclusion was based in part on the fact that calcium caused isolated chromaffin granules to aggregate in vitro.

The lipids of the chromaffin-granule membrane undergo a change in ordering at a rather high temperature range compared to other membranes (33–36°C). This change in lipid ordering affects the membrane permeability and the activity of membrane-bound enzymes. This ordering effect has been attributed to a lateral-phase segregation of cholesterol, or movement of cholesterol from certain portions of the membrane. The cholesterol-depleted, phospholipid-rich patches thus created would be considerably more fluid. It has been suggested that this segregation of membrane lipids is an early event leading to fusion of the granule membrane with the plasma membrane and subsequent exocytotic release of catecholamine (21,135). This hypothesis is made even more plausible by the observation that calcium ions induce a similar effect, possibly by increasing the temperature at which this change occurs (135). Since calcium is essential for the release of catecholamines, the segregation of the lipids of the granule membrane may be an essential early step in the release of catecholamines from the adrenal medulla.

When isolated chromaffin granules aggregate, electron micrographs show that there is an exclusion of membrane-intercalated particles from the site of intimate contact of opposing membranes. These particles are generally considered to be membrane proteins seen against the background of the lipid bilayer. Since these proteins do not normally aggregate in the membrane, they may be kept apart by similar ionic charges which would in turn interfere with close contact and fusion between opposing membranes. Therefore, Schober et al. (190) suggested that a first step in the exocytotic process is that calcium causes these particles to be excluded from certain areas of the membrane so that a more intimate contact is possible. However, Schuler et al. (192) presented evidence that indicates that these particles are "squeezed out" of certain areas of the membrane whenever there is close physical contact of the membranes in an ionic medium. The ionic medium (not necessarily calcium) provides a partial-charge screening so that the membrane particles (proteins) can be forced closer together. Thus, Schuler et al. suggest that segregation of membrane particles is the result of an aggregation of chromaffin granules rather than a necessary precondition for aggregation.

Morris et al. have recently studied these protein and lipid interactions further. They find that potassium will promote a dimerization of chromaffin granules, but divalent cations are required to promote higher orders of aggregation and fusion. Aggregation of isolated granule membranes occurs very rapidly, but phospholipid vesicles prepared from the lipids extracted from chromaffin granules aggregate much more slowly. Thus it appears that interactions between the chromaffin-granule proteins are very important in aggregation (89,147). This same group studied these protein–protein interactions further by differentially labeling chromaffin-granule proteins with fluorescent donors or acceptors (150). Very low concentrations of calcium (too low to cause aggregation) increased intramembrane association of proteins, suggesting that clustering or patching may occur as a prelude to aggregation, as previously suggested by Schober et al. (190). Calcium-induced aggregation led to extensive association of granule membrane proteins (about 75% of labeled proteins). This effect results primarily from association and exchange between granules of the more loosely bound peripheral proteins. Association of integral proteins is also involved. The rate of this protein association is considerably slower than the rate of calcium-induced aggregation, suggesting that this interaction is dependent on rearrangements of the proteins and lipids of the membrane secondary to aggregation (150). This would suggest that the protein–protein interactions studied here are not the cause of aggregation, but rather result from the aggregation.

In developing the concept of "stimulus–secretion coupling," Douglas and Rubin (63) noted many similarities between this process and excitation–contraction coupling in muscle. In recent years, evidence in support of this analogy has accumulated. Thus, adrenal medullary cells contain at least four of the most important contractile proteins. Bovine adrenal medulla contains two types of actin, both of which are slightly different from the actin found in skeletal muscle (123). As noted above, the actin is partially associated with the membrane of the catecholamine storage granules (12,76,124). The chromaffin-granule membrane also contains α-actinin which can serve as a binding site for actin (12,16). A role for actin in the release of catecholamines was suggested by recent experiments of Pollard et al. (178). They noted that isolated chromaffin-granule membranes increased the viscosity of actin solutions probably by providing binding sites which cross-linked the actin. These binding sites were protein in nature but probably not α-actinin. Their most interesting observation in this regard was that very low concentrations of calcium (0.1–1.0 μM) inhibited this binding of actin to the membranes. Pollard et al. (178) suggested that the calcium-induced inhibition of chromaffin-granule binding to actin may serve as an initial step in catecholamine release (step 2 in Figure 3). By freeing the granules from binding to the cytoskeleton, calcium would permit the granules to approach the plasma membrane. This interaction among actin, granule membranes, and calcium might also be important for the translocation of vesicles and for the process of membrane recovery after exocytosis.

The adrenal medullary cells also contain myosin, which is somewhat different in its properties from the myosin of striated muscle but similar to the myosin found in other nonmuscular tissue. The myosin appears to be somewhat concentrated in the region of the plasma membrane (49,91). This raises the interesting possibility that an interaction between the actin on the granules and the myosin on the plasma membrane could bring the storage granule close enough to the plasma membrane to permit fusion to occur. The analogy between excitation–contraction coupling and stimulus–secretion coupling continues with the demonstration that the adrenal medulla contains a calcium-binding protein which is very similar to, if not identical with, troponin-C of skeletal muscle. The troponin-C-like material of the adrenal medulla can account for at least 30% of the calcium-binding capacity in the cytosol and it undergoes a profound conformational change when it binds calcium, becoming more ordered, symmetrical, and compact (116,117). This then provides a molecular site of action for calcium in stimulus–secretion coupling. It is believed that in skeletal muscle, contraction is initiated by the calcium-induced conformational change in troponin-C, which is then transmitted to tropomyosin and other elements of the troponin system by a series of protein–protein interactions, which finally activates actomyosin ATPase. It is beginning to appear as if all of the elements necessary for this type of coupling exist in the adrenal medulla. In addition, Poisner (172) showed that the release of catecholamines from the adrenal medulla requires a source of metabolic energy and a calcium-activated ATPase activity. Finally, Aunis et al. (13) demonstrated that chromaffin granules could be seen in close association (separated by a gap of about 25 Å) with the inside of the plasma membrane. The gap between the two membranes was filled with an electron-dense material that appeared to be a cytoplasmic bridge between the two membranes. The investigators suggested that this was a proteinaceous material, but its nature is unknown. It might be the contractile proteins described above or some of the other proteins described below. There is also evidence indicating that elements of the cytoskeleton, especially the microtubules, are involved in catecholamine release from the adrenal medulla. It was suggested that the microtubles may be responsible for intracellular centrifugal movement of chromaffin granules to the region of the plasma membrane (45).

Creutz et al. (50) isolated and characterized a protein from the cytosol of bovine adrenal medulla that causes aggregation of chromaffin granules in the presence of physiological concentrations of calcium (but not magnesium, barium, or strontium). They called this protein "synexin" and showed that it was distinct from actin. The aggregation was temperature-dependent and stimulated by monovalent ions. Electron microscopic examination of the aggregates showed that the granules were flattened at the point of contact and that the contact was so close in some cases as to result in a pentalaminar membrane. However, the granules did not actually fuse to the point of having a common lumen. In the last few years a considerable amount of effort has gone into the study of synexin and its role in exocytosis. Immunofluorescent studies show that synexin is spread diffusely throughout the chromaffin cell but seems to be concentrated at the cell surface (177). The $K_{1/2}$ for calcium was very high, 200 μM. However, in the presence of 6 μM calcium, almost every chromaffin granule was associated with one or two others. Calcium concentrations of this magnitude are reasonable during activation of the cell, especially in the region of the plasma membrane (178). Calcium also induced self-association of synexin molecules in the absence of chromaffin granules. The molecular weight of synexin monomer is 47,000. In the presence of calcium, synexin polymerized into rods which were 100–150 Å long and 50 Å in diameter. These rods then joined themselves into parallel bundles (51). This reaction has the same $K_{1/2}$ and Hill coefficient for calcium as does the synexin-induced aggregation of chromaffin granules suggesting that the two phenomena may be related.

By binding chromaffin-cell-plasma membranes inside-out to polylysine-coated beads, Creutz et al. showed that there were calcium-sensitive binding sites for synexin on the inside of the plasma membrane. Other studies showed that there were binding sites on the outside of the chromaffin granule membrane (178). This provides strong support for a role of synexin in exocytosis (step 3 in Figure 3). Pollard and Scott (179) recently identified a cytosolic protein which competitively inhibits the synexin + calcium-induced aggregation of chromaffin granules. They called this protein "synhibin."

Meyer and Burger (141) isolated a protein from the plasma membrane of bovine adrenal medulla (note that synexin is a soluble protein) which also binds to chromaffin granules but not to adrenal medullary mitochondria or lysosomes. They presented evidence that this protein was distinct from synexin and suggested that it represented the site at which chromaffin granules bind to the plasma membrane during exocytosis. Recently, Zimmerberg et al. (242) demonstrated that incorporation of a membrane-associated calcium-binding protein into artificial lipid membranes greatly increased the sensitivity and specificity for calcium to facilitate membrane fusion. In their experiments, 10 μM calcium greatly increased the fusion of artifical phospholipid vesicles with membranes containing this protein.

A role for calmodulin has been suggested by the fact that several proteins in the chromaffin granule membrane bind calmodulin (79). Binding at some of these sites is increased by low concentrations of calcium; at other sites the binding is decreased by calcium. Binding of calmodulin to the chromaffin-granule membrane leads to the subsequent binding of several other cytosolic proteins to the granules. Since two of these proteins resemble the light chains of clathrin, Geisow and Burgoyne (79) suggested that this effect of calmodulin may be more important for endocytosis (membrane recovery) than exocytosis. Creutz (53) also identified several proteins in chromaffin cell cytosol which bind to granule membranes in the presence of calcium. Some of these proteins also promote granule aggregation. The molecular weight of four of these proteins coincide with the molecular weight of the cytosolic proteins identified by Geisow and Burgoyne.

Trifluoperazine inhibits synexin + calcium-induced granule aggregation. However, the specificity of this reaction for various phenothiazines was very different than the specificity of calmodulin. Thus calmodulin does not appear to be involved in this aggregation, but synexin appears to share some properties (sensitivity to phenothiazines) with calmodulin (178). Pollard et al. also reported that trifluoperazine inhibited catecholamine release from cultured chromaffin cells. They suggested that this was due to effects on the synexin-induced aggregation (178). It also appears that trifluoperazine inhibits the uptake of calcium by chromaffin cells in response to cholinergic agonists (222).

As noted above, synexin + calcium induces aggregation but not fusion of chromaffin granules. For exocytosis to occur, the chromaffin-granule membrane must fuse with the plasma membrane. In a search for something that would promote fusion of the membranes, Creutz (52) discovered that cis-unsaturated fatty acids have a specific action to cause fusion of previously aggregated chromaffin granules (step 4 in Figure 3). This fusion occurs quite rapidly with low concentrations of specific fatty acids. Arachidonic acid is the most effective, but conversion to prostaglandins or other products does not appear to be involved. In order for this fusion to occur, the vesicles must first be aggregated by synexin + calcium; aggregation by other compounds will not lead to fusion by arachidonic acid. Although calcium is required for the aggregation by synexin, it is not required for the fusion (52). The phospholipids of the chromaffin-granule membrane do contain a large percentage of arachidonic acid (237). The phospholipids of chromaffin cells can be labeled by incubating them with ^{3}H-arachidonic acid. When these cells are washed and then stimulated with secretogogues, there is a rapid release of labeled arachidonic acid into the medium (178). Thus, arachidonic acid–induced fusion of chromaffin-granule membranes to the plasma membrane may play an important role in exocytosis.

Once the granules have bound to and fused with the plasma membrane, Creutz, et al. have suggested that the granule actually releases its contents to the outside due to chemiosmotic lysis (175,176,178) (step 5 in Figure 3). According to this scheme, the membrane ATPase pumps hydrogen ions inside the granule. In the absence of an anion which can permeate the granule membrane (a permeant anion such as chloride or hydroxyl), a hydrogen ion gradient (inside acid), and membrane potential (inside positive) develop and this electrochemical gradient counterbalances the proton pump. The cytosol does not contain appreciable concentrations of anions which permeate the granule membrane but the extracellular fluid does contain such anions. When the granule membrane fuses with the plasma membrane, the granule membrane is exposed to these permeant anions. The anions are transported in by a specific carrier down their electrochemical gradient, thereby allowing more hydrogen ions to be pumped into the granule. Note that the anions are entering from the extracellular fluid whereas the hydrogen ions may be entering from the cytosol. This accumulation of hydrogen ions plus anions leads to an osmotic swelling and eventual rupture of the granule membrane. The point of rupture would most likely be at the most stressed point on the membrane, the site of fusion with the plasma membrane. This hypothesis is supported by several studies of the effect of various procedures on the lysis of isolated chromaffin granules induced by ATP-Mg^{+2} plus chloride, and on the catecholamine release from cultured chromaffin granules by veratridine and A23187 (a calcium ionophore). Both lysis of isolated granules and catecholamine release from cultured cells are: 1) increased by substitution of chloride with the more permeant anions bromide or iodide; 2) decreased by substitution of chloride with the less permeant anions isethionate or acetate; 3) decreased by an increase in the osmotic pressure of the medium; 4) decreased by the proton ionophore FCCP; and 5) decreased by inhibitors of specific anion transport such as probenecid and SITS (4-acetamido-4′-isothiocyanostilbene-2, 2′-disulfonic acid disodium) (177,178). Thus it appears that the proton pump ATPase plays a central role in the accumulation of catecholamines by the chromaffin granule and also in the rupture of the granule leading to catecholamine release.

The last two steps involved in exocytosis, namely sealing of the ruptured granule and recovery of the empty granule from fusion with the plasma membrane, remain a puzzle. Very little is known about the way in which the empty granule membrane is recovered and refilled for later reuse. This represents a vast frontier for future research.

REFERENCES

1. Abbs, M., and Phillips, J. (1980) Organization of the proteins of the chromaffin granule membrane. Biochim. Biohys. Acta 595, 200–221.
2. Aberer, W., Kostron, H., Huber, E., and Winkler, H. (1978) A characterization of the nucleotide uptake by chromaffin granules of bovine adrenal medulla. Biochem. J. 172, 353–360.
3. Aguirre, J., Pinto, J.E.B., and Trifaro, J.M. (1977) Calcium movements during the release of catecholamines from the adrenal medulla: Effects of methoxyverapamil and external cations. J. Physiol. (Lond.) 269, 371–394.
4. Ahkong, Q.F., Cramp, F.C., Fisher, D., Howell, J.I., and Lucy, J.A. (1972) Studies on chemically induced cell fusion. J. Cell Sci. 10, 769–787.
5. Ames, M.M., Lerner, P., and Lovenberg, W. (1978) Tyrosine hydroxylase. Activation by protein phosphorylation and end product inhibition. J. Biol. Chem. 253, 27–31.
6. Apps, D.K., and Schatz, G. (1979) An adenosine triphosphatase isolated from chromaffin-granule membranes is closely similar to F_1-adenosine triphosphatase of mitochondria. Eur. J. Biochem. 100, 411–419.
7. Apps, D.K., Pryde, J.G., and Phillips, J.H. (1980) Cytochrome b-561 is identical with chromomembrin B, a major polypeptide of chromaffin granule membranes. Neurosciences 5, 2279–2287.
8. Apps, D.K., Pryde, J.G., and Sutton, R., (1982) The H^+-translocating adenosine triphosphatase of chromaffin granule-membranes. N.Y. Acad. Sci. 402, 134–144.
9. Apps, D.K., Pryde, J.G., Sutton, R., and Phillips, J.H. (1980) Inhibition of adenosine triphosphatase, 5-hydroxytryptamine transport and proton-translocation activities of resealed chromaffin granule 'ghosts.' Biochem. J. 190, 273–282.
10. Archer, E.G., Breakfield, X.O., and Sharata, M.N. (1977) Transport of tyrosine, phenylalanine, tryptophan and glycine in neuroblastoma clones. J. Neurochem. 28, 127–135.
11. Aunis, D., Bouclier, M., Pescheloche, M., and Mandel, P. (1977) Properties of membrane-bound dopamine-β-hydroxylase in chromaffin granules from bovine adrenal medulla. J. Neurochem. 29, 439–447.
12. Aunis, D., Guerold, B., Bader, M.-F., and Cieselski-Treska, J. (1980) Immunocytochemical and biochemical demonstration of contractile proteins in chromaffin cells in culture. Neuroscience 5, 2261–2277.
13. Aunis, D., Hesketh, J.E., and Devillieus, G. (1979) Freeze-fracture study of the chromaffin cell during exocytosis: Evidence for connections between the plasma membrane and secretory granules and for movements of plasma membrane-associated particles. Cell Tissues Res. 197, 433–441.
14. Axelrod,J. (1962) Purification and properties of phenylethanol amine-N-methyl transferase. J. Biol. Chem. 237, 1657–1660.
15. Axelrod, J. (1975) Catechol-O-methyl transferase and other O-methyl transferases, In: H. Blaschko, G. Sayers, and A.D. Smith (eds.), Handbook of Physiology, Section 7: Endocrinology, Vol. 6: Adrenal Gland, Am. Physiol. Soc., Washington D.C., pp. 669–676.

16. Bader, M.-F., and Aunis, D. (1983) The 97-KD alpha -actinin-like protein in chromaffin granule membranes from adrenal medulla: Evidence for localization on the cytoplasmic surface and for binding to actin filaments. Neuroscience 8, 165–181.
17. Baker, P.F., and Knight, D.E. (1978) Calcium-dependent exocytosis in bovine adrenal medullary cells with leaky plasma membranes. Nature 276, 620–622.
18. Banks, P. (1965) The adenosine-triphosphatase activity of adrenal chromaffin granules. Biochem. J. 95, 490–496.
19. Banks, P. (1966) An interaction between chromaffin granules and calcium ions. Biochem. J. 101, 18c–20c.
20. Bashford, C.L., Casey, R.P., Radda, G.K., and Ritchie, G.A. (1976) Energy-coupling in adrenal chromaffin granules. Neuroscience 1, 399–412.
21. Bashford, C.L., Johnson, L.N., Radda, G.K., and Ritchie, G.A. (1976) Lipid ordering and enzymic activities in chromaffin granule membranes. Eur. J. Biochem. 67, 105–114.
22. Beers, M.F., Carty, S.E., Johnson, R.G., and Scarpa, A. (1982) H^+-ATPase and catecholamine transport in chromaffin granules. N.Y. Acad. Sci. 402, 116–132.
23. Berenbeim, D.M., Wong, D.L., Masover, S.J., and Ciaranello, R.D. (1979) Regulation of synthesis and degradation of rat adrenal phenylethanolamine N-methyltranferase. III. Stabilization of PNMT against thermal and tryptic degradation by S-adenosylmethionine. Molec. Pharmacol. 16, 482–490.
24. Biales, B., Dichter, M., and Tischler, A. (1976) Electrical excitability of cultured adrenal chromaffin cells. J. Physiol. (Lond.) 262, 743–753.
25. Bjerrum, O.J., Helle, K.B., and Bock, E. (1979) Immunochemically identical hydrophilic and amphiphilic forms of the bovine adrenomedullary dopamine β-hydroxylase. Biochem. J. 181, 231–237.
26. Blaschko, H. (1939) The specific action of L-Dopa decarboxylase. J. Physiol. (Lond.) 96, 50–51.
27. Blaschko, H., and Welch, A.D. (1953) Localization of adrenaline in cytoplasmic particles of the bovine adrenal medulla. Arch. exper. Pathol. Pharmakol. 219, 17–22.
28. Blaschko, H., Born, G.V.R., D'Iorio, A., Eade, N.R., (1956) Observations on the distribution of catechol amines and adenosinetriphosphate in the bovine adrenal medulla. J. Physiol. (Lond.) 133, 548–557.
29. Boonyaviroj, P., and Gutman, Y. (1977) Acetylcholine and cAMP in adrenal medulla: Indirect effect. Nauyn-Schmiedeberg's Arch. Pharmacol. 297, 241–243.
30. Borchardt, R.T., Olsen, J., Eiden, L., Schowen, R.L., and Rutledge, C.O. (1978) The isolation and characterization of the methyl acceptor protein from adrenal chromaffin granules. Biochem. Biophys. Res. Comm. 83, 970–976.
31. Brandt, B.L., Hagiwara, S., Kidokoro, Y., and Miyazaki, S. (1976) Action potentials in the rat chromaffin cell and effects of acetylcholine. J. Physiol. (Lond.) 263, 417–439.
32. Bruinvels, J. (1975) Role of sodium in neuronal uptake of monoamines and amino acid precursors. Nature 257, 606–607.
33. Bruinvels, J. (1977) Effects of sodium and potassium ions on the uptake of noradrenaline and its percursor tyrosine. Life Sci. 20, 437–444.
34. Buckland, R.M., Radda, G.K., and Shennan, C.D. (1978) Accessibility of phospholipids in the chromaffin granule membrane. Biochim. Biophys. Acta 513, 321–337.
35. Burke, W.J., Davis, J.W., Joh, T.H., Reis, D.J., Horenstein, S., and Bhagat, B.D. (1978) The effect of epinephrine on phenyl-ethanolamine N-methyltransferase in cultured explants of adrenal medulla. Endocrinology 103, 358–367.
36. Bygdeman, S., and Euler, U.S.v. (1958) Resynthesis of catechol hormones in the cat's adrenal medulla. Acta Physiol. Scand. 44, 375–383.
37. Carmichael, S.W., and Smith, D.J. (1978) Direct connections between mitochondria and catecholamine-storage vesicles demonstrated by high voltage electron microscopy in rat adrenal medulla. Cell Tiss. Res. 191, 421–432.
38. Carmichael, S.W., and Smith, D.J. (1978) High-voltage electron microscopy of adrenal

medulla: Direct connections between mitochondria and catecholamine-storage vesicles. Experientia 34, 391–392.

39. Casey, R.P., Njus, D., Radda, G.K., and Sehr, P.A. (1977) Active proton uptake by chromaffin granules: Observation by amine distribution and phosphorous-31 nuclear magnetic resonance techniques. Biochemistry 16, 972–976.
40. Christensen, H.N. (1969) Some special kinetic problems of transport. Adv. Enzymol. 32, 1–20.
41. Chubb, I.W., Preston, B.N., and Austin, L. (1969) Partial characterization of a naturally occurring inhibitor of dopamine β-hydroxylase. Biochem. J. 11, 243–244.
42. Cidon, S., and Nelson, N. (1983) A novel ATPase in the chromaffin granule membrane. J. Biol. Chem. 258, 2892–2898.
43. Cloutier, G., and Weiner, N. (1973) Further studies on the increased synthesis of norepinephrine during nerve stimulation of guinea-pig vas deferens preparation: Effect of tyrosine and 6,7-dimethyltetrahydropterin. J. Pharmacol. Exp. Ther. 186, 75–85.
44. Connett, R.J., and Kirshner, N. (1970) Purification and properties of bovine phenylethanolamine N-methyltransferase. J. Biol. Chem. 245, 329–334.
45. Cooke, P.H., and Poisner, A.M. (1979) The role of cytoskeleton in adreno-medullary secretion. Methods Archive. Exp. Pathol. 9, 137–146.
46. Costa, E., and Sandler, M. (eds.) (1972) Monoamine oxidases—New Vistas. Advances in Biomedical Psychopharmacology, Vol. 5, Raven Press, New York.
47. Coupland, R.E. (1975) Blood supply of the adrenal gland. In: H. Blaschko, G. Sayers, and A.D. Smith (eds), Handbook of Physiology, Section 7: Endocrinology, Vol. 6: Adrenal Gland, Am. Physiol. Soc., Washington, D.C., pp. 283–294.
48. Coupland, R.E., and Selby, J.E. (1976) The blood supply of the mammalian adrenal medulla: A comparative study. J. Anat. 122, 539–551.
49. Creutz, C.E. (1977) Isolation, characterization and localization of bovine adrenal medullary myosin. Cell Tissue Res. 178, 17–38.
50. Creutz, C.E., Pazoles, C., and Pollard, H.B. (1978) Identification and purification of an adrenal medullary protein (synexin) that causes calcium-dependent aggregation of isolated chromaffin granules. J. Biol. Chem. 253, 2858–2866.
51. Creutz, C.E., Pazoles, C.J., and Pollard, H.B. (1979) Self-association of synexin in the presence of calcium. J. Biol. Chem. 254, 553–558.
52. Creutz, C.E. (1981) cis-Unsaturated fatty acids induce the fusion of chromaffin granules aggregated by synexin. J. Cell. Biol. 91, 247–256.
53. Creutz, C.E. (1981) Secretory vesicle-cytosol interactions in exocytosis: Isolation by Ca^{2+}-dependent affinity chromatography of proteins that bind to the chromaffin granule membrane. Biochem. Biophys. Res. Comm. 103, 1395–1400.
54. Creveling, C.R., Daly, J.W., Witkop, B., and Udefriend, S. (1962) Substrates and inhibitors of dopamine-β-oxidase. Biochim. Biophys. Acta 64, 125–134.
55. Dairman, W., Christenson, J., and Udenfriend, S. (1973) Characterization of dopa decarboxylase. In: E. Usdin and S. Snyder (eds.), Frontiers in Catecholamine Research, Pergamon Press, New York-Toronto-Oxford-Sydney, pp. 61–67.
56. Dairman, W., Baird-Lambert, J., Marchelle, M., and Almgren, O. (1975) Studies on a potent inhibitor of aromatic-L-amino acid decarboxylase activity found in rat submaxillary gland: Development regulation, location and properties. In: O. Almgren, A. Carlsson, and J. Engel (eds.), Chemical Tools in Catecholamine Research, Vol. II, Elsevier, New York, pp. 73–79.
57. Daniels, A.J., Williams, R.J.P., and Wright, P.E. (1978) The character of the stored molecules in chromaffin granules of the adrenal medulla: A nuclear magnetic resonance study. Neuroscience 3, 573–585.
58. Daniels, A.J., Johnson, L.N., and Williams, R.J.P. (1979) Uptake of manganese by chromaffin granules in vitro. J. Neurochem. 33, 923–929.
59. Daniels, A.J., Dean, G., Viveros, D.H., and Dilberto, E.J. (1983) Secretion of newly

taken up ascorbic acid by adrenomedullary chromaffin cells originates from a compartment different from the catecholamine storage vesicle. Molec. Pharmacol. 23, 437–444.

60. Diliberto, E., and Allen, P. (1981) Mechanism of dopamine-β-hydroxylation. Semidehydroascorbate as the enzymic oxidation product of ascorbate. J. Biol. Chem. 256, 3385–3393.

61. Diliberto, E., Dean, G., Carter, C., and Allen, P. (1982) Tissue subcellular and submitochondrial distributions of semidehydroascorbate reductase: Possible role of semidehydroascorbate reductase in cofactor regulation. J. Neurochem. 39, 563–568.

62. Douglas, W.W. (1975) Secretomotor control of adrenal medullary secretion: Synaptic, membrane, and ionic events in stimulus-secretion coupling. In: H. Blaschko, G. Sayers and A.D. Smith (eds.), Handbook of Physiology, Section 7: Endocrinology, Vol. 6: Adrenal Gland, Am. Physiol. Soc., Washington, D.C., pp. 367–388.

63. Douglas, W.W., and Rubin, R.P. (1961) The role of calcium in the secretory response of the adrenal medulla to acetylcholine. J. Physiol. (Lond.) 159, 40–57.

64. Douglas, W.W., and Rubin, R.P. (1963) The mechanism of catecholamine release from the adrenal medulla and the role of calcium in stimulus-secretion coupling. J. Physiol. (Lond.) 167, 288–310.

65. Douglas, W.W., and Rubin, R.P. (1964) The effects of alkaline earths and other divalent cations on adrenal medullary secretion. J. Physiol. (Lond.) 175, 231–241.

66. Douglas, W.W., Kanno, T., and Sampson, S.R. (1967) Influence of the ionic environment on the membrane potential of adrenal chromaffin cells and on the depolarizing effect of acetylcholine. J. Physiol. (Lond.) 191, 107–121.

67. Douglas, W.W., Kanno, T., and Sampson, S.R. (1967) Effects of acetylcholine and other medullary secretagogues and antagonists on the membrane potential of adrenal chromaffin cells: An analysis employing techniques of tissue culture. J. Physiol. (Lond.) 188, 107–120.

68. Dreyfus, H., Aunis, D., Harth, S., and Mandel, P. (1977) Gangliosides and phospholipids of the membranes from bovine adrenal medullary chromaffin granules. Biochim. Biophys. Acta 489, 89–97.

69. Echeverria, O.M., Vazquez-Nin, G.H., and Chavez, B. (1977) Correlated ultrastructural and biochemical studies on the mechanisms of secretion of catecholamines. Acta Anat. 93, 313–324.

70. Echeverria, O.M., Vazquez-Nin, G.H., and Aguilar, R. (1978) Cytochemical study on the mechanism of secretion of catecholamines. Acta Anat. 100, 51–60.

71. Fenwick, E.M., Fajdiga, P.B., Howe, N.B.S., and Levitt, B.G. (1978) Functional and morphological characterization of isolated bovine adrenal medullary cells. J. Cell Biol. 76, 12–30.

72. Flatmark, T., Terland, O., and Helle, K.B. (1971) Electron carriers of the bovine adrenal chromaffin granules. Biochim. Biophys. Acta 226, 9–19.

73. Friedman, S., and Kaufman, S. (1965) 3,4-Dihydroxyphenylethylamine β-hydroxylase. Physical properties, copper content, and role of copper in the catalytic activity. J. Biol. Chem. 240, 4763–4773.

74. Friedman, S., and Kaufman, S. (1966) An electron paramagnetic resonance study of 3,4-dihydroxyphenylethylamine β-hydroxylase. J. Biol. Chem. 241, 2256–2259.

75. Fuxe, K., Goldstein, M., Hokfelt, M., and Joh, T.H. (1971) Cellular localization of dopamine-β-hydroxylase and phenylethanolamine-N-methyltransferase as revealed by immunohistochemistry. Prog. Brain Res. 34, 127–138.

76. Gabbiani, G., Da Prada, M., Richards, G., and Pletscher, A. (1976) Actin associated with membranes of monoamine storage organelles. Proc. Soc. Exp. Biol. Med. 152, 135–138.

77. Gabizon, R., Yetinson, T., and Schuldiner, S. (1982) Photoinactivation and identification of the biogenic amine transporter in chromaffin granules from bovine adrenal medulla. J. Biol. Chem. 257, 15145–15150.

78. Gagnon, C., Otten, U., and Thoenen, H. (1976) Increased synthesis of dopamine

β-hydroxylase in cultured rat adrenal medullae after in vivo administration of reserpine. J. Neurochem. 27, 259–265.

79. Geisow, M.J., and Burgoyne, R.D. (1983) Recruitment of cytosolic proteins to a secretory granule membrane depends on Ca^{2+}-calmodulin. Nature 301, 432–435.

80. Geissler, P., Martinek, A., Margolis, R.U., Margolis, RK., Skrivanek, J.A., Ledeen, R., Konig, P., and Winkler, H. (1977) Composition and biogenesis of complex carbohydrates of ox adrenal chromaffin granules. Neuroscience 2, 685–693.

81. Giraudat, J., Roisin, M.-P., and Henry, J.-P. (1980) Solubilization and reconstitution of the adenosine 5′-triphosphate dependent proton translocase of bovine chromaffin granule membrane. Biochemistry 19, 4499–4505.

82. Goldstein, M., Joh, T.H., and Garvey, T.Q. (1968) Kinetic studies on the enzymatic dopamine β-hydroxylation reaction. Biochemistry 7, 2724–2730.

83. Goldstein, M., Anagnoste, B., Freedman, L.S., Roffman, M., Ebstein, R.P., Park, D.H., Fuxe, K., and Hokfelt, T. (1973) Characterization, localization and regulation of catecholamine synthesizing enzymes. In: E. Usdin and S. Snyder (eds.), Frontiers in Catecholamine Research, Pergamon Press, New York-Toronto-Oxford-Sydney, pp. 69–78.

84. Granot, J., and Rosenheck, K. (1978) On the role of ATP and divalent metal ions in the storage of catecholamines. FEBS Lett. 95, 45–48.

85. Guidotti, A., and Costa, E. (1977) Trans-synaptic regulation of tyrosine 3-monooxygenase biosynthesis in rat adrenal medulla. Biochem. Pharmacol. 26, 817–823.

86. Guldberg, H.C., and Marsden, C.A. (1975) Catechol-O-methyl transferase: Pharmacological aspects and physiological role. Pharmacol. Rev. 27, 135–206.

87. Gutman, Y., and Boonyaviroj, P. (1979) Activation of adrenal medulla adenylate cyclase and catecholamine secretion. Naunyn-Schmiedebergs Arch. Pharmacol. 307, 39–44.

88. Gutman, Y., Lichtenberg, D., Cohen, J., and Boonyaviroj, P. (1979) Increased catecholamine release from adrenal medulla by liposomes loaded with sodium or calcium ions. Biochem. Pharmacol. 28, 1209–1211.

89. Haynes, D.H., Kolber, M., and Morris, S.J. (1979) Short-and long-range forces involved in cation-induced aggregation of chromaffin granule membranes. J. Theor. Biol. 87, 713–743.

90. Hersey, R.M. and DiStefano, V. (1979) Control of phenylethanolamine N-methyltranferase by glucocorticoids in cultured bovine adrenal medullary cells. J. Pharmacol. Exp. Therap. 209, 147–152.

91. Hesketh, J.E., Aunis, D., Pescheloch, M., and Mandel, P. (1977) Subcellular distribution of myosin (K+, EDTA)-ATPase in bovine adrenal medulla. FEBS Lett. 80, 324–328.

92. Hillarp, N.-A (1958) Enzymic systems involving adenosine-phosphatases in the adrenaline and noradrenaline containing granules of the adrenal medulla. Acta Physiol. Scand. 42, 144–165.

93. Hillarp, N.-A., Lagerstedt, S., and Nilson, B. (1953) The isolation of a granular fraction from the suprarenal medulla, containing the sympathomimetic catechol amines. Acta Physiol. Scand. 29, 251– 263.

94. Hochman, J., and Perlman, R.L. (1976) Catecholamine secretion by isolated adrenal cells. Biochim. Biophys. Acta 421 168–175.

95. Hoeldtke, R., Kaufman, S. (1977) Bovine adrenal tyrosine hydroxylase. Purification and properties. J. Biol. Chem. 252, 3160–3169.

96. Holz, R.W. (1978) Evidence that catecholamine transport into chromaffin vesicles is coupled to vesicle membrane potential. Proc. Nat. Acad. Sci. (U.S.A.) 75, 5190–5194.

97. Hortnagl, H. (1976) Membranes of the adrenal medulla: A comparison of membranes of chromaffin granules with those of the endoplasmic reticulum. Neuroscience 1, 9–18.

98. Hortnagl, H., Lochs, H., and Winkler, H. (1974) Immunological studies on the acidic chromogranins and on dopamine β-hydroxylase (EC 1.14.2.1) of bovine chromaffin granules. J. Neurochem. 22, 197–199.

99. Huber, E., Konig, P., Schuler, G., Aberer, W., Plattner, H., and Winkler, H. (1979) Characterization and topography of the glycoproteins of adrenal chromaffin granules. J. Neurochem. 32, 35–47.
100. Joh, T.H., and Goldstein, M. (1973) Isolation and characterization of multiple forms of phenylethanolamine N-methyltransferase. Mol. Pharmacol. 9, 117–129.
101. Johnson, R.G., and Scarpa, A. (1976) Ion permeability of isolated chromaffin granules. J. Gen. Physiol. 68, 601–631.
102. Jonasson, J., Rosengren, E., and Waldeck, B. (1964) Effects of some pharmacologically active amines on the uptake of arylalkylamines by adrenal medullary granules. Acta Physiol. Scand. 60, 136–140.
103. Kanner, B.I., Fishkes, H., Maron, R., Sharon, I., and Schuldiner, S. (1979) Reserpine as a competitive and reversible inhibitor of the catecholamine transporter of bovine chromaffin granules. FEBS Lett. 100, 175–178.
104. Katz, I.R., Yamauchi, T., and Kaufman, S. (1976) Activation of tyrosine hydroxylase by polyanions and salts. An electrostatic effect. Biochim. Biophys. Acta 429, 84–95.
105. Kaufman, S. (1973) Cofactors of tyrosine hydroxylase. In: E. Usdin and S. Snyder (eds.), Frontiers in Catecholamine Research, Pergamon Press, New York-Toronto-Oxford-Sydney, pp. 53–60.
106. Kayaalp, S.O., and Neff, N.H. (1979) Muscarinic receptor binding in the rat adrenal medulla. Eur. J. Pharmacol. 57, 255–257.
107. Kirshner, N. (1962) Uptake of catecholamines by a particulate fraction of the adrenal medulla. J. Biol. Chem. 237, 2311–2317.
108. Kirshner, N. (1975) Biosynthesis of catecholamines. In: H. Blaschko, G. Sayers, and A.D. Smith (eds.), Handbook of Physiology, Section 7: Endocrinology, Vol. 6: Adrenal Gland, Am. Physiol. Soc., Washington, D.C., pp. 341–355.
109. Kirshner, N., and Goodall, McC. (1957) The formation of adrenaline from noradrenaline. Biochim. Biophys. Acta 24, 658–659.
110. Kirshner, N., Kirshner, A.G., and Kamin, D.L. (1966) Adenosine triphosphatase activity of adrenal medulla catecholamine granules. Biochim. Biophys. Acta 113, 332–335.
111. Knoth, J., Handloser, K., and Njus, D. (1980) Electrogenic epinephrine transport in chromaffin granule ghosts. Biochemistry 19, 2938–2942.
112. Konig, P., Hortnagl, H., Kostron, H., Sapinsky, H., and Winkler, H. (1976) The arrangement of dopamine β-hydroxylase (EC 1.14.2.1) and chromomembrin B in the membrane of chromaffin granules. J. Neurochem. 27, 1539–1541.
113. Konings, F., and DePotter, W. (1983) Protein phosphorylation and the exocytosis-like interaction between adrenal medullary plasma membranes and chromaffin granules. Biochem. Biophys. Res. Comm. 110, 55–60.
114. Kostron, H., Winkler, H., Geissler, D., and Konig, P. (1977) Uptake of calcium by chromaffin granules in vitro. J. Neurochem. 28, 487–493.
115. Kuhar, M.J., and Zarbin, M.A. (1978) Synaptosomal transport: A chloride dependence for choline, GABA, glycine and several other compounds. J. Neurochem. 31, 251–256.
116. Kuo, I.C.Y., and Coffee, C.J. (1976) Purification and characterization of a troponin-C-like protein from bovine adrenal medulla. J. Biol. Chem. 251, 1603–1609.
117. Kuo, I.C.Y., and Coffee, C.J. (1976) Bovine adrenal medulla troponin-C. Demonstration of a calcium-dependent conformational change. J. Biol. Chem. 251, 6315–6319.
118. Laduron, P. (1972) N-Methylation of dopamine to epinine in adrenal medulla: A new model for the biosynthesis of adrenaline. Arch. Int. Pharmacodyn. 195, 197–208.
119. Laduron, P., and Belpaire, F. (1968) Tissue fractionation and catecholamines. II. Intracellular distribution patterns of tyrosine hydroxylase, dopa decarboxylase, dopamine-β-hydroxylase, phenethanolamine-N-methyltransferase and monoamine oxidase in adrenal medulla. Biochem. Pharmacol. 17, 1127–1140.
120. Lagercrantz, H. (1976) On the composition and function of large dense cored vesicles in sympathetic nerves. Neuroscience 1, 81–92.

121. Ledbetter, F.H., and Kirshner, N. (1975) Studies of chick adrenal medulla in organ culture. Biochem. Pharmacol. 24, 967–974.

122. Ledbetter, F.H., Kilpatrick, D., Sage, H.L., and Kirshner, N. (1978) Synthesis of chromogranins and dopamine β-hydroxylase by perfused bovine adrenal glands. Am. J. Physiol. 235, E475–E-486.

123. Lee, R.W.H., Mushyhski, W.E., and Trifaro, J.M. (1979) Two forms of cytoplasmic actin in adrenal chromaffin cells. Neuroscience 4, 843–852.

122. Lee, R., and Trifaro, J. (1981) Characterizaion of anti-actin antibodies and their use in immunocytochemical studies on the localization of actin in adrenal chromaffin cells in culture. Neuroscience 6, 2087–2108.

125. Lefebvre, Y.A., White, D.A., and Hawthorne, J.N. (1976) Diphosphoinositide metabolism in bovine adrenal medulla. Can. J. Biochem. 54, 746–753.

126. Letendre, C.H., Mac Donnell, P.C., and Guroff, G. (1977) The biosynthesis of phosphorylated tyrosine hydroxylase by organ cultures of rat adrenal medulla and superior cervical ganglia. Biochem. Biophys. Res. Comm. 74, 891–897.

127. Letendre, C.H., Mac Donnell, P. C., and Guroff, G. (1977) The biosynthesis of phosphorylated tyrosine hydroxylase by organ cultures of rat adrenal medulla and superior cervical ganglia: A correction. Biochem. Biophys. Res. Comm. 76, 615–617.

128. Levin, J.A. (1974) The uptake and metabolism of ^{3}H-*l*-and ^{3}H-*d,l*-norepinephrine by intact rabbit aorta and by isolated adventitia and media. J. Pharmacol. Exp. Therap. 190, 210–226.

129. Levitt, M., Spector, S., Sjoerdsma, A., and Udenfriend, S. (1965) Elucidation of the rate-limiting step in norepinephrine biosynthesis in the perfused guinea-pig heart. J. Pharmacol. Exp. Therap. 148, 1–8.

130. Liang, B.T., and Perlman, R.L. (1979) Catecholamine secretion by hamster adrenal cells. J. Neurochem. 32, 927–933.

131. Ljones, T., Skotland, T., and Flatmark, T. (1976) Purification and characterization of dopamine-β-hydroxylase from bovine adrenal medulla. Eur. J. Biochem. 61, 525–533.

132. Lloyd, T., and Kaufman, S. (1975) Evidence for the lack of direct phosphorylation of bovine caudate tyrosine hydroxylase following activation by exposure to enzymatic phosphorylating conditions. Biochem. Biophys. Res. Comm. 66, 907–913.

133. Lovenberg, W., Bruckwick, E.A., and Hanbauer, I. (1975) ATP, cyclic AMP and magnesium increase the affinity of rat striatal tyrosine hydroxylase for its cofactor. Proc. Nat. Acad. Sci. (USA) 72, 2955–2958.

134. Maron, R., Fishkes, H., Kanner, B.I., and Schuldiner, S. (1979) Solubilization and reconstitution of the catecholamine transporter from bovine chromaffin granules. Biochemistry 18, 4781–4785.

135. Marsh, D., Radda, G.K., and Ritchie, G.A. (1976) A spin-label study of the chromaffin granule membrane. Eur. J. Biochem. 71, 53–61.

136. Masover, S.J., Berenbeim, D.M., and Ciaranello, R.D. (1979) Regulation of synthesis and degradation of rat adrenal phenylethanolamine N-methyl transferase. IV. Synergistic stabilization of the enzyme against thermal and tryptic degradation by S-adenosylmethionine and biogenic amine substrates. Molec. Pharmacol. 16, 491–503.

137. Masserano, J.M., and Weiner, N. (1979). The rapid activation of adrenal tyrosine hydroxylase by decapitation and its relationship to a cyclic AMP-dependent phosphorylating mechanism. Molec. Pharmacol. 16, 513–528.

138. Matthews, E.K., Evans, R.J., and Dean, P.M. (1972) The ionogenic nature of the secretory-granule membrane. Biochem. J. 130, 825–832.

139. Meyer, S.E. (1980) Neurohumoral transmission and the autonomic nervous system. In: A.G. Gilman, L.S. Goodman, and A. Gilman (eds.), The Pharmacological Basis of Therapeutics, 6th Edition, Macmillan, New York, pp. 56–90.

140. Meyer, D.I., and Burger, M.M. (1976) The chromaffin granule surface. Localization of carbohydrate on the cytoplasmic surface of an intracellular organelle. Biochim. Biophys. Acta 443, 428–436.

141. Meyer, D.I., and Burger, M.M. (1979) Isolation of a protein from the plasma membrane of adrenal medulla which binds to secretory vesicles. J. Biol. Chem. 254, 9854–9859.

142. Molinoff, P.B., and Axelrod, J. (1971) Biochemistry of catecholamines. Ann. Rev. Biochem. 40, 465–500.

143. Molinoff, P.B., Brimijoin, S., Weinshilboum, R., and Axelrod, J. (1970) Neurally mediated increase in dopamine-β-hydroxylase activity. Proc. Nat. Acad. Sci. (USA) 66, 453–458.

144. Morgenroth, V.H., Boadle-Biber, M., and Roth, R.H. (1974) Tyrosine hydroxylase: Activation by nerve stimulation. Proc. Nat. Acad. Sci. (USA) 71, 4283–4287.

145. Morita, K., Oka, M., and Izumi, F. (1977) Activation by cyclic AMP of soluble tyrosine hydroxylase in bovine adrenal medulla. FEBS Lett. 76, 148–150.

146. Morita, K., Tachikawa, E., Oka, M., and Ohuchi, T. (1977) Activation of adrenal tyrosine hydroxylase by ATP and other nucleotides. FEBS Lett. 84, 101–104.

147. Morris, S.J., Chiu, V.K.C., and Haynes, D.H. (1979) Divalent cation-induced aggregation of chromaffin granule membranes. Membr. Biochem. 2, 162–202.

148. Morris, S.J., and Schovanka, I. (1977) Some physical properties of adrenal medulla chromaffin granules isolated by a new continuous iso-osmotic density gradient method. Biochim. Biophys. Acta 464, 53–64.

149. Morris, S.J., Schober, R., and Schultens, H.A. (1977) Correlation of physical and morphological parameters with release of catecholamines, ATP, and protein from adrenal medulla chromaffin granules. Biochim. Biophys. Acta. 464, 65–81.

150. Morris, S.J., Sudhof, T.C., and Haynes, D.H. (1982) Calcium-promoted resonance energy transfer between fluorescently labelled proteins during aggregation of chromaffin granule membranes. Biochim. Biophys. Acta. 693, 425–436.

151. Muller, T.W., and Kirshner, N. (1975) ATP-ase and phosphatidylinositol kinase activities of adrenal chromaffin vesicles. J. Neurochem. 24, 1155–1161.

152. Musacchio, J.M. (1968) Subcellular distribution of adrenal tyrosine hydroxylase. Biochem. Pharmacol. 17, 1470–1473.

153. Musacchio, J., Kopin, I.J., and Snyder, S. (1964) Effects of disulfiram on tissue norepinephrine content and subcellular distribution of dopamine, tyramine and their beta-hydroxylated metabolites. Life Sci. 3, 769–775.

154. Nagatsu, T., Levitt, M., and Undenfriend, S. (1964) Tyrosine hydroxylase. The initial step in norepinephrine biosynthesis. J. Biol. Chem. 239, 2910–2917.

155. Nagatsu, T., Hidaka, H., Kuzuya, H., and Takeya, K. (1970) Inhibition of dopamine β-hydroxylase by fusaric acid (5-butylpicolinic acid) in vitro and in vivo. Biochem. Pharmacol. 19, 35–44.

156. Nichols, J.W., and Deamer, D.W. (1976) Catecholamine uptake and concentration by liposomes maintaining pH gradients. Biochim. Biophys. Acta 455, 269–271.

157. Nikodijevic, O., Nikodijevic, B., Zinder, O., Yu, M.-Y. W., Guroff, G., and Pollard, H.B. (1976) Control of adenylate cyclase from secretory vesicle membranes by β-adrenergic agents and nerve growth factor. Proc. Nat. Acad. Sci. (USA) 73, 771–774.

158. Njus, D., Knoth, J., Cook, C., and Kelley, P.M. (1983) Electron transfer across the chromaffin granule membrane. J. Biol. Chem. 258, 27–30.

159. Njus, D., and Radda, G.K. (1978) Bioenergetic processes in chromaffin granules. A new perspective on some old problems. Biochim. Biophys. Acta 463, 219–244.

160. Njus, D., Knoth, J., and Zallakian, M. (1981) Proton-linked transport in chromaffin granules. Curr. Topics Bioenergetics 11, 107–147.

161. Njus, D., Sehr, P.A., Radda, G.K., Ritchie, G.A., and Seeley, P.J. (1978) Phosphorus-31 nuclear magnetic resonance studies of active proton translocation in chromaffin granules. Biochemistry, 17, 4337–4343.

162. O'Connor, D.T., Frigon, R.P., and Stone, R.A. (1979) Human pheochromocytoma dopamine-beta-hydroxylase: Purification and molecular parameters of the tetramer. Mol. Pharmacol. 16, 529–538.

163. de Oliveria Filgueiras, O.M., Van den Besselaar, A.M.P.H., and Van den Bosch, H. (1979) Localization of lysophosphatidylcholine in bovine chromaffin granules. Biochim. Biophys. Acta 558, 73–84.

164. Otten, U., Schwab, M., Gagnon, C., and Thoenen, H. (1977) Selective induction of tyrosine hydroxylase and dopamine β-hydroxylase by nerve growth factor: Comparison between adrenal medulla and sympathetic ganglia of adult and newborn rats. Brain Res. 133, 291–303.

165. Paton, D.M. (ed.) (1976) The mechanism of neuronal and extraneuronal transport of catecholamines. Raven Press, New York.

166. Peer, L.J., Winkler, H., Snider, S.R., Gibb, J.W., and Baumgartner, H. (1976) Synthesis of nucleotides in adrenal medulla and their uptake into chromaffin granules. Biochem. Pharmacol. 25, 311–315.

167. Perlman, R.L. (1976) The permeability of chromaffin granules to non-electrolytes. Biochem. Pharmacol. 25, 1035–1038.

168. Phillips, J.H. (1978) 5-Hydroxytryptamine transport by the bovine chromaffin granule membrane. Biochem. J. 170, 673–679.

169. Phillips, J.H., and Allison, Y.P. (1978) Proton translocation by the bovine chromaffin-granule membrane. Biochem. J. 170, 661–672.

170. Pinto, J.E.B., and Trifaro, J.M. (1976) The different effects of D-600 (methoxyverapamil) on the release of adrenal catecholamines induced by acetylcholine, high potassium or sodium deprivation. Br. J. Pharmacol. 57, 127–132.

171. Pletscher, A., Da Prada, M., Berneis, K.H., Steffen, H., Lutold, B., and Weder, H.G. (1974) Molecular organization of amine storage organelles of blood platelets and adrenal medulla. In: B. Ceccarelli, F. Clementi and J. Meldolesi (eds.), Advances in Cytopharmacology, Vol. 2, Raven Press, New York, pp. 257–264.

172. Poisner, A.M. (1970) Release of transmitters from storage: A contractile model. In: E. Costa and E. Giacobini (eds.), Advances in Biochemical Psychopharmacology, Vol. 2, Raven Press, New York, pp. 95–108.

173. Poisner, A.M. (1973) Mechanisms of exocytosis. In: E. Usdin and S. Snyder (eds.), Frontiers in Catecholamine Research, Pergamon Press, New York-Toronto-Oxford-Sydney, pp. 477–482.

174. Poisner, A.M., and Douglas, W.W. (1966) The need for calcium in adrenomedullary secretion evoked by biogenic amines, polypeptides, and muscarinic agents. Proc. Soc. Exp. Biol. Med. 123, 62–64.

175. Pollard, H.B., Zinder, O., Hoffman, P.G., and Nikodijevic, O. (1976) Regulation of the transmembrane potential of isolated chromaffin granules by ATP, ATP analogs and external pH. J. Biol. Chem. 251, 4544–4550.

176. Pollard, H.B., Pazoles, C.J., Creutz, C.E., Ramu, A., Strott, C.A., Ray, P., Brown, E.M., Aurbach, G.D., Tack-Goldman, K.M., and Shulman, N.R. (1977) A role for anion transport in the regulation of release from chromaffin granules and exocytosis from cells. J. Supramolec. Struct. 7, 277–285.

177. Pollard, H.B., Pazoles, C.J., and Creutz, C.E. (1981) Mechanism of calcium action and release of vesicle-bound hormones during exocytosis. Rec. Prog. Horm. Res. 37, 299–325.

178. Pollard, H.B., Creutz, C.E., Scott, F.J., and Pazoles, C.J. (1982) Calcium-dependent regulation of chromaffin granule movement, membrane contact, and fusion during exocytosis. Cold Spring Harbor Symp. Quant. Biol. 46, 819–834.

179. Pollard, H.B., and Scott, J.H. (1982) Synhibin: A new calcium-dependent membrane binding protein that inhibits synexin-induced chromaffin granule aggregation and fusion. FEBS Lett. 150, 201–206.

180. Price, H.C., and Yu, R.K. (1976) Adrenal medulla gangliosides. A comparative study of some mammals. Comp. Biochem. Physiol. 54B, 451–454.

181. Ravazzola, M. (1976) Intracellular localization of calcium in the chromaffin cells of the rat adrenal medulla. Endocrinology 98, 950–953.

182. Richelson, E. (1974) Studies on the transport of L-tyrosine into an adrenergic clone of mouse neuroblastoma. J. Biol. Chem. 249, 6218–6224.
183. Rimle, P., Morse, P.D., and Njus, D. (1983) A spin-label study of plasma membranes of adrenal chromaffin cells. Biochim. Biophys. Acta 728, 92–96.
184. Rink, T.J. (1977) The influence of sodium on calcium movements and catecholamine release in thin slices of bovine adrenal medulla. J. Physiol. (Lond.) 266, 297–325.
185. Roisin, M.P., Scherman, D., and Henry, J.P. (1980) Synthesis of ATP by an artificially imposed electrochemical proton gradient in chromaffin granule ghosts. FEBS Lett. 115, 143–147.
186. Roth, R.H., and Salzman, P.M. (1977) Role of calcium in the depolarization-induced activation of tyrosine hydroxylase. In: E. Usdin, N. Weiner and M.B.H. Youdim (eds.), Structure and Function of Monoamine Enzymes, Marcel Dekker, New York-Basel, pp. 149–168.
187. Scherman, D., and Henry, J.-P. (1983) The catecholamine carrier of bovine chromaffin granules. Form of the bound amine. Molec. Pharmacol. 23, 431–436.
188. Schneeweiss, F., Naquira, P., Rosenheck, K., and Schneider, A.S. (1979) Cholinergic stimulants and excess potassium ion increase the fluidity of plasma membranes isolated from adrenal chromaffin cells. Biochim. Biophys. Acta 555, 460–471.
189. Schneider, A., Herz, R., and Rosenbeck, K. (1977) Stimulus-secretion coupling in chromaffin cells isolated from bovine adrenal medulla. Proc. Nat. Acad. Sci. (USA) 74, 5036–5040.
190. Schober, R., Natsch, C., and Rinne, U. (1977) Calcium-induced displacement of membrane-associated particles upon aggregation of chromaffin granules. Science 195, 495–497.
191. Schuldiner, S., Fishkes, H., and Kanner, B. (1978) Role of a transmembrane pH gradient in epinephrine transport by chromaffin granule membrane vesicles. Proc. Nat. Acad. Sci (USA) 8, 3713–3716.
192. Schuler, G., Plattner, H., Aberer, W., and Winkler, H. (1978) Particle segregation in chromaffin granule membranes by forced physical contact. Biochim. Biophys. Acta 513, 244–254.
193. Schumann, H.J., and Brodde, O.-E. (1976) Lack of epinine formation in adrenal medulla and brain of rats during cold exposure and inhibition of dopamine β-hydroxylase. Naunyn-Schmiedeberg's Arch. Pharmacol. 293, 139–144.
194. Sedvall, G.C., and Kopin, I.J. (1967) Acceleration of norepinephrine synthesis in the rat submaxillary gland in vivo during sympathetic nerve stimulation. Life Sci. 6, 45–51.
195. Sen, R., Sharp, R.R., Domnio, L.E., and Domino, E.F. (1979) Composition of the aqueous phase of chromaffin granules. Biochim. Biophys. Acta 587, 75–88.
196. Sharman, D.F. (1975) The metabolism of circulating catecholamines. In: H. Blaschko, G. Sayers, and A.D. Smith (eds.), Handbook of Physiology, Section 7: Endocrinology, Vol. 6: Adrenal Gland, Am. Physiol. Soc., Washington, D.C., pp. 699–712.
197. Sharp, R.R., and Richards, E.P. (1977) Molecular mobilities of soluble components in the aqueous phase of chromaffin granules. Biochim. Biophys. Acta 497, 260–271.
198. Sharp, R.R., and Sen, R. (1978) Molecular mobilities in chromaffin granules. Magnetic field dependence of proton T_1 relaxation times. Biochim. Biophys. Acta 538, 155–163.
199. Shiman, R., Akino, M., and Kaufman, S. (1971) Solubilization and partial purification of tyrosine hydroxylase from bovine adrenal medulla. J. Biol. Chem. 246, 1330–1340.
200. Silsand, R., and Flatmark, T. (1974) Purification of cytochrome b-561. An integral heme protein of the adrenal chromaffin granule membrane. Biochim. Biophys. Acta 359, 257–266.
201. Skotland, T., and Ljones, T. (1980) Direct spectrophotometric detection of ascorbate free radical formed by dopamine-β-monooxygenase and by ascorbate oxidase. Biochim. Biophys. Acta 630, 30–35.

202. Skotland, T., Petersson, L., Backstrom, D., Ljones, T., Flatmark, T., and Ehrenberg, A. (1980) Electron paramagnetic resonance of the copper in dopamine β-monooxygenase. Eur. J. Biochem. 103, 5–11.

203. Slotkin, T.A. (1977) Hypothetical model of catecholamine uptake into adrenal medullary storage vesicles. Life Sci. 13, 675–683.

204. Slotkin, T.A., Anderson, T.R., Seidler, F.J., and Lau, C. (1975) Inhibition of epinephrine and metaraminol uptake into adrenal medullary vesicles by aralkylamines and alkylamines. Biochem. Pharmacol. 24, 1413–1419.

205. Snider, S.R., Miller, C., Prasad, A.L.N., Jackson, V., and Fahn, S. (1977) Is dopamine a neurohormone of the adrenal medulla? Naunyn-Schmiedeberg's Arch. Pharmacol. 297, 17–22.

206. Sourkes, T. (1977) Enzymology of aromatic amino acid decarboxylases. In: E. Usdin, N. Weiner, and M.B.H. Youdim (eds.), Structure and Function of Monoamine Enzymes, Marcel Dekker, New York-Basel, pp. 477–496.

207. Stjarne, L. (1972) The synthesis, uptake and storage of catecholamines in the adrenal medulla. The effect of drugs. In: H. Blaschko and E. Muscholl (eds.), Handbook of Experimental Pharmacology, XXXIII, Catecholamines, Springer-Verlag, Berlin-Heidelberg-New York, pp. 231–269.

208. Taugner, G., and Wunderlich, I. (1979) Partial characterization of a phosphoryl group transferring enzyme in the membrane of catecholamine storage vesicles. Naunyn-Schmiedeberg's Arch. Pharmacol. 309, 45–58.

209. Taugner, G., Wunderlich, I., and John, F. (1979) Distribution and metabolic fate of adenosine nucleotides in the membrane of storage vesicles from bovine adrenal medulla. Naunyn-Schmiedeberg's Arch. Pharmacol. 309, 29–43.

210. Terland, O., and Flatmark, T. (1975) Ascorbate as a natural constituent of the chromaffin granules from the bovine adrenal medulla. FEBS Lett. 59, 52–56.

211. Terland, O., Flatmark, T., and Kryvi, H. (1979) Isolation and characterization of noradrenalin storage granules of bovine adrenal medulla. Biochim. Biophys. Acta 553, 460–468.

212. Tipton, K.F., (1975) Monoamine oxidase. In: H. Blaschko, G. Sayers, and A.D. Smith (eds.), Handbook of Physiology, Section 7: Endocrinology, Vol. 6: Adrenal Gland, Am. Physiol. Soc., Washington, D.C., pp. 677–697.

213. Tirrell, J.G., and Westhead, E.W. (1979) The uptake of ascorbic acid and dehydroascorbic acid by chromaffin granules of the adrenal medulla. Neuroscience 4, 181–186.

214. Toll, L., Gundersen, C.B., Jr., and Howard, B.D. (1977) Energy utilization in the uptake of catecholamines by synaptic vesicles and adrenal chromaffin granules. Brain Res. 136, 59–66.

215. Treiman, M., Weber, W., and Gratzl, M. (1983) 3′,5′-Cyclic adenosine monophosphate and Ca^{2+}-calmodulin-dependent endogenous protein phosphorylation activity in membranes of the bovine chromaffin secretory vesicles: Identification of two phosphorylated components as tyrosine hydroxylase and protein kinase regulatory subunit type II. J. Neurochem. 40, 661–669.

216. Trifaro, J.M., Duerr, A.C., and Pinto, J.E.B. (1976) Membranes of the adrenal medulla: A comparison between the membranes of the Golgi apparatus and chromaffin granules. Mol. Pharmacol. 12, 536–545.

217. Uvnas, B., and Aborg, C.-H. (1977) The ability of ATP-free granule material from bovine adrenal medulla to bind inorganic cations and biogenic amines. Acta Physiol. Scand. 99, 476–483.

218. Van Dyke, K., Robinson, R., Urquilla, P., Smith, D., Taylor, M., Trush, M., and Wilson, M. (1977) An analysis of nucleotides and catecholamines in bovine medullary granules by anion exchange high pressure liquid chromotography and fluorescence. Pharmacology 15, 377–391.

219. Van Orden, L.S., Burke, J.P., Redick, J.A., Rybarczyk, K.E., Van Orden, D.E., Baker, H.A., and Hartman, B.K. (1977) Immunocytochemical evidence for particulate locali-

zation of phenylethanolamine-N-methyltransferase in adrenal medulla. Neuropharmacology 16, 129–133.

220. Vigny, A., Flamand, M.-F., and Henry, J.-P. (1978) Bovine adrenal medulla tyrosine hydroxylase: Separation of the native and aggregate forms. FEBS Lett. 86, 235–238.

221. Viveros, O.H. (1975) Mechanism of secretion of catecholamines from adrenal medulla. In: H. Blaschko, G. Sayers and A.D. Smith (eds.), Handbook of Physiology, Section 7: Endocrinology, Vol. 6: Adrenal Gland, Am. Physiol. Soc., Washington, D.C., pp. 389–426.

222. Wada, A., Yanagihara, N., Izumi, F., Sakuri, S., and Kobayashi, H. (1983) Trifluoperazine inhibits $^{45}Ca^{2+}$ uptake and catecholamine secretion and synthesis in adrenal medullary cells. J. Neurochem. 40, 481–486.

223. Wallace, E.F., Krantz, M.J., and Lovenberg, W. (1973) Dopamine β-hydroxylase: A tetrameric glycoprotein. Proc. Nat. Acad. Sci (USA) 70, 2253–2255.

224. Waymire, J.C., Gilmer-Waymire, K., Noritake, D., Gibson, G., Kitayama, D., and Haycock, J.W. (1979) Induction of tyrosine hydroxylase and dopamine β-hydroxylase in cultured mouse neuroblastoma by 8Br-cAMP. Mol. Pharmacol. 15, 78–85.

225. Weber, A., and Winkler, H. (1981) Specificity and mechanism of nucleotide uptake by adrenal chromaffin granules. Neuroscience 11, 2269–2276.

226. Weber, A., Westhead, E.W., and Winkler, H. (1983) Specificity and properties of the nucleotide carrier in chromaffin granules from bovine adrenal medulla. Biochem. J. 210, 789–794.

227. Weiner, N. (1970) Regulation of norepinephrine synthesis. In: H.W. Elliott (ed.) Annual Review of Pharmacology, Vol, 10, Annual Reviews, Palo Alto, pp. 273–290.

228. Weiner, N. (1980) Norepinephrine, epinephrine, and the sympathomimetic amines. In: A.G. Gilman, L.S. Goodman and A. Gilman (eds.), The Pharmacological Basis of Therapeutics, 6th edition, Macmillan, New York, pp. 138–175.

229. Weiner, N., and Rabadjija, M. (1968) The regulation of norepinephrine synthesis. Effect of puromycin on the accelerated synthesis of norepinephrine associated with nerve stimulation. J. Pharmacol. Exp. Ther. 164, 103–114.

230. Weiner, N., Cloutier, G., Bjur, R., and Pfeffer, R.I. (1972) Modification of norepinephrine synthesis in intact tissue by drugs and during short-term adrenergic nerve stimulation. Pharm. Rev. 24, 203–221.

231. Weiner, N., Lee, F.-L., Barnes, E., and Dreyer, E. (1977) Enzymology of tyrosine hydroxylase and the role of cyclic nucleotides in its regulation. In: E. Usdin, N. Weiner, and M.B.H. Youdim (eds.), Structure and Function of Monoamine Enzymes. Marcel Dekker, New York-Basel, pp. 109–148.

232. Wexler, B., and Katzman, R. (1975) Effects of dibutyryl cyclic AMP on tyrosine uptake and metabolism in neuroblastoma cultures. Exp. Cell Res. 92, 291–298.

233. White, T.D. (1976) Models for neuronal noradrenaline uptake. In: D.M. Paton (ed.), The Mechanism of Neuronal and Extraneuronal Transport of Catecholamines, Raven Press, New York, pp. 175–193.

234. Wilson, S.P., and Kirshner, N. (1977) The acetylcholine receptor of the adrenal medulla. J. Neurochem. 28, 687–695.

235. Winkler, H. (1976) The composition of adrenal chromaffin granules: An assessment of controversial results. Neuroscience 1, 65–80.

236. Winkler, H. (1977) The biogenesis of adrenal chromaffin granules. Neuroscience 2, 657–683.

237. Winkler, H., and Hortnagl, H. (1973) Composition and molecular organization of chromaffin granules. In: E. Usdin and S. Snyder (eds.), Frontiers in Catecholamine Research, Pergamon Press, New York-Oxford-Toronto-Sydney, pp. 415–421.

238. Winkler, H., Schneider, F.H., Rufener, C., Nakane, P.K., and Hortnagl, H. (1974) Membranes of adrenal medulla: Their role in exocytosis. In: F. Clementi and J. Meldolesi (eds.), Advances in Cytopharmacology, Vol. 2, Raven Press, New York, pp. 127–139.

239. Yamauchi, T., and Fujisawa, H. (1978) Evidence for phosphorylation of bovine adrenal tyrosine hydroxylase by cyclic AMP-dependent protein kinase. Biochem. Biophys. Res. Comm. 82, 514–517.

240. Yamauchi, T., and Fujisawa, H. (1979) In vitro phosphorylation of bovine adrenal tyrosine hydroxylase by adenosine 3′:5′-monophosphate-dependent protein kinase. J. Biol. Chem. 254, 503–507.

241. Yoshizaki, T. (1975) Effects of cholinergic drugs and their blockers on adrenaline release from rat adrenal. Biochem. Pharmacol. 24, 1401–1405.

242. Zimmerberg, J., Cohen, F.S., and Finkelstein, A. (1980) Micromolar Ca^{2+} stimulates fusion of lipid vesicles with planar bilayers containing a calcium-binding protein. Science 210, 906–908.

243. Zinder, O., Hoffman, P.G., Bonner, W.M., and Pollard, H.B. (1978) Comparison of chemical properties of purified plasma membranes and secretory vesicle membranes from the bovine adrenal medulla. Cell Tiss. Res. 188, 153–170.

RICHARD A. YEASTING, Ph.D.

SELECTED MORPHOLOGICAL ASPECTS OF HUMAN SUPRARENAL GLANDS

INTRODUCTION

The adrenal gland is a compound endocrine gland that is composed of two developmentally unrelated tissues. The outer, cortical tissue is related to the interrenal tissue of lower vertebrates. This tissue produces a group of closely related, cholesterol-derived steroid hormones such as cortisol, corticosterone, aldosterone, and the adrenal androgens, mainly dehydroepiandrosterone and dehydroepiandrosterone sulphate. Aldosterone is the major corticosteroid hormone involved in the regulation of body water and electrolyte balance and, thus, is the principle mineralocorticoid. Cortisol and corticosterone are involved in the overall regulation of carbohydrate metabolism and are grouped together as the principle glucocorticosteroids. The corticosteroids also have important activity in the inflammatory response, the reaction of the immune system, and general growth and maintenance of the body. The cortex also produces steroid compounds that possess androgenic and estrogenic properties. The cells producing the mineralocorticoid hormones are influenced by the concentration of the angiotensin II in the blood. The angiotensin II is in turn ultimately regulated by juxtaglomerular cells of the kidney which

From the Department of Anatomy, Medical College of Ohio, Toledo, Ohio.

react chiefly to alterations in blood pressure or blood volume. The cells secreting the glucocorticoids are primarily controlled by concentration of adrenocorticotrophic hormone (ACTH) released by the adenohypophysis. Adrenal androgen secretion is also controlled mainly by ACTH. Cells producing ACTH are in turn regulated by corticotrophin-releasing factor produced in cells of the hypothalamus.

The cells of the medulla of the human adrenal gland are a portion of the sympathochromaffin system of the body. As such, they produce the catecholamines norepinephrine and epinephrine. The medullary cells are controlled by direct cell-to-cell contact with preganglionic sympathetic neurons and thus function as a form of postganglionic sympathetic neuron. They differ from the usual postganglionic neuron in that the catecholamine secretory product is released into the blood stream instead of being released at a nerve terminal to affect an immediately subjacent effector cell.

GROSS ANATOMY

The paired human adrenal glands, more correctly named the suprarenal glands, are located superomedial to the cranial pole of the kidney (Figure 1). The suprarenal glands, which are situated in the perirenal adipose capsules of the kidneys, are within the retroperitoneal compartment

FIGURE 1. General location and major vascular supply of human suprarenal glands. **SSA** = superior suprarenal arteries; **MSA** = middle suprarenal arteries; **ISA** = inferior suprarenal arteries; **SV** = suprarenal vein; **RA** = renal artery; **Ao** = aorta; **IVC** = inferior vena cava.

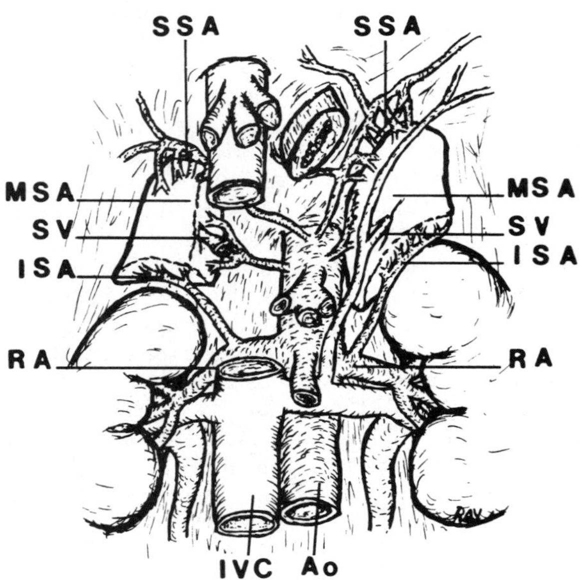

delimited by the renal fascia. The glands are separated from the kidney by a thin lamina of the renal fascia and a variable amount of areolar connective tissue. The glands are situated at the level of the eleventh or twelfth thoracic vertebra. The right gland rests against the right crus of the diaphragm. It abuts against or projects slightly posterior to the inferior vena cava. It is in close apposition to the bare area of the liver. The left gland is posterior to the omental bursa. It is in close apposition to the tail of the pancreas and the splenic artery.

The arterial supply of the suprarenal glands is usually derived from three groups of vessels. The superior suprarenal arteries arise from the inferior phrenic arteries, the middle suprarenal vessels arise directly from the abdominal aorta, and the inferior group of suprarenal arteries are branches of the renal arteries. The vessels branch as they approach the gland and form an anastomotic plexus of small arteries around the superior, medial, and inferior glandular margins. From this plexus of vessels, some forty to sixty vessels penetrate through the capsule to enter the substance of the gland.

One vein emerges from each gland. The right suprarenal vein is short and opens directly into the inferior vena cava. On the left side, the vein often joins the inferior phrenic vein of that side, which then enters the left renal vein. The suprarenal vein may enter the renal vein directly. The suprarenal gland receives a greater amount of blood per gram of tissue than any organ in the body, with the possible exception of the thyroid gland.

The innervation of the suprarenal gland is derived from the sympathetic portion of the autonomic nervous system. It reaches the gland primarily via the greater splanchnic nerve, the celiac ganglion, and the celiac and subsidiary plexuses. Although many of the nerve fibers approaching the gland appear to be nonmyelinated, they are functionally preganglionic. The nerve fibers predominately terminate on the pheochromaffin cells located in the suprarenal medulla. The pheochromaffin cells are, thereby, the functional equivalent of postganglion sympathetic neurons. Other fibers reaching, or to a small degree originating, in the gland are postganglionic in nature and terminate on the smooth muscle of the intraglandular arteries and veins. The importance of a possible parasympathetic innervation to the gland and the occasionally observed neural–cortical cell relationships is uncertain.

The suprarenal glands are not tightly tethered as they lie in the perirenal fascia. They are somewhat free to move slightly with the kidneys during changes in the position of the diaphragm during its inspiratory–expiratory excursions as well as during changes in body position. The glands however, are, somewhat restricted in their total potential to move because the surrounding vascular pattern and nerves tend to suspend them. Consequently, the suprarenal glands will remain in the usual position even if the related kidney undergoes ptosis. The laminae of renal fascia that surrounds the suprarenal glands are sufficient to trap injected air or gas to provide contrast in radiographic studies. The right suprarenal vein is short and thus does not offer much compliance to changes in vascular pressure. Possibly, this explains the higher incidence of hemorrhage in the right gland than in the left one, whose longer venous return pattern offers more compliance.

The suprarenal glands do not show marked sexual or racial variations although the glands in the female are often slightly larger than in the male. The female gland demonstrates some changes in relative amounts of tissue in the cortical zones dependent upon the season of the year and reproductive status of the individual (7).

At birth each suprarenal gland weighs approximately 4 g. With the loss of the fetal zone of the cortex, the weight decreases to about 1 g each at the end of the first year. The glands then increase in weight rather steadily into adulthood, with a slight adolescent growth spurt. The adult weight of an unstressed suprarenal gland is approximately 4 g. With ACTH stimulation produced by stresses of various types, i.e., illness, injury, etc., the cells of the gland's cortex will undergo hypertrophy and hyperplasia to produce an increased weight, averaging approximately 6 g.

Each suprarenal gland consists of a cortex accounting for some 90% of the glandular mass, and a medulla, accounting for the remaining 10%. The right gland is somewhat pyramidal in shape, as partially determined by the surrounding organs which are the inferior vena cava, liver, kidney, and diaphragm. The left gland is situated in a somewhat less confined area and tends to be crescentric or semilunare in appearance. Each gland presents a somewhat convoluted surface and has been likened in appearance to a shrunken leaf. The glands are flattened anteroposteriorly and have a thickness of about 10 mm. The superior–inferior dimension is approximately 50 mm while the mediolateral dimension is approximately 30 mm for each gland. When the fresh gland is sectioned and viewed macroscopically, the cortex and medulla can be distinguished with the cortex being more prominent. The outer major portion of the cortex is strikingly yellowish in color, while the inner, smaller portion of the cortex tends to be more reddish-brown. The yellowish color is produced by the lipochrome pigments and lipids contained with the cells. The medulla is pearl-gray, if it does not contain blood, or reddish in color if blood has been retained in the vessels. The fibrous connective tissue capsule and major connective tissue trabeculae extending into the cortex from it can be distinguished. The medullary tissue is not uniformly distributed throughout the inner aspect of the gland. It tends to be located in the head (medial) and body (middle) portions of the gland. The tail (lateral) portion and extreme margins of the gland consist solely of cortical tissue with no intervening medulla. (Figure 2) A brief summary of the developmental history of the gland can partially explain the microscopic appearance of the gland: During development, the total cortex is quite large and the medullary cells are aggregated around the major veins in the deepest areas of the cortex. The surface of the gland is smooth and the contours are generally rounded. After birth the deeper and largest regions of the cortex degenerate while the outer cortex temporarily retains the original circumference of the gland or even increases in size. The medullary cells become more compacted in the inner region of the gland and assume a

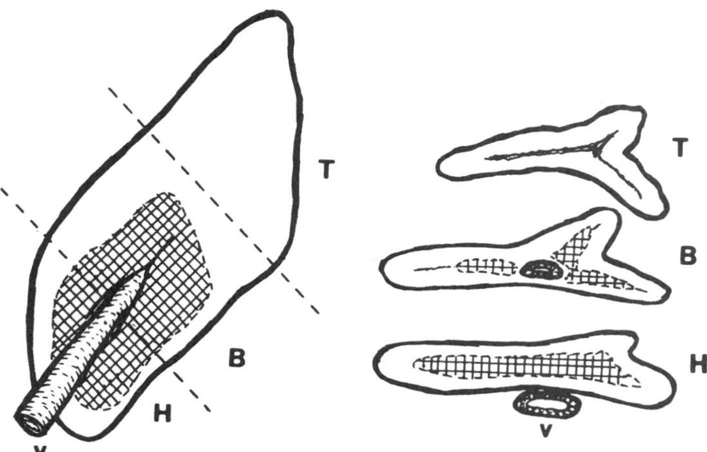

FIGURE 2. Schematic placement of medulla within left suprarenal gland. Crosshatched area represents medulla. **H** = head; **B** = body; **T** = tail; **v** = suprarenal vein.

somewhat medially eccentric position relative to the major transverse dimensions of the gland. With the loss of the inner cortical tissue, the outer, remaining cortex collapses inwardly without decreasing the surface area of the gland. These movements produce cortical folds (the tail and alae of the gland) that would not necessarily contain medullary tissue and create the image of a "small" medulla enveloped by an "overly large" and somewhat "crumpled" cortex.

MICROSCOPIC ANATOMY

Upon microscopic examination, the cortex usually is found to be divided into three zones (Figure 3). The boundaries are not clearly demarcated from each other, but do show differences in cell type and arrangement. The connective tissue stroma and vascular pattern both help define as well as reflect the arrangement of cells within each zone. The outermost zone has been named the zona glomerulosa because the cells in this region are arranged in clumps or clusters (Figure 3A). In humans the zona glomerulosa may be focally absent. It usually accounts for approximately 5% of total cortical thickness. The cells are small and have a high nuclear: cytoplasmic ratio. The cytoplasm contains abundant, somewhat elongated mitochondria with lamellar cristae, prominent Golgi, moderate amounts of granular and agranular endoplasmic reticulum, and abundant free ribosomes. Lipid-containing vacuoles are not a prominent feature of the cells. The cells within the clusters or glomeruli often demonstrate interdigitations and junctional complexes between adjacent cells. The perivascular surface of the cells often possess microvilli or folds. Each cluster of cells is surrounded by a layer of basal lamina.

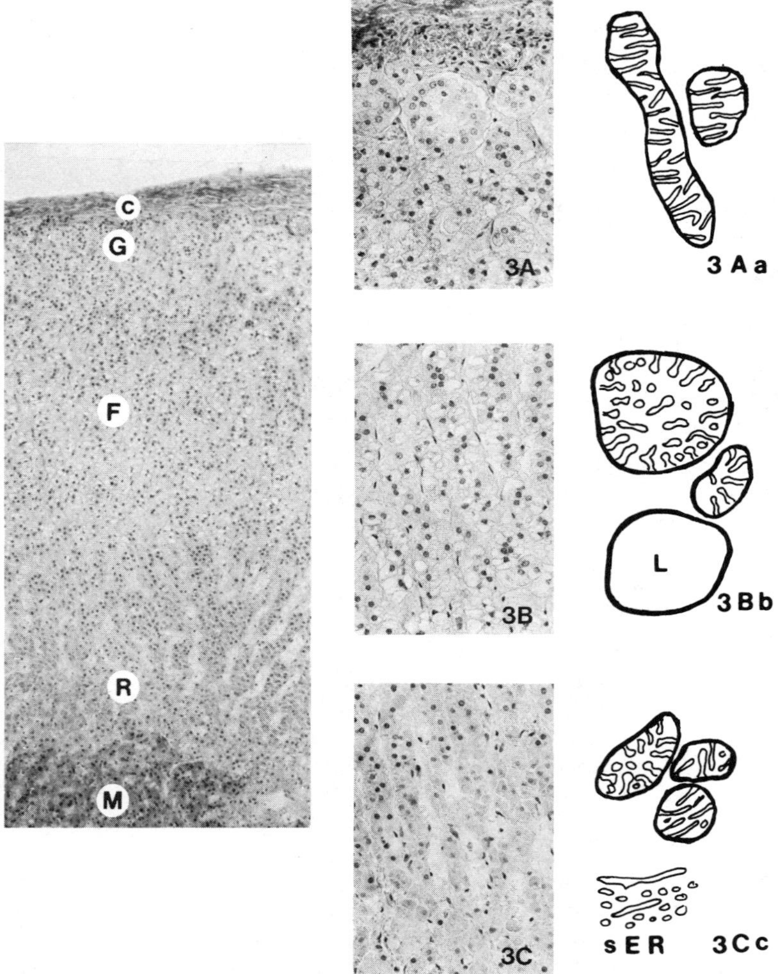

FIGURE 3. A. Light photomicrograph of human suprarenal cortex. **c** = capsule; **G** = zona glomerulosa; **F** = zona fasciculata; **R** = zona reticularis; **M** = medulla. **B**. Zona glomerulosa demonstrating typical clusters of cells. Zona fasciculata with typical columnar arrangement of cells containing large lipid vacuoles. **C.** Note small nuclei of endothelial cells and fibroblasts between columns of cells. **3Aa**. Zona reticularis with anastomosing columns of cells; **3Bb**. Schematic diagram of mitochondria typically found in zona glomerulosa cells. **3Cc**. Schematic diagram of mitochondria typically found in zona fasciculata and lipid vacuoles (**L**) that are characteristic features of cells within zone. Schematic diagram of mitochondria typically found in zona reticularis and smooth endoplasmic reticulum (**sER**) which is abundant in the cells of zone.

The zona glomerulosa merges with the more deeply lying zona fasciculata without a precise boundary. There are rather marked changes, however, in cellular arrangement and cell type as the zona fasciculata is entered. The zona fasciculata occupies approximately 70% of the normal, unstressed cortex. The cells are larger than those of the glomerulosa (Figure 3B). Large and abundant lipid vacuoles are a prominent feature of the cells of the zona fasciculata. Cholesterol and cholesterol esters are the predominant lipids to be stored in the vacuoles. The zona fasciculata is composed of two subsections. The cells of the outer section of the zona fasciculata possess the largest and most numerous lipid vacuoles. The mitochondria are rather small, oblong, and uniform in size. The cristae are tubulolamellar in configuration. The number of mitochondria per cell is less than that of the zona glomerulosa. The cells contain both agranular and granular endoplasmic reticulum. The clusters of granular endoplasmic reticulum account for basophilic staining of this region. In the inner section of the zona fasciculata, there is an increase in the amount of agranular (smooth) endoplasmic reticulum. The number and size of the lipid vacuoles are decreased. The mitochondria are increased in number and are of varied sizes. Many tend to be spherical and contain tubular cristae and internal tubulovesicular arrays. When the suprarenal gland is processed in preparation for examination by light microscopy, the lipid contained in the vacuoles is extracted. Thus, the cells of the zona fasciculata appear to have a frothy or spongy cytoplasm following routine processing. Hence, the cells of the fasciculata are sometimes called spongiocytes or clear cells. The zona fasciculata is so named because the cells are arranged in narrow fascicles or cord-like columns.

The inner section of the zona fasciculata merges with the next deeper region of the cortex, the zona reticularis. The cells of the zona reticularis are arranged in an anastomotic network (Figure 3C). The cells are smaller than those of the zona fasciculata, but larger than those of the zona glomerulosa. They lack the large numbers of lipid vacuoles found in the more superficial regions of the cortex and are often called compact cells. There is a greatly increased amount of smooth endoplasmic reticulum. The large amount of smooth endoplasmic reticulum helps produce the eosinophilic staining of the cells of the region. Many of the innermost cells in the reticularis contain numerous lipofuscin granules which produce the brownish color often seen in the unfixed gland. The mitochondria within the zona reticularis are numerous and contain cristae that are predominantly tubular as well as vesicular structures. Numerous microvilli are found on the vascular surface of the cells. The zona reticularis occupies approximately 25% of the normal cortex.

The cortical tissue is reflected into the inner aspect of the gland upon the surface of the suprarenal vein and its major tributaries. Although much thinner than the cortex in other areas of the gland, the three major cortical zones may be distinguished within this tissue known as the cortical cuff (Figure 4). The cortical cuff is interposed between the smaller arteries accompanying the suprarenal veins and the medullary tissue in a

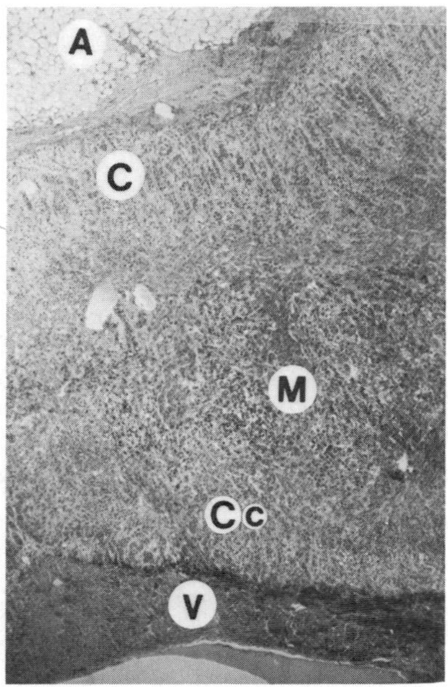

FIGURE 4. Light photomicrograph of human suprarenal gland demonstrating cortex (**C**), medulla (**M**), cortical cuff (**Cc**), and wall of intraglandular portion of suprarenal vein. **A** = adipose tissue.

similar fashion as the major areas of the cortex are interposed between the medullary cells and the primary arterial supply of the gland. Thus, the zona glomerulosa is nearest the vessels and zona reticularis is next to the medulla.

The suprarenal medulla arises from a totally separate tissue source, the neural crest, than does the cortex. The medullary cells are a portion of the sympathochromaffin (pheochromaffin) system of the body. Functionally, the cells of the medulla are somewhat similar to postganglionic sympathetic neurons in that they are innervated by preganglionic sympathetic neurons and produce catecholamines. The cells are rather large and epitheliod in appearance (Figure 5). They are arranged in clusters surrounded by the medullary venous plexus. The major morphological features of the cells are the storage–secretory vesicles or granules that contain either norepinephrine or epinephrine. The norepinephrine-containing granules are distinguished by having a very electron-dense core while those containing epinephrine appear to be more homogeneous in texture. Following stimulation of the cells, the contents of the vesicles appear to be released from the cells by exocytosis. The catecholamines, after separation from the storage–carrier substance, enter the blood in the capillaries surrounding the cells to be transported throughout the body.

As discussed earlier, the arterial blood supply to the suprarenal gland is derived from branches of three adjacent, but separate, major arteries. The

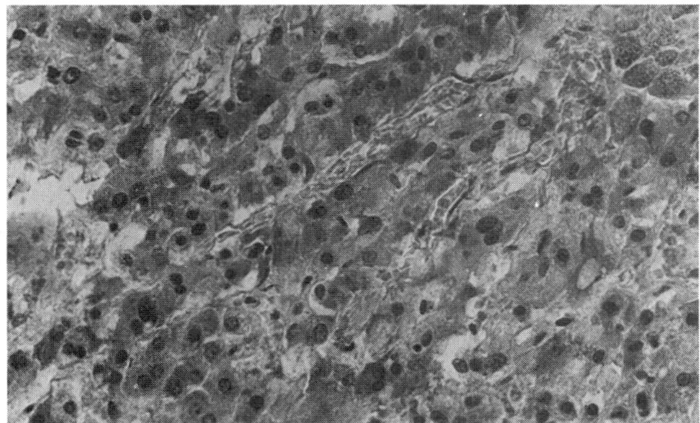

FIGURE 5. Light photomicrograph of suprarenal medullary cells. **R** = deepest cells of zona reticularis. **v** = vessels of medullary plexus containing RBCs.

small arteries tend to anastomose as they approach the gland and form a plexus on or near the surface of the capsule (Figure 6). From the capsular plexus, many smaller vessels enter the cortex. Although a number of these small arteries pass directly through the cortex to enter the medulla, the vast majority of the vessels emerging from the capsular plexus enter the cortical plexus. The cortical plexus in the zona glomerulosa region surrounds the clusters of cells found there and, therefore, is somewhat irregular in configuration. The plexus within the zona glomerulosa continues without interruption into the zona fasciculata. In this region, the capillaries enlarge and are often designated as sinusoids. The vessels within this portion of the cortical plexus are arranged in a radical pattern commensurate with the radical cord/column configuration of the fasiculata cells. Transverse anastomoses between the radial channels occur, but do not impose a significant branching pattern to this region of the plexus. However, as the zona reticularis, with its pattern of branching/anastomosing cords of cells, is entered, the pattern of the plexus is changed by an increase in the branching and anastomosing of the vessels that is produced or allowed by the altered parenchymal architecture.

Although the pattern of the cortical plexus varies commensurately with the enmeshed parenchymal cells, the predominant type of endothelial cell forming the plexus is similar throughout the plexus. These endothelial cells are primarily of the fenestrated type, with the fenestrae closed by a plasmalemmal diaphragm, as is found in other endocrine glands and areas that require or allow substances to pass through the endothelial layer quickly and easily.

The reticular portion of the cortical plexus coalesces into a large number of venules. These venules enter into either the medullary veins or the capillary plexus of the medulla. The medullary plexus, which receives direct arteries from the capsular arterial plexus in addition to the venules from the cortical plexus, ultimately forms tributaries to the medullary

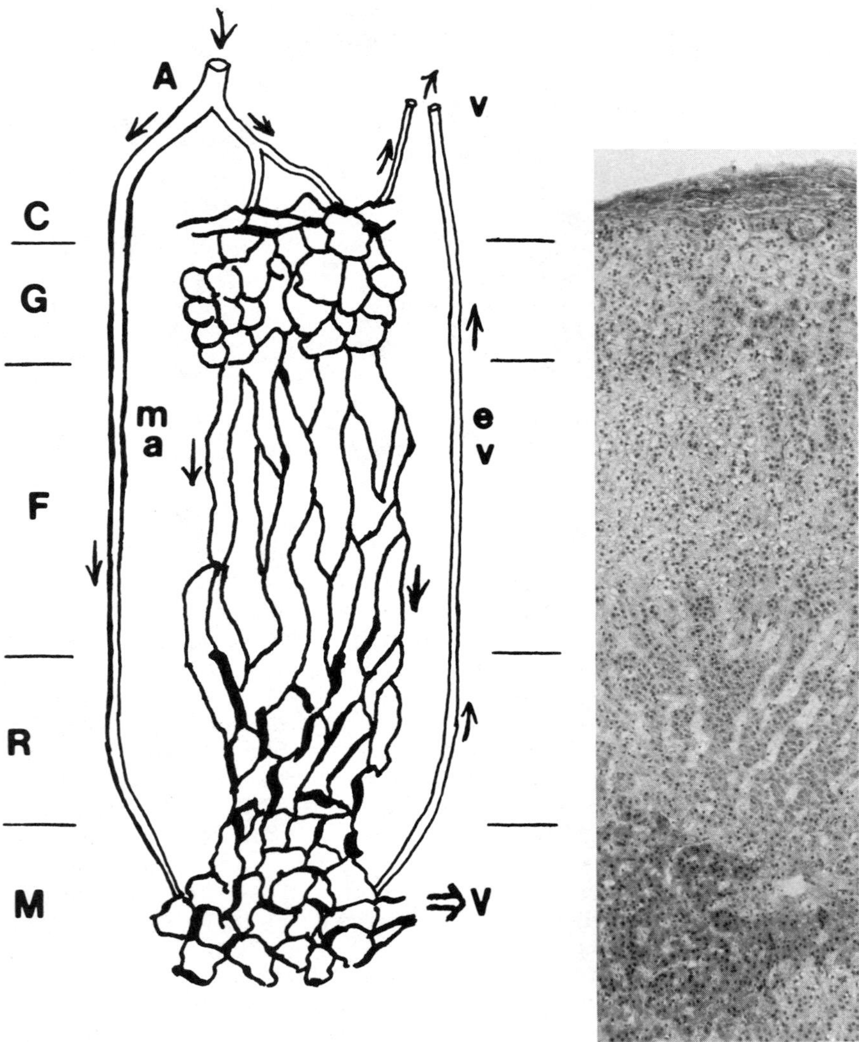

FIGURE 6. Schematic diagram of blood flow within suprarenal gland. **A** = small artery giving rise to either arterioles entering capsular plexus or medullary artery (**ma**) which penetrates directly to medulla; **C** = capsular plexus; **G** = plexus within zona glomerulosa; **F** = plexus within zona fasciculata—note parallel channels; **R** = plexus within zona reticularis with larger channels and more anastomoses than in F; **M** = medullary plexus which primarily drains via suprarenal vein (**V**); **ev** = emissary vein penetrating from medulla to surface of gland; **v** = small veins forming superficial plexus around gland.

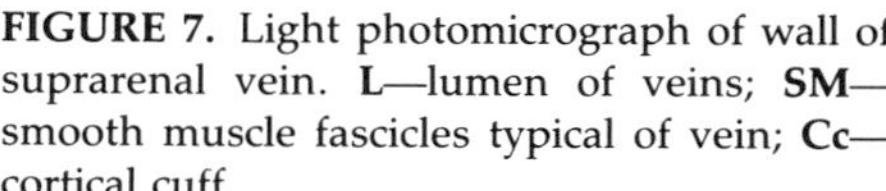

FIGURE 7. Light photomicrograph of wall of suprarenal vein. **L**—lumen of veins; **SM**—smooth muscle fascicles typical of vein; **Cc**—cortical cuff.

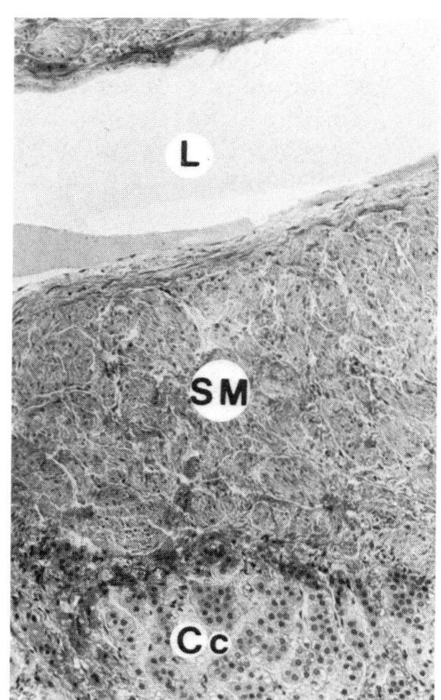

veins. The endothelial cells composing the medullary plexus are similar to those of the cortical plexus.

The suprarenal vein and its major tributaries, the medullary veins, possess prominent longitudinal bundles of smooth muscle in their walls (Figure 7). The bundles of smooth muscle are not uniformly distributed throughout the walls of the medullary veins, but are grouped as eccentric fascicles. The tributaries of the medullary veins pass through the clusters of smooth-muscle fascicles to enter the larger vein. The state of contraction of the smooth-muscle fascicles helps to control the flow of blood from the parenchyma of the gland into its major veins. The occlusion of the vessels draining the cortical and medullary plexuses would impede the flow of blood through the plexus. The parenchymal cells related to the respective plexuses would thereby be exposed to substances within the blood for a somewhat prolonged time interval and in higher concentrations of the substance than normal. The most physiologically important substances in the blood related to the function of the suprarenal gland include ACTH from the hypophysis to stimulate the cortical cells, hormones secreted by the outer zona fasciculata which may influence the activity of cells in that zone and in the inner zona fasciculata and zona reticularis (6), and corticosteroids produced in the cortex that will influence the synthetic pattern in the medullary cells to produce norepinephrine or epinephrine (11). With the exception of the blood that enters the medullary plexus via the direct medullary arteries, all of the blood exiting the gland in the suprarenal vein has traversed the cortex or cortical cuff and the medulla in a continuous vascular system.

A small quantity of venous return from the gland is derived from the capsular plexus and immediately subjacent cortex. Emissary veins passing from the medulla through the cortex to the surface of the gland form a small but potentially important subsidiary route of venous return from the gland. The rate of flow through the intraglandular vasculature is determined by the sympathetic tone in the arterioles and veins as well as potentially by the activity of prostaglandins produced intracortically by the metabolism of arachidonic acid. The rate of blood flow through each human suprarenal gland may reach 10 mm/minute.

ANATOMIC–PHYSIOLOGIC CORRELATIONS

The cells of the adrenal cortex are all derived from the same embryonic tissue source, mesoderm from the dorsal coelomic wall, and thus have features that are common among themselves and similar to the steriodogenic cells of the glands, which share a closely related origin. Although the adult suprarenal cortex displays the three zones that have been mentioned, the functional differences between the zones may be more apparent than real. The secretory cells of the cortex do not store the secretory products, the corticosteroid hormones. Rather, the cells tend, if possible, to store the precursor substances used in the synthesis of the hormones. Because there are no stored secretory products, the cells must synthesize the secretory products upon stimulation and almost immediately release their secretions. Therefore, they demonstrate a longer time delay between stimulation and appearance of the secretory products than cells that contain stored products. The zona fasciculata and zona reticularis most likely are functionally one unit with the cellular configuration demonstrating the differences in cellular activity. In this concept, the lipid-rich outer zona fasciculata cells would function primarily as rather inactive cells containing surplus stores of the necessary precursors to form the glucocorticoids. The inner zona fasciculata and zona reticularis cells would thereby be the cells actively producing the glucocorticoids and sex steroids produced by the gland. This is implied because of the increased endoplasmic reticulum, more active mitochondrial configurations, and decreased stores of cholesterol. The relative thickness of the respective zone varies, depending upon the physiological status of the individual. Following appropriate ACTH stimulation, the cells of the inner zona fasciculata become like those found in the zona reticularis. Consequently, the relative size of the zones change, with reticularis seeming to increase at the expense of the fasciculata. With further continued stimulation by ACTH, it is possible to convert all of the zona fasciculata cells to cells similar in appearance to those of the zona reticularis, i.e., greatly decreased amounts of stored lipid, increased amount of organelles involved in steroid hormone synthesis and metabolism, and altered mitochondrial configuration indicative of increased general cellular metabolic acitivity and steroidal metabolism. In addition, the altered morphological configuration of the zona fasciculata and reticularis produced by ACTH stimulation is reflected in changes in the amounts of biochemical constituents found in the cells and the total hormone output of the gland.

It is important to realize that the conversion from the lipid-rich, clear cells of the outer zona fasciculata to the more compact cells of the inner zona fasciculata and zona reticularis usually occurs in a rather uniform, centrifugal manner. In some instances, however, the changes may occur in radially disposed columns extending to the zona glomerulosa or in randomly arranged, isolated areas. Thus, it is possible to find the more active compact cells dispersed among the more inactive clear cells. As the cells are stimulated by ACTH, they tend to hypertrophy as well as undergo the configurational changes from the clear to compact cell types. This hypertrophy and the physiologically induced hyperemia contribute to the increased size and weight of the stimulated gland. With continued ACTH stimulation, as produced by very stressful stimuli, the cells may begin to separate from each other and thus produce the appearance of degeneration in the gland. This cellular retraction would be similar to that seen in vitro (8,10).

The cellular population within the various cortical regions is maintained by cellular proliferation within the respective zones, as evidenced by the appearance of mitotic figures throughout the cortex. The "cellular escalatory;" with cells being produced in the zona glomerulosa, progressing into the zona fasciculata, and ultimately degenerating in the zona reticulum, probably does not have a major physiological basis. However, in normal human postnatal development and in regenerative repair found in lower animals following injury to the gland, either physiologically or surgically, the major source of the cells to form the cortex appears to be the most peripheral (subcapsular) cells or the zona glomerulosa. Cells produced within that zone move centripetally to produce the cellular population necessary for the more deeply lying zones. The cells within the deeper zones then demonstrate a differentiation process to ultimately produce the morphological and physiological zonation apparent in the normal adult gland. The zonation produced in the normal or reconstituted gland is such that the zona glomerulosa is closest to the arterial supply of the gland and the reticularis is the furthest cortical area from the arterial supplies. The human gland does not seem to have a high regenerative capacity within the parameters usually seen.

The cellular function within cortex and medulla is determined not only by external influences such as the renin–angiotensin system, ACTH, and innervation acting on the various regions of the gland, but also by the microenvironment developed within the respective areas. If the cells of the cortex are dissociated, as in tissue culture, they revert to a single type. Thus, cells originally derived from the zona glomerulosa (rat) initially produced aldosterone when in culture. They later, however, transform into cells that are essentially similar in appearance and posses the functional attributes of zona fasciculata cells (4). Further in vitro observations introducing known amounts of exogenous steroids indicate that glucocorticoids, at essentially physiological levels, inhibit aldosterone production by zona glomerulosa cells (5).

However, the cells in the intact suprarenal cortex are not functioning in isolation, but are closely interrelated to each other by centripetal flow of blood through the gland. The following pattern suggests one hypothesis for the structural and functional integration of the gland. The cells on the outermost aspect of the gland are the first to be contacted by the arterial blood from the capsular plexus. This blood would have very low concentrations of cortical hormones and medullary secretions. The cells in this region produce many of the cortical hormones, but aldosterone production predominates. As the blood passes through the outer levels of cells, the concentration of aldosterone and corticosterone, etc., increases significantly. The increasing concentration of glucocorticoids may inhibit more deeply located cells from producing aldosterone (5). These more deeply located cells begin to change from ones that are actively producing mineralocorticoids to a type that is producing glucocorticoids. These somewhat less active cells are in a position that enables them to gain cholesterol from the passing blood and store it intracellularly in the form of lipid vacuoles. Thus, the appearance of the cell and the contained organelles becomes that of the zona fasciculata. As the blood continues more deeply into the cortex, the concentration of the glucocorticoids increases and that of the cholesterol decreases. The more deeply located cells, thereby, would not be able as easily to absorb more cholesterol than is used in the production of the steroid hormones. As the decreased stores of lipid and perhaps somewhat increased hormone production occurs, the cellular configuration is altered from the lipid-rich "clear" cell to the "compact" cell of the inner zona fasciculata and zona reticularis. As the concentration of glucocorticoids continues to increase, the synthetic activities of some of the deepest cortical cells are shifted away from the glucocorticoid pattern. Instead, if the hormone–cell interactions described in the fetus by Kahri et al. (6) apply to the adult, the high concentration of glucocorticoids, especially corticosterone, enhances sex hormone production in the deepest cortical cells of the zona reticularis.

As the adrenocortical hormone-rich blood continues centripetally from the cortex into the medulla, it comes in contact with the medullary cells. Here the high concentration of glucocorticoids provides the stimulus for the induction and maintenance of phenylethanolamine-N-methyl transferase, the enzyme necessary for the conversion of norepinephrine to epinephrine in the chromaffin cells.

In summary, the suprarenal gland is a very delicately integrated unit. The component positions are controlled, not only by extrinsic mechanisms, but also by intraglandular, intrinsic relationships. The cortex is composed of cells capable of steroidogenesis. Which steroid hormone any given cortical cell will ultimately produce is determined not only by the extraglandular stimuli of ACTH, the renin–angiotensin system, etc., but also by the intracortical position of the cell and its corticosteroidal microenvironment (9). The medulla is composed of catecholamine-producing cells that are developmentally and functionally unrelated to the cortex that surrounds them. However, the physiology of each chromaffin cell is influenced by the corticosteroidal microenvironment that surrounds it.

DEVELOPMENTAL ANATOMY

The steroid secretory cells of the suprarenal cortex develop from the epithelium of the embryonic coelom, and thus share a common tissue origin with elements of the gonads. The medullary cells are derived from the neural crest tissue, and thus are closely related to the postganglionic sympathetic neurons of the body. The suprarenal rudiment begins its development in the medial coelomic bay which is located between the dorsal mesogastrium and the mesonephros. Thus, the suprarenal gland is developing somewhat cranial to the gonads. The first indication of suprarenal development is an increased mitotic rate in the coelomic mesothelium that is medial to the urogenital ridge. This occurs about day 25 of development in the human. The proliferating cells invade the very vascular, adjacent mesenchyme. At about day 30 of human development, mesenchymal cells from the mesonephric capsule migrate medially and intermingle with the suprarenal primordium. These mesenchymal cells apparently will give rise to the cortical stroma and capsule of the gland. A second migration of coelomic mesothelial cells into the suprarenal anlage occurs at approximately day 35. These cells merge and intermingle with the cells of the developing cortex that took part in the initial migration. Thus, the embryonic cortex which shows two regions, the fetal zone of the precursor of the definitive cortex, is most likely formed as a result of the intermingling of the two mesothelial contributions and not by a discrete, orderly compartmentalization of the two cell populations (1,3). The gland continues to receive contributions from the coelomic epithelium until about day 45. Mitotic activity is found within the outer cortical region during the remainder of embryonic developmental and fetal life. The resulting cells contribute to the peripheral, definitive zone, as well as move centripetally into the inner fetal zone (1).

The sympathochromaffin cells that will become the medulla migrate from the neural crest toward the vicinity of the suprarenal primordium around day 25. They make contact with and enter the cortical primordia at about day 40 and ultimately become located near the major venous structure by day 45 (12). However, a unified compact medulla is not created until after the postnatal changes within the gland.

The primitive vascular pattern within the gland is established early in its development. The primordium invades a well-vascularized area of mesenchyme that receives its arterial supply from paired lateral, nonsegmental branches of the aorta. The intraglandular vascular pattern is established as the cortex proliferates and the medullary chromaffin cells become situated in the more central regions of the gland (Figure 8). During this time, the more central vessels, i.e., the future veins, undergo changes in patterns that ultimately produce three major venous channels within the gland and one major vein emerging from the gland. The single

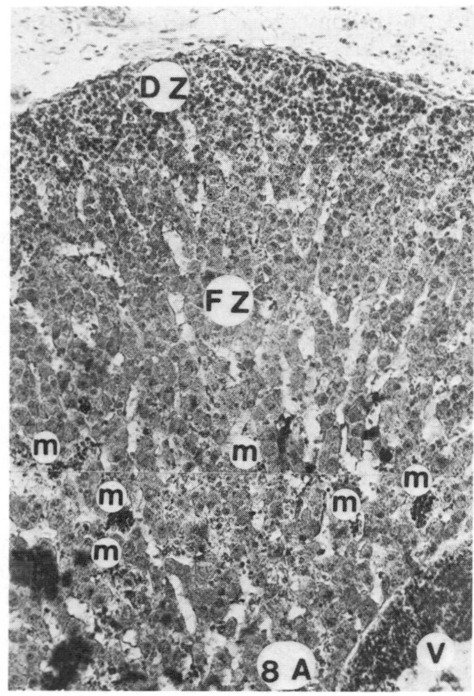

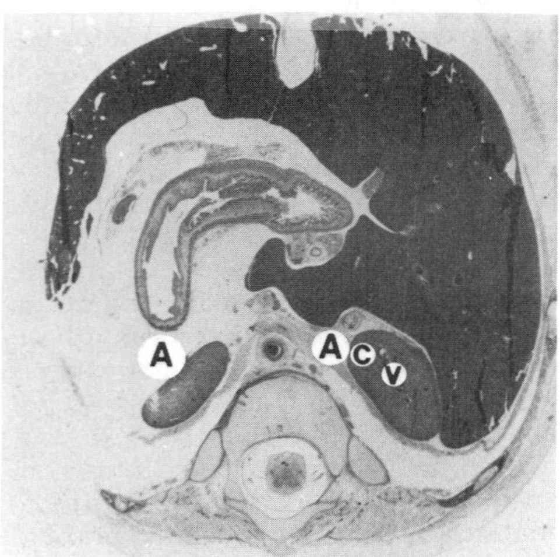

FIGURE 8. A. Suprarenal glands in transverse section of 75-mm human embryo. **A** = suprarenal glands; **c** = cortex; **v** = developing suprarenal vein. **B.** Light photomicrograph of embryonic suprarenal gland. **DZ** = peripheral definitive zone (precursor of adult cortex); **FZ** = fetal zone; **m** = clusters of cells destined to become medullary cells; **V** = developing suprarenal vein.

suprarenal vein will enter the major vessels that result from the transformation of the subcardinal venous system.

The prenatal suprarenal gland increases in size rapidly. During the second trimester of development, the gland is in direct proportion to total body weight at a ratio of approximately 4 g/kg. During the third trimester, the growth rate slows and ultimately produces a gland that weighs a little more than 4 g or a gland to total body weight ratio of 2.5 g/kg.

When the prenatal suprarenal gland is examined microscopically, it is found to consist of an outer region of small cells that characteristically possess poorly differentiated endoplasmic reticulum, numerous free ribosomes, and numerous glycogen particles, and a much larger inner, more darkly staining region of cells that possess well-differentiated granular and agranular endoplasmic reticulum, well-developed Golgi, lipid droplets, and mitochondria with tubular cristae. Within the inner or fetal zone, are found isolated groups of medullary cells. The medullary cells tend to be located near the larger venous structures. The cells within the fetal zone are arranged in radially oriented columns that are separated by vascular channels, much like the arrangement within the adult cortex.

The prenatal gland is involved in steroidogenesis and is controlled to an extent by the fetal hypophysis. It must be remembered, however, that many of the maternal adrenal hormones are allowed to pass through the placental membrane and, thus, influence the fetal hypophyseal–suprarenal axis. The primary effect would be one of seemingly suppressing the secretory activity of the suprarenal gland because of perceived normal plasma hormonal levels. Thus, the outer zone of the prenatal cortex, the portion that will develop ultimately into the definitive cortex, is seen to contain cells that for the most part demonstrate a rather low level of secretory activity. These cells are thought to be producing the C-21 hormones of the fetus.

The inner, or fetal zone, of the prenatal gland morphologically indicate a rather high degree of secretory activity. These cells are producing the fetal C-19 compounds. The major one being produced is dehydroepiandrosterone sulphate (DHEA-S). The nonsulfated form of this hormone is a potent androgen, but its activity as the sulfated form is much reduced. The hormone is produced by the fetal zone cells and circulates to the placenta. The placental tissues then metabolize it to produce the estrogenic compounds essential for controlling the pregnancy. Thereby, the fetal zone of the suprarenal gland, the syncytiotrophoblastic tissue of the placenta and the fetal liver function as an integrated unit to produce and metabolize the major steroid hormones necessary for proper fetal development and maintenance of the pregnancy.

Decreased activity of any of the tissues would almost automatically lead to an altered hormonal balance within the system. An example of this phenomena is found in the anencephalic fetus. In these fetuses, the hypothalamus and usually the hypophysis is poorly developed because of the massive malformaton of the cephalic central nervous system. Due to lack of appropriate ACTH stimulation, the fetal zone of the suprarenal gland is hypoplastic and hypoactive. (If stimulated by exogenous ACTH, the zone will respond by increasing in size and related activity.) Due to the reduced production of DHEA-S the placental estrogen levels are lowered. The lowered estrogenic hormone levels do not produce the appropriate alterations in the uterine and other maternal physiology that seem to signal the appropriate termination of pregnancy (2). Thus, the anencephalic-producing pregnancy is usually significantly longer than normal. Other alterations in the fetal suprarenal–placental axis, such as enzyme deficiencies, may also affect the course of pregnancy.

Shortly before birth, cells of the fetal zone of the suprarenal gland begin to demonstrate degenerative changes. These changes continue after birth and result in cellular death, degradation, and ultimate loss of the fetal zone. With the loss of the fetal zone cells, the gland is structurally reorganized. The sympathochromaffin cells that had previously been scattered in clumps throughout the inner region of the fetal zone are collected to form the definitive medulla. The outer, definitive cortex slumps or collapses inward with the disappearance of the originally deeper fetal zone. Although the secretory cells of the fetal zone disappear, the connective tissue stromal elements do not. As the cortex collapses inward toward the medulla, the fetal zone stromal elements are compressed into a zone of connective tissue, the "medullary capsule." If the glandular reorganization occurs too rapidly, the radially arranged vascular channels can become relatively unsupported and may rupture, producing intraglandular hemorrhage. The definitive cortical zone differentiates into the functioning postnatal cortex and at about the time of puberty, the zona reticularis type of cell begins to be found in the deeper regions of the cortex. At that time, the typical, nonstressed cortical zonation is complete and the adult glandular configuration has been obtained.

Accessory suprarenal gland tissue is often found in regions remote from the normal gland. Although the accessory glands may contain both representations of cortical and medullary tissue, they most often consist only of cortical tissue. Common remote locations are within the broad ligament near the ovary and in the epididymis near the testis. These locations can be explained easily because of the movement of the gonads following their organogenesis within the urogenital ridge. The suprarenal cortex originates from the coelomic mesothelium, just medial and cranial to the developing gonad and, thus, aberrant suprarenal tissue is often carried with the tissue surrounding the gonad. Other accessory glands found near the normally positioned suprarenal gland are the result of misdirected migratory movements as the mesothelial and neural crest cells approach the area of the primordium development.

REFERENCES

1. Crowder, R.E. (1957) Development of adrenal gland in man, with special reference to origin and ultimate location of cell types, and evidence in favor of cell "migration" theory. Contrib. Embryol. Carnegie Instit. 36, 195.
2. France, J.T., Seddon, R.J., and Liggins, G.C. (1973) A study of a pregnancy with low estrogen production due to placental sulfatase deficiency. J. Clin. Endocrinol. 36, 1.

3. Gruenwald, P. (1946) Embryonic and postnatal development of the adrenal cortex, particularly the zona glomerulosa and accessory nodules. Anat. Rec. 95, 391.
4. Hornsby, P.J., O'Hare, M.J., and Neville, A.M. (1974) Functional and morphological observations on rat adrenal zona glomerulosa cells in monolayer culture. Endocrinology 90, 1240.
5. Hornsby, P.J., and O'Hare, M.J. (1977) The roles of potassium and corticosteroids in determining the pattern of metabolism of (^{3}H) deoxycorticosterone by monolayer cultures of rat adrenal glomerulosa cell. Endocrinology 101, 997.
6. Kahri, A.T., Voutilainen, R., and Salmenpera, M. (1979) Different biological action of corticosteroids, corticosterone and cortisol as a base of zonal function of adrenal cortex. Acta Endrocrinol. (Copenh.) 91, 329.
7. MacKinnon, I.L., and MacKinnon, P.C.B. (1958) Seasonal rhythm in the morphology of the suprarenal cortex in women of childbearing age. J. Endocrinol. 17, 456–467.
8. Neville, A.M., and O'Hare, M.J. (1978) Cell culture and Histopathology of the human adrenal cortex in relation to hypercorticalism. In: V.H.T. James, M. Serio, G. Guisti, and L. Marti (eds). The Endocrine Function of the Human Adrenal Cortex. Academic Press, New York-London, p. 229.
9. Neville, A.M., and O'Hare, M.J. (1982) The human adrenal cortex—pathology and biology—an integrated approach. Springer-Verlag, New York, pp. 108–111.
10. O'Hare, M.J., and Neville, A.M. (1973) Morphological responses to corticotrophin and cyclic AMP by adult rat adrenocortical cells in monolayer culture. J. Endocrinol. 56, 529.
11. Wurtman, R.J., and Pohorecky, L.A. (1971) Adrenocortical control of epinephrine synthesis in health and disease. Adv. Metab. Disord. 5, 53–76.
12. Zuckerkandl, E. (1912) The development of the chromaffin organs and the suprarenal glands. In: Keibel and Mall's Manual of Human Embryology, Vol. II, Chapter 15, Philadelphia.

JOHN P. RAPP, D.V.M., Ph.D.

ADRENAL STEROID BIOSYNTHESIS AND METABOLISM

BIOSYNTHESIS OF ADRENAL STEROIDS

Adrenal steroids are derived from cholesterol (20,51,101) and are made in the cortex of the adrenal. Adrenal cortical cholesterol originates both from plasma cholesterol and from cholesterol synthesized from acetate by the adrenal (38,51). Plasma cholesterol esters enter the adrenal cell in combination with plasma low-density lipoprotein by the binding of lipoprotein at a high affinity receptor site. The cholesterol esters are hydrolyzed in lysosomes to provide cholesterol for corticosteroid biosynthesis (49). Figure 1 shows the numbering system for the carbon atoms in cholesterol and the steroids derived from it.

The first step in steroid biosynthesis is the cleavage of the cholesterol side chain between carbons 20 and 22 to produce pregnenolone. This is a complex reaction, the initial steps of which involve the addition of hydroxyl groups to the side chain. An explanation of mechanism of hydroxylation, therefore, is given first.

From the Departments of Medicine and Pathology, Medical College of Ohio, Toledo, Ohio.

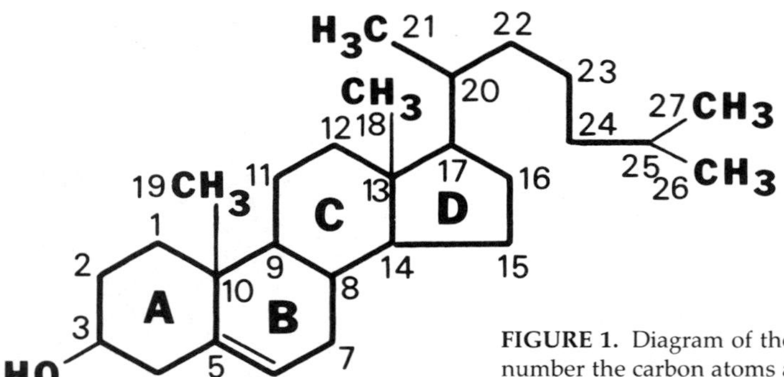

FIGURE 1. Diagram of the system used to number the carbon atoms and rings of cholesterol and adrenal steroids.

Electron Transport and Steroid Hydroxylation in Adrenal Cortical Mitochondria

Figure 2 shows the electron transport sequence that is common to all mitochondrial steroid hydroxylation reactions (3). NADPH reduces a flavoprotein (adrenodoxin reductase), which in turn reduces a non-heme-iron protein. The latter was discovered in 1965 (65,88) and is also referred to as adrenodoxin, adrenal ferrodoxin, or adrenal iron-sulfur protein. Adrenodoxin serves to reduce the enzyme cytochrome P-450. Cytochrome P-450 is a heme containing enzyme and is depicted in Figure 2 by Fe, representing the various oxidation states of the heme iron. The specificity of the reaction in terms of the substrate (steroid) attacked and the position on the substrate, which is hydroxylated, resides with the cytochrome P-450. These cytochromes also have been referred to as hydroxylases, mixed function oxidases, or monooxygenases.

The components of this enzyme system are contained in adrenal cortical mitochondria. Mitochondrial cytochrome P-450 is membrane bound and is probably contained in the inner mitochondrial membrane (76,105), though it has also been reported to be localized in the outer membrane (7). The components of this hydroxylase system are easily separated by centrifugation of sonicated mitochondria. The membrane bound cytochrome P-450 (so called cytochrome P-450 particles) can be sedimented by differential centrifugation leaving the flavoprotein and adrenodoxin in the supernatant (65). Both the flavoprotein and adrenodoxin have been isolated and characterized (15,91).

Adrenodoxin and the flavoprotein form a 1:1 complex (16). Initially, neither adrenodoxin nor the flavoprotein were found to form a complex with cytochrome P-450. Recent reports, however, present evidence for a 1:1 complex between adrenodoxin and cytochrome P-450, and suggest that the presence of substrate (43) (cholesterol, in the case of cytochrome P-450 for cholesterol side chain cleavage) or an excess of adrenodoxin (78) are necessary for such a complex to form. Thus, it appears very likely that

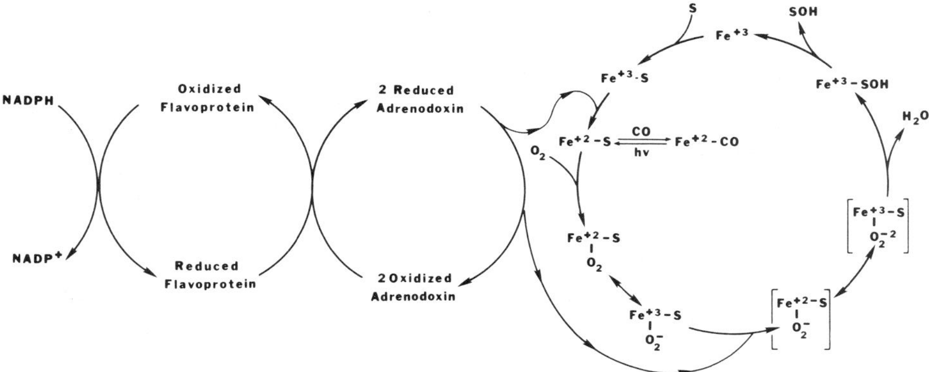

FIGURE 2. Electron transport chain and cytochrome P-450 mediated steroid hydroxylation. Reducing energy is supplied by NADPH at the left of the diagram and electrons transported via flavoprotein to adrenodoxin. Steroid substrate (S) enters the reaction at the top right by reacting with oxidized cytochrome P-450. The oxidation states of cytochrome P-450 are represented by oxidation states of iron (Fe) contained in cytochrome P-450. Electrons and oxygen are sequentially added to the P-450–substrate complex in the order shown, internal arrangements occur and water and the hydroxylated steroid substrate (SOH) are formed, leaving the P-450 free for another cycle. The reaction of reduced (Fe^{+2}) cytochrome P-450 with carbon monoxide and the reversal of this reaction by light (hv) are also indicated. [Redrawn from ref. 22]

the electron transport enzymes, cytochrome P-450 and substrate bind in some manner into functional complexes.

Figure 2 indicates that reduced adrenodoxin is thought to interact with cytochrome P-450 in two ways: First, to reduce the heme iron after binding of the steroid substrate; then, to provide a second reducing equivalent after the addition of oxygen to the cytochrome P-450–substrate-complex. The first reducing equivalent can be provided by a number of chemical reducing agents, but reduced adrenodoxin is specifically required to provide the second equivalent (37).

Like all cytochromes, cytochrome P-450 contains a iron-porphyrin moiety. In the case of bacterial and liver cytochrome P-450 enzymes, this group is protoporphyrin IX (55,107). The exact nature of porphyrin groups in adrenal cytochromes P-450 is unknown. Cytochromes are inactivated by binding to carbon monoxide (CO), because CO competes with O_2 for binding to the enzyme. The absorption spectra of the cytochromes involved in steroidogenesis when reduced and bound to CO have a maximum at about 450 nm and the enzymes, therefore, are called P-450, P standing for pigment. The CO binding is photosensitive, that is, the P-450·CO complex is disassociated by light. The efficiency of this disassociation is dependent on wave length with maximum effect at 450 nm (103,104). Besides the spectral changes induced by CO, addition of steroid substrates to cytochrome P-450 also induces spectral changes in light absorption and electron paramagnetic resonance (14,19).

The cytochrome P-450 from adrenocortical mitochondrial has been separated into two distinct enzymes (40,73,82,87): a) P-450_{scc} for cholesterol side chain cleavage, and b) P-$450_{11\beta}$ for 11β-hydroxylation. Each enzyme catalyzes its reaction with specificity for substrate and positions hydroxylated, and the two enzymes can be differentiated immunologically (87).

Cholesterol Side Chain Cleavage

Figure 3 shows a scheme for the formation of pregnenolone from cholesterol (i.e., cholesterol side chain cleavage), which is compatible with existing data. Cholesterol is hydroxylated at the 22R position followed by a second hydroxylation at 20α to form 20α,22R-dihydroxycholesterol. The latter is cleaved between carbons 20 and 22 to yield pregnenolone. It has been suggested that an alternative pathway, changing the order of hydroxylation, could also exist: cholesterol → 20α-hydroxycholesterol → 20α,22R-dihydroxycholesterol → pregnenolone. This idea is controversial because though adrenals do convert 20α-hydroxycholesterol into the dihydroxy compound and pregnenolone, the step cholesterol → 20α-hydroxycholesterol is quantitatively very small (see refs. 9 and 80 for reviews).

Pure P-450_{scc} has been isolated (82,90,99). The enzyme appears to be composed of two subunits present in stoichiometric amounts of 1:1. One of these subunits is associated with the iron-porphyrin and the other is not. The active form of the enzyme may exist as a complex of 16 subunits, eight of each type (83,94).

The evidence shows that a single molecular species of cytochrome P-450 cleaves the side chain of cholesterol and that hydroxylated products are intermeates. P-450_{scc} must be responsible for hydroxylations at both the 20α and 22R positions, by mechanisms shown in Figure 2, but the

FIGURE 3. Intermediate hydroxylation steps in the side chain cleavage of cholesterol to yield pregnenolone. The solid arrows indicate well estalbished steps, but the dashed arrow indicates a less well established step.

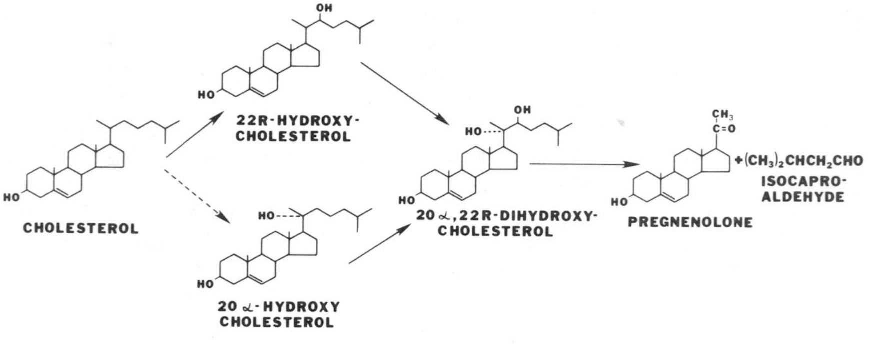

exact molecular mechanism by which the carbon–carbon bond between carbons 20 and 22 is broken remains obscure.

Studies with isotopes of oxygen have established that the hydroxyl groups at positions 20α and 22R are introduced from two different molecules of oxygen. This is compatible with the sequential hydroxylation of the side chain (10). The oxygen in the 20 keto group of pregnenolone is derived from the oxygen introduced into the 20-hydroxyl group of cholesterol (89). The oxygen in the isocaproaldehyde side product is probably derived from the oxygen introduced at C-22. The oxygen in isocaproaldehyde exchanges rapidly with water, and this process may be catalyzed by the P-450_{scc} (21).

The stoichiometry involved is as follows:

$$\textit{Cholesterol} + 3\ \textit{NADPH} + 3\ H^+ + 3\ O_2 \rightarrow \textit{pregnenolone} + \textit{isocaproaldehyde} + 3\ \textit{NADP}^+ + 4\ H_2O.$$

It takes 2 NADPH: 2 O_2 : 2 H^+ to form pregnenolone from 20α-hydroxycholesterol and 1 NADPH : 1 O_2 : 1 H^+ to form pregnenolone from 20α,22R-dihydroxycholesterol (84). The latter is especially interesting, because it means that NADPH and O_2 are still required for cleavage of the carbon–carbon bond following hydroxylations at carbons 20 and 22.

Alternate mechanisms for cholesterol side chain cleavage have been proposed. In these schemes the side-chain–hydroxylated derivatives of cholesterol are considered to be reaction side products, rather than obligatory intermediates (36,50). Some of the compounds suggested as intermediates involve double bond (olefin) and epoxy configurations between carbons 20 and 22 (50). Although such compounds are converted to pregnenolone by crude enzyme preparations, they do not yield pregnenolone with the purified side-chain–cleavage system (92). This suggests that crude preparations contain double-bond reductases and epoxide hydratases, which convert the olefins and epoxides to compounds that can then be converted to cholesterol, and that the 20(22)-olefins and 20,22-epoxides are not, in fact, intermediates for side chain cleavage.

Adrenal mitochondria contain a substance that activates cholesterol side chain cleavage. The adrenal activator stimulates pregnenolone synthesis from the hydroxylated intermediates of cholesterol side chain cleavage, as well as from cholesterol (93). The activator is heat stable, nondialyzable and partially inactivated by trypsin. This substance binds to cholesterol, but has little or no affinity for pregnenolone or other steroid hormones (42). There is a carrier protein in liver that binds squalene and sterol precursors of cholesterol (75,79). This liver protein also stimulates cholesterol side chain cleavage in adrenal preparations in vitro (42). Antibodies against the purified liver-sterol–binding protein show the presence of cross reactive material in many tissues, including the adrenal (2).

Conversions from Pregnenolone

3β-Hydroxysteroid dehydrogenase. This enzyme catalyzes the conversion of the 3β-hydroxy configuration to a 3 keto group. As shown in

Figure 4, the immediate product formed from pregnenolone by 3β-hydroxysteroid dehydrogenase is Δ^5-pregnenedione. This is the first step on the important pathway for the conversion of pregnenolone to progesterone. A similar conversion is carried out on 17α-hydroxy-pregnenolone to yield 17α-hydroxy-Δ^5-pregnenedione as the first step on the conversion of 17α-hydroxy-pregnenolone to 17α-hydroxy-progesterone (Figure 4).

The 3β-hydroxysteroid dehydrogenase is located in the adrenal microsomal fraction (6,39,59) and requires NAD^+ as a hydrogen acceptor(6). Whether or not there is one or more than one such adrenal enzyme is controversial (34,62).

Δ^5-3-Ketosteroid isomerase. This enzyme catalyzes the conversion of a 3-ketosteroid with a Δ^5 double bond into a 3-ketosteroid with a Δ^4 double bond. It is the second enzyme necessary for the conversion of pregnenolone to progesterone or for the conversion of 17α-hdyroxy-pregnenolone to 17α-hydroxy-progesterone (Figure 4). The Δ^5-3-ketosteroid isomerase is associated with the 3β-hydroxysteroid dehydrogenase in adrenal micro-somes (39,59,64,100).

There is a question as to the number of isomerase enzymes present in adrenals. It was possible to separate bovine adrenal isomerase into fractions, each showing different specificity for different substrates (23,24).

FIGURE 4. Biosynthetic pathways for steroids in the adrenal zona fasiculata-reticularis.

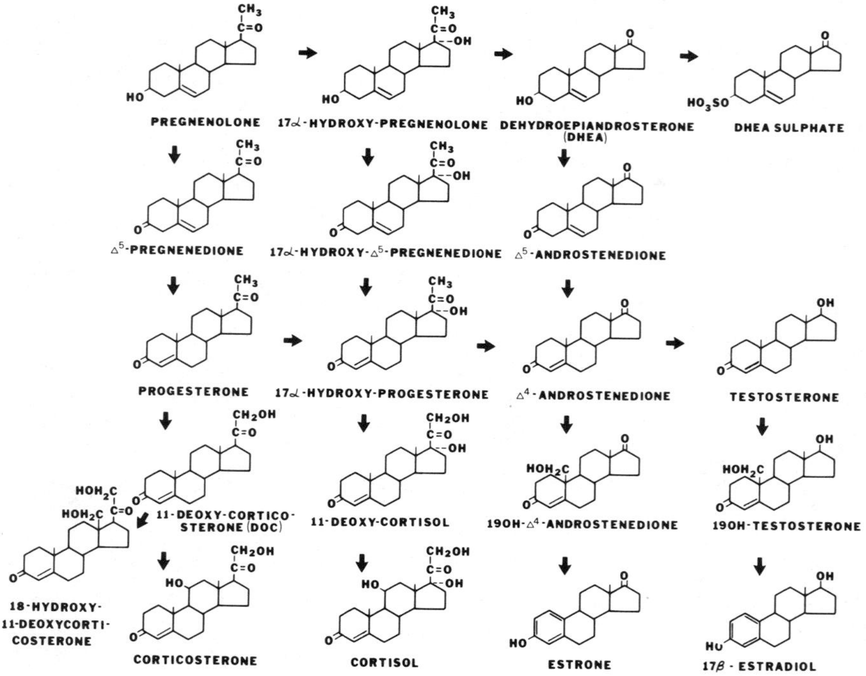

PREGNENOLONE
17α-HYDROXY-PREGNENOLONE
DEHYDROEPIANDROSTERONE (DHEA)
DHEA SULPHATE
Δ^5-PREGNENEDIONE
17α-HYDROXY-Δ^5-PREGNENEDIONE
Δ^5-ANDROSTENEDIONE
PROGESTERONE
17α-HYDROXY-PROGESTERONE
Δ^4-ANDROSTENEDIONE
TESTOSTERONE
11-DEOXY-CORTICOSTERONE (DOC)
11-DEOXY-CORTISOL
19OH-Δ^4-ANDROSTENEDIONE
19OH-TESTOSTERONE
18-HYDROXY-11-DEOXYCORTICOSTERONE
CORTICOSTERONE
CORTISOL
ESTRONE
17β-ESTRADIOL

The Δ^5-3 ketosteroid isomerase does not require cofactors, but both NAD^+ and NADH activate the enzyme probably by binding to the enzyme at a site other than the catalytic site (64).

17α-Hydroxylation. The properties of this enzyme have not been studied extensively. The enzyme requires NADPH for hydroxylation (106) and it is contained in the adrenal cortical microsomal fraction (39).

The amount of 17α-hydroxylation can vary greatly between species. The adrenal of the rat makes virtually no 17α-hydroxylated steroids and corticosterone, therefore, is the major glucocorticoid formed. In humans, 17α-hydroxylation is an important reaction and cortisol is the major glucocorticoid, though some corticosterone is also produced (Figure 4). In early studies (35) with a perfused bovine adrenal preparation, progesterone was shown to be converted to 17α-hydroxy-progesterone on the pathway to cortisol formation. Using radioactive labeled steroids it was shown that pregnenolone was also 17α-hydroxylated to form 17α-hydroxy-pregnenolone, which could be converted by the 3β-hydroxy-steroid Δ^5-3 ketosteroid isomerase catalyzed reactions to 17α-hydroxy-progesterone and, thus, to cortisol (Figure 4).

Thus, there are two competing pathways from pregnenolone to 17α-hydroxy-progesterone: pregnenolone → progesterone → 17α-hydroxy-progesterone or pregnenolone → 17α-hydroxy-pregnenolone → 17α-hydroxy-progesterone, depending on the order of 3β-hydroxysteroid isomerase and 17α-hydroxylase reactions. Although the existence of both pathways is easy to demonstrate, their relative importance is difficult to establish (see ref. 31 for review).

21-Hydroxylation

The steroids that are substrates for 21-hydroxylase are progesterone and 17α-hydroxy-progesterone, which yield 11-deoxy-corticosterone and 11-deoxy-cortisol, respectively (Figure 4). Steroids are hydroxylated at carbon 21 by a mixed function oxidase in adrenal cortical microsomes (39). The overall stoichiometry is (18)

$$Steroid + NADPH + H^+ + O_2 \rightarrow 21\text{-}hydroxy\text{-}steroid + NADP^+ + H_2O.$$

The mechanism of 21-hydroxylation, in principle, is similar to that shown in Figure 2, but there are some important differences between microsomal 21-hydroxylation and mitochondrial hydroxylations. First, adrenodoxin does not function in the electron transport chain from NADPH for 21-hydroxylation. Antibodies against adrenodoxin inhibit adrenal mitochondrial hydroxylations but not 21-hydroxylation (4). Also, immunologic studies have demonstrated that the flavoprotein for electron transport in 21-hydroxylation is different from the flavoprotein involved in electron transport in mitochondrial hydroxylations (57).

The involvement of a cytochrome P-450 in 21-hydroxylation has been demonstrated by inhibition of the reaction by CO. Such inhibition is reversed by light, and the action spectrum of reversal is identical to the spectrophotometric difference spectrum of CO-bound microsomal cytochrome (66).

There is some question as to whether or not adrenals contain one 21-hydroxylase for both 17-deoxy and 17α-hydroxy C_{21} steroids, or two 21-hydroxylases, one for 17-deoxy and one for 17α-hydroxy compounds. Studies with inhibitors of steroidogenesis showed different degrees of inhibition for cortisol and corticosterone production (41). Partial purification of adrenal 21-hydroxylase resulted in a greater increase in specific activity toward 17α-hydroxy-progesterone than for progesterone or pregnenolone as substrate (54). In a study of the competition of progesterone and 17α-hydroxy-progesterone for 21-hydroxylase Orta-Flores et al. (67) interpreted their data as suggesting two active sites for 21 hydroxylation, but not necessarily two different enzymes.

11β- and 18-Hydroxylase System

The final step in the production of the major glucocorticoids, corticosterone and cortisol is the 11β-hydroxylation of the 21-hydroxylated precursors 11-deoxy-corticosterone and 11-deoxy-cortisol (Figure 4). This reaction takes place in the adrenal mitochondria and proceeds by the mechanism given in Figure 2 (61,66,104). The cytochrome P-450 for 11β-hydroxylation (P-$450_{11\beta}$), however, is distinct from the cholesterol side chain cleavage enzyme (P-450_{scc}), though both are contained in adrenal mitochondria. P-$450_{11\beta}$has been isolated free of cholesterol side chain cleavage activity (87).

Early studies with adrenal mitochondrial cytochrome P-450 particles that possessed 11β-hydroxylase activity with 11-deoxy-corticosterone as substrate also showed 18-hydroxylase activity toward the same substrate. Studies with carbon monoxide inhibition of 11β- and 18-hydroxylase have shown that the two activities were identically inhibited (74). A wide variety of experimental conditions (pH, buffer concentration, or addition of metopirone, which is an inhibitor of 11β-hydroxylation) also influenced the two activities in parallel (8). Moreover, the existence of a genetic mutant of P-450 affecting both 11β- and 18-hydroxylase activities and their sensitivity to carbon monoxide inhibition strongly suggested that both activities were related to the same enzyme [74]. When cytochrome P-450 with 11β-hydroxylase activity was purified, 18-hydroxylase copurified with it and the ratio of 11β-: 18-hydroxylase activity was the same in the crude as in the pure preparation (87). Antibodies to this P-$450_{11\beta}$ showed a single precipitin line on double diffusion plates and the antibodies inhibited both 18- and 11β-hydroxylase activities equally in crude solubilized extracts, again suggesting a single enzyme for hydroxylations at both positions (87).

Purified bovine P-$450_{11\beta}$ in vitro catalyzes the 11β-hydroxylation of steroids containing 21 carbon atoms (11-deoxy-corticosterone, 11-deoxy-cortisol). It also catalyzes 11β- and 19-hydroxylation of steroids with 19 carbon atoms (testosterone, 4-androstene-3,17-dione) (77). It is evident, therefore, that the single cytochrome P-$450_{11\beta}$ hydroxylates steroids at more than one position. It is noteworthy that the carbon 18 and carbon 19 methyl groups jut out from the planar steroid ring structure on the same side as and close to the 11β position. This proximity may account for multiple hydroxylations by the same enzyme. There is no evidence that P-$450_{11\beta}$ hydroxylates a single molecule at more than one position. For example 11-deoxy-corticosterone is either 11β- *or* 18-hydroxylated by P-$450_{11\beta}$ and the 11β, 18-dihydroxylated compound, that is 18-hydroxy-corticosterone has not been observed to be formed by P-$450_{11\beta}$ (77). The formation of 18-hydroxy-corticosterone is catalyzed by a different enzyme in the zona glomerulosa and is discussed below.

The ratio of 11β- : 18-hydroxylase activity was dependent on the species from which the P-450 particles were derived. Although 11β-hydroxylase was always greater than 18-hydroxylase activity, the rat and pig showed more 18-hydroxylase activity than the human or ox (61). It is emphasized that the 18-hydroxylated product of 11-deoxy-corticosterone (i.e., 18-hydroxy-11-deoxy-corticosterone) is produced in only small amounts by the human adrenal (58). The product expected from 18-hydroxylation of 11-deoxy-cortisol (i.e., 18-hydroxy-11-deoxy-cortisol) has not been reported (or looked for) with human adrenal tissue and therefore, is not shown in Figure 4.

Formation of Aldosterone

The formation of aldosterone takes place only in the mitochondria of the adrenal zona glomerulosa. The biosynthetic pathway for aldosterone is corticosterone → 18-hydroxy-corticosterone → aldosterone (25,63,69, 72,98). The conversion of radioactive corticosterone → aldosterone is readily demonstrated, but the conversion of exogenous radioactive 18-hydroxy-corticosterone to aldosterone, though demonstrable, goes at a much slower rate (63) (see ref. 60 for review). Exogenous 18-hydroxy-corticosterone probably forms an 18,20-cyclic hemiketal, thus, its conversion to aldosterone with in vitro systems is difficult to demonstrate (63). It has also been suggested that once formed, 18-hydroxy-corticosterone either remains associated with an enzyme complex to be converted to aldosterone or disassociates from the enzyme to yield 18-hydroxy-corticosterone (30).

Clearly, there are two steps between corticosterone and aldosterone, with 18-hydroxy-corticosterone as an intermediate, because each step has been found to be individually defective in congenital disorders in humans (95). Although the first step (formation of 18-hydroxy-corticosterone) is certainly a hydroxylation, the second step has in the past been assumed to be a dehydrogenation of the 18-hydroxyl to yield aldosterone. This is unlikely because the conversion of 18-hydroxy-corticosterone to aldosterone requires NADPH and oxygen (56).

The formation of aldosterone from corticosterone involves cytochrome P-450, because the reaction is inhibited by carbon monoxide and this inhibition is maximally reversed by light at 450 nm (30). The two steps in the conversion of corticosterone → aldosterone can be differentiated by their sensitivity to carbon monoxide, suggesting that two cytochrome P-450 steps are involved (74). A genetic mutant in the rat has been shown to alter the first cytochrome P-450 step (18-hdyroxylation of corticosterone) without any effect on the second (74).

Figure 5 shows a likely sequence of events on the basis of existing data. Corticosterone is probably hydroxylated twice at carbon 18 to yield 18, 18-dihydroxy-corticosterone (74,95): this configuration is unstable and decomposes into aldosterone and water.

Pathways alternate to the above have been described for aldosterone production (25,81,98). A minor pathway, most easily demonstrated in the rabbit adrenal, appears to circumvent 18-hydroxy-corticosterone as an obligatory intermediate by utilizing the steps corticosterone → 11-dehydro-corticosterone → 18-hydroxy-11-dehydro-corticosterone → 11-dehydro-aldosterone → aldosterone. This pathway depends on the known ability of adrenals to interconvert the 11β-hydroxyl ⇄ 11-keto (26). The physiologic significance of this alternate pathway for aldosterone is not established.

Figure 6 reviews the steroidogenic sequences from cholesterol to aldosterone and cortisol. The cofactor requirements for each step are given and the subcellular location of each step is illustrated.

Formation of Androgens and Estrogens

The adrenal cortex is capable of removing the two carbon side chain of 17α-hydroxy-pregnenolone to form dehydroepiandrosterone (DHEA) (Figure 4). This compound is sulfated at the hydroxyl group on carbon 3 and secreted largely as the sulfate (102). Smaller amounts of 4-androsten-3, 17-dione and still smaller amounts of testosterone, estrone and possibly 17β-estradiol are also formed by the adrenal (1,32,52,102) (Figure 4).

METABOLISM OF ADRENAL STEROIDS

The main metabolic pathways for inactivation of adrenal steroids will be illustrated with cortisol as a model compound. The metabolism of aldosterone, which has some unique features, will also be given.

FIGURE 5. Biosynthesis of aldosterone from corticosterone. These steps occur only in mitochondria of adrenal zona glomerulosa cells.

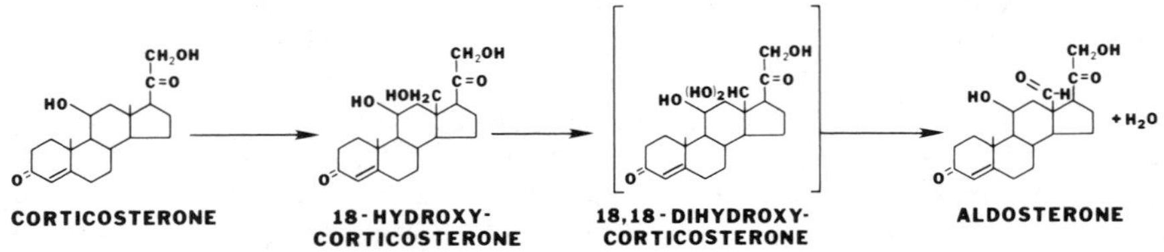

CORTICOSTERONE → 18-HYDROXY-CORTICOSTERONE → 18,18-DIHYDROXY-CORTICOSTERONE → ALDOSTERONE + H_2O

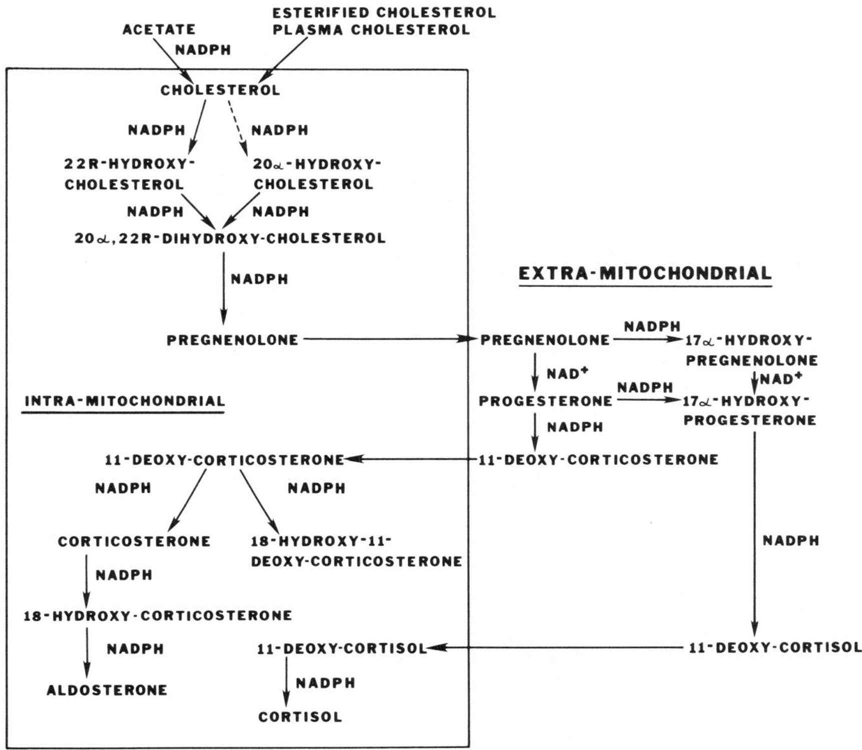

FIGURE 6. Subcellular localization of adrenal steroidogenic steps. The intramitochondrial steps probably take place on the inner mitochondrial membrane [76,105]. Extramitochondrial steps probably take place on the smooth-surfaced endoplasmic reticulum [39]. [Redrawn from ref 80]

Metabolism of Cortisol

Figure 7 shows the main metabolic conversions of cortisol by nonadrenal tissues. The interconversion of cortisol $\rightleftarrows$ cortisone takes place in many tissues but the liver and kidney have the highest activities (11). The enzyme involved, 11β-hydroxysteroid dehydrogenase, is contained in microsomes. It works more efficiently with NADP(H) than NAD(H), and the reaction is reversible (12). The 11β-hydroxysteroid dehydrogenase requires a planar structure between rings A and B of the steroid, that is, Δ^4-3-ketosteroids and steroids with a 5α hydrogen are good substrates. Steroids with a nonplanar structure between rings A and B (i.e., 5β hydrogen) react little (12, 47).

The main metabolic inactivation of adrenal steroids occurs through reduction of the Δ^4 double bond (addition of two hydrogen atoms to yield "dihydro" compounds) followed by the reduction of the 3-keto group (addition of two additional hydrogen atoms to yield "tetrahydro" com-

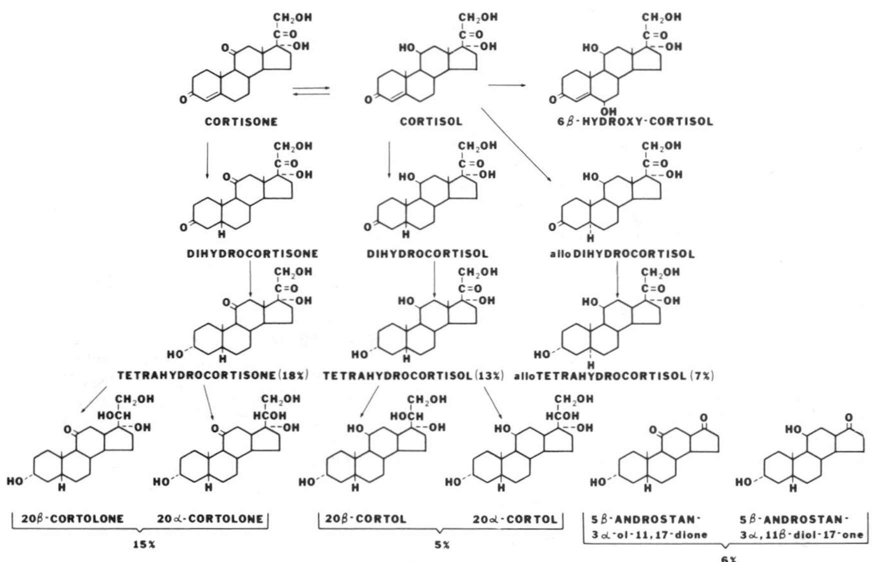

FIGURE 7. Metabolism of cortisol. The percentages indicate the proportion of a dose of cortisol recovered as urinary metabolites. [Redrawn from Fotherby and James [28] and based on the work of Fukushima et al [29]].

pounds). The reduction of the Δ^4 double bond can occur in two stereospecific ways, such that the hydrogen at carbon 5 is either 5α (referred to as "allo" compounds) or 5β (referred to as "normal" compounds). The conversion of 3-keto to 3-hydroxyl can yield either 3α- or 3β-hydroxyl configurations. Thus, there are four possible tetrahydro configurations: 3α,5α; 3α,5β; 3β,5α; 3β,5β. Enzymes that reduce the Δ^4 double bond to the 5β configuration and another enzyme that reduces the 3-keto group of dihydro compounds have been partially purified from rat liver (5). The main metabolite of cortisol in humans has the 3α,5β configuration, although significant amounts of 3α,5α configuration are also formed (Figure 6) (29). Most of the tetrahydro metabolites are conjugated with glucuronic acid, which increases their water solubility, and the conjugates are excreted in urine.

In addition to the reduction of the Δ^4-3-keto group to form tetrahydro derivatives, the 20-keto group is also reduced to a 20-hydroxyl configuration. The 20-hydroxyl can be in either of two isomeric forms 20α or 20β. Such derivatives of cortisol are known as cortols, and such derivatives of cortisone are called cortolones (Figure 7). The side chain of cortols and cortolones can be cleaved between carbons 17 and 20 to yield 5β-androstan-3α,11β-diol-17-one and 5β-androstan-3α-ol-11,17-dione, the structures of which are given in the lower right side of Figure 7 (29).

The liver is capable of hydroxylating the steroids at positions 6α,6β,7α, and 15α and 16α (17,27). In man 6β-hydroxycortisol is produced from cortisol by the liver and may account for small amounts (up to 2%) of the cortisol excretion in normal humans (28,68). The liver hydroxylating systems are microsomal enzymes containing cytochrome P-450 (17).

Metabolism of Aldosterone

Aldosterone probably exists in vivo as the 11 → 18 hemiacetal and its metabolic products retain this ring structure (Figure 8). Because the 11β-hydroxyl is involved in this ring closure it is not available for conversion by 11β-hydroxy-steroid dehydrogenase (48). The Δ^4-3-keto group is reduced much as in the case of cortisol and three of the four possible configurations at carbons 3 and 5 have been found to be urinary metabolites of aldosterone in humans. These are 3α,5α; 3α,5β; and 3β,5β (44,46, 70,96). Rat liver in vitro (48) also produces the 3β,5α isomer.

In addition, two bicyclic acetal metabolites of aldosterone have been isolated from human urine following large doses of tritiated aldosterone (45,46). These compounds are shown at the bottom of Figure 8 and could

FIGURE 8. Metabolism of aldosterone.

ALDOSTERONE

ALDOSTERONE 11→18 HEMIACETAL

ISOMERS OF DIHYDRALDOSTERONE

ISOMERS OF TETRAHYDROALDOSTERONE

BICYCLIC ACETAL METABOLITES OF ALDOSTERONE

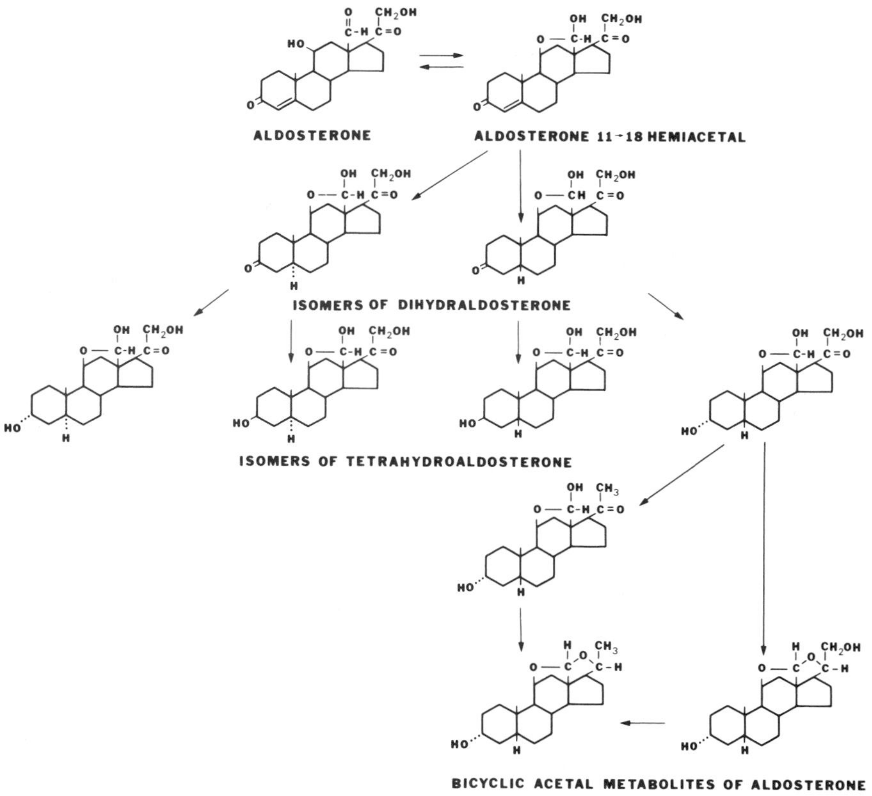

arise as indicated. These bicyclic acetals account for about 10% of aldosterone metabolites; tetrahydro compounds account for about 30% (46).

Tetrahydro aldosterone is excreted as a conjugate with glucuronic acid. In addition, there is an acid labile conjugate of aldosterone in urine (71,97), which has been identified as a glucuronide at the hydroxyl on carbon 18 of the hemiacetal structure (13). This conjugate is probably made in the kidney (53,85). Small amounts of aldosterone (less than 1%) are excreted in the urine as aldosterone-21-monosulfate (33).

REFERENCES

1. Baird, D.T., Uno, A., and Melby, J.C. (1969) Adrenal secretion of androgens and estrogens. J. Endocrinol. 45, 135–136.
2. Baker, H.N., and Dempsey, M.E. (1978) Preparation and use of antibodies to liver squalene and sterol carrier protein. Fed. Proc. 37,1663, Abstr. 2167.
3. Baron, J. (1976) Immunochemical studies on adrenal ferredoxin: Involvement of adrenal ferredoxin in the cholesterol side-chain cleavage reaction of mammalian adrenals. Arch. Biochem. Biophys. 174, 226–238.
4. Baron, J., Taylor, W.E., and Masters, B.S.S. (1972) Immunochemical studies on electron transport chains involving cytochrome P-450. The role of the iron-sulfur protein, adrenodoxin, in mixed function oxidation reactions. Arch. Biochem. Biophys. 150, 105–115.
5. Berseus, O. (1967) Conversion of cholesterol to bile acids in rat: Purification and properties of a Δ^4-3-ketosteroid 5β-reductase and a hydroxysteroid dehydrogenase. Eur. J. Biochem. 2, 493–502.
6. Beyer, K.F., and Samuels, L.T. (1956) Distribution of steroid-3β-o1-dehydrogenase in cellular structures of the adrenal gland. J. Biol. Chem. 219, 69–76.
7. Billiay, R.B., Alousi, M.A., Knappenberger, M.H., and Little, B. (1971) Distribution of cholesterol side-chain cleavage and 11β-hydroxylase in the mitochondria of bovine adrenal cortex: Release by phospholipase A. Arch. Biochem. Biophys. 144, 30–50.
8. Björkhem, I., and Karlmar, K. (1977) Common characteristics of cytochrome P-450 system involved in 18- and 11β-hydroxylation of deoxycorticosterone in rat adrenals. J. Lipid Res. 18, 595–603.
9. Burnstein, S., and Gut, M. (1971) Biosynthesis of pregnenolone. Recent Prog. Hormone Res. 27, 303–345.
10. Burnstein, S., Middleditch, B.S., and Gut, M. (1975) Mass spectrometric study of the enzymatic conversion of cholesterol to (22R)-22-hydroxycholesterol, (20R, 22R)-20, 22-dihydroxycholesterol, and prednisone, and of (22R)-22-hydroxycholesterol to the glycol and pregnenolone in bovine adrenocortical preparations. J. Biol. Chem. 250, 9028–9037.
11. Burton, A.F., and Turnell, R.W. (1968) 11-Dehydrocorticoids in tissues of mice. Can. J. Biochem. 46, 497–502.
12. Bush, I.E., Hunter, S.A., and Meigs, R.A. (1968) Metabolism of 11-oxygenated steroids. Metabolism in vitro by preparations of liver. Biochem. J. 107, 239–258.
13. Carpenter, P.C., and Mattox, V.R. (1976) Isolation, determination of structure and synthesis of the acid-labile conjugate of aldosterone. Biochem. J. 157, 1–14.
14. Cheng, S.C., and Harding, B.W. (1973) Substrate induced difference spectral, electron paramagnetic resonance, and enzymatic properties of cholesterol-depleted mitochondrial cytochrome P-450 of bovine adrenal cortex. J. Biol. Chem. 248, 7263–7271.
15. Chu, J-W., and Kimura, T. (1973) Studies on adrenal steroid hydroxylases. Molecular and catalytic properties of adrenodoxin reductase (a flavoprotein). J. Biol. Chem. 248, 2089–2094.

16. Chu, J.W., and Kimura, T. (1973) Studies on adrenal steroid hydroxylases. Complex formation of the hydroxylase components. J. Biol. Chem. 248, 5183–5187.
17. Conney, A.H., Levin, W., Ikeda, M., Kuntzman, R., Cooper, D.Y., and Rosenthal, O. (1968) Inhibitory effect of carbon monoxide on the hydroxylation of testosterone by rat liver microsomes. J. Biol. Chem. 243, 3912–3915.
18. Cooper, D.Y., Estabrook, R.W., and Rosenthal, O. (1963) The stoichiometry of C_{21} hydroxylation of steroids by adrenocortical microsomes. J. Biol. Chem. 238, 1320–1323.
19. Cooper, D.Y., Narashimhulu, S., Slade, A., Raich, W., Foroff, O., and Rosenthal, O. (1965) Hemoprotein content and activity of solubilized steroid 11β-hydroxylase preparations from adrenocortical mitochondria. Life Sci. 4, 2109–2114.
20. Dailey, R.E., Swell, L., and Treadwell, C.R. (1962) Utilization of free and esterified cholesterol-4-C^{14} for corticoid biosynthesis by hog adrenal homogenates. Proc. Soc. Exp. Biol. Med. 110, 571–574.
21. Duque, C., Morisaki, M., Ikekawa, N., Shikita, M., and Tamoki, B. (1978) The final step of side-chain cleavage of cholesterol by adrenal cortical cytochrome P-$450_{(scc)}$ studied with [22-^{18}O] 20,22-dihydroxy-cholesterols, [^{18}O] isocaproaldehyde, [^{18}O] water and atmospheric [^{18}O] oxygen. Biochem. Biophys. Res. Commun. 85, 317–325.
22. Estabrook, R.W., Mason, J.I., Baron, J., Lambeth, D., and Waterman, M. (1973) Drugs, alcohol, and sex hormones: A molecular perspective of the receptivity of cytochrome P-450. Ann. N.Y. Acad. Sci. 212, 27–47.
23. Ewald, W., Werbin, H., and Chaikoff, I.L. (1964) Evidence for two substrate specific Δ^5-3-ketosteroid isomerases in beef adrenal glands and their separation from 3β-hydroxysteroid dehydrogenase. Biochem. Biophys. Acta 81, 199–201.
24. Ewald, W., Werbin, H., and Chiacoff, I.L. (1965) Evidence for the presence of 17-hydroxy-pregnenedione isomerase in beef adrenal cortex. Biochem. Biophys. Acta 111, 306–312.
25. Fazekas, A.G., and Sandor, T. (1969) Unusual pathways of aldosterone biosynthesis in the rabbit adrenal. Steroids 14, 161–177.
26. Fazekas, A.P., Sandor, T., and Lanthier, A. (1970) Conversion of corticosterone to 11-dehydrocorticosterone by adrenal gland preparations of different animal species. Endocrinology 86, 438–440.
27. Ford, H.C., Lee, E., and Engel, L.G. (1979) Circannual variation and genetic regulation of hepatic testosterone hydroxylase activities in inbred strains of mice. Endocrinology 104, 857–861.
28. Fotherby, K., and James, F. (1972) Metabolism of synthetic steroids. Advances in Steroid Biochemistry and Pharmacology 3, 67–165.
29. Fukushima, D.K., Bradlow, H.L., Hellman, L., Zumoff, B., and Gallagher, T.F. (1960) Metabolic transformation of hydrocortisone-4-C^{14} in normal men. J. Biol. Chem. 235, 2246–2252.
30. Greengard, P., Phychoyos, S., Tallen, H.H., Cooper, D.Y., Rosenthal, O., and Estabrook, R.W. (1967) Aldosterone synthesis by adrenal mitochondria III. Participation of cytochrome P-450. Arch. Biochem. Biophys. 121, 298–303.
31. Griffiths, K., and Cameron, E.H.D. (1970) Steroid biosynthetic pathways in the human adrenal. Advances in Steroid Biochemistry and Pharmacology 2, 223–265.
32. Griffiths, K., and Giles, C.A. (1965) Metabolism of testosterone by adrenal tissue of the golden hamster and identification of 19-hydroxylated steroids. J. Endocrinol. 33, 333–334.
33. Grose, J.H., Nowaczynski, W., Kuchel, O., and Genest. J. (1973) Isolation of aldosterone urinary metabolites, glucuronides and sulfate. J. Ster. Biochem. 4, 551–556.
34. Handler, R.P., and Brandsome, E.D. (1969) Guinea pig adrenal 3β-hydroxy-steroid dehydrogenase: Is there more than one enzyme? J. Clin. Endocrinol. Metab. 29, 1117–1119.
35. Hector, O., and Pincus, G. (1954) Genesis of the adrenocortical secretion. Physiol. Rev. 34, 459–496.

36. Hochberg, R.B., McDonald, P.D., Feldman, M., and Lieberman, S. (1974) Studies on the biosynthetic conversion of cholesterol into pregnenolone. Side chain cleavage of some 20-p-tolyl analogs of cholesterol and 20α-hydroxy-cholesterol. J. Biol. Chem. 249, 1277– 1285.

37. Huang, J.J., and Kimura, T. (1971) A specific role of reduced adrenodoxin in adrenal mitochondrial steroid hydroxylases. Biochem. Biophys. Res. Commun. 44, 1065–1070.

38. Ichii, S., Kobayashi, S., Yago, N., and Omata, S. (1967) Role of plasma cholesterol in rat-adrenal corticosteroidogenesis in vitro. Endocrinologia Japonica 14, 138–142.

39. Inano, H., Inano, A., and Tamaoki, B-I. (1969) Submicrosomal distribution of adrenal enzymes and cytochrome P-450 related to corticosteroidogenesis. Biochim. Biophys. Acta 191, 257–271.

40. Jefcoate, C.R., Hume, R., and Boyd, G.S. (1970) Separation of two forms of cytochrome P-450 adrenal cortex mitochondria. FEBS Lett. 9, 41–44.

41. Kahnt, F.W., and Nehr, R. (1972) On adrenocortical steroid biosynthesis in vitro. Part v. activators and inhibitors. Evidence for the presence of substrate-specific 21-hydroxylases. Acta Endocrinol. 70, 315–330.

42. Kan, K.W., and Ungar, F. (1973) Characterization of an adrenal activator for cholesterol side chain cleavage. J. Biol. Chem. 248, 2868–2875.

43. Katagiri, M., Takikawa, O., Sato, N., and Suhara, K. (1977) Formation of a cytochrome $P\text{-}450_{scc}$-adrenodoxin complex. Biochem. Biophys. Res. Commun. 77, 804–809.

44. Kelly, W.G., Bandi, L., and Lieberman, S. (1962) Isolation and characterization of human urinary metabolites of aldosterone: III. Three isomeric tetrahydro metabolites. Biochemistry 1, 792–803.

45. Kelly, W.G., Bandi, L. and Lieberman, S. (1963) Isolation and characterization of human urinary metabolites of aldosterone: IV. The synthesis and sterochemistry of two bicyclic acetal metabolites. Biochemistry 2, 1243–1249.

46. Kelly, W.G., Bandi, L., Shoolery, J.N., and Lieberman, S. (1962) Isolation and characterization of aldosterone metabolites from human urine: Two metabolites bearing a bicyclic acetal structure. Biochemistry 1, 172–181.

47. Koerner, D.R. (1969) Assay and substrate specificity of liver 11β-hydroxy-steroid dehydrogenase. Biochim. Biophys. Acta. 176, 377–382.

48. Kohler, H., Hesse, R.H., and Pechet, M.M. (1964) The metabolism of aldosterone. Metabolic pathway, isolation characterization, and synthesis of metabolites. J. Biol. Chem. 239, 4117–4123.

49. Kovanen, P.T., Faust, J.R., Brown, M.S., and Goldstein, J.L. (1979) Low density lipoprotein receptors in bovine adrenal cortex. I. receptor-mediated uptake of low density lipoprotein and utilization of its cholesterol for steroid synthesis in cultured adrenocortical cells. Endocrinology 104, 599–609.

50. Kraaipoel, R.J., Degenhart, H.J., van Beek, V., de Leeuw-Boon, H., Abeln, G., Visser, H.K.A., and Leferink, J.G. (1975) Evidence for 20,22-epoxy-cholesterol as an intermediate in side chain cleavage 22R-OH cholesterol by adrenal cortex mitochondria. FEBS Lett. 54, 172–179.

51. Krum, A.A., Morris, M.D., and Bennett, L.L.. (1964) Role of cholesterol in the in vitro biosynthesis of adrenal steroids by the dog. Endocrinology 74, 543–547.

52. Lawrence, J.R., and Griffiths (1966) Oestrogen biosynthesis in vitro by adrenal tissue from the golden hamster. Biochem. J. 99, 27C–28C.

53. Luetscher, J.A., Hancock, E.W., Camargo, C.A., Dowdy, A.J. and Nokes, G.W. (1965) Conjugation of 1,2-^{3}H aldosterone in human liver and kidneys and renal extraction of aldosterone and labeled conjugates from blood plasma. J. Clin. Endocrinol. 25, 628.

54. Mackler, B., Haynes, B., Tattoni, D.S., Tippit, D.F., and Kelly, V.C., (1971) Studies of adrenal steroid hydroxylation. 1. Purification of the microsomal 21-hydroxylase system. Arch. Biochem. Biophys. 145, 194–198.

55. Maines, M.D., and Anders, M.W. (1973) Characterizatoin of the heme of cytochrome P-450 using gas chromatography/mass spectometry. Arch. Biochem. Biophys. 159, 201–205.

56. Marusic, E.T., White, A., and Aedo, A.R. (1973) Oxidative reactions in the formation of an aldehyde group in the biosynthesis of aldosterone. Arch. Biochem. Biophys. 157, 320–321.

57. Masters, B.S.S., Baron, J., Taylor, W.E., Isaacson, E.L., and LoSpalluto, J. (1971) Immunochemical studies on electron transport chains involving cytochrome P-450. J. Biol. Chem. 246, 4143–4150.

58. Melby, J.C., Dale, S.L., Gerkin, R.J., Gaunt, R., and Wilson, T.E. (1972) 18-hydroxy-11-deoxycorticosterone (180H-DOC) secretion in experimental and human hypertension. Recent Prog. Hormone Res. 28:287–339.

59. Moustafa, A.M., and Koritz, S.A. (1975) Concerning the subcellular distribution of 3β-hydroxysteroid dehydrogenase/isomerase in the rat adrenal. Proc. Soc. Ex. Biol. Med. 149, 823–825.

60. Müller, J. (1971) Regulation of Aldosterone Biosynthesis. Springer Verlag, New York, p.4.

61. Nakamura, Y., Otsuka, H., and Tamaoki, B. (1966) Requirement of a new flavo-protein and non-heme iron containing protein in the 11β-and 18-hydroxylase system. Biochim. Biophys. Acta 122, 34–42.

62. Neville, A.M., Orr, J.C., and Engle, L.L. (1969) The Δ^5-3β-hydroxysteroid dehydrogenase of bovine adrenal microsomes. J. Endocrinol. 43, 599–608.

63. Nicolis, G.L., and Ulich, S. (1965) Role of 18-hydroxylation in the biosynthesis of aldosterone. Endocrinology 76, 514–521.

64. Oleinick, N.L., and Koritz, S.B. (1966) The activation of the Δ^5-3-keto steroid isomerase in rat adrenal small particles by diphosphopyridine nucleotides. Biochemistry 5, 715–724.

65. Omura, T., Sanders, E., Estabrook, R.E., Cooper, D.Y., and Rosenthal, O. (1969) Isolation from adrenal cortex of a nonheme iron protein and a flavoprotein functional as a reduced triphosphopyridine nucleotide-cytochrome P-450 reductase. Arch. Biochem. Biophys. 117, 660–673.

66. Omura, T., Sato, R., Cooper, D.Y., Rosenthal, O., and Estabrook, R.W. (1965) Function of cytochrome P-450 microsomes. Proc. 24, 1181–1189.

67. Ora-Flores, Z., Cantu, J.M., and Dominguez, O.V. (1976) Reciproal interactions of progesterone and 17α-OH-progesterone as exogenous substrates of rat adrenal 21-hydroxylase. J. Steroid Biochem. 7, 761–767.

68. Pal, S.B. (1978) 6-hydroxylation of cortisol and urinary 6β-hydroxycortisol. Metabolism 27, 1003–1011.

69. Pasqualini, J.R. (1964) Conversion of tritiated-18-hydroxy-corticosterone to aldosterone by slices of human cortico-adrenal gland and adrenal tumor. Natare 201, 501–502.

70. Pasqualini, J.R., Legrand, J.C., and Jayle, M.F. (1963) Separation and evaluation of tetrahydroaldosterone by paper chromatography. Acta Endocrinol. 43, 67–71.

71. Pasqualini, J.R., Uhrich, F., and Jayle, M.F. (1965) Contribution to the study of the structure of the aldosterone-conjugate isolated from human urine. Biochim. Biophys. Acta 104, 515–523.

72. Raman, P.B., Sharma, D.C., Dorfman, R.I., and Gabrilove, J.L. (1965) Biosynthesis of C-18-oxygenated steroids by an aldosterone-secreting human adrenal tumor. Metabolism of [4-^{14}C] progesterone, [1,2,-^{3}H] 11-deoxycorticosterone and [4-^{14}C] pregnenolone. Biochemistry 4, 1376–1385.

73. Ramseyer, J., and Harding, B.W. (1973) Solubilization and properties of bovine adrenal cortical cytochrome P-450 which cleaves the cholesterol side chain. Biochim. Biophys. Acta 315, 306–316.

74. Rapp, J.P., and Dahl, L.K. (1976) Mutant forms of cytochrome P-450 controlling both 18- and 11β-steroid hydroxylation in the rat. Biochemistry 15, 1235–1242.

75. Ritter, M.C., and Dempsey, M.E. (1971) Specificity and role in cholesterol biosynthesis of a squalene and sterol carrier protein. J. Biol. Chem. 246, 1536–1547.

76. Rydstrom, J., Gufstafsson, J.A. Ingelman-Sundberg, M., Montelius, J., and Ernster, L.

(1976) The topology of the mitochondrial 11β-hydroxylase system in bovine adrenal cortex. Biochem. Biophys. Res. Commun. 73, 555–561.

77. Sato, H., Ashida, N., Suhara, K., Itagaki, E., and Takemori, S. (1978) Properties of an adrenal cytochrome P-450 (P-$450_{11\beta}$) for the hydroxylations of corticosteroids. Arch. Biochem. Biophys. 190, 307–314.

78. Seybert, D.W., Lambeth, J.D., and Kamin, H. (1978) The participation of a second molecule of adrenodoxin in cytochrome P-450-catalyzed 11β-hydroxylation. J. Biol. Chem. 253, 8355–8358.

79. Scallen, T.J., Schuster, M.W., and Dhar, A.K. (1971) Evidence for a non-catalytic carrier protein in cholesterol biosynthesis. J. Biol. Chem. 246, 224–230.

80. Schulster, D. (1974) Adrenocorticotrophic hormone and the control of adrenal corticosteroidogenesis. Advances in Steroid Biochemistry and Pharmacology 4, 233–295.

81. Sharma, D.C. (1970) Studies on aldosterone biosynthesis in vitro. Acta Endocrinol. 63, 299–312.

82. Shikita, M., and Hall, P.F. (1973) Cytochrome P-450 from bovine adrenocortical mitochondria: An enzyme for the side chain cleavage of cholesterol. I. Purification and properties. J. Biol. Chem. 248, 5598–5604.

83. Shikita, M., and Hall, P.F. (1973) Cytochrome P-450 from bovine adrenocortical mitochondria: An enzyme for the side chain cleavage of cholesterol. II. Subunit structure. J. Biol. Chem. 248, 5605–5609.

84. Shikita, M., and Hall, P.F. (1974) The stoichiometry of the conversion of cholesterol and hydroxycholesterols to pregnenolone (3β-hydroxypregn-5-en-20-one) catalysed by adrenal cytochrome P-450. Proc. Natl. Acad. Sci. 71, 1441–1445.

85. Siegenthaler, W.E., Dowdy, A.J., and Luetscher, J.A. (1962) Determination of the secretion rate of aldosterone in normal man by use of 7-H^3-d-aldosterone and acid hydrolysis of urine. J. Clin. Endocrinol. 22, 172–177.

86. Simpson, E.R., and Boyd, S.S. (1967) The cholesterol side chain cleavage system of bovine adrenal cortex. Eur. J. Biochem. 2, 275–285.

87. Suhara, K., Gomi, T., Sato, H., Itagaki, E., Takemori, S., and Katagiri, M. (1978) Purification and immunochemical characterization of the two adrenal cortex mitochondrial cytochrome P-450-proteins. Arch. Biochem. Biophys. 190, 290–299.

88. Suzuki, K., and Kimura, T. (1965) An iron protein as a component of steroid 11β-hydroxylase complex. Biochem. Biophys. Res. Commun. 19, 340–345.

89. Takemoto, C., Nakano, H., Sato, H., and Tamaoki, B. (1968) Fate of molecular oxygen required by endocrine enzymes for the side chain cleavage of cholesterol. Biochim. Biophys. Acta 152, 749–757.

90. Takikawa, O., Gomi, T., Suhara, K., Itagaki, E., Takemori, S., and Katagiri, M. (1978) Properties of an adrenal cytochrome P-450 (P-450_{scc}) for the side chain cleavage of cholesterol. Arch. Biochem. Biophys. 190, 300–306.

91. Tanaka, M., Haniu, M., Yasunobu, K.T., and Kimura, T. (1973) The amino acid sequence of bovine adrenodoxin. J. Biol. Chem. 248, 1141–1157.

92. Teicher, B.A., Koizumi, N., Koreeda, M., Shikita, M., and Talalay, P. (1978) Biosynthesis of pregnenolone from cholesterol by mitochondrial enzymes of bovine adrenal cortex. The question of the participation of the 20(22)-olefins and 20,22-epoxides of cholesterol. Eur. J. Biochem. 91, 11–19.

93. Teicher, B.A., Shikita, M., and Talalay, P. (1978) Effects of adrenal steroid activator protein on the conversion of various 20- and 22-hydroxy-cholesterols to pregnenolone by adrenal mitochondrial enzymes. Biochem. Biophys. Res. Commun. 83, 1436–1441.

94. Tilley, B.E., Watanuki, M., and Hall, P.F. (1976) Cytochrome P-450 from bovine adrenocortical mitochondria: Two species of subunit. Biochem. Biophys. Res. Commun. 70, 1303–1307.

95. Ulick, S. (1976) Diagnosis and nomenclature of the disorders of the terminal portion of the aldosterone biosynthesis pathway. J. Clin. Endocrinol. Metab. 43, 92–96.

96. Ulick, S., Vetter, K.K., and August, J.T. (1962) Identification of 2 C_{18} oxygenated cortisteroids isolated from human urine. J. Biol. Chem. 237, 3364–3373.

97. Underwood, R.H., and Tait, J.F. (1964) Purification, partial characterization and metabolism of an acid labile conjugate of aldosterone. J. Clin. Endocrinol. Metab. 24, 1110–1124.

98. Vecsei, P., Lommer, D., and Wolff, H.P. (1968) The intermediate role of 18-hydroxycorticosteroids in aldosterone biosynthesis. Experientia 24, 1199–1291.

99. Wang, H-P., and Kimura, T. (1976), Purification and characterization of adrenal cortex mitochondrial cytochrome P-450 specific for cholesterol side chain cleavage activity. J. Biol. Chem. 251, 6068–6074.

100. Ward, M.G., and Engle, L.L. (1966) Reversibility of steroid Δ-isomerase? J. Biol. Chem. 241, 3147–3153.

101. Werbin, H., and Chaikoff, I.L. (1961) Utilization of adrenal gland cholesterol for synthesis of cortisol by the intact normal and the ACTH-treated Guinea pig. Arch. Biochem. Biophys. 93, 476–482.

102. Wieland, R.G., Levy, R.P., Katz, D., and Hirschmann (1963) Evidence for secretion of 3β-hydroxy-androst-en-17-one sulfate by measurement in normal human adrenal venous blood. Biochem. Biophys. Acta 78, 566–568.

103. Wilson, L.D., and Harding, B.W. (1970) Studies on adrenal cortical cytochrome P-450. IV. Effects of carbon monoxide and light on cholesterol side chain cleavage. Biochemistry 9, 1621–1625.

104. Wilson, L.D., and Harding, B.W. (1970) Studies on adrenal cortical cytochrome P-450. III. Effects of carbon monoxide and light on steroid 11β-hydroxylation. Biochemistry 9, 1615–1621.

105. Yago, N., and Ichii, S. (1969) Submitochondrial distribution of components of the steroid 11β-hydroxylase and cholesterol side chain-cleaving enzyme systems in hog adrenal cortex. J. Biochem. 65, 215–224.

106. Young, R.B., Bryson, M.J., and Sweat, M.L. (1965) Preparation of a soluble progesterone 17α-hydroxylating system. Arch. Biochem. Biophys. 109, 233–240.

107. Yu, C-A., and Gunsalus, I.C. (1974) Cytochrome $P\text{-}450_{cam}$ III. Removal and replacement of ferriprotoporphyrin IX. J. Biol. Chem. 249, 107–110.

RICHARD P. McPARTLAND, Ph.D.

METABOLIC AND PHARMACOLOGIC ACTIONS OF GLUCOCORTICOIDS

INTRODUCTION

In recent years an impressive amount of research has led to the development of a proposal for the mechanism of action of steroid hormones. The androgens, estrogens, progestins, and corticocoids all appear to act by binding to specific cellular receptors. The characterization of specific receptors for glucocorticoids has been discussed in detail elsewhere in this book. The specific interactions of the hormone–receptor complex and nuclei appear necessary for the initiation of biological events. However, the precise interaction between the steroid–receptor complex and nuclear processes, leading to biological activity, remains unclear. Recent developments provide evidence that the steroid can induce increased or decreased levels of specific messenger-RNA synthesis and protein synthesis (32,101).

The biological actions of glucocorticoids appear to have diverse effects on hepatic and extrahepatic tissues. Glucocorticoids promote gluconeogenesis and glycogen deposition in liver while they have "catabolic-like" effects on extrahepatic tissues. This chapter reviews the metabolic actions

From the Wampole Laboratories, a division of Carter-Wallace, Inc., Cranbury, New Jersey.
Formerly of the Department of Medicine, Medical College of Ohio, Toledo, Ohio.

of glucocorticoids by describing the effects of steroids on glucose, lipid, and protein metabolism in general, and then discusses the actions of glucocorticoids on major target tissues. The effects of mineralocorticoids and glucocorticoids on water and electrolyte balance are discussed separately in Ch. 8. Where possible, the proposed mechanism of glucocorticoid action on the organ is also discussed, as are the pharmacological actions of glucocorticoids as antiinflammatory agents.

EFFECTS OF ADRENOCORTICOID DEFICIENCY

A great deal of knowledge about the role of glucocorticoids has come from studies using adrenalectomized subjects or from subjects with adrenal insufficiency. The vigor and appetite of animals following adrenalectomy is markedly depressed. Growth is actually impaired unless the animals are force-fed (17). Patients usually have a loss of appetite, reduced production of gastric HCl and pepsin, and insufficient reabsorption of fat (75). Blood glucose decreases to extremely low levels and liver glycogen becomes depleted following brief periods of starvation in adrenalectomized subjects. Following a period of exercise, blood glucose levels become markedly depleted. The level of free fatty acids in plasma also fails to increase during periods of exercise in the adrenalectomized rat (143). This indicates that in the absence of glucocorticoids, lipid mobilization from fat depots is impaired. The decrease in blood glucose levels is apparently independent of insulin levels because similar results have been reported in fasted-depancreatized rats (87). Insulin levels have been shown to be slightly lower following adrenalectomy (140). The insulin response to a glucose challenge is also depressed in adrenalectomized rats, indicating that glucocorticoids may play some role in glucose-stimulated insulin secretion (144) (i.e., pharmacological levels of glucocorticoids can elevate insulin secretion). On the other hand, adrenalectomized rats are more sensitive to an insulin challenge than intact rats. The adrenalectomized dog shows severe hypoglycemia following insulin administration. The liver fails to release glucose despite depressed plasma glucose levels indicating that the adrenalectomized animal has deficiencies in the pathways which led to glucose production.

The normal hyperglycemic response to epinephrine is also markedly suppressed in adrenalectomized dogs. Surprisingly, perfused livers isolated from adrenalectomized rats are more sensitive than livers from intact rats to stimulation by glucagon or epinephrine using cyclic AMP (cAMP) as a measure of stimulation. However, epinephrine or glucagon stimulation of gluconeogenesis is not enhanced in the absence of glucocorticoids. The administration of large amounts of dibuteryl AMP also failed to induce gluconeogenesis in adrenalectomized rat livers, indicating that there must be a glucocorticoid-dependent step in the pathway at a point that follows the activation of adenylate cyclase (33). This may mean that the conversion of inactive to active phosphorylase induced by epinephrine may be glucocorticoid-dependent. Activation of phosphorylase is required for the conversion of glycogen to glucose. Liver from adrenalectomized rats also shows depressed levels of the active form of glycogen synthetase, although this effect may be insulin-dependent since glycogen synthetase failed to respond to cortisol in alloxan-diabetic rats (60).

Adrenalectomy also has dramatic effects upon the circulatory system. The absence of mineralocorticoids causes a loss in the salt-conserving ability of the animal. For an adrenalectomized animal on a normal sodium diet, daily sodium excretion exceeds intake. This can lead to volume depletion, increased blood viscosity, reduced heart rate, reduced cardiac output, and hypotension. Glomerular filtration rate (GFR) drops and plasma renin increases in an attempt to compensate for sodium depletion. Failure to restore adequate sodium levels can eventually result in circulatory collapse. Animals provided with free access to saline water maintain adequate blood volume. In addition to the threat of cardiovascular collapse, the low levels of blood glucose associated with adrenalectomy do not provide the animal with adequate supplies of glucose during conditions of stress. Survival despite stress appears to be more dependent upon the presence of glucocorticoids than mineralocorticoids. Deoxycorticosterone is less effective than cortisol in prolonging survival of individuals with Addison's disease (28). Stress creates other difficulties for the animal. Normally, epinephrine is secreted in response to stress to act on liver to release glucose and on vascular tissue to maintain vascular tone. Since glucocorticoids appear to play a role in the mediation of the actions of epinephrine, the response to stress is not adequate. The adrenalectomized animal is also less responsive to renin and angiotensin II, which further reduces vascular tone. Chronic administration of mineralocorticoid potentiates the effects of renin and angiotensin II (129).

Other effects have been observed in situations of adrenal insufficiency, including increased growth of lymphoid tissues, weakness and fatigue, hypercalcemia, excessive pigmentation of the skin (especially in normally pigmented areas, intensification of inflammatory responses and hypersensitivity reactions), and increased influx of polymorphonuclear lymphocytes. Additional effects of adrenalectomy are discussed when specific target tissues are mentioned.

EFFECTS OF GLUCOCORTICOIDS ON GLUCOSE METABOLISM

Cortisol administration to adrenalectomized-fasted animals restores blood glucose to normal after 2–3 hours via a mechanism of gluconeogenesis. Liver glycogen also rises, but the maximal increase in liver glycogen has a lag period of 24–48 hours when compared with fed control rats (88). Under conditions of prolonged glucocorticoid excess, steroid-diabetes can occur, including glucosuria, with an increase in urinary nitrogen excretion as well. The elevated blood glucose levels stimulate a rise in insulin levels. This reduces the sensitivity of the animal to exogenously administered insulin, making the animal insulin-resistant. Some species, like man, are somewhat refractory to steroid-induced diabetes, while the rat is sensitive to glucocorticoid-induced diabetes.

The question can be raised, how do glucocorticoids manage to raise blood glucose levels and eventually increase liver glycogen content? Part of the glucocorticoid effect may be due to the inhibitory actions of glucocorticoids on glucose and amino acid uptake by extrahepatic tissues, such as the thymus gland and adipose tissue. Glucocorticoids also increase the release of precursors required for the synthesis of glucose, such as the glucogenic and branched-chained amino acids from skeletal muscle. The lipolytic action of catecholamines, which require glucocorticoids, causes the release of fatty acids from adipose tissue. These fatty acids can be metabolized to form the precursors for glucose production. A decrease in extrahepatic tissue uptake of glucose explains only partially the elevation in blood glucose level. This is because glucose uptake is not significantly inhibited in skeletal muscle which comprises a large proportion of total body mass (97). It appears that a large amount of glucose is generated by the liver itself after its machinery for glucoenogenesis has been turned on by glucocorticoids. Friedmann et al. (44) have shown in perfused liver studies that epinephrine can stimulate glucose release from livers treated with dexamethasone despite the fact that these livers were depleted of their glycogen stores. By contrast, glucose release was insensitive to glucagon in adrenalectomized rats. Thus, glucocorticoids appear to mediate the actions of epinephrine and glucagon on the release of glucose from liver. The block appears to be beyond the induction of cAMP since both glucagon and epinephrine can stimulate cAMP in the liver of adrenalectomized rats.

Schaeffer et al. (132) found that glucocorticoids were required for the epinephrine-stimulated conversion of inactive to active glycogen phosphorylase. Active phosphorylase acts on glycogen to release glucose 1-phosphate which can be converted to glucose 6-phosphate. There is also evidence that the enzyme, glucose 6-phosphatase, increases following glucocorticoid treatment (151–153). This is consistent also with an increase in the conversion of glucose 6-phosphate to glucose, which can be released by the liver. Nordlie et al. (105) indicate that increased activity of glucose 6-phosphatase may be due to an activation of the membrane-bound enzyme rather than due to an increase in the synthesis of new enzyme molecules. They found that 5 mM deoxycholate could mimic the activation of glucose 6-phosphatase and could obliterate the glucocorticoid-induced activation of the enzyme.

Seitz et al. (134) found both intact and adrenalectomized rat livers respond to starvation in a similar manner. Plasma glucagon and liver cAMP increase along with the coordinated increase in hepatic pyruvate carboxylase, phosphoenolpyruvate carboxykinase, and fructose 1,6 diphosphatase. However, phosphoenolpyruvate and 3-phosphoglyceric acid levels were elevated in intact (in the presence of glucocorticoids) but not in the adrenalectomized rat. This indicates that cAMP and glucocorticoids may act in concert to stimulate the flow of pyruvate to phosphoenolpyruvate. The increased levels of phosphoenolpyruvate may be due to glucocorticoid stimulation of the breakdown of triglycerides into fatty acids and protein into amino acids that are being shunted to the liver from extrahepatic tissues.

Kreutner and Goldberg (74) presented evidence that cortisol elevated the active form of glycogen synthase to enhance glycogen deposition. Presumably, this effect was mediated through insulin since alloxan-diabetic rats failed to show an increase in glycogen synthesis unless insulin was also administered. Chronic insulin deprivation, however, resulted in the failure of both insulin and cortisol to increase the levels of glycogen synthase. In fetal liver, glucocorticoids may have a more direct action on glycogen synthesis. Adrenal steroids are required for fetal liver glycogen storage (64,65). The activity of synthase phosphatase increases five fold on the 19th day of gestation corresponding with a rise in fetal glucocorticoid levels (140) The enzyme can also develop prematurely following glucocorticoid administration. Synthase phosphatase converts inactive synthase to active glycogen synthase.

In the adult liver, glycogen production is largely believed to be insulin-dependent. Glucocorticoids, however, are required to maximally stimulate glycogen deposition. Liver glycogen synthase phosphatase has been found to be quite low in adrenalectomized-fasted rats. Glucocorticoids or glucose can restore the activity of synthase phosphatase that will stimulate the conversion of inactive to active glycogen synthase. Phosphorylase A has been shown to inhibit synthase phosphatase. Thus, in situations of maximal glycogenolysis, high levels of phosphorylase A should shut down glycogen deposition. Glucocorticoids appear to relieve the inhibitory effect of phosphorylase A on glycogen synthase phosphatase. Glucocorticoids also appear to increase the activity of phosphorylase phosphatase, which converts active phosphorylase to inactive phosphorylase. These data appear to conflict with the stimulatory effect that glucocorticoids have on glucagon-stimulation of glycogenolysis, which is mediated through phosphorylase A. Perhaps other factors are required to determine whether phosphorylase A is stimulated or inhibited. It is proposed (140) that a glucocorticoid-dependent protein factor may decrease the inhibitory effects of phosphorylase A on glycogen synthase phosphatase.

EFFECTS OF GLUCOCORTICOIDS ON GLUCOSE UPTAKE

Normally, glucose uptake by tissues is dependent upon the blood glucose levels, which are dependent upon the absorption of glucose from the gut and the release of glucose from liver. Insulin secretion plays a major role in determining the blood levels of glucose, and glucocorticoids inhibit glucose uptake by peripheral tissues (i.e., lymphoid and adipose tissue). It is thought that some of the inhibitory effects of glucocorticoids on glucose uptake may be attributed to the effects of glucocorticoids on fat mobilization. Glucocorticoid treatment in insulin-maintained pancreatectomized rats caused severe hyperlipemia, ketosis, and fatty livers (132). Glucocorticoids had no effect in insulin-deficient fat-depleted animals.

Randle et al. (116) and Park (108) indicated that free fatty acids made available by glucocorticoid-stimulated lipid mobilization may provide a source of energy for the cells of extrahepatic tissues, thus reducing their glucose requirements. Growth hormone and glucocorticoids can act additively on isolated hearts to reduce glucose uptake. Both hormones also reduce the uptake of glucose by rat diaphragm induced by low levels of insulin but they cannot inhibit glucose uptake in the face of high levels of insulin (94). This effect of insulin may be dependent upon free fatty acids since the in vitro addition of fatty acids has been shown to reduce insulin stimulation of glucose transport (108). The release of free fatty acids from triglycerides produces an increase in acetyl CoA, which then enters the citric acid cycle to generate increased intracellular citrate concentrations. Citrate can inhibit the enzyme phosphofructokinase resulting in elevated glucose 6-phosphate levels. Glucose 6-phosphate can act as a feedback inhibitor to inhibit glucose phosphorylation and glucose uptake by cells. Inhibition of glucose phosphorylation can also be mediated by elevated adenosine diphosphate (ADP) levels. These overall effects could decrease phosphorylation of glucose and therefore reduce glucose uptake. Additional aspects of the effects of glucocorticoids on glucose uptake will be described later when individual tissues are discussed.

ACTIONS OF GLUCOCORTICOIDS ON LIPID MOBILIZATION AND GLUCOSE METABOLISM IN ADIPOSE TISSUE

Glucocorticoids have direct actions on adipose tissue. Glucocorticoids inhibit glucose uptake in white adipose cells while glucocorticoids have virtually no effect upon glucose uptake by brown adipose tissue. This is despite the fact that brown adipose tissue has specific glucocorticoid receptors (39). Brown adipose tissue is responsive to glucocorticoids since inhibition of uridine incorporation into RNA can be observed following glucocorticoid administration. However, glucocorticoids have no effect upon the activity of the enzyme phosphoenolpyruvate carboxykinase, lipolysis, or glucose metabolism in brown adipose tissue. Thus, brown adipose tissue appears to have lost most of its responsiveness to glucocorticoids.

In white adipose tissue, the inhibitory effects of glucocorticoids on glucose oxidation appear to decline as a function of age in the rat, while basal levels of glucose uptake remain essentially unchanged in the aging rat. This decline in the action of glucocorticoids parallels a decline in specific glucocorticoid receptor binding in fat cells (125). Thus, the inhibition of glucose uptake by adipose cells appears to be mediated by specific steroid receptors.

The inhibitory effects of cortisol on glucose oxidation in adipose tissue is blocked by actinomycin D, an inhibitor of RNA synthesis. If actinomycin D is added 1 hour after the administration of dexamethasone, the inhibitory effect of glucocorticoids is diminished (20). If actinomycin D is added 2 hours after dexamethasone treatment, it has no effect upon the inhibition of glucose uptake and metabolism. If dexamethasone is washed from the cells within 2.5 hours, the inhibitory effects of steroids are reversed. However, this "wash-out" effect is also blocked by actinomycin D, indicating that RNA synthesis is required to reverse the inhibitory effects of dexamethasone. Cycloheximide, an inhibitor of protein synthesis, also inhibits glucose oxidation and, in essence, mimicks the inhibitory effects of glucocorticoids (35). Cycloheximide even demonstrates a 1–2-hour lag period (20) similar to the inhibitory lag period exhibited by glucocorticoids. Thus, glucocorticoids may act to inhibit glucose uptake in fat cells by inhibiting the synthesis of protein(s) required for transport processes.

Insulin has been shown to have antilipolytic effects and acts as an antagonist of glucocorticoids. Lundquist (89) found that cortisol inhibited the stimulation of glucose uptake and metabolism by adipose tissue induced by submaximal doses but not maximal doses of insulin. Czech and Fain (21) found that cortisol inhibited the response of adipose cells to maximal doses of insulin under low concentrations of glucose (0.1–0.05 mM glucose) but no inhibition was observed in the presence of high glucose concentrations (1 mM) in the presence of a maximal dose of insulin. In a more recent study (86) a low concentration of dexamethasone (0.1 μM) gave a characteristic lag period of 1–2 hours for the inhibition of glucose uptake. The action of dexamethasone could be blocked by actinomycin C. Cycloheximide by itself (0.1 mM) could inhibit glucose uptake and mimic the action of glucocorticoids. The V_{max} for the uptake process decreases without much of an effect upon the K_m for glucose. Hexokinase activity and adenosine triphosphate (ATP) levels are not affected by glucocorticoid treatment. The uptake of 3-O-methyl glucose is also reduced by glucocorticoids indicating that phosphorylation of the sugar is not required and that the site of inhibition involved the transport of glucose into the cell. Fucose uptake is not affected by glucocorticoids indicating that fucose may be transported by a different mechanism (34). At high concentrations of 3-O-methyl glucose (10 mM), the inhibitory effect of glucocorticoids is reduced. Insulin overcomes the inhibitory effects of dexamethasone only when the concentration of sugar is high (5 mM). In contrast to the work of Lundquist, maximal stimulation of fat cells by insulin does not completely correct the inhibitory effects of dexamethasone on glucose or 3-O-methyl glucose uptake when low concentrations of sugar are used (86). Dexamethasone has no effect upon the biological responsiveness (receptors) of the fat cells for insulin. This is in agreement with Bennet and Cuatrecasas (8), who found no change in insulin binding to adipocytes following short-term corticosteroid treatment.

The lipolytic action of glucocorticoids is dependent upon the presence of the pituitary. Glucocorticoids are effective when administered in combination with growth hormone, adrenocorticotrophic hormone (ACTH) or thyroxine. Glucocorticoids appear to potentiate the effects of these lipolytic hormones (catecholamines, thyroid hormone, growth hormone, and ACTH) which cause ketosis and release of fatty acids while insulin can antagonize the lipolytic effects of glucocorticoids. The release of fatty acids by glucocorticoids has a lag period of 1–2 hours (36). Dexamethasone in combination with ACTH has an additional effect upon fatty acid release. The release of free fatty acids can be accounted for, in part, by a reduction in the reesterification of fatty acids into triglycerides. The glucocorticoid-induced inhibition of glucose uptake could be involved in this effect upon lipolysis, as discussed earlier. Inhibition of glucose uptake impairs the formation of α-glycerol phosphate, which is a precursor for triglyceride formation. This helps reduce reesterification processes and favors an increase in free fatty acids. Others find increased release of both fatty acids and glycerol following glucocorticoid administration, indicating that lipase activity may also be involved in triglyceride breakdown. Divakaran and Friedman (27) found that the addition of dexamethasone to perfused livers results in an increased release of free fatty acids and glycerol within 30 minutes. The addition of glucagon also increased the release of fatty acids, but the effect was not additive with the effect of glucocorticoids. Curiously, actinomycin D by itself increased the release of free fatty acids from perfused livers suggesting that the action of glucocorticoids may be mediated by the inhibition of RNA synthesis. Part of the glucagon-induced increase in fatty acid release was attributed to a hormone-sensitive lipase originally described by Soderline et al. (138). Thus, lipolysis may be due to a decrease in reesterification processes and to an increase in lipase activity resulting in the release of fatty acids and glycerol.

Fain and Czech (35) have shown a 20% increase in adenylate cyclase activity in response to norepinephrine after treatment with 0.02 μg/ml dexamethasone. Part of this effect may be due to a slight inhibition of phosphodiesterase caused by glucocorticoids. However, the primary effects of glucocorticoids were attributed to events not directly related to cAMP accumulation. Lamberts et al. (76) found in fat cells a significant increase in the cAMP-dependent phosphorylation of histone protein by protein kinase following dexamethasone treatment. There was no increase in basal protein kinase activity in the absence of cAMP. Long-term treatment with cortisol resulted in a 33% increase in protein kinase activity. This increase in total protein kinase due to glucocorticoid in the presence of cAMP could explain the potentiation of the lipolytic effects of cAMP in the presence of glucocorticoids. This enzyme is involved in the activation of inactive to active lipase.

The effects of glucocorticoids on phosphodiesterase activity appear to be somewhat controversial. Some investigators believe that phosphodiesterase activity is inhibited by glucocorticoids while others find that glucocorticoids have no effect upon phosphodiesterase activity. Ross et al. (123) identified at least three enzymes with phosphodiesterase activity in cultured hepatoma cells. Dexamethasone decreased the activities of EI and EII after 72 hours, but had no effect upon EIII (which has a low K_m for cAMP). In cells incubated with cAMP and theophylline, EIII activity doubled in 14 hours, indicating that glucocorticoids and cAMP are acting on different phosphodiesterases. These results may explain the conflicting results of other investigators.

The long-term effects of methyl prednisolone (16 weeks) on lipid metabolism were recently described (49). Plasma triglycerides and cholesterol were elevated in the rabbit following chronic glucocorticoid therapy. Plasma prostaglandin A and E were converted to prostaglandin B by alkaline treatment and PGB was measured by RIA. There was a significant increase in plasma prostaglandin levels following chronic glucocorticoid treatment. These effects are probably due to the increased levels of free fatty acids induced by glucocorticoids. Arachidonic acid is a substrate for prostaglandin biosynthesis. The investigators (49) speculate that the increased levels of prostaglandins may induce avascular necrosis of bone, which is associated with long-term glucocorticoid therapy.

Others have found that glucocorticoids inhibit the synthesis of prostaglandins (40). Danon and Assouline (22) have found that inhibition of prostaglandin synthesis by cortisol in rat renal papilla required both RNA and protein synthesis with a classic 20–40-minute lag period following glucocorticoid administration. Flower and Blackwell (41) gave evidence that the inhibition of prostaglandin synthesis by glucocorticoids was mediated by the induction of an inhibitor of the enzyme, phospholipase A_2. This enzyme is required for the release of arachidonic acid from triglycerides. Inhibition of this enzyme would block the supply of substrate required for the production of prostaglandins. Dexamethasone blocked the release of thromboxane A_2 from guinea pig lung with a lag period of 40 minutes. The effect of dexamethasone was blocked by actinomycin D, cycloheximide, and puromycin. Chandrabose et al. (15) also found that dexamethasone inhibited the stimulation of phospholipase activity by thrombin and bradykinin in cultured fibroblasts. However, steroid did not inhibit basal activity of phospholipase. In fact, steroid-treated cells showed a greater conversion of arachidonic acid into prostaglandins in resting nonstimulated cells. They also found the activity of the cyclooxygenase enzyme enhanced in steroid-treated cells. They propose that prostacyclin (PGI), a potent inhibitor of platelet adenylate cyclase and platelet phospholipase activity, could be acting as feed-back inhibitor in steroid-treated cells to inhibit further release of arachidonic acid from phospholipids.

This discrepancy between increases and decreases in prostaglandin production caused by chronic versus acute administration of glucocorticoids has not yet been resolved. Differences may also arise due to different effects of glucocorticoids in vivo versus in vitro.

Foster and Perkins (42) have shown that glucocorticoids potentiate the responsiveness of cultured astrocytoma cells to PGE_1. The potency of PGE_1 increased five-fold in the presence of glucocorticoids. This indicates that glucocorticoids may regulate the synthesis of prostaglandins and the sensitivity of some cells to prostaglandins.

EFFECTS OF GLUCOCORTICOIDS ON PROTEIN METABOLISM

In liver, glucocorticoids have been shown to stimulate RNA and protein synthesis including the specific induction of enzymes involved in gluconeogenesis. Cortisol causes an increase in total serum protein including albumin, increased liver weight, increased liver protein, and increased liver RNA. There is also a slight increase in DNA content (136). Henderson et al. (58) found in fed rats that short-term cortisol treatment causes an increase in liver weight and liver protein content, but only a slight increase in liver RNA and a slight decrease in DNA content. Long-term cortisol therapy (16 days) causes decreases in body weight, liver weight, DNA, RNA, and protein content compared with control animals. Kim and Kim (71) have shown that pharmacological doses of steroid can decrease protein accumulation even in liver. In time-course studies, the early effects of glucocorticoids show a decrease and then an increase in protein synthesis. Chronic injection of glucocorticoids produces a net decrease in protein synthesis. Other workers have found that both DNA and protein synthesis are inhibited by glucocorticoids in rapidly growing liver (58) and regenerating liver (31). The inhibition of DNA synthesis may be related to reduced activity of DNA polymerase. Inhibition of DNA synthesis appears to be a common action of glucocorticoids in liver and other tissues. Extrahepatic tissues generally exhibit glucocorticoid-induced inhibition of RNA, DNA, and protein synthesis. A number of investigators have found decreased incorporation of amino acids into protein (46,110,146).

In diaphragm muscle, glucocorticoids decrease the incorporation of labeled-histidine into protein (156). Similar results were found in heart and thymocytes. The decreased uptake and incorporation of amino acids into extrahepatic tissues provide these amino acids as precursors for gluconeogenesis by the liver.

Mayer and Rosen (96) recently reviewed the actions of glucocorticoids on muscle. They indicate that glucocorticoids can stimulate alkaline-neutral proteases in muscle which may be responsible for the muscle-wasting processes caused by glucocorticoid administration, starvation, tumor growth and muscular dystrophy. These proteases degrade protein into amino acids which could then be used as precursors for gluconeogenesis.

BIOCHEMICAL CHANGES IN TARGET TISSUES

Lymphoid Tissues

Glucocorticoids suppress the size and weight of the thymus gland, bursae of Fabricus, lymph nodes, spleen, and Peyer's patches. Circulating lymphocytes and bone marrow lymphocytes are also depressed (100). White et al. (154) initially demonstrated that adrenal steroids caused a loss of cellular protein from lymphoid tissues. Glucocorticoid treatment also caused a depression in the incorporation of labeled-thymidine into DNA, indicating that DNA synthesis was depressed. The effects of glucocorticoids on lymphoid tissues have been studied using thymus glands, isolated thymus cells, and various lymphoid tumor lines as model systems. The P1798-sensitive lymphosarcoma cells carried in mice regress significantly following glucocorticoid therapy while the P-1798-resistant cells remain unaffected by steroid therapy. The P-1798-sensitive cells demonstrate glucocorticoid-induced inhibition of the incorporation of thymidine into DNA, while thymidine incorporation is not inhibited in the P-1798-resistant cells (121). The inhibitory action of glucocorticoids may be acting at sites affecting thymidine uptake and the conversion of thymidine into nucleosides and nucleotides.

In thymus cells the concentration of thymidine is important. At high concentrations of labeled thymidine (1 mM), cortisol did not inhibit thymidine uptake and incorporation into DNA, while at low concentrations of thymidine, incorporation was cortisol-dependent. Glucocorticoids appear to be specific for the inhibitory effect. Testosterone, desoxycorticosterone acetate, and estrogen had no inhibitory effect upon thymidine incorporation into DNA (122).

Five to ten minutes after cortisol administration to rats, inhibition of RNA synthesis was observed by Kidson (69). Borthwick and Bell (7,14) found that the activities of thymus DNA polymerase, RNA polymerase A, and RNA polymerase B were all decreased 1 hour after in vivo treatment with glucocorticoids. This was also found by Fox and Gabourel (43). When similar experiments were performed in vitro using isolated thymus cells, RNA polymerase A declined in a fashion similar to the in vivo results. RNA polymerase B, however, actually increased during the first 10 minutes following glucocorticoid addition to the cells and this elevation lasted for about 30 minutes before RNA polymerase B activity declined below control levels. Kidson (70) also found that protein synthesis actually was increased 15–20 minutes after steroid administration followed by an inhibition of protein synthesis. Thus, although the overall effect of glucocorticoids is to inhibit RNA and protein synthesis, glucocorticoids may actually induce specific RNA and protein synthesis to promote the biochemical actions of glucocorticoids.

The effects of glucocorticoids on the inhibition of RNA synthesis appeared to precede the inhibition of protein synthesis. These effects include decreased synthesis of RNA, decreased purine nucleotide biosynthesis (38), and decreased uridine incorporation into 18S and 28S ribosomal RNA (142). Inhibition of uridine incorporation into RNA in thymus cells was observed within 30 minutes after in vivo administration of cortisol (103). Inhibition of ribosomal RNA synthesis could impair the machinery required for protein synthesis. The P-1798-glucocorticoid-sensitive cells also showed impaired uridine uptake and incorporation into RNA and (^{14}C) leucine incorporation into protein 3 hours after cortisol administration (122), while only small changes in leucine incorporation into protein were seen in P-1798-resistant cells. Inhibition of uridine uptake was small but signficant even in the resistant cells indicating that inhibition of uridine uptake may not be a crucial event in P-1798 lymphocytolysis.

Inhibition of protein synthesis by glucocorticoids may be mediated by a decrease in messenger RNA production with a concomitant decrease in protein synthesis. However, glucocorticoids also appear to have a direct inhibitory effect upon microsomal machinery involved in protein synthesis. Steroid effects upon microsomes varied from 3–18 hours after glucocorticoid treatment as reviewed by Rosen and Milholland (120). Gabourel and Fox (46) found a decrease in polysome aggregation 6–12 hours after cortisol administration. Uete (147) found that glucocorticoid-induced inhibition of amino acid incorporation into protein was reduced in nuclei, mitochondria, and microsomes of treated thymus cells.

Cortisol also has an effect upon glucose uptake by the thymus cells. Fifteen to 20 minutes following cortisol administration glucose uptake was decreased (97,98). The inhibition of glucose uptake preceded the inhibitory effects of cortisol on the incorporation of nucleotides into DNA and RNA and the incorporation of amino acids into protein. Munck (99) proposed that inhibition of glucose uptake may be a primary effect of glucocorticoid action. In P1798 cells, in the absence of glucose in the media, the inhibitory effects of cortisol on thymidine incorporation, uridine incorporation, and leucine incorporation were markedly reduced. Therefore, glucose may be required for transport and phosphorylation of uridine by P1798 cells (122).

Young (157) found that glucose is also required to maintain maximal incorporation of amino acids into protein in thymus cells. The reduced levels of glucose induced by glucocorticoids could reduce cellular ATP levels. This reduction in ATP may deprive the cell of energy, resulting in reduced uptake of glucose and amino acids and, ultimately, result in cell death and lysis. Evidence by Nordeen and Young (104) indicates that the actions of glucocorticoids are not totally dependent upon glucose uptake. Adenosine can support glycolytic and oxidative ATP production and therefore can replace glucose as an energy source. Glucocorticoid treatment of thymus cells maintained on adenosine, however, still demonstrate inhibition of protein synthesis, inhibition of uridine uptake, and decreased levels of ATP. Glucocorticoid-induced nuclear fragility of thymocytes (48) and glucocorticoid-induced inhibition of aminobutyric acid transport also does not require glucose.

It was proposed that the inhibitory effect of cortisol on sugar uptake is mediated through the induction of a protein inhibitor (93). This effect can be blocked by actinomycin D and cycloheximide. Actinomycin D and cycloheximide have no effect upon basal 2-deoxyglucose uptake in the absence of steroid. By contrast, Rosen et al. (122) found that cycloheximide inhibited 2-deoxyglucose uptake, even in the absence of glucocorticoid, indicating that constant protein synthesis may be required for glucose transport in P1798 cells. These discrepancies between the results in thymus and P1798 cells may be due either to specific differences between P1798 and thymus cells or to differences in the media used by the investigators. Glucocorticoid-induced inhibition of glucose uptake can be blocked by actinomycin D only when given within 5 minutes after cortisol is administered. Actinomycin D does not block the effect of cortisol when added after 5 minutes. Likewise, if cortisol is added to cells for 5 minutes and then the cells are washed free of steroid, the glucocorticoid effect still occurs. Cycloheximide, on the other hand, only blocks the effect of cortisol on glucose metabolism starting 15 minutes after cortisol administration. This is the time when inhibition of glucose uptake and metabolism is usually observed (56). These data suggest that an inhibitor(s) of glucose uptake is induced by glucocorticoids. The inhibitor(s) may act on membrane transport systems involved in glucose and amino acid transport (56,93).

Kaiser and Edelman (67) discovered that Ca^{+2} may play a role in lymphocytolysis. The synthetic glucocorticoid, triamcinolone acetonide, and the Ca^{+2} ionophore, A23187, have similar effects upon the inhibition of uridine uptake and lysis of thymus cells. Removal of Ca^{+2} from the media diminished the inhibitory effects of triamcinolone acetonide and virtually eliminated the action of A23187. Cell viability was also inversely related with ^{45}Ca uptake by these cells. They proposed that lysis by Ca^{+2} may be mediated by inhibition of (NA^+, K^+), ATPase, or by inhibition of the electron transport chain, which would reduce the phosphorylation of ADP. This would ultimately reduce ATP levels. This result could fit the model proposed by Nordeen and Young (104). The effects of glucocorticoids and Ca^{+2} on lymphocytolysis warrant further investigation.

Glucocorticoids also have effects on the activity of various enzymes in the thymus gland. Alanine α-ketoglutarate transaminase activity is increased in both thymus and liver following glucocorticoid administration (119). Elevations of ribonuclease, β-glucuronidase, acid phosphatase, and deoxyribonuclease II have also been observed, as reviewed by Rosen and Milholland (120). Increases in these enzymes may be due to an increase in the release of lysosomal material induced by glucocorticoids. Whether these enzymes are involved in cellular lysis remains unclear (103).

In summary, glucocorticoids inhibit glucose metabolism, the incorporation of amino acids into protein and the incorporation of nucleotides into RNA and DNA. Ultimately these effects can induce lymphocytolysis using rat or mouse lymphoid tissues. The action of glucocorticoids on lymphoid tissues have made them useful as immunosuppressive agents and as antineoplastic agents for the treatment of various lymphoid tumors.

Glucocorticoid Effects on Liver

Liver is a major target organ for glucocorticoids. Glucocorticoids stimulate gluconeogenesis and glycogen deposition in liver. Contrary to their stimulation of lipolysis in extrahepatic tissues, glucocorticoids produce an increase in triglyceride synthesis in liver. Most of these effects were discussed above. Glucocorticoids appear to increase the activities of various enzymes involved in the gluconeogenic pathway (112). Alanine aminotransferase, aspartate aminotransferase, histidine aminotransferase, and ornithine aminotransferase increase 1 day after cortisol treatment. Leucine aminotransferase, tryptophan oxygenase, and tyrosine aminotransferase increased in activity 3–5 hours after steroid therapy. Pyruvate carboxylase also appears to be responsive within 6 hours.

Slower responding enzymes include fructose 1,6-diphosphatase, arginase, histidase, serine dehydratase, and phosphoenolpyruvate carboxykinase. Fructose 1,6-diphosphatase, pyruvate carboxylase, and phosphoenolpyruvate carboxykinase utilize amino acid precursors which are first converted to pyruvate and transforms them into glucose (112). Glucocorticoid-specific induction of proteins in cultured rat hepatoma cells has also been shown using two-dimensional gel electrophoresis (62).

The effects of glucocorticoids on the enzyme glycogen synthase is unclear. Fetal liver glycogen synthetase activity increases two- to threefold following in utero hormone administration (112), while adult glycogen synthase is not responsive to glucocorticoids. As mentioned earlier, Kreutner and Goldberg (74) indicate that glycogen synthesis is dependent upon insulin. It was also mentioned earlier that glucocorticoids create a "diabetic-like state." Kahn et al. (66) found that the administration of either ACTH or dexamethasone to rats results in an insulin-resistant state. The insulin response decreased by 50%−60%. They correlated the decline in insulin sensitivity with the number of liver insulin receptor sites and found that glucocorticoids did not change the number of insulin receptor sites but did decrease the affinity of the receptor for insulin. Adrenalectomy resulted in an increase in sensitivity and binding affinity. The effect of dexamethasone on insulin receptor binding is in agreement with the results of Olefsky (106,107), but differs from the results of Bennet and Cuatrecasas (8), who found no change in insulin binding in adipocytes following short-term steroid treatment.

Despite the general anabolic effects of glucocorticoids on liver, the steroid also exerts antianabolic effects. DNA synthesis is inhibited by glucocorticoids in regenerating liver (31). This decline in DNA synthesis has been associated with a decrease in the activity of DNA polymerase (58). The inhibition of DNA synthesis appears to be a common link between the effects of glucocorticoids on liver and extrahepatic tissues.

Glucocorticoids actually enhanced liver uptake of nucleotides for the synthesis of RNA. Within hours after glucocorticoid administration, RNA polymerase activity almost doubled in the adult liver (5,135). Hanoune and Feigelson (57) found that steroids increased the formation of both ribosomal and messenger RNA. Presumably specific messenger RNA is synthesized which leads to the synthesis of specific proteins. However, care must be taken when interpreting hormone-induced increases in enzyme activity. The increase in activity following glucocorticoid therapy can be the result of an increase in the number of enzyme molecules, increased enzyme activity by a modification of the kinetic properties of the enzyme, and by decreased enzyme degradation.

The activity of alkaline phosphatase, for example, increases tenfold when HeLa cells are treated with glucocorticoids. These effects can be blocked by actinomycin D and cycloheximide. It appears to be a clear case for specific glucocorticoid induction involving the synthesis of specific messenger RNA and protein. However, recent evidence indicates that the number of enzyme molecules is not altered by steroid therapy (19,53). Glucocorticoids appeared to induce a more active form of the enzyme (higher v_{max}). The formation of this activated enzyme appears to be dependent upon the synthesis of RNA and a specific protein, which somehow activates alkaline phosphatase. Thus, this enzyme's activity is a secondary effect of glucocorticoid action, as reviewed by Thompson and Lippman (145).

Tyrosine aminotransferase is an example of an enzyme that appears to be specifically induced by glucocorticoids in liver and hepatoma cells (5). That is, the number of newly synthesized enzyme molecules is increased following glucocorticoid treatment. Recently, Voigt et al. (150) showed that the formation of new tyrosine amonotransferase molecules could be detected 25 minutes after hormone administration. This characteristic lag time is usually associated with the biological actions of glucocorticoids. The in vivo induction of tyrosine aminotransferase by glucocorticoids could be blocked to some extent by deoxycorticosterone, indicating a fairly high degree of steroid specificity (119). In more recent studies, the steroid specificity for the induction of tyrosine aminotransferase has been well characterized in hepatoma cells (130).

Tyrosine aminotransferase activity also increases following changes in cAMP levels (155). Both insulin and glucagon can induce tyrosine aminotransferase activity in vivo and in perfused livers. The action of insulin and glucagon are independent of the effects of glucocorticoids. The cAMP-induced stimulation of tyrosine aminotransferase activity is also shown to be additive with glucocorticoid induction indicating separate mechanisms for induction.

More recent evidence casts some doubt as to whether separate mechanisms are involved. In isolated liver cells using dextran–charcoal-treated or Sephadex G25-treated serum (to remove endogenous hormones), the induction of tyrosine aminotransferase was found to require the presence of both glucocorticoids and a source of cAMP (32). The induction of tyrosine aminotransferase gave a 2-hour-lag period associated with glucocorticoid induction. Both glucagon and dexamethasone were also required to maintain tyrosine aminotransferase activity at induced levels. Enzyme induction was associated with increased synthesis of new enzyme molecules and was not simply an activation of the enzyme. Preincubation of the liver cells with dexamethasone followed by the addition of glucagon significantly decreased the lag time for enzyme induction. Ernest and Feigelson (32) speculate that glucocorticoids are the rate limiting step for enzyme induction. Glucocorticoids stimulate the production of increased amounts of specific messenger RNA for tyrosine aminotransferase, while cAMP may control the processing of messenger for specific translation of tyrosine aminotransferase messenger RNA. However, they do not believe that cAMP only acts as a translation control since they find increased amounts of functional hepatic messenger for tyrosine aminotransferase following cAMP treatment.

Phosphoenolpyruvate carboyxlase is another enzyme regulated by glucocorticoids and cAMP. In one study it was found that the induction of phosphoenolpyruvate carboxykinase in response to cAMP is caused by the stabilization of messenger RNA (63).

Thompson and Lippman (145) recently reviewed whether the actions of glucocorticoids are mediated by cAMP. They concluded that glucocorticoids and cAMP can act to induce a common enzyme but that the actions of glucocorticoids do not require cAMP as an intermediate (second messenger). The finding of Ernest and Feigelson (32) may modify their conclusions. Recently, however, Gehring and Coffin (47) found in S49.1 mouse lymphocytes that resistance to glucocorticoids and cAMP develop independently of each other. This further strengthens the argument that glucocorticoids and cAMP act by different mechanisms. Liu and Greengard (85) have identified a protein which is phosphorylated by cAMP and is regulated by steroids. Perhaps this protein (SCARP) is involved in the induction of tyrosine aminotransferase mediated by both glucocorticoids and cAMP. Thus, additional information is needed to clarify the role of cAMP and glucocorticoids as enzyme inducers.

The effects of glucocorticoids on tryptophan oxygenase activity has also recently been reviewed (101). Glucocorticoid-stimulated increases in tryptophan oxygenase activity corresponds with an increase in specific messenger RNA production. The increase in specific messenger RNA could then be characterized in an in vitro cell-free system to translate the RNA into protein. Specific antibodies for tryptophan oxygenase demonstrate that increased levels of enzyme molecules are translated into protein from the messenger RNA. Removal of steroid results in a decrease in both messenger RNA and in the activity of tryptophan oxygenase.

Thus, by turning on specific enzymes in liver, glucocorticoids can increase the synthesis of enzymes involved in the metabolism of amino acids. These metabolites can then serve as precursors for glucose and glycogen biosynthesis in the liver.

Glucocorticoid Effects on Muscle

Adrenalectomy produces a decrease in net protein degradation in muscle, yet muscle weakness is a symptom of adrenalectomy. The work capacity of the gastrocnemius muscle declines in the adrenalectomized rat. This effect can be reversed by glucocorticoids that increase the work capacity of the muscle almost sixfold. However, prolonged hypercorticoidism can also cause muscle weakness. This effect is attributable partly to a loss of cellular potassium, causing an increase in resting membrane potential. However, synthetic glucocorticoids with little mineralocorticoid activity can also induce myopathy, indicating that other factors must be involved in muscle weakness. Steroid-induced myopathy may be due to increased protein catabolism in muscle tissue. Glucocorticoids can stimulate alkaline-neutral proteases, which may be responsible for muscle wasting (96). Muscle wasting occurs predominantly in nonworking muscle (i.e., denervated muscle) rather than in working muscle (i.e., cardiac and diaphragm) (50,51).

Mineralocorticoids can restore extracellular electrolyte balance but cannot completely restore work capacity, indicating the glucocorticoids must also be required. Part of the decline in work capacity may be due to reduced blood supply to the muscle. Restoring blood pressure, for example, with norepinephrine can restore muscle contraction in an exhausted animal. The administration of glucocorticoids can also restore the blood pressure response to norepinephrine, which again improves muscle contractility (115).

As mentioned earlier (72) glucocorticoids were found to reduce amino acid uptake by muscle to further deplete the muscle of the precursors required for the build-up of muscle. This includes a decrease in muscle glycogen, lipid, and amino acids. However, glucocorticoids do not inhibit glucose uptake in muscle. Munck (97) concluded that skeletal muscle is not a prime target for cortisol action with respect to glucose utilization.

Other effects of glucocorticoids on muscle include altered mitochondrial morphology, decreased function of contractile elements, decreased membrane excitability of type II fibrils, and increased sensitivity of phosphorylase to activation by epinephrine and cAMP (115).

Glucocorticoid Effects on the Lung

Glucocorticoids appear to play a role in the maturation of the fetal lung (26,73). Adrenalectomy inhibits normal fetal lung development (11). Glucocorticoids stimulate the production of surfactants which prevent the collapse of the neonatal lung when first expanded in air (37,146). Surfactants are a mixture of phospholipids, neutral lipids, and specific proteins that act to reduce surface tension at the air–aqueous interface. Glucocorticoids stimulate the activity of the enzyme choline phosphotransferase, which increases the incorporation of leucine into lecithin in the fetal lung. Glucocorticoids also increase the activity of phosphatidic acid phosphatase (PAPase) in fetal lung (1). This enzyme converts phosphatidic acid to 1,2 diacyl-SN-glycerol, which is a precursor for lecithin formation. The activity of the enzyme almost doubles 24 hours after steroid administration (1). Induction of PAPase activity corresponds with an increase in lamellar bodies and alveolar lecithin (3). In the absence of surfactants, respiratory distress syndrome (RDS) can occur resulting in the death of a large number of premature infants. Injection of betamethasone into pregnant women with premature labor resulted in fivefold reduction in neonatal death and a lower incidence of RDS (84). Injection of glucocorticoids into newborns with RDS, however, was not effective. Apparently the action of glucocorticoids must take place in utero. (2), where proper maturation processes of the lung require glucocorticoids during specific developmental events (111).

Glucocorticoid Effects on Vascular Tissues

As mentioned earlier, adrenal insufficiency can result in circulatory collapse. Part of this effect is due to sodium depletion caused by the removal of mineralocorticoids. This will result in volume depletion and hyposention. Glucocorticoids also play a role in maintaining vascular tone: glucocorticoids enhance the response of vascular tissues to catecholamines. Bohr and Cummings (13) found that both mineralocorticoids and glucocorticoids potentiate the contraction of isolated smooth muscle by epinephrine while the steroids have no direct effect on the contraction of smooth muscle. The mechanism for this effect has not been completely elucidated. Bohr (12) has proposed that calcium uptake by smooth muscle cells is involved. Another hypothesis involves a change in the affinity of receptors for catecholamines induced by glucocorticoids (9). Kalsner (68) proposed that glucocorticoids potentiate the effects of catecholamines by inhibiting their metabolism presumably by inhibiting the enzyme, catecholamine O-methyl transferase. The changes in cellular and extracellular sodium and potassium may also alter smooth muscle vascular reactivity to catecholamines.

In whole-animal studies, mineralocorticoids also potentiate the pressor effects of epinephrine and norepinephrine. Raab (114) has proposed that the accumulation of sodium by cells in vascular tissue responsive to catecholamines may potentiate the actions of catecholamines on these vascular tissues. Sodium chloride also plays a role in the storage of norepinephrine in storage granules. High sodium levels decrease the storage capacity of granules for norepinephrine thus raising their circulating levels (25). Glucocorticoid administration to intact rats, either acutely or chronically, did not potentiate the pressor effects of catecholamines (77).

The pressor response to renin and angiotensin is also steroid-dependent. Adrenalectomized animals are insensitive to angiotensin. Chronic administration of mineralocorticoids potentiates the pressor effects of renin and angiotensin. The acute administration of steroid, however, failed to potentiate the effects of renin and angiotensin. This may be explained by the fact that mineralocorticoid-induced sodium retention suppresses renin secretion. This reduces endogenous renin and angiotensin levels. The number of unoccupied angiotensin II receptor sites increases. Thus, when renin or angiotensin is administered the unoccupied receptor sites can be filled, producing a larger biological response, i.e., a potentiation of the vasoconstrictor effects of renin and angiotensin.

Glucocorticoid Effects on the Heart

Adrenalectomy reduces the pumping capability of the heart. There are a number of changes that may account for the decreased contractility of the heart. 1) Cardiac glycogen is decreased. Glucocorticoid replacement causes an increase in cardiac glycogen concentrations. Changes in cardiac glycogen, however, may not be too important since the primary source of energy for the heart comes from fatty acid metabolism. 2) Cardiac potassium and water are altered. These changes may be reflected by electrocardiogram changes which are frequently observed in adrenalectomized animals. However, even after potassium levels have been normalized the electrocardiogram changes persist (23). Elevation of plasma potassium levels in adrenalectomized animals to levels found in intact animals also failed to mimic the electrocardiogram changes associated with adrenal insufficiency (79), indicating that electrolyte changes are only partially responsible for electrocardiogram changes. 3) There is a decreased response to catecholamines. 4) ATPase activity is decreased. Rovetto et al. (127) found a 40% decrease in myofibrillar calcium-dependent ATPase activity in the hearts of adrenalectomized cats. This decline could be prevented by the administration of dexamethasone. The decrese in ATPase activity may be the reason why adrenalectomized animals are more sensitive to cardiac glycosides (79,148). By contrast, glucocorticoids have been shown to inhibit the contractile response of cardiac glycosides in the heart and smooth muscle (80). Others have failed to demonstrate these antagonistic effects (82). The inhibitory effects of glucocorticoids on the actions of cardiac glycosides may be related to an increase in cardiac ATPase activity following glucocorticoid administration.

In vitro, low concentrations of aldosterone appear to have weak inotropic activity in papillary muscles (78) of cats, guinea pigs, and monkeys. Deoxycorticosterone and 9α-fluorocortisol also have cardiotonic effects. The inotropic effects show a latent period of 20–60 minutes indicating that protein synthetic processes may be involved (30). Cortisol had been shown to stimulate chick heart fragments (18), and the endurance of rat heart–lung preparations (131). For the most part, however, glucocorticoids show little or no cardiotonic activity. Since the synthetic glucocorticoids did not have any cardiotonic activity, it may be that cardiotonic activity is mediated by mineralocorticoid activity (79).

Positive inotropic effects of glucocorticoids have been shown in some in vivo studies. Dexamethasone increased the contractile force of the heart by 70% (79). Additional studies will have to be performed to confirm this effect. The steroid-induced increase in contractility may be due to the depressed contractile force caused by anesthesia.

It may be concluded that glucocorticoids probably do not exert significant inotropic effects especially in in vitro studies.

As was mentioned earlier, glucocorticoids have less of an effect upon muscle wasting processes in heart than in skeletal muscle.

Guideri et al (54) found that prednisone, and to a lesser extent deoxycorticosterone, sensitizes a rat to cardiac arrhythmias induced by isoproterenol. This finding could have serious clinical implications.

Based upon the information described above it is difficult to ascribe a specific function for glucocorticoids on the heart. Additional work needs to be done in this area.

Glucocorticoids as Antiinflammatory Agents and Immunosuppressive Agents

The actions of glucocorticoids as antiinflammatory and immunosuppressive agents is quite complex. Glucocorticoids have multiple actions on cells involved in antibody formation and the cells involved in inflammatory responses. Parrillo and Fauci (109) have recently reviewed the mechanism of glucocorticoids' actions as immunosuppressants and as antiinflammatory agents. Therefore, these actions of glucocorticoids shall be discussed briefly.

For many years, it was proposed that the antiinflammatory effects of glucocorticoids were mediated by stabilization of lysosomal membranes. Lysosomes contain hydrolytic enzymes that would be released by synovial cells to promote degradative processes. Glucocorticoids also block histamine-induced release of lysosomal enzymes involved in the erosion of cartilage (10,16) There are some contradictions, however, concerning membrane stabilization. High steroid levels are usually required to stabilize lysosomal membranes. In a few studies, physiological levels of steroids reduced (139) the release of lysosomal enzymes and reduced other toxic effects, as reviewed by Thompson and Lippman (145). However, not all lysosomal systems are stabilized (61) and there is a lack of steroid specificity. Both cortisone and cortisol stabilize lysosomes in vitro, but only cortisol is an active glucocorticoid in terms of binding to specific glucocorticoid receptors. Cortisone must be metabolized to cortisol before becoming biologically active. Therefore, the actions of glucocorticoids on lysosomes may be possible but these effects are probably not mediated by interaction with specific glucocorticoid receptors.

The effects of glucocorticoids on lymphoid tissues has already been discussed. In a glucocorticoid-sensitive species such as the rat, glucocorticoids have cytolytic effects. This effectively reduces the number of thymus-derived T-lymphocytes from the circulation. In a glucocorticoid-resistant species (such as humans), glucocorticoids cause a redistribution of lymphocytes from the circulation into other body compartments. Once again, the T-lymphocytes are affected to a greater extent than the lymphocytes derived from bone marrow or B cells. Twenty-four hours after glucocorticoid administration, lymphocyte levels return to normal. Following each administration of glucocorticoid, the redistribution of lymphocytes occurs. Glucocorticoids have a greater depletion effect upon T-cells with Fc receptors for IgM than on cells with Fc-receptors for IgG. Glucocorticoids also appear to affect the binding of Fc-receptors on macrophages to antibody-coated cells.

Glucocorticoids also induce eosinopenia probably by mechanisms similar to the removal of lymphocytes from circulation.

Glucocorticoids reduce the number of monocyte macrophages and polymorphonuclear leukocytes 4–6 hours after glucocorticoid administration (117). This is important since macrophages are thought to initiate antibody production by ingesting the antigen and processing this antigen into information that the lymphocyte uses to initiate synthesis of specific antibodies. Therefore, decreases in the number of macrophages and polymorphonuclear leukocytes is an important step in the prevention of or blockage of the inflammatory response. Large doses of glucocorticoids also appear to interfere with the phagocytic processes of the macrophage to ingest the antibody (61,62). The migration of macrophages and polymorphonuclear leukocytes into the inflamed area is also inhibited by glucocorticoids. Glucocorticoids also induce a plasma factor that decreases neutrophilic granulocyte adherence to vascular tissue and neutralizes adherence factors found in inflammatory diseases (91,92). The reduced adherence of cellular elements to the vascular endothelium reduces the accumulation of these cells in the inflamed area. Glucocorticoids also antagonize the actions of migration inhibitory factor (MIF), which is usually released by sensitized lymphocytes (4,24). This results in reduced recruitment of neutrophils and monocyte-macrophages following glucocorticoid treatment.

The release of neutrophils from bone marrow is enhanced by glucocorticoids. However, glucocorticoids inhibit neutrophil accumulation at inflammatory sites. This reduces the body's defenses against invasive microorganisms.

Glucocorticoids also have a suppressive effect upon lymphocyte proliferation. Glucocorticoids are more effective against antigen-stimulated proliferation than mitogen-induced proliferation. Yet, glucocorticoids are required for maximal production of Ig. This may involve the formation of Ig-producing cells from B cells.

Cortisol has been shown to reduce the number and alter the structure of mast cells which contain histamines. Cortisol can also inhibit histamine release which may be involved in vascular leakage. Histamines can increase vascular permeability. Inhibition of histamine release could help reduce exudate fluid formation in inflammation. The activity of the enzyme, histaminase, has been shown to decrease in adrenalectomized animals and increase in glucocorticoid-stimulated animals thereby reducing histamine levels. Glucocorticoids have also been shown to inhibit the production of plasmin activator by cultured macrophages. Activation of plasmin could enhance proteolysis of vascular structures, which would result in extravasation of cells and fluid into the inflamed area (149).

The effects of glucocorticoids on prostaglandins has been discussed earlier.

Thus, glucocorticoids act at a multitude of sites involved in inflammatory responses. One overall effect of glucocorticoids may be the altering of the cell surface of lymphocytes and monocytes to change their binding properties. However, it is unlikely that one can determine a specific mechanism for the antiinflammatory actions of glucocorticoids. It is rather the unification of all these effects which make glucocorticoids such potent antiinflammatory agents.

Glucocorticoid Effects on the Pituitary

It is well recognized that under conditions of glucocorticoid excess, either by glucocorticoid therapy or because of high endogenous levels of adrenal steroids, ACTH secretion from the pituitary is suppressed. Recent studies indicate that glucocorticoids may be acting as feedback inhibitors via a receptor mechanism, since specific receptors for glucocorticoids have been isolated from the pituitary gland. Nakanishi et al. (102) have shown that the level of messenger RNA coding for immunoprecipitable ACTH is increased three- to sixfold following adrenalectomy and is suppressed following dexamethasone administration. Progesterone and aldosterone failed to demonstrate a suppressive effect on ACTH messenger RNA levels, indicating that the effect was specific for glucocorticoids. Another interesting finding is that the protein produced from ACTH messenger RNA has molecular weights of 33,000 and 22,000 daltons, which is considerably higher than the molecular weight of ACTH (102). It was subsequently determined by Mains and Eipper (92) and Roberts and Herbert (118) that the high molecular weight form of ACTH was actually a precursor form of ACTH. This precursor form actually contains the sequence of ACTH and β-lipotropin. This is an interesting finding because an endogenous morphine-like peptide (β-endorphin) has been sequenced and identified as a fragment of β-lipotropin. This morphine-like peptide has been shown to compete for specific opiate receptors (83,113).

The regulation of the precursor molecule for ACTH and β-lipotropin has recently been examined. Clones of mouse pituitary tumor cells AtT-20/D1 show a common precursor for the synthesis of ACTH and β-endorphin (128). The amount of β-endorphin generated by these cells is inversely related to the dose of steroid incubated with these cells. Steroid had no effect upon the growth rate of these cells. Dexamethasone, cortisol, corticosterone, and aldosterone were effective inhibitors of β-endorphine production, in order of decreasing potency. Testosterone, progesterone, and 17β-estradiol had no effect upon the production of β-endorphin. It is implied that the inhibitory effects observed were mediated by a reduction in the concentration of messenger RNA specific for ACTH and β-endorphin (128). Holaday et al. (59) also found a relationship between β-endorphin activity and the adrenal gland. The intravenous potency of β-endorphin was markedly enhanced by adrenalectomy possibly because of high endogenous levels. This effect could be reversed by dexamethasone administration. J. Rossier et al. (124) have also shown that adrenalectomy increased pituitary levels of β-endorphin.

If the regulation of ACTH and β-endorphin are under the feedback control of glucocorticoids, then the metabolic action of glucocorticoids appears to be expanding into the regulation of endorphin action. Beta endorphins have been shown to increase the plasma levels of somatotropin by six- to tenfold when given as an intraventricular dose of 2 μg. Beta endorphins also cause a release of prolactin when injected by the intraventricular route (29). However, β-endorphin has no effect upon the release of vasopressin, growth hormone, and prolactin in vitro, indicating that the effects of β-endorphin may not be direct (55). It has been demonstrated (136) that morphine-like peptides can initiate adrenal steroid biosynthesis. Thus, there is still a great deal to learn about the relationship between endorphin and glucocorticoid activity. As more information is made available, the role of glucocorticoids as effectors of endorphins may be modified. One could speculate that the anxiety and psychosis syndromes associated with adrenalectomy and glucocorticoid excess may be related to the levels of endogenous morphine-like substances acting on the brain.

Although glucocorticoids retard growth in vivo, there is a substantial amount of evidence that glucocorticoids increase growth hormone production by cultured pituitary cells (96). Glucocorticoids stimulate specifically the synthesis of messenger RNA coding for growth hormones. Pituitary cells grown in the absence of thyroid hormone are not responsive to glucocorticoid induction of growth hormone. T_3 alone can restore partially increased production of growth hormone. However, T_3 and dexamethasone combined act synergistically to stimulate growth hormone production.

Glucocorticoid Effects on Bone

Glucocorticoids decrease bone formation rates by inhibiting osteoblastic function and increasing bone resorption by stimulating osteoclastic activity (1a). The increased bone resorption may well be due to the increased serum parathyroid levels which in turn may result from decreased intestinal calcium absorption and increased renal excretion of calcium produced by glucocorticoid therapy (47a). In animals the increased osteoclastic activity can be prevented by parathyroidectomy. The elevated parathormone activity could directly stimulate renal 1α-hydroxylase activity resulting in a greater synthesis of $1,25(OH_2)D_3$. Furthermore, the direct effect of glucocorticoids on bone cells sensitizes the cells to the bone-resorbing actions of parathormone and $1,25(OH_2)D_3$.

Long-term treatment with supraphysiological doses of glucocorticoids may result in severe bone loss and subsequent spontaneous fractures. The osteopenia caused by glucocorticoids is more severe in bones with a high content of trabecular bone, such as ribs and vertebrae, and is less severe in the long bones which are mainly composed of the less metabolically active cortical bone. As a consequence, compression fractures of vertebrae and rib fractures are frequent in patients on long-term, high-dose glucocorticoid therapy. This complication may be accelerated in those patients with underlying bone disease, as may be present in patients with rheumatoid arthritis. Children have a high bone turnover rate and rapid skeletal remodeling that predispose them to rapid severe bone loss and delayed skeletal growth, while postmenopausal women have a low bone mass which can be further lowered by steroids to a clinically significant level for development of fractures. This topic is reviewed in detail by Avioli (1a).

Since secondary hyperparathyroidism from steroid inhibition of intestinal calcium absorption appears to be the cause of increased bone resorption, increasing intestinal calcium absorption should reverse the hyperparathyroidism. Calcium supplements plus vitamin D have been administered to patients on large dose prednisone with conflicting results (116a). Alternate day therapy may lessen the osteopenia induced by glucocorticoids.

More recently, an oxazoline derivative of prednisolone called deflazacort, has been shown to have markedly reduced effects on bone. In one study in which deflazacort was compared with prednisone administration for 30 dyas, there was a striking difference (47a). Prednisone significantly increased serum levels of parathyroid hormone, and alkaline phosphatase, and urinary excretion of calcium, phosphate, hydroxyproline, and nephrogenous cyclic AMP, while deflazacort induced minimal or no change in these variables. Deflazacort has a weaker inhibitory effect on intestinal calcium absorption and thus less tendency to induce secondary hyperparathyroidism.

CONCLUSIONS

The actions of glucocorticoids are multifaceted. The physiological effects vary, depending upon the target organ involved. There are a few unifying concepts, however. 1) Most actions of glucocorticoids appear to be dependent upon the presence of glucocorticoid receptors in target tissues. A decline in receptor levels can lead to steroid resistance. 2) Most glucocorticoid effects appear to be mediated by an increase or decrease of specific messenger RNA leading to the production of specific proteins. These proteins could be specific enzymes like those involved in gluconeogenesis or the proteins may be regulators of other processes, such as glucose transport. 3) Glucocorticoids also appear to regulate the activity of other hormones, either as potentiators of antagonists. Our knowledge about the mechanism of action for these effects is still not completely known (52,126).

REFERENCES

1. Ariyoshi, Y. and Plager, J.E. (1970) Relationships between the influence of cortisol on tissue amino acid accumulation and amino acid incorporation into protein and the cortisol inhibition of substrate metabolism. Endocrinology 86, 996–1003.

1a. Avioli, L.V. (1984) Effects of chronic corticosteroid therapy on mineral metabolism and calcium absorption. Adv. in Exp. Biol. and Med. 171, 81–90.

2. Baden, M., Bauer, C.R., Colle, E., Klein, G., Taeusch, H.W., Jr., and Stein, L. (1972) A controlled trial of hydrocortisone therapy in infants with respiratory distress syndrome. Pediatrics 50, 526–534.

3. Ballard, P.L. (1979) Glucocorticoids and differentiation. In: J.D. Baxter and G.G. Rousseau (eds.), Monographs on Endocrinology Glucocorticoid Hormone Actions. Springer-Verlag, Berlin, Heidelberg, and New York, pp. 493–515.

4. Balow, J.E., and Rosenthal, A.S. (1973) Glucocorticoid suppression of macrophage migration inhibitory factor. J. Exp. Med. 137, 1031–1041.

5. Barnabei, O., Romano, B., DiBitonto, G. and Tomasi, V. (1966) Factors influencing the glucocorticoid-induced increase of ribonucleic acid polymerase activity in rat liver. Arch. Biochem. Biophys. 113, 478–486.

6. Baxter, J.D., and Tomkins, G.M. (1970) The relationship between glucocorticoid binding and tyrosine aminotransferase induction in hepatoma tissue culture cells. Proc. Nat. Acad. Sci (USA) 65, 709–715.

7. Bell, P.A., and Borthwick, N.M. (1976) Glucocorticoid effects on DNA-dependent RNA polymerase activity in rat thymus. J. Steroid Biochem. 7, 1147–1150.

8. Bennet, G.V., and Cuatrecasas, P. (1972) Insulin receptor of fat cells in insulin-resistant metabolic states. Science 176, 805–806.

9. Besse, J.C., and Bass, A.D. (1966) Potentiation by hydrocortisone of responses to catecholamines in vascular smooth muscle. J. Pharmacol. Exp. Therapeut. 154, 224–238.

10. Bitensky, L., Butcher, R.G., Johnstone, J.J., and Chayen, J. (1974) Effect of glucocorticoids on lysosomes in synovial lining cells in human rheumatoid arthritis. Ann. Rheum. Dis. 33, 57–61.
11. Blackburn, W.R., Travers, H., and Potter, D.M. (1972) The role of the pituitary-adrenal-thyroid axis in lung differentiation. I. Studies of the cytology and physical properties of anencephalic fetal rat lung. Lab. Invest. 26, 306–318.
12. Bohr, D.F. (1964) Contraction of vascular smooth muscle. Can. Med. Assoc. J. 90, 174–179.
13. Bohr, D.F., and Cummings, G. (1958) Comparative potentiating action of various steroids on the contraction of vascular smooth muscle. Fed. Proc. 17, 17.
14. Borthwick, N.M., and Bell, P.A. (1975) Early glucocorticoid-dependent stimulation of DNA-dependent RNA polymerase activity in rat thymus cells. FEBS Lett. 60, 396–399.
15. Chandrabose, K.A., Lapetina, E.G., Schmitges, C.J., Siegel, M.I., and Cuatrecases,P. (1978) Action of corticosteroids in regulation of prostaglandin biosynthesis in cultured fibroblasts. Proc. Natl. Acad. Sci. (USA) 75, 214–217.
16. Chayen, J., Bitensky, L., Butcher, R.G., Poulter, L.W., and Ubhi, G.S., (1970) Methods for the direct measurement of anti-inflammatory action on human tissue maintained in vitro. Br. J. Dermatol. 82 (Suppl. 6), 62–81.
17. Cohen, C., Shrago, E., and Joseph, D. (1955) Effect of food administration on weight gains and body composition of normal and adrenalectomized rats. Am. J. Physiol. 180, 503–507.
18. Cornman, I., MacDonald, M., and Trams, E. (1957) Reversal of desoxycorticosterone inhibition of heart beat by serum factors. Comparison with known factors. Am. J. Physiol. 189, 350–354.
19. Cox, R.P., and Elson, N.A. (1971) Hormonal induction of alkaline phosphatase activity by an increase in catalytic efficiency of the enzymes. J. Mol. Biol. 58, 197–215.
20. Czech, M.P., and Fain, J.N. (1971) Dactinomycin inhibition of dexamethasone action on glucose metabolism in white fat cells. Biochim. Biophys. Acta 230, 185–193.
21. Czech, M.P., and Fain, J.N. (1972) Antagonism of insulin action of glucose metabolism in white fat cells by dexamethasone. Endocrinology 91, 518–522.
22. Danon, A., and Assouline, G. (1978) Inhibition of prostaglandin biosynthesis by corticosteroids requires RNA and protein synthesis. Nature 273, 552–554.
23. Da Vanzo, J.P., Crossfield, H.C., and Swingle, W.W. (1958) Effect of various adrenal steroids on plasma magnesium and the electrocardiogram of adrenalectomized dogs. Endocrinology 63, 825–830.
24. David, J.R., Al-Askari, S., Lawrence, H.S., and Thomas, L. (1964) Delayed hypersensitivity in vitro. I. The specificity of inhibition of cell migration by antigens. J. Immunol. 93, 264–273.
25. de Champlain, J., Krakoff, L.R., and Axelrod, J. (1968) Relationship between sodium intake and norepinephrine storage during the development of experimental hypertension. Circ. Res. 23, 479–491.
26. De Lemos, R.A., Shermeta, D.W., Knelson, J.H., Kotas, R., and Avery, M.E., (1970) Acceleration of appearance of pulmonary surfactant in fetal lamb by the administration of corticosteroids. Am. Rev. Respir. Dis. 102, 459–461.
27. Divakaran, P., and Friedman, N. (1976) A fast in vitro effect of glucocorticoids on hepatic lipolysis. Endocrinology 98, 1550–1553.
28. Dunlop, D. (1963) Eighty-six cases of Addison's disease. Br. Med. J. 2, 887–891.
29. Dupont, A., Cusan, L., Garon, M., Labrie, F., and Li, C.H. (1977) β-Endorphin: Stimulation of growth hormone release in vivo. Proc. Natl. Acad. Sci. (USA) 74, 358–359.
30. Edelman, I.S., Bogoroch, R., and Porter, G.A. (1963) On the mechanism of action of aldosterone on sodium transport: The role of protein synthesis. Proc. Natl. Acad. Sci. (USA) 50, 1169–1177.

31. Einhorn, S.L., Hirschberg, E., and Gellhorn, A. (1954) The effects of cortisone on regenerating rat liver. J. Gen. Physiol. 37, 559–568.
32. Ernest, M.J., and Feigelson, P. (1979) Multihormonal control of tyrosine aminotransferase in isolated liver cells. In: J.D. Baxter and G.G. Rousseau (eds.), Monograph on Endocrinology. Glucocorticoid Hormone Action. Springer-Verlag, Berlin, Heidelberg, New York, pp. 219–241.
33. Exton, J.H., Mallette, L.E., Jefferson, L.S., Wong, E.H., Friedman, N., and Clark, C.R. (1970) Role of cyclic AMP in the control of gluconeogenesis. Am. J. Clin. Nutr. 23, 993–1003.
34. Fain, J.N. (1964) Effects of dexamethasone and 2-deoxy-D-glucose on fructose and glucose metabolism by adipose tissue. J. Biol. Chem. 239, 958–962.
35. Fain, J.N., and Czech, M.P. (1975) Glucocorticoid effects on lipid mobilization and adipose tissue metabolism. In: H. Blaschko, G. Sayers, A.D. Smith (eds.), Handbook of Physiology, Vol. 6, Adrenal Gland, American Physiology Society, Washington, (D.C.) pp 169–189.
36. Fain, J.N., Scow, R.O., and Chernick, S.S. (1963) Effects of glucocorticoids on metabolism of adipose tissue in vitro. J. Biol. Chem. 238, 54–58.
37. Farrell, P.M. (1977) Fetal lung development and the influence of glucocorticoids on pulmonary surfactant. J. Steroid Biochem. 8, 463–470.
38. Feigelson, M., and Feigelson, P. (1966) Relationships between hepatic enzyme induction, glutamate formation, and purine nucleotide biosynthesis in glucocorticoid action. J. Biol. Chem. 241, 5819–5826.
39. Feldman, D. (1978) Evidence that brown adipose tissue is a glucocorticoid target organ. Endocrinology 103, 2091–2097.
40. Floman, Y., and Zor, U. (1976) Mechanism of steroid action in inflammation. Inhibition of prostaglandin synthesis and release. Prostaglandins 12, 403–413.
41. Flower, R.I., and Blackwell, G. (1979) Anti-inflammatory steroids induce biosynthesis of a phospholipase A_2 inhibitor which prevents prostaglandin generation. Nature 278, 456–459.
42. Foster, S.J., and Perkins, J.R., (1977) Glucocorticoids increase the responsiveness of cells in culture to prostaglandin E_1. Proc. Natl. Acad. Sci. (USA) 74, 4816–4820.
43. Fox, K.E., and Gabourel, J.D. (1972) Effect of cortisol on the activity and distribution of two DNA-dependent RNA polymerases extractable from rat thymus. Endocrinology 90, 1388–1390.
44. Friedmann, N., Exton, J.H., and Park, C.R. (1967) Interaction of adrenal steroids and glucagon on gluconeogenesis in perfused rat liver. Biochem. Biophys. Res. Commun. 29, 113–119.
45. Gabourel, J.D., and Comstock, J.P. (1964) Effect of hydrocortisone on amino acid incorporation by microsomes isolated from mouse lymphoma ML-388 cells and rat thymus. Biochem. Pharmacol. 13, 1369–1376.
46. Gabourel, J.D., and Fox, K.E. (1965) Effect of hydrocortisone on the size of rat thymus polysomes. Biochem. Biophys. Res. Commun. 18, 81–86.
47. Gehring, U., and Coffin, P. (1977) Independent mechanisms of cyclic AMP and glucocorticoid action. Nature 268, 167–168.
47a. Gennari, C., Imbimbo, B., Montagnani, M., Bernini, M., Nardi, P., and Avioli, L.V. (1984) Effects of prednisone and deflazacort on mineral metabolism and parathyroid hormone activity in humans. Calcified Tissue Intl. 36, 245–252.
48. Giddings, S.J., and Young, D.A. (1974) An in vitro effect of physiological levels of cortisol and related steroids on the structural integrity of the nucleus in rat thymic lymphocytes as measured by resistance to lysis. J. Steroid Biochem. 5, 587–595.
49. Gold, E.W., Fox, O.D., and Edgar, P.R. (1978) The effect of long-term corticosteroid administration on lipid and prostaglandin levels. J. Steroid Biochem. 9, 313–316.
50. Goldberg, A.L. (1969) Effects of denervation and cortisone on protein catabolism in skeletal muscle. J. Biol. Chem. 244, 3223–3229.

51. Goldberg, A.L., and Goodman, H.M. (1969) Relationship between cortisone and muscle work in determining muscle size. J. Physiol. (Lond.) 200, 667–675.
52. Granner, D.K. (1976) Restoration of sensitivity of cultured hepatoma cells to cyclic nucleotides shows permissive effect of dexamethasone. Nature 259, 572–573.
53. Griffin, M.J., and Cox, R.P. (1966) On the mechanism of hormone induction of alkaline phosphatase in human cell culture II. Rate of enzyme and properties of base levels and induced enzymes. Proc. Natl. Acad. Sci. (USA) 56, 946–953.
54. Guideri, G., Green, M., and Lehr, D. (1978) Potentiation of isoproterenol cardiotoxicity by corticoids. Res. Commun. Chem. Pathol. Pharmacol. 21, 197–212.
55. Guillemin, R. (1978) β-lipotropin and endorphins. Implications of current knowledge. Hosp. Prac. (Nov.), 53–60.
56. Hallahan, C., Young, D.A., and Munck, A. (1973) The time course of early events in the action of glucocorticoids on the rat thymus cells in vitro. Synthesis and turnover of a hypothetical cortisol-induced protein inhibitor of glucose metabolism as a presumed ribonucleic acid. J. Biol. Chem. 248, 2922–2927.
57. Hanoune, J., and Feigelson, P. (1970) Turnover of protein and RNA of liver ribosomal components in normal and cortisol-treated rats. Biochim. Biophys. Acta 199, 214–223.
58. Henderson, I.C., Fischel, R.E., and Loeb, J.N. (1971) Suppression of liver DNA synthesis by cortisone. Endocrinology 88, 1471–1476.
59. Holaday, J.W., Law, P.Y., Tseng, L.F., Loh, H.H., and Li, C.H. (1977) β-endorphin: Pituitary and adrenal glands modulate its actions. Proc. Natl. Acad. Sci. 74, 4628–4632.
60. Hornbrook, K.R. (1970) Synthesis of liver glycogen in starved alloxan diabetic rats. Diabetes 19, 916–923.
61. Ignarro, L.J. (1971) Dissimilar effects of anti-inflammatory drugs on stability of lysosomes from peritoneal and circulating leukocytes and liver. Biochem. Pharmacol. 20, 2861–2870.
62. Ivarie, R.D., and O'Farrell, P.H. (1978) The glucocorticoid domain. Steroid mediated changes in the rate of synthesis of rat hepatoma proteins. Cell 13, 41–50.
63. Iynedjian, P.B., and Hanson, R.W. (1977) Increase in level of functional messenger RNA coding for phosphoenolpyruvate carboxykinase (GTP) during induction by cyclic AMP. J. Biol. Chem. 252, 655–662.
64. Jost, A., and Picon, L. (1970) Hormonal control of fetal development and metabolism. Adv. Metab. Disord. 4, 123–184.
65. Jost, A. (1966) Problems of fetal endocrinology: The adrenal gland. Rec. Prog. Horm. Res. 22, 541–574.
66. Kahn, C.R., Goldfine, I.D., Neville, Jr., D.M., and DeMeyts, P. (1978) Alterations in insulin binding induced by changes in vivo in the levels of glucocorticoids and growth hormone. Endocrinology 103, 1054–1066.
67. Kaiser, N., and Edelman, I.S. (1977) Calcium dependence of glucocorticoid-induced lymphocytolysis. Proc. Natl. Acad. Sci. (USA) 74, 638–642.
68. Kalsner, S.(1969) Mechanism of hydrocortisone potentiation of responses to epinephrine and norepinephrine in rabbit aorta. Circ. Res. 24, 383–395.
69. Kidson, C. (1965) Kinetics of cortisol action on RNA synthesis. Biochem. Biophys. Res. Commun. 21, 283–289.
70. Kidson, C. (1967) Cortisol in the regulation of RNA and protein synthesis. Nature 213, 779–782.
71. Kim, Y.S., and Kim, Y. (1975) Glucocorticoid inhibition of protein synthesis in vivo and in vitro. J. Biol. Chem. 250, 2293–2298.
72. Kostyo, J.L., and Redmond, A.F. (1966) Role of protein synthesis in the inhibitory action of adrenal steroid hormones on amino acid transport by muscle. Endocrinology 79, 531–540.
73. Kotas, R.V., and Avery, M.E. (1971) Accelerated appearance of pulmonary surfactant in the fetal rabbit. J. Appl. Physiol. 30, 358–361.

74. Kreutner, W., and Goldberg, N.D. (1967) Dependence on insulin of the apparent hydrocortisone activation of hepatic glycogen synthetase. Proc. Natl. Acad. Sci. (USA) 58, 1515–1519.

75. Labhart, A., and Alexis (1974) Clinical Endocrinology—Theory and Practice. Springer-Verlag, Berlin, Heidelberg, New York, pp. 312–332.

76. Lamberts, S.W.J., Timmermans, H.A.T., Kramer-Blankenstijn, M., and Birkenhager, J.C. (1975) The mechanism of the potentiating effect of glucocorticoids on catecholamine-induced lipolysis. Metabolism 24, 681–689.

77. Lefer, A.M. (1966) Corticosteroid antagonism of the positive inotropic effect of ouabain. J. Pharmacol. Exp. Ther. 151, 294–299.

78. Lefer, A.M. (1967) Factors influencing the inotropic effect of corticosteroids. Proc. Soc. Exptl. Biol. Med. 125, 202–205.

79. Lefer, A.M. (1975) Corticosteroids and circulatory function. In: H. Blaschko, G. Sayers, A.D. Smith (eds.) Handbook of Physiology, Vol. 6, Adrenal Gland. American Physiology Soc., Washington, D.C., pp. 191–207.

80. Lefer, A.M., Manwaring, J.L., and Verrier, R.L. (1966) Effect of corticosteroids on the cardiovascular responses to angiotensin and norepinephrine. J. Pharmacol. Exp. Ther. 154, 83–91.

81. Leung, K., and Munck, A. (1975) Peripheral actions of glucocorticoids. In: J.H. Comroe (ed.), Annual Review of Physiology, Vol. 37, Annual Rev., Inc. Palo Alto, Calif., pp. 245–272.

82. Levy, J.V., and Richards, V. (1963) Effect of aldosterone on ouabain-induced potassium loss from isolated rabbit atria. Proc. Soc. Exp. Biol. Med. 114, 280–283.

83. Li, C.H., Yamashiro, D., Tseng, L.F., and Loh, H.H. (1977) Synthesis and analgesic activity of human β-endorphin. J. Med. Chem. 20, 325–328.

84. Liggins, G.C., and Howie R.N. (1972) A controlled trial of antepartum glucocorticoid treatment for prevention of the respiratory distress syndrome in premature infants. Pediatrics 50, 515–525.

85. Liu, A.Y.C., and Greengard, P. (1976) Regulation by steroid hormones of phosphorylation of specific proteins common to several target organs. Proc. Natl. Acad. Sci. (USA) 73, 568–572.

86. Livingston, J.N., and Lockwood, D.H. (1975) Effect of glucocorticoids on the glucose transport system of isolated fat cells. J. Biol. Chem. 250, 8353–8360.

87. Long, C.N.H., and Lukens, F.D.W. (1935) Effect of adrenalectomy and hypophysectomy upon experimental diabetes in the rat. Proc. Soc. Exp. Biol. Med. 32, 743–745.

88. Long, C.H., Smith, O.K., and Fry, E.G. (1960) Actions of cortisol and related compounds on carbohydrate and protein metabolism. In: G.E.W. Wolstenholm and M. O'Connor (eds.)., Metabolic Effects of Adrenal Hormones. Churchill, London, pp. 4–19.

89. Lundquist, I. (1968) On the significance of serum dilution and cortisol antagonism in the rat fat pad bioassay of insulin. Acta Endocrinol. 58, 11–26.

90. MacGregor, R.R. (1977) Granulocyte adherence changes induced by hemodialysis, endotoxin, epinephrine and glucocorticoids. Ann. In. Med. 86, 35–39.

91. MacGregor, R.R., (1976) The effect of anti-inflammatory agents and inflammation on granulocyte adherence. Evidence for regulation by plasma factors. Am. J. Med. 61, 597–607.

92. Mains, R.E., and Eipper, B.A. (1978) Coordinate synthesis of corticotropins and endorphins by mouse pituitary tumor cells. J. Biol. Chem. 253, 651–655.

93. Makman, M.N., Dvorkin, B., and White, A. (1971) Evidence for induction by cortisol in vitro of a protein inhibitor of transport and phosphorylation processes in rat thymocytes. Proc. Natl. Acad. Sci. (USA) 68, 1269–1273.

94. Manchester, K.L., Randle, P.J., and Young, F.G. (1959) The effect of growth hormone and cortisol on the response of isolate rat diaphragm to the stimulating effect of insulin on glucose uptake and on incorporation of amino acids into protein. J. Endocrinol. 18, 395–408.

95. Martial, J.A., Seeburg, P.H., Matulich, D.T., Goodman, H.M., and Baxter, J.D. (1979) In: J.D. Baxter and G.G. Rousseau (eds.), Monograph on Endocrinology. Glucocorticoid Hormone Action. Springer-Verlag, Berlin, Heidelberg, New York, pp. 279–289.

96. Mayer, M., and Rosen, F. (1977) Interaction of glucocorticoids and androgens with skeletal muscle. Metabolism 26, 937–962.

97. Munck, A. (1965) Steroid concentration and tissue integrity as factors determining the physiological significance of effects of adrenal steroids in vitro. Endocrinology 77, 356–360.

98. Munck, A. (1968) Metabolic site and time course of cortisol action on glucose uptake, lactic acid output, and glucose 6-phosphate levels of rat thymus cells in vitro. J. Biol. Chem. 243, 1039–1042.

99. Munck, A. (1971) Glucocorticoid inhibition of glucose uptake by peripheral tissues: Old and new evidence, molecular mechanisms, and physiological significance. Perspect. Biol. Med. 14, 265–289.

100. Munck, A., and Young, D.A (1975) Corticosteroids and lymphoid tissue. In: H. Blaschko, G. Sayers, A.D. Smith (eds.), Handbook of Physiology, Vol. 6, Adrenal Gland. American Physiology Society, Washington, D.C., USA. pp. 231–243.

101. Murthy, L.R., Colman, P.D., and Feigelson, P. (1975) Studies on the glucocorticoid receptor and hormonal modulation of messenger RNA for tryptophan oxygenase. In: D.M. Klachko, L.R. Forte, J.M. Franz (eds.), Advances in Experimental Medicine and Biology, Vol. 96. Plenum Press, New York, London, pp. 73–100.

102. Nakanishi, S., Kita, T., Taii, S., Imura, H., and Numa, S. (1977). Glucocorticoid effect on level of corticotropin messenger-RNA activity in rat pituitary. Proc. Natl. Acad. Sci. (USA) 74, 3283–3286.

103. Nakawana, S., and White, A. (1968) Acute decrease in RNA polymerase activity of rat thymus in response to cortisol injection. Proc. Natl. Acad. Sci. (USA) 55, 900–904.

104. Nordeen, S.K., and Young, D.A. (1976) Glucocorticoid action on rat thymic lymphocytes. J. Biol. Chem. 251, 7295–7303.

105. Nordlie, R.C., Arion, W.J., and Glende, Jr. E.A. (1965) Liver microsomal glucose 6-phosphatase, inorganic pyrophosphatase, and pyrophosphate-glucose phosphotransferase. IV. Effects of adrenalectomy and cortisone administration on the activities assayed in the absence and presence of deoxycholate. J. Biol. Chem. 240, 3479–3484.

106. Olefsky, J.M. (1975) Effect of dexamethasone on insulin binding, glucose transport and glucose oxidation of isolated rat adipocytes. J. Clin. Invest. 56, 1499–1508.

107. Olefsky, J.M., Johnson, J., Liu, F., Jen, P., and Reaven, G.M. (1975). The effects of acute and chronic dexamethasone administration on insulin binding to isolated rat hepatocytes and adipocytes. Metabolism, 24, 517–527.

108. Park, C.R. (1964) Some factors regulating the utilization of carbohydrate in muscle. Intern. Union Biochem. Sci. 32, 711–712.

109. Parrillo, J.E., and Fauci, A.S. (1979) Mechanisms of glucocorticoid action on immune processes. In: R. George, R. Okun, A.K. Cho (eds.), Annual Review of Pharmacology and Toxicology. Annual Review, Inc., Palo Alto, Calif., pp. 179–201.

110. Pena, A., Dvorkin, B., and White, A. (1964) Acute effect of a single in vivo injection of cortisol on in vitro amino acid incorporating activity of rat liver and thymic preparations. Biochem. Biophys. Res. Commun. 16, 449–454.

111. Pettit, B.R., and Fry, D.E. (1978) Corticosteroids in aminotic fluid and their relationship to fetal lung maturation. J. Steroid Biochem. 9, 1245–1249.

112. Pitot, H.C., and Yatvin, M.B. (1973) Interrelationships of mammalian hormones and enzyme levels in vivo. Physiol. Rev. 53, 228–325.

113. Queen, G., Pinsky, C., and LaBella, F. (1976) Subcellular localization of endorphin activity in bovine pituitary and brain. Biochem. Biophys. Res. Commun. 72, 1021–1027.

114. Raab, W. (1959) Transmembrane cationic gradient and blood pressure regulation: Interaction of corticoids, catecholamines and electrolytes on vascular cells. Am. J. Cardiol. 4, 752–774.

115. Ramey, E.R. (1975) Corticosteroids and skeletal muscle. In: H. Blaschko, G. Sayers,

A.D. Smith (eds.), Handbook of Physiology, Vol. 6, Adrenal Gland, American Physiology Society, Washington, D.C., pp. 245–261.

116. Randle, P.J., Garland, P.B., Hales, C.N., Newsholme, E.A., Denton, R.M., and Pogson, C.I. (1966) Interactions of metabolism and the physiological role of insulin. Rec. Prog. Horm. Res. 22, 1–44.

116a. Rickers, H., Deding, A., Christiansen, C., and Rødbro, P. (1984) Mineral loss in cortical and trabecular bone during high dose prednisone treatment. Calcif. Tissue Intl. 36, 269–273.

117. Roberts, B.V., Jessop, J.D., and Dore, J. (1973) Effects of gold salts and prednisolone on inflammatory cells. II. Suppression of inflammation and phagocytosis in the rat. Ann. Rheum. Dis. 32, 301–307.

118. Roberts, J.L., and Herbert, E. (1977) Characterization of a common precursor to corticotriopin and β-lipotropin: Identification of β-lipotropin peptides and their arrangement relative to corticotropin in the precursor synthesized in a cell-free system. Proc. Natl. Acad. Sci. (USA) 74, 5300–5304.

119. Rosen, F., Harding, H.R., Milholland, R.J., and Nichol, C.A. (1963) Glucocorticoids and transaminase activity. VI. Comparison of the adaptive increase of alanine and tyrosine-α-ketoglutarate transaminase. J. Biol. Chem. 238, 3725–3729.

120. Rosen, F., and Milholland, R.J. (1975) Mechanism of Action of Glucocorticoids. In: A.C. Sartorelli, D.G. Johns (eds.), Handbook of Experimental Pharmacology, Vol. 38 (2), Springer-Verlag, Berlin, Heidelberg, New York, pp. 86–103.

121. Rosen, J.M., Rosen, F., Milholland, R.J., and Nichol, C.A. (1970) Effects of cortisol on DNA metabolism in the sensitive and resistant lines of mouse lymphoma P1798. Cancer Res. 30, 1129–1136.

122. Rosen, J.M., Fina, J. Milholland, R.J., and Rosen, F. (1972) Inhibitory effect of cortisol in vitro on 2-deoxyglucose uptake and RNA and protein metabolism in lymphosarcoma P1798. Cancer Res. 32, 350–355.

123. Ross, P.S., Manganiello, V.C., and Vaughn, M. (1977) Regulation of cyclic nucleotide phosphodiesterases in cultured hepatoma cells by dexamethasone and N^6, O^2-dibutyryl adenosine. J. Biol. Chem. 252, 1448–1452.

124. Rossier, J., Vargo, T.M., Minick, S., Ling, N., Bloom, F.E., and Guillemin, R. (1977) Regional dissociation of β-endorphin and enkephalin contents in rat brain and pituitary. Proc. Natl. Acad. Sci. (USA) 74, 5162–5165.

125. Roth, G.S., and Livingston, J.N. (1976) Reductions in glucocorticoid inhibition of glucose oxidation and presumptive glucocorticoid receptor content in rat adipocytes during aging. Endocrinology 99, 831–839.

126. Rousseau, G.G., and Werenne, J. (1976) Possible mechanisms for the permissive action of glucocorticoid hormones: Studies on cyclic AMP dependent protein kinase activity of rat liver and of mouse L1210 cells. J. Steroid Biochem. 7, 1131–1134.

127. Rovetto, M.J., Murphy, R.A., and Lefer, A.M. (1970) Cardiac impairment in adrenal insufficiency: Reduced ATPase activity of myocardial contractile proteins. Circ. Res. 26, 419–428.

128. Sabol, S.L. (1978) Regulation of endorphin production by glucocorticoids in cultured pituitary tumor cells. Biochem. Biophys. Res. Commun. 82, 560–567.

129. Salmoiraghi, G.C., and McCubbin, J.W. (1954) Effect of adrenalectomy on pressor responsiveness to angiotensin and renin. Circ. Res. 2, 280–283.

130. Samuels, H.H., and Tomkins, G.M. (1970) Relation of steroid structure to enzyme induction in hepatoma tissue culture cells. J. Mol. Biol. 52, 57–74.

131. Sayers, G., and Soloman, N. (1960) Work performance of rat heart-lung preparation: Standardization and influence of corticosteroids. Endocrinology 66, 719–730.

132. Schaeffer, L.D., Chenoweth, M., and Dunn, A. (1969) Adrenal corticosteroid involvement in the control of phosphorylase in muscle. Biochim. Biophys. Acta 192, 304–309.

133. Scow, R.D., and Chernick, S.S. (1960) Hormonal control of protein and fat metabolism in the pancreatectomized rat. Rec. Prog. Horm. Res. 16, 497–541.

134. Seitz, H.J., Kaiser, M., Krone, W., and Tarnowski, W. (1976) Physiological significance of glucocorticoids and insulin in the regeneration of hepatic gluconeogenesis during starvation in rats. Metabolism 25, 1545–1555.

135. Sereni, F., and Barnabei, O. (1967) Nuclear ribonucleic acid polymerase activity, rate of ribonucleic acid synthesis and hydrolysis during development. The role of glucocorticoids. In: G. Weber (ed.), Advanced Enzyme Regulation, Vol. 5. Pergamon Press, Oxford, pp. 165–177.

136. Shanker, G., and Sharma, R.K. (1979) β-Endorphin stimulates corticosterone synthesis in isolated rat adrenal cells. Biochem. Biophys. Res. Comm. 86, 1–5.

137. Silber, R.H., and Porter, C.C. (1953) Nitrogen balance, liver protein repletion and body composition of cortisone treated rats. Endocrinology 52, 518–525.

138. Soderlin, T.R., Corbin, J.D., and Park, C.R. (1973) Regulation of adenosine 3,5-monophosphate-dependent protein kinase. II. Hormonal regulation of the adipose tissue enzyme. J. Biol. Chem. 248, 1822–1829.

139. Sollott, S.J., Galvin, M.J., and Lefer, A.M. (1979) Glucocorticoid induced protection in experimental traumatic shock. Proc. Soc. Exp. Biol. Med. 160, 317–320.

140. Stalmans, W., and LaLoux, M. (1979) Glucocorticoids and hepatic glycogen metabolism. In: J.D. Baxter and G.G. Rousseau (eds.), Monograph on Endocrinology. Glucocorticoid Hormone Action. Springer-Verlag, Berlin, Heidelberg, New York, pp. 517–533.

141. Steele, R. (1975) Influences of corticosteroids on protein and carbohydrate metabolism. In: H. Blaschko, G. Sayers, A.D. Smith, R.O. Greep, E.B. Astwood, S.R. Geiger (eds.), Handbook of Physiology, Vol. 6, Adrenal Gland. American Physiology Society Washington, D.C., pp. 135–167.

142. Stevens, J., Mashburn, L.T., and Hollander, V.P. (1969) Effect of 9α-fluoroprednisolone and L-asparaginase on uridine incorporation into ribosomal RNA of P1798 lymphosarcoma. Biochim. Biophys. Acta 186, 332–339.

143. Struck, P.J., and Tipton, C.M. (1974) Effect of acute exercise on glycogen levels in adrenalectomized rats. Endocrinology 95, 1385–1391.

144. Sutter, B.C.J., Strosser, M.T., and Mialhe, P. (1969) Permissive action of adrenal cortical hormones on insulin secretion in the rat. Diabetologia 5, 55–61.

145. Thompson, E.B., and Lippman, M.E. (1974) Mechanism of action of glucocorticoids. Metabolism, 23, 159–202.

146. Torday, J.S., Smith, B.T., and Giroud, C.J.P. (1975) The rabbit fetal lung as a glucocorticoid target tissue. Endocrinology 96, 1462–1467.

147. Uete, A. (1968) Mode of action of adrenal cortical homones. I. Effect of corticosteroids on amino acid incorporation into proteins of thymus and liver subcellular components in cell-free systems. J. Biochem. 63, 176–185.

148. Unterman, D.A., DeGraff, A.C., and Kupperman, H.S. (1955) Effect of hypoadrenalism and excessive doses of desoxycorticosterone acetate upon response of the rat to ouabain. Circ. Res. 3, 280–284.

149. Vassalli, J., Hamilton, J., and Reich, E. (1976) Macrophage plasminogen activation. Modulation of enzyme production by antiinflammatory steroids, mitotic inhibitors and cyclic nucleotides. Cell. 8, 271–281.

150. Voigt, J., Wieland, T., and Sekeris, C.E. (1978) Initial steps in the induction by glucocorticosteroids of rat liver tryptophan oxygenase and tyrosine aminotransferase. Arch. Biochem. Biophys. 191, 101–109.

151. Weber, G., and Singhal, R.L. (1964) Role of enzymes in homeostasis VI. Effect of triamcinolone and other steroids on enzymes involved in gluconeogenesis. Biochem. Pharmacol. 13, 1173–1187.

152. Weber, G., Singhal, R.L., and Srivastara, S.K. (1965) Action of glucocorticoids as inducer and insulin as suppressor of biosynthesis of hepatic gluconeogenic enzymes. In: G. Weber (ed.), Advances in Enzyme Regulation, Vol. 3. Pergamon Press, London, pp. 43–75.

153. Weber, G. (1967) Hormonal regulation and liver enzymes. Gastroenterology 53, 984–988.
154. White, A., Hoberman, H.D., and Szego, C.M. (1948) Influence of adrenalectomy and fasting on the incorporation of isotonic nitrogen into tissues of mice. J. Biol. Chem. 174, 1049–1050.
155. Wicks, W.P., Kenney, F.T., and Lee, K.L. (1969) Induction of hepatic enzyme synthesis in vivo by adenosine 3,5-monophosphate. J. Biol. Chem. 244, 6008–6013.
156. Wool, I.G., and Weinshelbaum, E.I. (1959) Incorporation of ^{14}C-amino acids into protein of isolated diaphragms: Role of the adrenal steroids. Am. J. Physiol. 197, 1089–1092.
157. Young, D.A. (1969) Glucocorticoid action of rat thymus cells. Interrelationships between carbohydrate, protein, and adenine nucleotide metabolism and cortisol effects on these functions. J. Biol. Chem. 244, 2210–2217.

MURRAY SAFFRAN, Ph.D.

CONTROL MECHANISMS IN THE PITUITARY–ADRENAL SYSTEM

INTRODUCTION

This chapter will describe the control mechanisms involved in the stimulation of the formation of glucocorticoids by the adrenal cortex in response to stress. A complete review of the subject would occupy this entire volume; therefore, only selected areas are discussed. Within each topic one or a few pioneering papers are reviewed in detail. Then selected recent papers are reviewed to bring the subject up to date. The connecting papers are left for specialized reviews.

In outline, the events that lead to an increased formation of glucocorticoids are shown in Figure 1.

Details of many of these events are still lacking. In the last few years, dramatic advances have been made in two areas: the nature of one of the major neurohormones of the hypothalamus, the corticotropin releasing factor (CRF) (event 3), is now known and the biosynthetic precursor of ACTH has been identified (event 6). While this chapter will concentrate on a description of these two recent advances, I will also discuss other areas and try to identify those in which important information is still lacking.

From the Department of Biochemistry, Medical College of Ohio, Toledo, Ohio.

1. STRESS → DETECTION BY CENTRAL NERVOUS SYSTEM →
2. STIMULATION OF A HYPOTHALAMIC CENTER →
3. RELEASE OF NEUROHORMONE(S) INTO THE HYPOPHYSIAL PORTAL VESSELS →
4. CARRIAGE BY BLOOD TO ADENOHYPOPHYSIS →
5. BINDING OF NEUROHORMONE(S) BY RECEPTOR ON CELL SURFACE →
6. STIMULATION OF SECRETION AND BIOSYNTHESIS OF ACTH →
7. RELEASE OF ACTH INTO CIRCULATION →
8. BINDING OF ACTH BY ADRENOCORTICAL CELL RECEPTOR →
9. STIMULATION OF ADENYLATE CYCLASE →
10. STIMULATION OF CONVERSION OF CHOLESTEROL TO PREGNENOLONE →
11. CONVERSION OF PREGNENOLONE TO GLUCOCORTICOIDS →
12. RELEASE OF GLUCOCORTICOIDS INTO CIRCULATION →
13. CARRIAGE OF GLUCOCORTICOIDS BY CORTICOSTEROID BINDING GLOBULIN (CBG) →
14. BINDING OF GLUCOCORTICOIDS BY RECEPTORS ON ADENOHYPOPHYSIAL ACTH-PRODUCING CELL →
15. FEEDBACK INHIBITION OF THE RELEASE OF ACTH →
16. BINDING OF GLUCOCORTICOIDS BY RECEPTORS ON HYPOTHALAMIC CRF-PRODUCING CELLS →
17. FEEDBACK INHIBITION OF THE RELEASE OF CRF.

FIGURE 1. Outline of the events by which stress stimulates steroidogenesis by the adrenal cortex.

NEURAL EVENTS

The role of the pituitary–adrenal system seems to be the adjustment of the metabolic economy of the organism in response to stress, where stress is defined as any deviation from the accustomed environment. A stress can therefore be as tangible as tissue damage by injury, or as subtle as a strange sound or sight. Stress can include a change in temperature, up or down, or any other sources of physical discomfort; stress may be a chemical change due to external or metabolic agents; stress can result from psychological or emotional discomforts, such as an examination, an interview, or anxiety over the unknown. In spite of the large variety of stimuli that constitute stress, the acute response of the pituitary–adrenal system is the same—an increased production of glucocorticoids.

Most of the stresses are detected by neural mechanisms, such as pain endings, the eye, the ear, the organs of smell and taste, and neural detectors of psychologic and emotional discomforts, whatever they may be. All of these stimuli are apparently processed by a higher center in the brain before the information is passed on to the hypothalamus. Some stresses, such as changes in blood composition, the presence of toxic agents, etc., may also be detected in the nervous system, but there is always the possibility that such changes may act directly on the hypothalamic center, rather than on higher centers of the brain.

It is beyond the scope of this review to survey the voluminous literature dealing with the putative pathways connecting the organs that detect stress with the hypothalamus (85). Here it suffices to say that the signals from such stimuli eventually are funneled to the hypothalamus.

The late G. W. Harris, in a little volume called *Neural Control of the Pituitary Gland*, succinctly summarized the evidence from his own and others' work that the connection between the hypothalamus and the adenohypophysis was blood-borne, rather than neuronal (52). He marshalled the evidence for the secretion of neurohormones by the hypothalamus into a portal circulation to the pituitary gland, where they evoke the secretion of the adenohypophysial hormones.

NEUROHORMONES

In 1955 there were several candidate neurohormones in the control of the release of ACTH. Epinephrine (adrenaline) was first proposed as a stimulant of ACTH-release by Vogt (147) on the basis of her observation that intravenous infusion of epinephrine was followed almost immediately by an increase in the secretion of adrenocortical hormones. Vogt's suggestion was supported vigorously by Long (79) because of the similarity of the stimuli that provoked the secretion of epinephrine and ACTH.

The role of epinephrine as the sole effector of the response to stress was questioned by Fortier (41) when he observed that the response to stress persisted in rats subjected to removal of the adrenal medulla, the major source of epinephrine. However, the response to stress was attenuated by adrenalmedullectomy, suggesting that epinephrine did play some role in the release of ACTH after stress. But Fortier's experiments changed the focus of the search for the mediator of the reponse to stress from the adrenal medulla to the brain, as suggested by Harris.

One of the early candidates as a neural mediator of stress was the posterior pituitary antidiuretic hormone, vasopressin. The presence of powerful hormones in the neural lobe of the pituitary gland was demonstrated in the opening years of the twentieth century by observations that injection of posterior pituitary extracts produced an increase in blood pressure, a decrease in urine formation, ejection of milk from the lactating mammary gland, and increased contractions of the uterus. The agents responsible for these biological effects were identified and subsequently synthesized by du Vigneaud and his colleagues in the late 1940s and early 1950s as nonapeptides that differed in only two of the nine amino acids. Oxytocin was responsible for inducing contractions of the uterus and ejection of milk from the lactating mammary gland, and vasopressin was shown to be the substance responsible for the elevation of blood pressure and the inhibition of the formation of urine (antidiuresis).

Early evidence for the involvement of vasopressin in the release of ACTH by stress came from experiments by Mirsky et al. (92). They found that stress resulted in the appearance of an antidiuretic substance in the blood of rats. Their work was supported by others who noted that the administration of vasopressin preparations was followed by signs of the increased formation of corticosteroids like those elicited by stress (86, 137). However, doubt was cast on the role of vasopressin as the *sole* mediator in the response to stress by the work of Nagareda and Gaunt (95), who found that the administration of large doses of water, which inhibited the release of vasopressin, also elicited signs of the release of ACTH. In spite of this negative evidence, the notion that vasopressin is a mediator in the response to stress persists to this day. Newer evidence for the role of vasopressin will be discussed later.

The suggestion by Harris and others that a hypothalamic factor was an obligatory mediator in the pituitary–adrenal response to stress naturally led to attempts to detect and identify such a substance. Because both epinephrine and vasopressin were found in or near the hypothalamus, they had strong appeal as candidates for the hypothalamic mediator. Nevertheless, the objections that arose to epinephrine and vasopressin as the sole mediators stimulated the search for other ACTH-releasing agents in the hypothalamus. The earliest report of an active extract of the hypothalamus was by Slusher and Roberts (136), who found that lipid and lipoprotein preparations of bovine posterior hypothalamus injected into intact rats caused signs characteristic of the stimulation of the release of ACTH. Unfortunately, they used intact rats for the assay of their extracts, and it is therefore possible that the materials in the extract acted directly upon the hypothalamus to release the factor, instead of containing the factor itself. Attempts by de Wied (24) to reproduce the effects of lipid and lipoprotein hypothalamic fractions on the release of ACTH under more specific conditions led to the conclusion that the extracts stimulated the release of the ACTH-releasing substance from the hypothalamus. Unfortunately, little work was carried out on the fractionation of the lipids and lipoproteins to determine the nature of the active materials. Did the lipid extract contain prostaglandins, which might have stimulated the hypothalamus? Did the lipoprotein fraction serve as a carrier for circulating ACTH-releasing hormone? Methods of fractionating these extracts are available today that should allow the purification and identification of the active principles with a modest amount of effort.

The first steps towards the detection and subsequent identification of the corticotropin-releasing principle of the hypothalamus were taken by the design of in vitro assays that were insensitive to the nonspecific nature of the response to stress of in vivo assays. Two groups of investigators simultaneously used in vitro assays for the detection of the ACTH-releasing activity in neural extracts and soon were able to announce the demonstration of such activity in the hypothalamus and the neurohypophysis: Saffran and Schally (117) and Guillemin and Rosenberg (47).

Saffran and Schally used anterior pituitary fragments from normal rats as the test tissue in an incubation of 1 to 2 hours. The ACTH released from the anterior pituitary fragments was assayed by an in vitro method using quartered rat adrenals as the test tissue. The index of response was the steroid formed by the adrenal quarters; the steroid was measured by the absorbance of ultraviolet light at 240 nm by a methylene chloride extract of the adrenal incubation medium. In contrast, Guillemin and Rosenberg used organ cultures of rat anterior pituitary tissue over several days as the detector of the ACTH-releasing activity. The ACTH released into the tissue culture medium was estimated by the in vivo bioassay of Sayers et al. (125), in which the sample is injected intravenously into hypophysectomized rats, and the decrease in adrenal ascorbic acid is estimated by the chemical determination of the ascorbic acid.

While differing in detail, the two methods have an important principle in common—they both depend upon the exposure of pituitary tissue in vitro to the sample containing the ACTH-releasing substance. In this way, the nonspecific release of ACTH by the stress of the assay in vivo is avoided. The name "corticotropin-releasing factor," or CRF, was given to the putative active principle by Saffran et al. (119).

The identification of CRF (Figure 2) was accomplished in 1981 by Spiess et al. (138). Why did it take so long to progress from the detection of the activity in neural tissues to the identification of CRF as a 41-amino-acid linear peptide? The reasons lie in the many factors that enter into the process of identifying a natural product. These include the development of a specific, sensitive, and relatively rapid assay for CRF, the limited amount of CRF in the tissue, the amount of tissue available, the availability of methods for the efficient separation of the active agent from other components of the tissue, the ability of the investigator to adapt to unexpected findings, etc. Each of these factors played a significant role in delaying the identification of CRF for over a quarter of a century. The slow, inaccurate assays of Saffran and of Guillemin gave way to the use of pituitary cell cultures, with the subsequent radioimmunoassay of the ACTH released from the cells. The procedures for the separation of tissue components improved from the slow paper and column chromatography to the fast HPLC (High Pressure Liquid Chromatography). The techniques for amino acid sequencing improved in sensitivity and accuracy by several orders of magnitude. Also, investigators finally shed the blinkers of believing that CRF had to be a small peptide, like vasopressin (because vasopressin itself has considerable ACTH-releasing activity), and accepted the evidence that it may be as large as ACTH (Figure 3). In fact, CRF is accompanied by ACTH in hypothalanic extracts, a fact that complicated the search because, in the past, the workers in the field tended to set aside as useless the fractions that contained ACTH.

The synthetic peptide with the structure in Figure 2 shares all the biological activities of the material isolated from the ovine hypothalamus (146). The CRF of the rat has recently been identified (107). It is also

FIGURE 2. Primary structure of ovine CRF.

H-Ser-Gln-Glu-Pro-Pro-Ile-Ser-Leu-Asp-Leu-Thr-Phe-His-Leu-
Leu-Arg-Glu-Val-Leu-Glu-Met-Thr-Lys-Ala-Asp-Glu-Leu-Ala-
Gln-Gln-Ala-His-Ser-Asn-Arg-Lys-Leu-Leu-Asp-Ile-Ala-NH_2

41-amino acid residues long and it differs only slightly (17%) from the sequence of the ovine peptide. The biological activities are identical.

The messenger RNAs of the sheep hypothalamus and a synthetic DNA corresponding to a 14-amino-acid sequence of CRF were used to isolate clones with the DNA sequence of the CRF precursor (42). These were used to prepare the messenger RNA for the precursor, which contains 1098 nucleotide residues, corresponding to a protein with 366 amino acids. The first 72 nucleotides code for a 24-amino-acid signal sequence characteristic of a secreted peptide. Nucleotide residues 442–564 code for the 41-amino-acid sequence of ovine CRF. The amino terminus region of the CRF sequence is preceded by Arg–Lys–Arg–Arg–, which is a site for proteolytic cleavage in the processing of the precursor to the active peptide. It is interesting that the non-CRF portion of the precursor contains amino acid sequences that have strong resemblance to the sequences contained in the vasopressin–neurophysin precursor and to the ACTH precursor.

The availability of synthetic CRF will facilitate the solution of several outstanding problems in the control of the release of ACTH. The physiological role of vasopressin is still uncertain. There is no doubt that vasopressin is a powerful releaser of ACTH, both in vitro and in vivo. Antidiuresis seems to be a common occurrence under conditions of stress. However, the pituitary–adrenal response to stress can still occur in the absence of vasopressin. The old observation by Nagareda and Gaunt (95), that a large dose of water is at the same time an inhibitor of the release of vasopressin and a stress, is joined by more recent evidence that vasopressin can be suppressed and yet the pituitary–adrenal response to stress persists. Treatment of rats with a vasopressin analogue that is an inhibitor of the biological activities of vasopressin did not prevent the increase in plasma ACTH and corticosterone levels in rats exposed to the stress of a novel environment (93). Some residual pituitary–adrenal response due to vasopressin seems to persist in most of these experiments. This has been ascribed to a secondary pathway for the response to a stress involving the paraventricular nucleus of the hypothalamus, in which vasopressin is synthesized (12). CRF and vasopressin may act by different mechanisms. CRF induces an increase in pituitary cyclic AMP at the same time that it releases ACTH, while vasopressin releases ACTH without increasing cyclic AMP (1).

To add to the complexity of the picture, there is good evidence that vasopressin enhances the response of the pituitary cell to the action of CRF. This was first demonstrated using extracts of rat median eminence as the source of CRF (45) and later confirmed with pure CRF when it became available (44).

The release of ACTH may therefore be under multiple control (118, 114). The 41-amino-acid peptide CRF may act under most circumstances of stress involving stimulation of the central nervous system, such as after psychological, sensory, and chemical stimuli, while vasopressin may release ACTH under conditions involving fluid and electrolyte disturbances (e.g., hemorrhage). Other ACTH secretogogues, such as epinephrine, may predominate under other conditions, still to be defined. By funneling stimuli arising from every possible source into the same end response, the release of ACTH and the stimulation of the adrenal cortex, the organism is assured of a metabolic response to meet every kind of threat.

ACTH

ACTH, adrenocorticotropic hormone, is a 39-amino-acid peptide hormone (Figure 3) that is found in highest amounts in the anterior lobe of the pituitary gland (109).

ACTH was first detected in pituitary tissue by Collip et al. in 1933 (19) after extraction with dilute acid solutions. Very few proteins would have survived the conditions of extraction, yet the first "pure" preparations of ACTH announced in 1943 by Li et al. (76) and Sayers et al. (124) were proteins with a molecular weight in the order of 25,000! One of these "pure" preparations of ACTH was selected as the first International Standard for ACTH with a defined potency of 1 unit/mg. The true structures of the ACTHs of various species were found in the period 1953–1959 by several groups of investigators (149,4,77,134).

The long delay between the first demonstration of ACTH in pituitary extracts and its identification can be attributed to the intervention of World War II in 1939–1945. But the war also served as a stimulant to the first "purifications" of ACTH in 1943 because of the rumor that German pilots were able to fly at unusually high altitudes after treatment with adrenal steroids or with ACTH. Another reason for the delay is the frustrating tendency of ACTH to stick to surfaces, such as glass, and to other proteins and peptides. Only the evolution of powerful methods of

FIGURE 3. Amino acid sequence of human ACTH.

1	2	3	4	5	6	7	8	9	10	11	12	13	14	15	16	17	18	19	20	21	22	23	24
S	Y	S	M	E	H	F	R	W	G	K	P	V	G	K	K	R	R	P	V	K	V	Y	P

← α-MSH →

25	26	27	28	29	30	31	32	33	34	35	36	37	38	39
D	A	G	E	D	Q	S	A	E	A	F	P	L	E	F

The first 24 amino acids of ACTH are the same in all species and are required for full biological activity. The last 15 amino acids show some variation among species but can be shorn from the molecule without loss of activity.

The amino acid sequence of α-MSH is identical with that of the first 13 amino acids of ACTH. In α-MSH the serine (S) at the amino terminus (number 1) is acetylated.

The single letter code for the amino acids is:

A, alanine; C, cyteine; D, aspartic acid; E, glutamic acid; F, phenylalanine; G, glycine; H, histidine; I, isoleucine; K, lysine, L, leucine; M, methionine; N, asparagine; P, proline; Q, glutamine; R, arginine; S, serine; T, threonine; V, valine; W, trytophan; Y, tyrosine.

separation, such as partition and ion exchange chromatography, made possible the purification of ACTH. The "stickiness" of ACTH still plagues investigators who try to localize ACTH in extrapituitary tissues and those who try to study ACTH receptors.

The elucidation of the details of the mechanism of protein synthesis and its control in the last 30 years made clear that the primary products synthesized on the ribosomes of the anterior pituitary cell were much larger than the 39-amino-acid hormone that is secreted into the blood. The first well-characterized example of a large precursor of a peptide hormone was the discovery of proinsulin by Steiner and Oyer in 1967 (139). ACTH is also synthesized as a large precursor molecule in the pituitary cell (27). Although ACTH is a simple peptide of 39 amino acid residues, the precursor has a molecular weight of about 31,000 and contains carbohydrate residues.

Even before the ACTH precursor was discovered, the ACTH molecule was found to include in its structure the 13-amino-acid sequence of the intermediate pituitary lobe hormone α-melanocyte stimulating hormone, or α-MSH (Figure 3). In human adult pituitaries, in which there is no intermediate lobe, an MSH of different structure, β-MSH, is found (53). β-MSH contains 17 amino acid residues. The ACTH precursor contains the amino acid sequences of both ACTH and β-MSH. The β-MSH sequence is itself a portion of the sequence of a large peptide that was named β-lipotropin (β-LPH) because of its ability to mobilize fatty acids in certain species (74). For a decade, β-lipotropin was a hormone looking for a function. In 1975, a sharp-eyed chemist noted that the amino acid sequence of the newly discovered enkephalins was included in the β-LPH molecule (Hughes et al., 62). This led to the testing of lipotropin itself and fragments derived from it for opioid activity like that of the enkephalins. Some of the lipotropin fragments were found to be very active; the most active was the 32-amino-acid residue fragment called β-endorphin (75) (Figure 4).

The ACTH precursor is made in the corticotroph cells of the anterior pituitary, where peptidases split the molecule at sites containing pairs of basic amino acids, such as arg–arg or lys–arg, to liberate ACTH and other products. When the anterior pituitary is stimulated by CRF, ACTH and β-endorphin are released together from the gland (49). There is some evidence that the fragments of proopiomelanicortin, the ACTH precursor, may function as potentiators of the adrenocortical response to ACTH (100).

ACTH precursor is also made in the cells of the intermediary lobe of the pituitary gland, where the main product of enzymatic cleavage is α-MSH. In cells of the nervous system, the same precursor is split differently, to yield β-endorphin as the main active component. The wide distribution of the ACTH precursor may explain the early observation that the hypothalamus contains substantial amounts of ACTH, and α- and β-MSH (48). The ACTH in the hypothalamus contributed, as already noted, to the delay in the isolation and characterization of CRF.

The mRNA for the ACTH precursor was isolated and cloned by

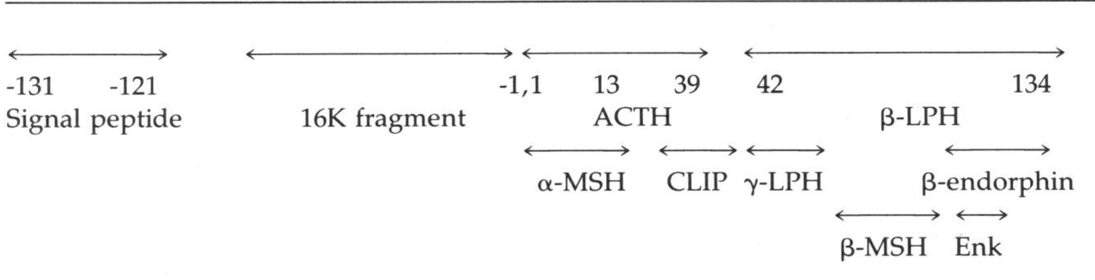

CLIP = corticotropin-like intermediary lobe peptide
Enk = enkephalin
LPH = lipotropin
MSH = melanocyte-stimulating hormone

FIGURE 4. The ACTH precursor, proopiomelanocortin, or POMC.

Nakanishi et al. in 1979 (96), permitting the translation of the first precursor peptide formed on the ribosomes. The first product is 256 amino acid residues long. Approximately the first 20 residues consist of a signal peptide, which is lost before the peptide leaves the ribosomes. The newly formed peptide is then glycosylated and further processed. The processing, as was already noted, depends upon the tissue in which synthesis takes place, accounting for the different products formed in different tissues (Figure 4).

ADRENAL ACTH RECEPTOR

The first step in the activation of a target cell by a peptide or protein hormone is binding by a receptor on the cell surface. An adrenocortical ACTH receptor was first detected by Lefkowitz et al. in 1970 (72). They used "pure monoiodo ACTH-^{125}I," which was claimed to be biologically active, and membranes prepared from a transplantable adrenal tumor in mice to show specific binding of the labeled hormone by the tissue preparation. The bound, labeled hormone was displaced from the membranes by a series of ACTH preparations in approximate order of their biological activity. The biological activity of the labeled hormone was measured by its ability to stimulate the production of 3′,5′-cyclic AMP by adrenocortical membrane preparations. Some assays were also done in hypophysectomized rats by measuring the increase in plasma corticosterone after injection of the hormone.

Confirmation of these findings in plasma membrane preparations of bovine adrenals soon came from Finn et al. (40). In this case, the ACTH preparation used was a synthetic, biologically active $^{14}C-Phe^{7}ACTH_{1-20}$ amide. The labeled hormone was displaced by porcine ACTH and various ACTH fragments and analogues. The membrane preparation was demonstrated to contain an ACTH-sensitive adenylate cyclase. However, there was no stimulation of the cyclase by the isotopically labeled analogue.

The binding of ACTH by a membrane preparation was soon put to practical use by Wolfsen et al. (150), who designed an assay for ACTH based on the displacement of ^{125}I-ACTH from binding to a solubilized receptor preparation made from adrenal membranes of the rat, sheep, or rabbit. The useful range of the method was between 1 and 10 pg/tube. However, only 20% of the bound ACTH could be displaced from the receptor preparation by excess unlabeled ACTH, indicating that most of the binding was "nonspecific." Nevertheless, the values for plasma ACTH obtained by the method matched the conditions of the subject. The administration of dexamethasone decreased the plasma ACTH to virtually nondetectable levels, while greater-than-normal levels were found after administration of metyrapone, after insulin hypoglycemia, in Cushing's disease, and in Addison's disease. Unfortunately, the membrane preparation was tricky to make. Only tissue from animals killed under controlled laboratory conditions yielded active preparations; slaughterhouse tissues could not be used.

Binding of ^{125}I-ACTH to isolated rat adrenocortical cells was demonstrated by McIlhinney and Schulster (90). The labeled ACTH retained about 50% of the steroidogenic activity of the native ACTH. Binding of the labeled hormone by the isolated cells was rapid, reaching a maximum in about 6 minutes at 37°C. Displacement of the labeled hormone by various ACTH and other preparations was approximately proportional to steroidogenic activity. A plateau in steroidogenic response was reached long before the ACTH receptors were saturated, illustrating the presence of "spare receptors" on the adrenocortical cells. Once more, there was evidence for the presence of a substantial amount of nonspecific binding of the labeled ACTH. McIlhinney and Schulster did not study the effect of the binding of ACTH on the production of 3′,5′-cyclic AMP in this paper.

In contrast, Ways et al. (148) studied the binding of ^{125}I-ACTH$_{1-24}$ by rat adrenal membrane particles and correlated it with the activation of adenylate cyclase in the tissue preparation. They prepared a series of synthetic peptides representing various other regions of the human ACTH molecule and found that none of them had the ability to stimulate the adenylate cyclase of rat adrenal membranes like the 1–24 peptide. However, some of the fragments were inhibitors of the stimulation of adenylate cyclase by ACTH$_{1-39}$ and ACTH$_{1-24}$. Moreover, there was an excellent correlation between the ability of an analogue to displace labeled ACTH from binding to adrenal particles and the ability of the analogue to inhibit the stimulation of adenylate cyclase by ACTH.

In spite of this promising start on the characterization of the adrenal ACTH receptor, relatively little progress has been made recently in learning more about it. Part of the reason for lack of progress was the relatively large nonspecific component of ACTH-binding by the preparations. Another partial explanation was the inconsistent recovery of biologic activity of the ACTH after iodination. In spite of care to ensure only monoiodination of the tyrosyl residue in ACTH, conditions of iodination are such that a mixture of mono- and diiodinated molecules is obtained. The disubstituted ACTH is devoid of biologic activity. An average iodine uptake of 1 atom/molecule may therefore represent monoiiodination of all the molecules, or diiodination of half of the molecules. The problem of inconsistent iodination was solved by Buckley et al. (11). Iodination causes loss of biologic activity by oxidation of the methionyl residue and the iodination of the Tyr^2 of the ACTH molecule. However, even diiodination of the Tyr^{23} of ACTH causes relatively little loss of activity. Therefore, Buckley et al. synthesized an ACTH analogue in which the Tyr^2 was replaced by Phe and the Met^4 was replaced by Norleucine (Nle). The analogue, $Phe^2,Nle^4\text{-}ACTH_{1-38}$, was iodinated and the mono- and diiodinated derivatives were easily separated by HPLC. The monoiodinated analogue had the same activity as native ACTH in an assay based on steroidogenesis by isolated rat adrenocortical cells. The monoiodinated analogue was then used as the labeled ligand in a radioimmunoassay for ACTH (9). It was also used by Buckley and Ramachandran (10) to study the ACTH receptor on isolated rat adrenocortical cells. They found good correlation between binding of the analogue and production of 3′,5′-cyclic AMP at concentrations between 0.1 and 1000 nM. Moreover, they observed that the analogue stimulated steroidogenesis maximally at a concentration of 60 pM. Because of the very high specific radioactivity obtainable with the analogue, they could also demonstrate binding of the analogue to adrenocortical cells at concentrations between 10 and 60 pM, in the range of concentration in which steroidogenesis was stimulated by the analogue. Stimulation of 3′,5′-cyclic AMP production needed about a thousand times as much ACTH as did stimulation of steroidogenesis by isolated adrenal cells. More than 85% of the bound iodinated ACTH

TABLE 1. Affinity Constants of the ACTH Receptor and Number of Binding Sites per Adrenocortical Cell

	Authors		
	Lefkowitz et al.	**McIlhinney and Schulster**	**Buckley and Ramachandran**
Year	1971	1975	1981
Reference	71	90	10
Tissue preparation	Mouse tumor membranes	Rat cells	Rat cells
Ligand	^{125}I-ACTH	^{125}I-ACTH	^{125}I-ACTH analog
Low affinity:			
K_d	3.3×10^{-8}	1.0×10^{-8}	none
Sites per cell	360,000	30,000	none
High affinity:			
K_d	1.1×10^{-12}	2.5×10^{-10}	1.4×10^{-9}
Sites per cell	60	3,000	3840

analogue was displaced by ACTH, in contrast with the relatively high nonspecific binding obtained by previous workers!

Persistent activation of rat adrenocortical cells was achieved by exposing the cells to the photoreactive derivative of ACTH, [(2-nitro-5-azidophenylsulfenyl)Trp^9]-ACTH, in the presence of ultraviolet light. Both 3′,5′-cyclic AMP and corticosterone production were stimulated by photocoupling of the ACTH analogue to adrenocortical cells (103).

The availability of a stable and biologically active ACTH analogue with high radioactive specific activity should allow the further purification and characterization of the adrenocortical ACTH receptor in the near future. So far, the evidence points to the existence of a common receptor for both stimulation of steroidogenesis and activation of adenylate cyclase. A summary of the affinities for ACTH and the number of binding sites per adrenocortical cell is in Table 1.

According to most recent figures, there are approximately 4000 binding sites for ACTH on each separated adrenocortical cell, with a K_d of about 10^{-9}, a higher value than those obtained by earlier investigators. Nevertheless, the K_d of about 10^{-9} agrees with the concentration of ACTH to give half-maximal production of 3′,5′-cyclic AMP by isolated rat adrenocortical cells (10).

ADRENOCORTICAL MEMBRANE

The ACTH receptor is located, like other peptide hormone receptors, on the outer surface of the adrenocortical cell membrane, where it can combine with the ACTH in the blood. Does binding of ACTH by the receptor result in changes in the properties of the cell membrane? This possibility has been investigated in two ways: changes in electrical properties of the membrane and changes in the phospholipids of the membrane.

While the electrophysiological properties of nerve and muscle cells have been well studied, the electrical properties of adrenocortical cells were relatively little studied. In 1959, Kruskemper and Reichertz (70) found changes in the "electrogram" of the adrenal gland after intravenous injection of ACTH in the anesthetized rat. The electrical changes were detected by an apparatus akin to the electrocardiograph, using surface electrodes which received signals from many cells. In 1967, Matthews and Saffran (87) used an intracellular microelectrode to record the transmembrane potential of a single cell of an adrenal gland removed from a newborn rabbit. The resting membrane potential was in the order of -70 mV; this value can be compared with the -80 to -90 mV recorded in nerve and muscle cells. Exposure of the tissue to ACTH did not alter the transmembrane potentials, even though corticosteroid production increased. However, the cells could be depolarized, i.e., the membrane potential difference was decreased, by increasing the external concentration of potassium, without affecting the steroidogenic response to ACTH. The authors concluded that stimulation of the adrenal cortex and the electrical properties of the adrenocortical cell were not related.

However, in the next year the same authors reported (88) that when the adrenocortical cells were first exposed to a medium virtually devoid of potassium ions, causing hyperpolarization to a transmembrane potential of -80 mV, the addition of ACTH was followed by a progressive depolarization to values from around -50 mV to less than -25 mV, accompanied by the appearance of trains of depolarizations, similar in form to action potentials seen in stimulated nerve cells. Although the resting membrane potential of adrenocortical cells seemed to be generated largely by the difference in concentration of potassium between the interior and exterior of the cell, the waves of depolarization in response to ACTH are probably generated by movements of calcium ions, since they were inhibited by calcium chelators, and unaffected by sodium-ion transport inhibitors (89). Most of the work on adrenocortical membrane potentials was done on tissue taken from laboratory animals, but similar findings were reported by Lymangrover et al. (81) with human tissue.

In the rat adrenal gland, the resting membrane potential changes with age. The potential is highest in newborn and very young animals, and decreases steadily to about half the maximum value in aged animals (82). Contrary to findings in other species, the addition of ACTH results in depolarization of the adrenocortical cells of the mouse with development of action-potential-like changes, even in medium with a normal concentration of potassium (80).

The significance of the electrical changes of the membrane in response to ACTH is unknown. So far the evidence for a direct connection with binding of the ACTH by the receptor is weak. Further study is needed to understand the reasons for depolarization of the membrane (which reflects a decreased barrier to potassium ions) and for the appearance of "action potentials" (which probably reflects a movement of calcium ions).

PHOSPHOLIPIDS

Because the cell membrane is largely made up of phospholipids, changes in adrenocortical phospholipid composition and properties in response to ACTH were sought. An early study by Hokin et al. (60) of the incorporation of ^{32}P-phosphate into phospholipids of rat adrenal tissue, incubated in vitro with and without ACTH, concluded that there was no influence of ACTH. In contrast, the same paper showed that the addition of a CRF preparation to rat pituitary tissue in vitro stimulated the incorporation of ^{32}P-phosphate into the phosphoinositide, phosphatidylcholine, and phosphatidic acid fractions. The greatest change was in the phosphoinositide and phosphatidic acid fractions. The investigators concluded that increased turnover of phospholipid phosphate occurred only when a tissue was stimulated to secrete a peptide or protein product. Such a change apparently did not accompany the increased formation of a steroid.

This early observation was virtually lost sight of, even though similar work by Hokin and Hokin (59) on the turnover of phospholipid phosphorus in the acinar pancreas is acknowledged to be the original observation of a correlation of phospholipid metabolism and stimulation of cellular function. In the middle 1970s, the phospholipid response in the pancreas was found to be the result of a rapid hydrolysis of phosphatidylinositol by phospholipase-C, yielding 1,2-diacylglycerol and phosphatidic acid (3). Resynthesis of phosphatidylinositol accounted for the increased uptake of ^{32}P-phosphate into the phospholipid.

In 1979 Farese and Sabir (33) reported that cardiolipin, a phospholipid found in large amounts in mitochondrial membranes, stimulated steroidogenesis. Similar ACTH-like activity was found with other lipids containing multiple phosphate groups (34), such as the phosphatidylinositol phosphates (Figure 5). These observations prompted them to reexamine the effect of ACTH on adrenocortical phospholipids (36). Both in vivo and

FIGURE 5. Polyphosphophospholipids.

```
Cardiolipin
        O⁻            OH            O⁻
        |             |             |
      O=P-O-CH2—CH-CH2—O-P=O
        |                           |
        O                           O
        |                           |
        CH2                         CH2
        |                           |
      H-C-O-CO-R                  H-C-O-CO-R
        |                           |
        CH2—O-CO-R                  CH2—O-CO-R

                         CHOH
Polyphosphoinositide    /    \          O
                       /      \         ||
                    CHOH    CH-O-P-O-    )
                     |       |      |    |
                     |       |      O⁻   |  Two adjacent
        O⁻           |       |           |  negatively charged groups
        |            |       |      O⁻   |
        |            |       |      |    |
      O=P-O-CH           CH-O-P- O⁻      )
        |      \        /       ||
        |       \      /        O
        O        CHOH
        |
        CH2
        |
        CH-O-CO-R
        |
        CH2-O-CO-R
```

R = fatty acid hydrocarbon chains, which may be different.

in vitro stimulation of steroidogenesis with ACTH was accompanied by an increased concentration of di- and triphosphoinositides in the adrenal tissue. The time course of the increase was similar in shape to the increase in adrenal content of corticosterone in the rat. The concentration of diphosphoinositide increased with the dose of ACTH. The effect of ACTH on diphosphoinositide was abolished by treatment of the rat with the inhibitor of protein synthesis, cycloheximide. 3′,5′-Cyclic AMP also increased the diphosphoinositide concentration of rat adrenal quarters or separated cells. The response to the cyclic nucleotide was abolished by cycloheximide and by the omission of calcium from the incubation medium.

The apparent discrepancy between the early observations of Hokin et al. (60) and those of Farese and Sabir (33) is probably due to differences in experimental conditions. Hokin et al. used the incorporation of ^{32}P from phosphate into phosphoinositides as the index of phospholipid turnover, while Farese and his co-workers actually measured the net increase in the amount of phosphoinositides. Should the biosynthesis of new phosphoinositides take place without dipping into the phosphate ion pool, then stimulation of synthesis would result in a decrease in the incorporation of phosphate due to dilution of the labeled material. In fact, a slight decrease was actually observed in (60).

The lipids of the bovine adrenal gland were characterized by Seltzman et al. (129) in 1975. A preparation enriched in plasma membranes was obtained by zonal centrifugation. The lipids were extracted with chloroform-methanol and were separated and characterized by thin-layer and column chromatography. The plasma membrane preparation consisted of about 40% protein and 55% lipid. Phospholipids were about three-fourths of the lipid. Of the phospholipids, phosphatidylcholine is most prevalent, about 46%, phosphatidylethanolamine, next, with 22%, phosphatidylserine, 9%, and phosphatidylinositol, 4%. Phosphatidic acid is about 1% of the adrenal lipids in the cow. The phospholipids apparently involved in hormonal stimulation were not the major components of the plasma membrane.

The specificity of the effect of hormonal stimulation on phospholipid turnover was further complicated by Farese et al. (35), who reported that both ACTH and 3′,5′-cyclic AMP increased the incorporation of ^{3}H-labeled glycerol and ^{14}C-labeled palmitate into phosphatidic acid and its derivatives, phosphatidylcholine and phosphatidylethanolamine, as well as into the phosphoinositides.

There are several sites in the control of steroidogenesis at which phospholipids can play a role. The plasma membrane is composed largely of phospholipids and any ACTH-induced alteration in the ratio of the phospholipids can lead to an alteration in the properties of the membrane, such as membrane potential, permeability to ions, and the activity of enzymes associated with the plasma membrane (29). The observation that cyclic AMP's effects on steroidogenesis also involve phospholipids strongly suggests that the participation of the phospholipids occurs inside the cell, rather than within or on the plasma membrane. The ability of polyphospholipids to mimic the effects of ACTH on mitrochondrial preparations points to a role in the mitochondria. In fact, the mitochondrial membrane is rich in polyphosphophospholipids. The presence of adjacent phosphate groups on the inositol of polyphosphoinositide (Figure 5) makes it capable of binding Ca ions and, by dephosphorylation, capable of releasing Ca ions. The role of Ca ions in the control of steroidogenesis will be discussed later. It is also possible that phospholipids can function at multiple sites in the adrenocortical cell: at the plasma membrane level, to shuttle Ca ions in and out of the cell; within the plasma membrane, to control the activity of membrane-bound enzymes; within the cell, in the intracellular transport of cholesterol, the precursor of the steroid hormones; and at the mitochondrial level, in the transfer of Ca ions and/or cholesterol from the cytosol.

PROSTAGLANDINS

Phospholipase c catalyzes the removal of fatty acids from the phospholipids of the plasma and mitochondrial membranes. When polyunsaturated fatty acids, like arachidonic acid, are liberated from phospholipids, they can serve as precursors of the prostaglandins and other derivatives, which may be regulators of cellular functions (5). The effect of prostaglandins on adrenal function was first studied by Ramwell et al. (104) and by others in the 1960s, with variable results. With the availability of pure preparations of the prostaglandins and other arachidonic acid derivatives, the problem was reinvestigated in recent years. In vivo, the implantation of pellets of indomethacin, an inhibitor of prostaglandin formation, into the hypothalamus reduced the pituitary–adrenal response to stress (144), suggesting that prostaglandins play a role in the release and/or synthesis of CRF. At the adrenal level, prostacyclin, another derivative of archidonic acid, was found to stimulate steroidogenesis (28). However, more recent in vitro experiments with separated zones or cells of the adrenal gland failed to support the idea that the prostaglandins influence directly the production of glucocorticoids (135,142). The contradictory observations of the effects of the prostaglandins prevent a definite statement of their role in the pituitary–adrenal system at the present time. However, as their role in other tissues becomes better known, the knowledge will feed back into an understanding of how they act in the pituitary–adrenal system.

CALCIUM IONS

According to the current view, peptide hormones stimulate target cells at the plasma membrane level, but further transmission of the stimulus in the cell is via a second messenger system. The most widely distributed second messengers are 3′5′-cyclic AMP and Ca ions. There is evidence that both cyclic AMP and Ca ions are involved in the stimulation of steroidogenesis in the adrenal cortex by ACTH.

The demonstration that calcium ions participated in the stimulation of steroidogenesis by ACTH was made possible by the development by Saffran et al. (115,112) in 1952 of an in vitro system for studying the response of the adrenal cortex to ACTH. The first report that calcium ions participated in the action of ACTH was the classic paper by Birmingham et al. (6) in 1953. They observed that when a precipitate formed in the phosphate-buffered medium recommended by Saffran et al. (115,112), the addition of ACTH resulted in relatively little increase in steroidogenesis. Replacement of the phosphate buffer by a bicarbonate buffer abolished the precipitation and gave consistently good effects of ACTH. They concluded that the precipitate was calcium phosphate. To prove that calcium was involved, Birmingham et al. incubated adrenal tissue with ACTH in calcium-free medium and in medium with increasing concentrations of calcium. The effect of ACTH was uniformly less in calcium-free medium. As little as 0.5 M calcium was effective in restoring the full effect of ACTH (the "normal" concentration of calcium in the medium is 2.5 M). The authors speculated that either calcium allowed "freer access of ACTH to the cellular mechanisms involved in steroid production, or . . . calcium is a cofactor . . . in steroid formation".

The need for calcium for optimal stimulation by ACTH was confirmed by Peron and Koritz (101) in 1958, who found that higher-than-normal concentrations of potassium could replace the missing calcium. They suggested that the role of calcium might be in controlling the entry of potassium into the adrenocortical cell. Indeed, Birmingham et al. (8) found in 1960 that calcium in the medium does increase the potassium content of incubated adrenocortical tissue, but there was no correlation between the potassium content of the tissue and the ability to respond to ACTH. They also concluded that calcium did not seem to play a role in the binding of ACTH to its receptors, because exposure to ACTH in calcium-containing or in calcium-free medium gave the same stimulation of steroidogenesis in subsequent incubations in calcium-containing medium. However, the full expression of the stimulation of steroidogenesis by cyclic AMP required calcium. Birmingham et al. (8) postulated that the site of action of calcium was between the elaboration of cyclic AMP and the reactions leading to increased steroidogenesis. In 1973, Leier and Jungman (73) reported that both ACTH and cyclic AMP increased the uptake of calcium ions by rat adrenal glands. This is evidence for serial

$$\text{(ACTH} \rightarrow \text{cyclic AMP} \rightarrow \text{calcium ions} \rightarrow \text{steroidogenesis)}$$

rather than parallel

$$\text{(ACTH} \begin{array}{l} \rightarrow \text{cyclic AMP} \rightarrow \\ \rightarrow \text{calcium ions} \rightarrow \end{array} \text{steriodogenesis)}$$

roles for cyclic AMP and calcium ions as second messengers in the adrenocortical response to ACTH.

Calcium has been implicated in adrenal protein synthesis and steroid biosynthesis (30). Although broken cell preparations (e.g., homogenates) of the adrenal cortex no longer respond to ACTH, most of the corticosteroid-producing reactions (see chapter by Rapp in this volume) can be demonstrated to occur. Calcium ions are needed for maximal steroid production by rat adrenal homogenates (68). The stimulatory effect of calcium on steroidogenesis was best seen with homogenates prepared from adrenals taken from ACTH-treated rats (31). The calcium effect was localized to the ACTH-sensitive reaction, the conversion of cholesterol to pregnenolone (31).

The steroidogenic effect of prostacyclin on cat adrenal cells is also dependent on calcium (111); the permissive action of calcium on stimulation by both prostacyclin and ACTH was inhibited by the calcium antagonist, TMB-8.

Recently, the binding and release of Ca^{++} by the protein, calmodulin, has been implicated in many of the actions of calcium (91). A possible role for calmodulin in the adrenal cortex was investigated by Carsia et al. (14). They added the calmodulin antagonist, chlorpromazine, to rat adrenocortical cells and found that ACTH-stimulated steroidogenesis was inhibited. The kinetics of the inhibition matched the characteristics of the binding of chlorpromazine by calmodulin. Chlorpromazine also inhibited the stimulation of cyclic AMP production by ACTH as well as the stimulation of steroidogenesis by cyclic AMP.

The possible role of calcium in the binding of ACTH by its receptor was reopened by Cheitlin et al. (15) in 1983, who used the ACTH analogue of Buckley and Ramachandran (10). They found that separated rat adrenocortical cells did not respond to the ACTH analogue when the medium contained the calcium chelator, EGTA. Neither did the cells bind the analogue. Photolytic binding of an ACTH analogue with the receptor only occurred when the cells were illuminated in the presence of calcium. Both binding and increased steroidogenesis were restored by the addition of calcium. This new finding has yet to be reconciled with the older observations, by more indirect means, that calcium is not involved in the binding of ACTH to the receptor [e.g. (8)].

CYCLIC NUCLEOTIDES

There is now a large body of evidence that 3′,5′-cyclic AMP is a second messenger in the steroidogenic response of the adrenal cortex to ACTH. Most of the evidence comes from work carried out on in vitro systems.

The first traces of the trail that led to the discovery of a role for cyclic AMP in the adrenal cortex actually antedate the discovery of cyclic AMP itself. In 1953, Reiss et al. (105) found that the stimulation by ACTH of oxygen consumption by cow adrenal slices was significantly enhanced in the presence of glucose in the medium. That same year, Schonbaum et al. (127) observed that the stimulation by ACTH of steroidogenesis by rat adrenal tissue was enhanced by the addition of glucose to the medium. The first guesses for the role of glucose were that glucose was a precursor of the corticosteroids, or that glucose served as an energy source for the adrenocortical cell. But glucose could also serve as the source of reducing activity to make NADPH available to hydroxylating reactions in the biosynthesis of corticosteroids (55). The "beneficial" effect of glucose was followed by the observation in 1955 that adrenal glycogen was depleted by the administration of ACTH or by the imposition of a stress to the animal (98). By this time, the role of epinephrine and glucagon as stimulators of the breakdown of glycogen by activation of glycogen phosphorylase was known. In 1957, cyclic AMP was identified (21) and recognized as the agent responsible for the activation of glycogen phosphorylase by Sutherland and Rall (141). Soon afterward, a series of three papers by Haynes et al. (55,54,56) established that ACTH activated adrenal phosphorylase, and that the addition of cyclic AMP to rat adrenals in vitro stimulated steroidogenesis.

Utilizing the information available to them at that time, Haynes et al. (58) suggested that 1) ACTH stimulated the enzyme, adenyl cyclase, to form additional amounts of cyclic AMP from ATP; 2) the resulting cyclic AMP stimulated adrenal phosphorylase to break down adrenal glycogen to glucose-1-phosphate, and then to glucose-6-phosphate; and 3) the glucose-6-phosphate entered the hexose monophosphate shunt to result in the formation of NADPH, which was then used to hydroxylate precursors to the finished corticosteroids (Figure 6).

The Haynes hypothesis has not withstood the test of time in all details, but the role of cyclic AMP as a second messenger in the action of ACTH has resisted many attempts to discredit it (108, Ch. 9). The complete acceptance of cyclic AMP as the second messenger was delayed by lack of correspondence between steroidogenesis and increase in cyclic AMP in response to increasing concentrations of ACTH (130). However, in other cyclic-AMP-sensitive systems, cyclic AMP acts by binding to a receptor

FIGURE 6. Haynes's hypothesis for the mechanism of action of ACTH (59).

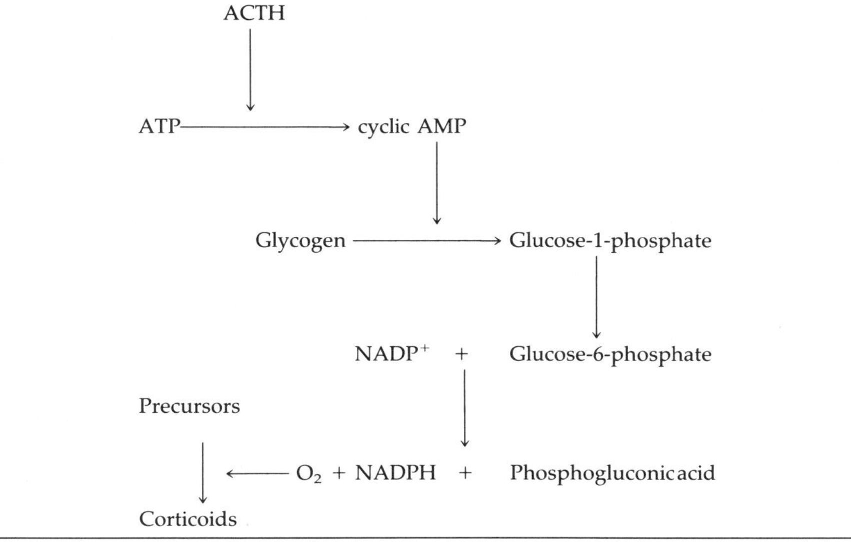

subunit of an enzyme, displacing an active catalytic subunit. When receptor-bound cyclic AMP was plotted against the concentration of ACTH, there was good agreement with the stimulation of corticosteroidogenesis by ACTH (Sala et al., 120).

Another doubt about the role of cyclic AMP was generated by observations by Sharma et al. (130) that concentrations of cyclic GMP increased in isolated rat adrenocortical cells at lower concentrations of ACTH than those that increased the levels of cyclic AMP. These observations were confirmed by Sala et al. (120) who noticed that the temporal relationship between cyclic GMP increase and steroidogenesis was not as good a fit as that between receptor-bound cyclic AMP and steroidogenesis. Therefore, they dismissed cyclic GMP as a primary second messenger in the adrenal cortex. In the intervening years, the role of cyclic guanine nucleotides was being clarified in other hormonal systems. Guanine nucleotides play an important role in the coupling of receptor binding of the hormone and the activation of adenylate cyclase, the enzyme that forms cyclic AMP from ATP (2). The adenylate cyclase complex is made up of at least three components: 1)the hormone receptor; 2) the catalytic unit; and 3) a guanine-nucleotide-binding regulatory unit. The guanine nucleotide involved in the complex is probably GTP rather than cyclic GMP. A role for cyclic GMP has not yet been defined (97). Neither has the guanine nucleotide scheme been unequivocally extended to the adrenal cortex.

The role of cyclic AMP in metabolic control is exerted via the activation of enzymes that phosphorylate other enzymes to either activate or inhibit them. Proof for such a role in the adrenal cortex is not complete, but cyclic-AMP-activated protein kinase activity has been detected in plasma membranes from bovine adrenal glands by Reitherman et al. (106). Moreover, one of the adrenal proteins phosphorylated by such an enzyme is a mitochondrial cytochrome P-450 active in a key reaction in adrenal steroidogenesis (22).

Figure 7 summarizes the current concept of the role of cyclic AMP in adrenal steroidogenesis.

"LABILE PROTEIN"

Because one of the effects of long-term administration of ACTH to an animal is adrenocortical hyperplasia, there were early attempts to find a stimulation of protein synthesis by ACTH. In 1957, Koritz et al. (69) incubated rat adrenal tissue with ^{14}C-glycine with and without ACTH. To their surprise, there was an *inhibition* of incorporation into adrenal proteins in the presence of a large dose of ACTH. The inhibition by ACTH of the incorporation of radioactive amino acid into protein has been amply confirmed by others (e.g., 51).

In 1963 Ferguson (37) reported that the antibiotic, puromycin, added in vitro to rat adrenal tissue, prevented the increase in steroidogenesis after the addition of either ACTH or cyclic AMP. Puromycin is an inhibitor of protein synthesis. However, if ACTH was added to the tissue before puromycin, stimulation did occur. Ferguson suggested that protein syn-

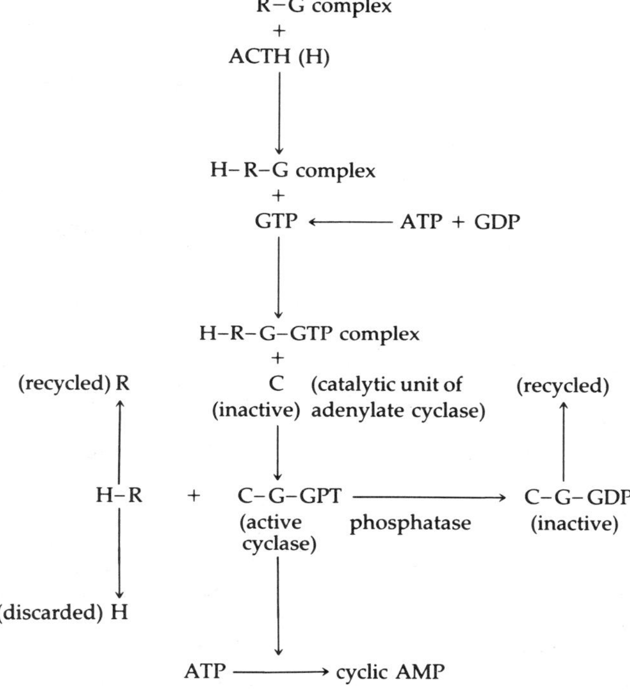

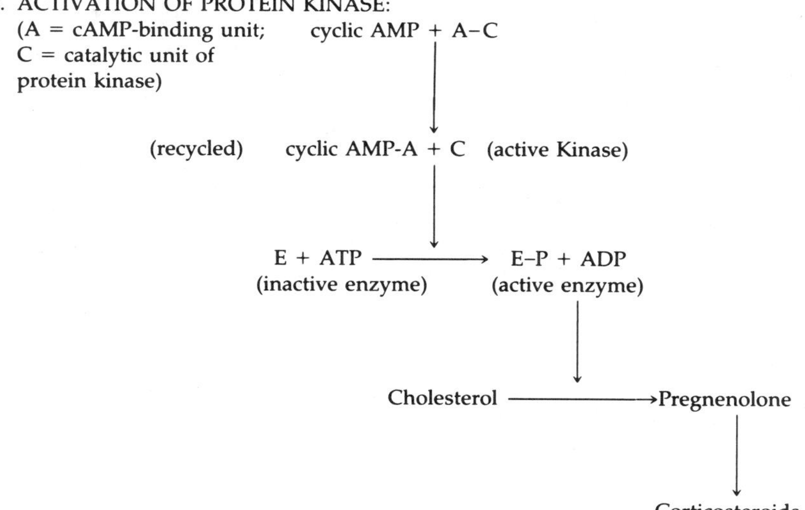

FIGURE 7. Current concept of the role of cyclic AMP in the control of adrenal steroidogenesis. Compare with Figure 6.

thesis was needed as part of the response to a stimulant of steroidogenesis. He then added the antibiotic actinomycin D to adrenal tissues, without any effect on the action of ACTH (38). Actinomycin D is an inhibitor of RNA synthesis. Now the site of action of ACTH was localized to the translation of mRNA into protein, rather than in the synthesis of new RNA on the DNA template. The conclusion was reinforced by experiments in which other inhibitors of translation, notably cycloheximide, reproduced the inhibition caused by puromycin (43).

The difference in steroidogenesis when cycloheximide was added before or after the stimulant (either ACTH or cyclic AMP) was very clearly displayed in an adrenal superfusion system in which the production of corticosterone by rat adrenal tissue was monitored continuously (116). The same system was able to show that the addition of ACTH was followed by a lag period of about 2 minutes before the stimulation of steroidogenesis began (99). The lag period was attributed to the time needed for the synthesis of a protein mediator of steroidogenesis (99). However, Schulster et al. (128) suggested that a protein mediator with a short half-life was continuously synthesized in the adrenal cortical cell, and that secretogogues, like ACTH and cyclic AMP, activated the protein to stimulate steroidogenesis. Their interpretation was based upon consideration of the different modes of action of puromycin and cycloheximide. Puromycin stops protein synthesis by prematurely terminating the growing polypeptide chain, while cycloheximide slows the rate of translation. If the lag time for the stimulation by ACTH represents the time needed to manufacture a new protein, then cycloheximide should increase the lag time by slowing translation, while puromycin should abolish the response to ACTH altogether. Instead, lower doses of both inhibitors increased the lag time. This was interpreted as evidence that both inhibitors decreased the supply of a labile protein, which is activated by ACTH.

An activation step undergone by the labile protein may be phosphorylation (see Figure 7). Cochet et al. (18) and Reitherman et al. (106) have recently examined a variety of protein kinases in the adrenal cortex, both cyclic-AMP-dependent and cyclic-AMP-independent, but none of the kinases nor their substrates has so far been identified with the "labile protein." However, Doherty et al. (25), using cultures of an ACTH-sensitive mouse adrenal tumor cell line, found that cyclic AMP, over the concentration range 10^{-8} to 10^{-6} M, increased protein kinase activity in the cytosol of the cells. The possibility that an enzyme involved in the turnover of polyphosphoinositides is the "labile protein" was explored in 1980 by Farese et al. (36) but not proved, when they found that the turnover was abolished by cycloheximide.

Other adrenocortical proteins may be candidates for the critical "labile protein." One of these is actin. Cheitlin and Ramachandran (16) found that ACTH causes a 20% decrease in the actin content of cultured rat adrenocortical cells. However, the decrease in actin takes place over the course of hours, while the stimulation of steroidogenesis occurs in minutes. Perhaps the actin plays a role in the growth response to ACTH.

WHICH REACTION IN STEROID BIOSYNTHESIS IS STIMULATED?

The early studies by Stone and Hechter (140) of the conversion of isotopic precursors to corticosteroids by perfused bovine adrenal glands showed that the site of action of ACTH was probably located between the precursors, acetate or cholesterol, and the first of the steroid substances formed, pregnenolone (see Chapter 3 by Rapp, this volume). They predicted that the rate-limiting reaction, and therefore the reaction most likely to be controlled, was the conversion of cholesterol to pregnenolone. The same conclusion was reached by many others since, working with other systems, such as adrenal slices or cells (e.g., 64).

The localization of the site of action of ACTH to an area involving cholesterol was not surprising because of the well-characterized depletion of adrenal cholesterol stores by ACTH or by stimuli that provoked the secretion of ACTH (122).

Stimulation of cholesterol→ pregnenolone can theoretically occur as the result of the removal of a substance that inhibits the reaction, as the result of an increase in the availability of a cofactor, by an increase in the activity of the enzyme system, or by an increased availability of cholesterol, or by a combination of two or more of these mechanisms. All of the possibilities have been explored.

We shall examine the first suggestion, that stimulation can occur by removal of an inhibitor. Pregnenolone is a powerful inhibitor of its own formation from cholesterol (67). The conversion occurs in the mitochondria of the adrenocortical cell, and, theoretically, high concentrations of pregnenolone can be formed quickly from cholesterol. A possible mode of action of a stimulant of steroidogenesis would therefore be to facilitate the removal of pregnenolone from the mitochondria (step [1], Figure 8). Such a mechanism was proposed by Koritz (66). Experimental proof of the hypothesis would require that stimulation of steroidogenesis should decrease the pregnenolone content of the mitochondria of the adrenal gland. But the contrary happens. The pregnenolone content of mitochondria from stimulated tissue is higher than the pregnenolone in mitochondria prepared from resting tissue (61).

The conversion of cholesterol to pregnenolone requires NADPH as a cofactor (Figure 6). In broken-cell preparations, in which the concentration of NADPH is reduced by dilution, the addition of NADPH or an NADPH-generating system is needed to boost the rate of the reaction to its maximum (50). However, in the intact cell, the supply of NADPH is not rate-limiting.

Attention has turned recently to the third explanation of the stimulation of steroidogenesis, that the activity of the enzyme system is increased. The possibility that the cholesterol→ pregnenolone enzyme system is activated by phosphorylation has already been mentioned (Figure 7 and discussion). Substantiation of this explanation of the effect of ACTH awaits the unequivocal demonstration that a component of the choles-

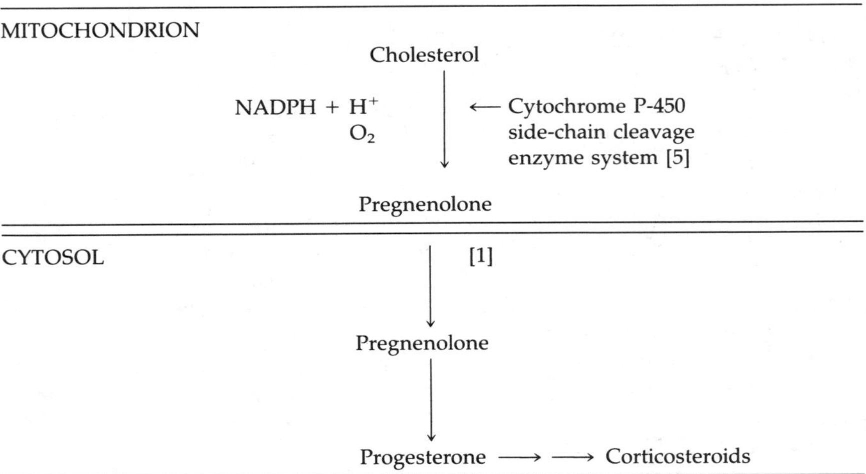

[1]. . . Transport of pregnenolone from mitochondria to cytosol for the next step in steroidogenesis.

FIGURE 8. Pregnenolone transport as a possible site of control of adrenal steroidogenesis.

terol side-chain cleaving enzyme system is indeed activated by phosphorylation by a cyclic-AMP-dependent kinase.

The rate of conversion of cholesterol to pregnenolone may be dependent upon the rate of movement of cholesterol into the mitochondria, where the converting enzyme system is located (Figure 9, steps [4] and [5]). Cholesterol is available internally in adrenocortical cells in the form of intracellular droplets of cholesterol esters [7] and externally as lipoprotein cholesterol [6] in the blood plasma. In either case, cholesterol must be freed from its companions, either carrier apoproteins or fatty acids, and transported across one or two membrane barriers into the mitochondria. It is conceivable that the mobilization (step [3]) and/or transport of cholesterol (step [2]) is under control of ACTH. Nakamura et al. (118) recently reported that the mouse adrenal tumor cell line, Y-1, treated with aminoglutethimide or incubated anaerobically to prevent the conversion of cholesterol to pregnenolone, responded to incubation with either ACTH or dibutyryl cyclic AMP with an increase in the cholesterol content of the inner mitochondrial membrane. The inhibition of the side-chain cleavage of cholesterol was necessary to demonstrate the accumulation of cholesterol.

Pretreatment of rats with aminoglutethimide was used by Farese et al. (32) to show that not only does ACTH increase the amount of cholesterol in lipid particles in the adrenal cortex, but ACTH also increases the formation of pregnenolone from cholesterol.

If stores of intraadrenal cholesterol are in the form of droplets of cholesterol esters, then another way in which ACTH can enhance the availability of cholesterol is to accelerate the hydrolysis of the esters to fatty acids and free cholesterol (Figure 9, step [3]). In 1965, Macho and

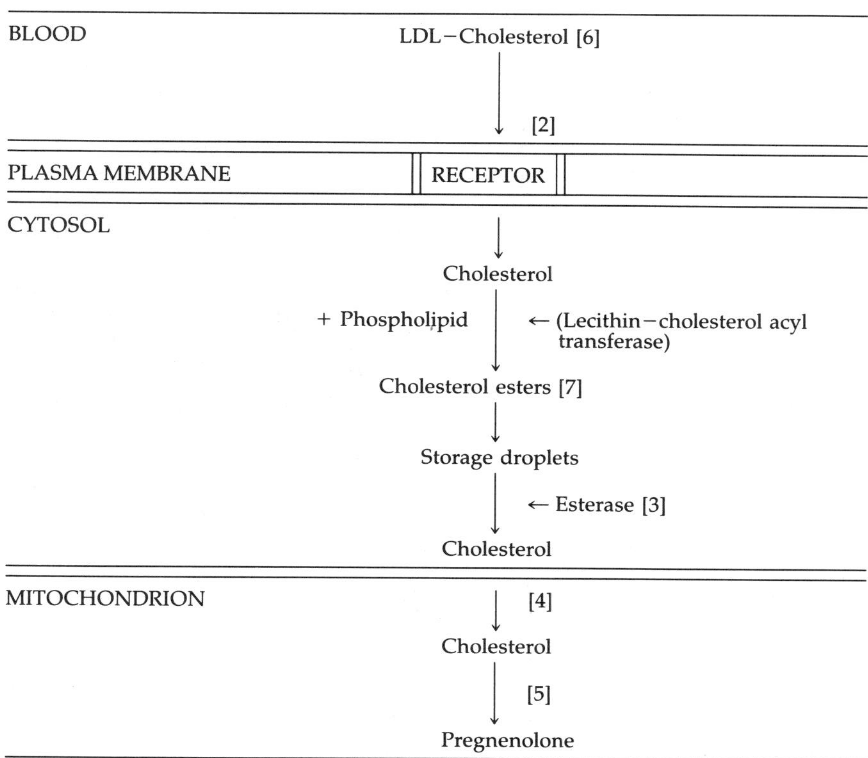

[2]. . . Binding of LDL–cholesterol by surface receptor
[3]. . . Hydrolysis of stored cholesterol esters
[4]. . . Cholesterol transport into mitochondrion
[5]. . . Side-chain cleavage, inhibited by aminoglutethimide

FIGURE 9. Cholesterol transport as a possible site of control of adrenal steroidogenesis by ACTH and cyclic AMP.

Palkovic (83) reported that ACTH increased the activity of rat adrenal lipase, both in vivo and in vitro. Moreover, ACTH stimulated the release of fatty acids from adrenal tissue in vitro (84). The same or a similar lipase is responsible for the hydrolysis of cholesterol esters (20).

In Stone and Hechter's classical experiments on adrenal steroidogenesis in the perfused bovine adrenal gland (140), they used ^{14}C-labeled acetate as a precursor of the corticosteroids. They observed incorporation of the isotope into cortisol and enhanced incorporation when the gland was stimulated by ACTH. In bovine and porcine adrenal slices, Haynes et al. (57) found that ACTH doubled the incorporation of labeled acetate into cortisol. Acetate is a common precursor to cholesterol and cortisol; according to the usual scheme of steroid biosynthesis, acetate carbons would pass through cholesterol to the corticosteroids (see Ch. 3, this volume). Mevalonic acid is an intermediate in the conversion of acetate to cholesterol. Isolated rat adrenal cells incorporated isotope from ^{3}H-labeled mevalonic acid equally into both corticosterone and cholesterol only when stimulated with ACTH. In the absence of ACTH, no isotope was incorporated into either corticosterone or cholesterol (122). The incorporation of isotope into corticosterone was stopped by the addition of cycloheximide, but not the incorporation into cholesterol. In the same paper, the authors found that 4-^{14}C-cholesterol was traced to corticosterone at the same rate in the absence and presence of ACTH. These results seem to imply that corticosterone biosynthesis can take place by a pathway independent of that to cholesterol, but parallel to it. Moreover, stimulation by ACTH occurs in both pathways. If ACTH stimulates the synthesis of cholesterol from mevalonic acid or "acetate," then the accumulation of extra cholesterol when ACTH is added in the presence of aminoglutethimide can be explained on the basis of Figure 10.

ASCORBIC ACID

The purification of ACTH was made possible by the application of an accurate bioassay for ACTH based upon the depletion of ascorbic acid in the adrenals of hypophysectomized rats (125). The adrenal glands were known to contain higher concentrations of ascorbic acid than any other tissue (46). When Sayers et al. (123) were studying the depletion of

FIGURE 10. Cholesterol synthesis as a possible site of control of adrenal steroidogenesis.

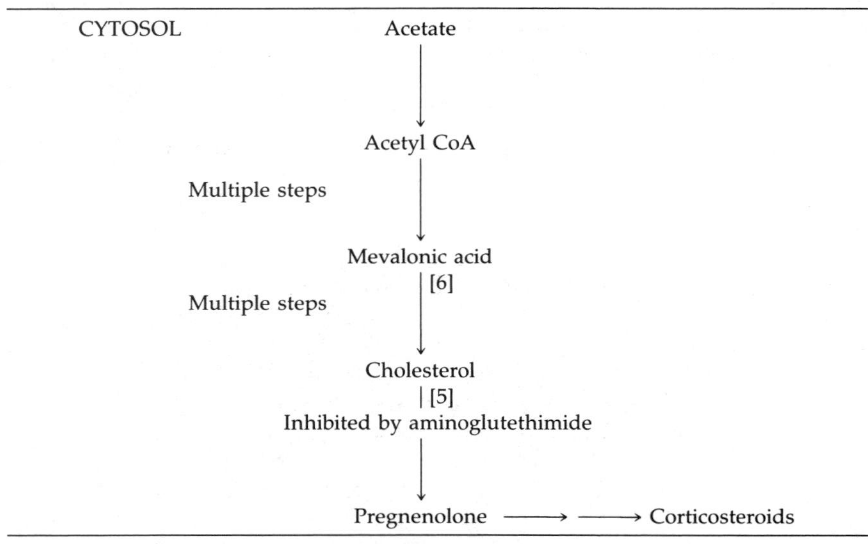

[5]. . . Side-chain cleavage enzyme (Fig. 8)
[6]. . . De novo synthesis of cholesterol

cholesterol ester stores in the rat adrenal by ACTH, they chose ascorbic acid as a "control" adrenal substance. To their surprise, adrenal ascorbic acid was also depleted, even more quickly than the adrenal cholesterol. The phenomenon was quickly converted into the bioassay (125). The Sayers adrenal ascorbic acid depletion assay for ACTH was for many years the official and universal assay for ACTH, yet the role of ascorbic acid in the response to ACTH was unknown, and remains unknown to this day.

Because ascorbic acid is a strong reducing agent, it seemed logical to assign to it the role of a source of reducing equivalents for the hydroxylations occurring in steroidogenesis (see chapter 3 by Rapp, this volume). Staudinger and his colleagues (65) observed that the addition of ascorbic acid to adrenal homogenates stimulated corticoid formation, especially after exposure of the incubation mixture to ultraviolet light. Steroidogenesis in adrenal homogenates is inhibited by dilution of the cellular contents, and restored by the addition of NADPH-generating systems. Apparently ascorbic acid can also serve to restore the reducing activity of homogenates.

The addition of ACTH in vitro to adrenal tissue resulted in relatively little depletion of ascorbic acid (113). This was attributed to the extremely quick loss of ascorbic acid from the tissue into the incubation medium. A portion of the ascorbic acid remained associated with the tissue and could not be discharged. This agreed with the observations in vivo in which a maximum of about 25% of the ascorbic acid was depleted (123).

When ^{14}C-labeled ascorbic acid became available, Johnstone et al. (1963 et seq.) found that ascorbic acid was transported *into* adrenal cells by an energy-requiring sodium-dependent system (132,133,23,17). ACTH inhibited the transport into the cells, resulting in a net loss of ascorbic acid from the tissue. The inhibition of transport was attributed to the corticosterone that was formed by the rat adrenals in response to ACTH. The action of ACTH could be mimicked by exposure of the tissue to corticosterone (133).

The existence of two pools of ascorbic acid in bovine adrenal cells was recently postulated by Finn and Johns (39). The transport of ascorbate into the cell seems to be mediated by a saturable carrier; the transport requires calcium.

The presence of such high concentrations of ascorbate in the adrenocortical cells, coupled with the sensitivity of the concentration to ACTH and corticosteroid makes it difficult to dismiss ascorbic acid as an accidental component of the cell. Adrenal ascorbic acid remains as a tempting target for research.

FEEDBACK CONTROL

One of the first hypotheses suggested for control of the release of ACTH in response to stress involved negative feedback control of ACTH secretion by the level of corticosteroids in the blood. This hypothesis, eloquently defended by Sayers in 1951 (121), was based upon the observation that adrenalectomy resulted in an immediate and large increase in the secretion of ACTH by the pituitary gland. According to the hypothesis, stress would cause the peripheral tissues to "utilize" corticosteroids at a more rapid rate, resulting in a fall in the blood levels of corticosteroids. The pituitary gland would then respond to the decreased blood level by secreting more ACTH. However, critics soon pointed out that in chronic stress the levels of both corticosteroids and ACTH are high. Then Sayers demolished his own hypothesis by showing that the imposition of stress to an adrenalectomized animal drove the high levels of circulating ACTH even higher (143). Therefore, control of ACTH secretion was possible without involvement of the adrenal gland.

Nevertheless, administration of corticosteroids *did* decrease the secretion of ACTH. The very potent artificial corticosteroids are very powerful suppressors of the secretion of ACTH. The *dexamethasone suppression test* is a very useful tool in the differential diagnosis of diseases of the pituitary–adrenal system (78). All components of the hypothalamo–pituitary–adrenal system are targets for the corticosteroids in feedback inhibition.

Birmingham and Kurlents showed in 1958 (7) that corticosteroids, added to rat adrenal tissue in vitro, suppressed the formation of corticosterone. This observation has been confirmed by others (102,13). The mechanisms of the inhibition are still uncertain, although Morrow et al. (1967) showed that adrenal protein synthesis is inhibited by corticosteroids in vitro (94).

The physiological significance of auto-feedback inhibition of steroidogenesis by corticosteroids added in vitro to adrenal tissue is doubtful because the experimental conditions do not duplicate conditions in vivo in which the adrenocortical products are continually washed away by the circulation. The effective concentrations, about 10^{-5}M, are beyond the physiological or pharmacological limits.

The anterior pituitary gland is a more likely physiological site of feedback control of ACTH secretion by corticosteroids. The definitive experiment awaited the availability of pure CRF. Donald et al. (26) in vivo in sheep and Vale et al. (145), in vitro using cultured isolated rat pituitary cells, found that the sensitivity of the pituitary gland to CRF was diminished by corticosteroids in a dose-dependent manner. Feedback inhibition may occur between the binding of CRF by receptors on the pituitary cell and the stimulation of formation of cyclic AMP (110). Although most evidence points to an acute effect of corticosteroids on the *release* of ACTH from stores in the pituitary, there is evidence that corticosteroids also inhibit the *synthesis* of ACTH by interfering with the formation of the mRNA for proopiomelanocortin, the precursor of ACTH (126).

Sites of feedback control by corticosteroids may exist in the hypothalamus (63) and other parts of the CNS. In addition, there may be so-called "short-loop" feedback inhibition by ACTH on its own production at the pituitary, hypothalamic or other CNS levels. CRF may also participate in feedback inhibition. However, these possibilities are not nearly as well documented as the feedback by corticosteroids and will not be considered here.

SUMMARY

Control of the hypothalamo–pituitary–adrenocortical system is complex and subject to modification at multiple levels. While major strides have been made in its understanding, the control mechanism contains significant areas of unknown that are fruitful targets for research.

REFERENCES

1. Aguilera, G., Harwood, J.P., Wilson, J.X., Morell, J., Brown, J. H., and Catt, K.J. (1983) Mechanisms of action of corticotropin-releasing factor and other regulators of corticotropin release in rat pituitary cells. J. Biol. Chem. 258, 8039–8045.
2. Aurbach, G.D. (1982) Polypeptide and amine hormone regulation of adenylate cyclase. Ann. Rev. Physiol. 44, 653–666.
3. Banschbach, M.W., Geison, R.L., and Hokin-Neaverson, M. (1974) Acetylcholine increases the level of diglyceride in mouse pancreas. Biochem. Biophys. Res. Commun. 58, 714–718.
4. Bell, P.H. (1954) Purification and structure of B-corticotropin. J. Am. Chem. Soc. 76, 5565–5567.
5. Bergstrom, S., Danielsson, H., and Samuelsson, B. (1964) The enzymatic formation of prostaglandin E_2 from arachidonic acid. Biochim. Biophys. Acta 90, 207–210.
6. Birmingham, M.K., Elliott, F.H., and Valere, P.H.L. (1953) The need for the presence of calcium for the stimulation in vitro of rat adrenal glands by adrenocorticotrophic hormone. Endocrinology 53, 687–689.
7. Birmingham, M.K., and Kurlents, E. (1958) Inactivation of ACTH by isolated rat adrenals and inhibition of corticoid formation by adrenocortical hormones. Endocrinology 62, 47–60.
8. Birmingham, M.K., Kurlents, E., Lane, R., Muhlstock, B., and Traikov, H. (1960) Effects of calcium on the potassium and sodium content of rat adrenal glands, on the stimulation of steroid production by adenosine 3′,5′-monophosphate, and on the response of the adrenal to short contact with ACTH. Can. J. Biochem. Physiol. 38, 1078–1085.
9. Buckley, D.I., Hagman, J., Ramachandran, J. (1981) A sensitive radioimmunoassay for corticotropin using a fully biologically active ^{125}I-labeled ligand. Endocrinology 109, 10–16.
10. Buckley, D.I., and Ramachandran, J. (1981) Characterization of corticotropin receptors on adrenocortical cells. Proc. Natl. Acad. U.S.A. 78, 7431–7334.
11. Buckley, D.I., Yamashiro, D., and Ramachandran, J. (1981) Synthesis of a corticotropin analog that retains full biological activity after iodination. Endocrinology 109, 5–9.
12. Carlson, D.E., Dornhorst, A., Seif, S.M., Robinson, A.G., and Gann, D.S. (1982) Vasopressin-dependent and -independent control of the release of adrenocorticotropin. Endocrinology 110, 680–682.
13. Carsia, R.V., and Malamed, S. (1979) Acute self-suppression of corticosteroidogenesis in isolated adrenocortical cells. Endocrinology 105, 911–914.
14. Carsia, R.V., Moyle, W.R., Wolff, D.J., and Malamed, S. (1982) Acute inhibition of corticosteroidogenesis by inhibitors of calmodulin action. Endocrinology 111, 1456–1461.
15. Cheitlin, R., Buckley, D.I., and Ramachandran, J. (1983) Calcium is required for the binding of ACTH to receptors on adrenocortical cells. Proc. Endocrinol. Soc. 1983, p. 273 (Abs).
16. Cheitlin, R., and Ramachandran, J. (1981) Regulation of actin in rat adrenocortical cells by corticotropin. J. Biol. Chem. 256, 3156–3158.
17. Clayman, M., Tsang, D., deNicola, A.F., and Johnstone, R.M. (1970) Specificity of action of adrenocorticotrophin in vitro on ascorbate transport in rat adrenal glands. Biochem. J. 118, 283–289.

18. Cochet, C., Job, D., Pirollet, F., and Chambaz, E.M. (1980) Adenosine 3′,5′-monophosphate-independent protein kinase activities in the bovine adrenal cortex cytosol. Endocrinology 106, 750–757.
19. Collip, J.B., Anderson, E.M., and Thomson, D.L. (1933) The adrenotropic hormone of the anterior pituitary lobe. Lancet 2, 347–348.
20. Cook, K.G., Lee, F.-T., and Yeaman, S.J. (1981) Hormone-sensitive cholesterol ester hydrolase of bovine adrenal cortex. Identification of the enzyme protein. FEBS Lett. 132, 10–14.
21. Cook, W.H., Lipkin, D., and Markham, R. (1957) Formation of a cyclic dianhydrodiadenylic acid by the alkaline degradation of adenosine-5′-triphosphoric acid. J. Am. Chem. Soc. 79, 3607–3608.
22. Defaye, G., Monnier, N., Guidicelli, C., and Chambaz, E.M. (1982) Phosphorylation of purified mitochondrial cytochromes P-450 (cholesterol desmolase and 11B-hydroxylase) from bovine adrenal cortex. Mol. Cell. Endocrinol. 27, 157–168.
23. deNicola, A.F., Clayman, M., and Johnstone, R.M. (1968) Hormonal control of ascorbic acid transport in rat adrenal glands. Endocrinology 82, 436–446.
24. de Wied, D. (1957) The effect of autonomic blockade on the release of corticotrophin from the hypophysis, as induced by a hypothalamus extract. Acta Endocrinol. 24, 200–208.
25. Doherty, P.J., Tsao, J., Schirmmer, B.P., Mumby, M.C., and Beavo, J.A. (1981) cAMP-dependent protein kinase and regulation of adrenocortical functions: A genetic evaluation. In: O.M. Rosen and E.G. Krebs (Eds.), Protein Phosphorylation, Book A, Cold Spring Harbor Conferences on Cell Proliferation, Vol. 8. Cold Spring Harbor Laboratory, Cold Spring, NY, pp. 211–225.
26. Donald, R.A., Redekopp, C., Cameron, V., Nicholls, M.G., Bolton, J., Livesey, J., Espiner, E.A., Rivier, J., and Vale, W. (1983) The hormonal actions of corticotropin-releasing factor in sheep: Effect of intravenous and intracerebroventricular injection. Endocrinology 113, 866–870.
27. Eipper, B.A., Mains, R.E., and Guenzi, D. (1976) High molecular weight forms of adrenocorticotropic hormone are glycoproteins. J. Biol. Chem. 251, 1421–1426.
28. Ellis, E.F., Shen, J.C., Schrey, M.P., Carchman, R.A., and Rubin, R.P. (1978) Prostacyclin: A potent stimulator of adrenal steroidogenesis. Prostaglandins 16, 483–490.
29. Farese, R.V., Bidot-Lopez, P., Sabir, M.A., and Larson, R.E. (1981) The phosphatidate-polyphosphoinositide cycle: Activation by parathyroid hormone and dibutyryl-cAMP in rabbit kidney cortex. Ann. N.Y. Acad. Sci. 372, 539–551.
30. Farese, R.V., and Prudente, W.J. (1977) Localization of the metabolic processes affected by calcium during corticotropin action. Biochim. Biophys. Acta 497, 386–395.
31. Farese, R.V., and Prudente, W.J. (1978) On the role of calcium in adrenocorticotropin-induced changes in mitochondrial pregnenolone synthesis. Endocrinology 103, 1264–1271.
32. Farese, R.V., Prudente, W. J., and Chuang, L.T. (1980) Non-esterified cholesterol-rich adrenal lipid fractions. Preparation, properties and preferential utilization for cholesterol side-chain cleavage by corticotropin-stimulated adrenal mitochondria. Biochem. J. 186, 145–152.
33. Farese, R.V., and Sabir, A.M. (1979) Polyphosphorylated glycerolipids mimic adrenocorticotropin-induced stimulation of mitochondrial pregnenolone synthesis. Biochim. Biophys. Acta 575, 299–304.
34. Farese, R.V., and Sabir, A.M. (1980) Polyphosphoinositides: Stimulator of mitochondrial cholesterol side chain cleavage and possible identification as an adrenocorticotropin-induced, cycloheximide-sensitive, cytosolic steroidogenic factor. Endocrinology 106, 1869–1879.
35. Farese, R.V., Sabir, M.A., and Larson, R.E. (1981) Adrenocorticotropin and adenosine 3′,5′-monophosphate stimulate de novo synthesis of adrenal phosphatidic acid by a cycloheximide-sensitive, Ca^{++}-dependent mechanism. Endocrinology 109, 1895–1901.

36. Farese, R.V., Sabir, A.M., Vandor, S.L., and Larson, R.E. (1980) Are polyphosphoinositides the cycloheximide-sensitive mediator in the steroidogenic actions of adrenocorticotropin and adenosine-3′,5′-monophosphate? J. Biol. Chem. 255, 5728–5734.
37. Ferguson, J.J., Jr. (1963) Protein synthesis and adrenocorticotropin responsiveness. J. Biol. Chem. 238, 2754–2759.
38. Ferguson, J.J., Jr., and Morita, Y. (1964) RNA synthesis and adrenocorticotrophic responsiveness. Biochim. Biophys. Acta 87, 348–350.
39. Finn, F.M., and Johns, P.A. (1980) Ascorbic acid transport by isolated bovine adrenal cortical cells. Endocrinology 106, 811–817.
40. Finn, F.M., Widnell, C.C., and Hofmann, K. (1972) Localization of an adrenocorticotropic hormone receptor on bovine adrenal cortical membranes. J. Biol. Chem. 247, 5695–5702.
41. Fortier, C. (1951) Dual control of ACTH release. Endocrinology 49, 782–788.
42. Furutani, Y., Morimoto, Y., Shibahara, S., Noda, M., Takahashi, H., Hirose, T., Asai, M., Inayama, S., Hayashida, H., Miyata, I., and Numa, S. (1983) Cloning and sequence analysis of cDNA for ovine corticotropin-releasing factor precursor. Nature 301, 537–540.
43. Garren, L.D., Ney, R.L., and Davis, W.W. (1965) Studies on the role of protein synthesis in the regulation of corticosterone production by adrenocorticotrophic hormone in vivo. Proc. Natl. Acad. Sci. U.S.A. 53, 1443–1450.
44. Giguere, V., and Labrie, F. (1982) Vasopressin potentiates cyclic AMP accumulation and ACTH release induced by corticotropin-releasing factor (CRF) in rat anterior pituitary cells in culture. Endocrinology 111, 1752–1754.
45. Gillies, G., and Lowry, P. (1979) Corticotrophin releasing factor may be modulated vasopressin. Nature 278, 463–464.
46. Giroud, A., Leblond, C.P., Ratismamanga, R., and Gero, E. (1938) Le taux normal en acide ascorbique. Bull. Soc. Chim. Biol. 20, 1079–1087.
47. Guillemin, R., and Rosenberg, B. (1955) Humoral hypothalamic control of anterior pituitary: A study with combined tissue cultures. Endocrinology 57, 599–607.
48. Guillemin, R., Schally, A.V., Lipscomb, H.S., Anderson, R.N., and Long, J.M. (1962) On the presence in hog hypothalamus of beta-corticotropin releasing factor, alpha- and beta-melanocyte stimulating hormones, adrenocorticotropin, lysine-vasopressin and oxytocin. Endocrinology 70, 471–477.
49. Guillemin, R., Vargo, R., Rossier, J., Minick, S., Ling, N., Rivier, C., Vale, W., and Bloom, F. (1977) Beta-endorphin and adrenocorticotropin are secreted concomitantly by the pituitary gland. Science 197, 1367–1369.
50. Halkerston, I.D.K., Eichhorn, J., and Hechter, O. (1961) A requirement for reduced triphosphopyridine nucleotide for cholesterol side-chain cleavage by mitochondrial fractions of bovine adrenal cortex. J. Biol. Chem. 236, 374–380.
51. Halkerston, I.D.K., Feinstein, M., and Hechter, O. (1965) Further observations on the inhibition of adrenal protein synthesis by ACTH in vitro. Endocrinology 76, 801–802.
52. Harris, G.W. (1955) Neural Control of The Pituitary Gland. Edward Arnold, London.
53. Harris, J.I. (1959) Structure of a melanocyte-stimulating hormone from the human pituitary gland. Nature (Lond.) 184, 167–169.
54. Haynes, R.C., Jr. (1958) The activation of adrenal phosphorylase by the adrenocorticotrophic hormone. J. Biol. Chem. 233, 1220–1222.
55. Haynes, R.C., Jr., and Berthet, L. (1957) Studies on the mechanism of action of the adrenocorticotrophic hormone. J. Biol. Chem. 225, 115–124.
56. Haynes, R.C., Jr., Koritz, S.B., and Peron, F.G. (1959) Influence of adenosine 3′,5′-monophosphate on corticoid production by rat adrenal glands. J. Biol. Chem. 234, 1421–1423.
57. Haynes, R., Savard, K., and Dorfman, R.I. (1952) An action of ACTH on adrenal slices. Science 116, 690–691.

58. Haynes, R.C., Jr., Sutherland, E.W., and Rall, T.W. (1960) The role of cyclic adenylic acid in hormone action. Rec. Prog. Hormone Res. 16, 121–138.

59. Hokin, L.E., and Hokin, M.R. (1953) Enzyme secretion and the incorporation of P^{32} into phospholipides of pancreas slices. J. Biol. Chem. 203, 967–977.

60. Hokin, M.R., Hokin, L.E., Saffran, M., Schally, A.V., and Zimmerman, B.U. (1958) Phospholipides and the secretion of adrenocorticotropin and of corticoids. J. Biol. Chem. 233, 811–813.

61. Holzbauer, M. (1981) Effect of ACTH on the subcellular distribution of steroids in the adrenal gland. J. Steroid Biochem. 14, 1189–1195.

62. Hughes, J., Smith, T.W., Kosterlitz, H.W., Fothergill, L.A., Morgan, B.A., and Morris, H.R. (1975) Identification of two related pentapeptides in brain with potent opiate agonist activity. Nature (Lond.) 258, 577–579.

63. Jones, M.T., Hillhouse, E.W., and Burden, J.L. (1977) Structure-activity relationships of corticosteroid feedback at the hypothalamic level. J. Endocrinol. 74, 415–424.

64. Karaboyas, G.C., and Koritz, S.B. (1965) Identity of the site of action of 3′,5′-adenosine monophosphate and adrenocorticotropic hormone in corticosteroidogenesis in rat adrenal and beef adrenal cortex slices. Biochemistry 4, 462–468.

65. Kersten, H., Kersten, W., and Staudinger, H.J. (1955) Stoffwechsel der Nebennierenrinde und Biosynthese der Corticosteroide. IX. Mitteilung. Weiterer Beitrag zum Mechanismus der Ascorbinsaurewirkung. Biochem. Z. 327, 284–291.

66. Koritz, S.B. (1968) On the regulation of pregnenolone synthesis. In: K.W. McKerns (ed.), Functions of the Adrenal Cortex, Vol. 1, Appleton-Century-Crofts, New York, pp. 27–48.

67. Koritz, S.B., and Hall, P.F. (1964) End-product inhibition of the conversion of cholesterol to pregnenolone in an adrenal extract. Biochemistry 3, 1298-1304.

68. Koritz, S.B., and Peron, F.F. (1959) The stimulation in vitro by Ca^{++}, freezing, and proteolysis of corticoid production by rat adrenal tissue. J. Biol. Chem. 234, 3122–3128.

69. Koritz, S.B., Peron, F.G., and Dorfman, R.I. (1957) Influence of adrenocorticotropic hormone on corticoid production and glycine-1-C^{14} incorporation into protein by rat adrenals. J. Biol. Chem. 226, 643–650.

70. Kruskemper, H.L., and Reichertz, P. (1959) Andrungen des Elektrogramms der Nebennieren nach intravenoser Injektion von Corticotrophin. Acta Endocr. (Copenh.) 30, 197–204.

71. Lefkowitz, R.J., Roth, J., and Pastan, I. (1971) ACTH-receptor interaction in the adrenal: A model for the initial step in the action of hormones that stimulate adenyl cyclase. Ann. N.Y. Acad. Sci. 185, 195–207.

72. Lefkowitz, R.J., Roth, J., Pricer, W., and Pastan, I. (1970) ACTH receptors in the adrenal: Specific binding of ACTH-^{125}I and its relation to adenyl cyclase. Proc. Natl. Acad. Sci. U.S.A. 65, 745–752.

73. Leier, D.J., and Jungman, R.A. (1973) Adrenocorticotropic hormone and dibutyryl–adenosine–cyclic monophosphate–mediated Ca^{2+} uptake by rat adrenal glands. Biochim. Biophys. Acta 329, 196–210.

74. Li, C.H., Barnafi, L., Chretien, M., and Chung, D. (1965) Isolation and amino acid sequence of beta-LPH from sheep pituitary glands. Nature (Lond.) 208, 1093–1094.

75. Li, C.H., and Chung, D. (1976) Isolation and structure of an untriakontapeptide with opiate activity from camel pituitary gland. Proc. Natl. Acad. Sci. U.S.A. 73, 1145–1148.

76. Li, C.H., Evans, H.M., and Simpson, M.E. (1943) Adrenocorticotropic hormone. J. Biol. Chem., 149, 413–424.

77. Li, C.H., Geschwind, I.I., Cole, R.D., Raacke, I.D., Harris, J.I., and Dixon, J.S. (1955) Amino-acid sequence of alpha-corticotropin. Nature 176, 687–689.

78. Liddle, G.W. (1960) Test of pituitary–adrenal suppressibility in the diagnosis of Cushing's syndrome. J. Clin. Endocrinol. 20, 1539–1560.

79. Long, C.N.H. (1952) Regulation of ACTH Secretion. Rec. Prog. in Horm. Res. 7, 75–97.

80. Lymangrover, J.R., Matthews, E.K., and Saffran, M. (1982) Membrane potential changes of mouse adrenal zona fasciculata cells in response to adrenocorticotropin and adenosine 3′,5′-monophosphate. Endocrinology 110, 462–468.
81. Lymangrover, J.R., Pearlmutter, A.F., Franco-Saenz, R., and Saffran, M. (1975) Transmembrane potentials and steroidogenesis in normal and neoplastic human adrenocortical tissue. 41, 697–706.
82. Lymangrover, J.R., Saffran, M., and Matthews, E.K. (1978) Developmental changes in rat adrenocortical membrane potential. Mechanisms Ageing Develop. 8, 377–382.
83. Macho, L., and Palkovic, M. (1965) The effect of corticotropin hormone on lipolytic activity in the adrenal glands of the rat. Physiol. Bohemoslov. 14, 563–565.
84. Macho, L., and Saffran, M. (1967) Metabolism of fatty acids in the rat adrenal gland. Endocrinology 81, 179–185.
85. Makara, G.B., Stark, E., Rappay, G., Karteszi, M., Kiss, J.Z., Antoni, F.A., and Palkovits, M. (1982) The hypothalamic path of corticoliberin (CRF) containing fibres in central nervous organization and the endocrine motor system. In: A.J. Baertschi and J.J. Dreifuss (eds.), Neuroendocrinology of Vasopressin, Corticoliberin and Opiomelanocortins, Academic Press, New York, pp. 107–115.
86. Martini, L., and Morpurgo, C. (1955) Neurohumoral control of the release of adrenocorticotrophic hormone. Nature 175, 1127–1128.
87. Matthews, E.K., and Saffran, M. (1967) Steroid production and membrane potential measurement in cells of the adrenal cortex. J. Physiol. (Lond.) 189, 149-161.
88. Matthews, E.K., and Saffran, M. (1968) Effect of ACTH on the electrical properties of adrenocortical cells. Nature (Lond.) 219, 1369–1370.
89. Matthews, E.K., and Saffran, M. (1973) Ionic dependence of adrenal steroidogenesis and ACTH-induced changes in the membrane potential of adrenocortical cells. J. Physiol. (Lond.) 234, 43–64.
90. McIlhinney, R.A.J., and Schulster, D. (1975) Studies on the binding of ^{125}I-labelled corticotrophin to isolated rat adrenocortical cells. J. Endocrinol. 64, 175–184.
91. Means, A.R., and Dedman, J.R. (1980) Calmodulin in endocrine cells and its multiple roles in hormone action. Mol. Cell. Endocrinol. 19, 215–227.
92. Mirsky, I.A., Stein, M., and Paulisch, G. (1954) The secretion of an antidiuretic substance into the circulation of rats exposed to noxious stimuli. Endocrinology 54, 491–505.
93. Mormede, P. (1983) The vasopressin receptor antagonist, dPTyr(Me)AVP, does not prevent stress-induced ACTH and corticosterone release. Nature (Lond.) 302, 345–346.
94. Morrow, L.B., Burrow, G.N., and Mulrow, P.J. (1967) Inhibition of adrenal protein synthesis by steroids in vitro. Endocrinology 80, 883–888.
95. Nagareda, C.S., and Gaunt, R. (1951) Functional relationship between the adrenal cortex and posterior pituitary. Endocrinology 48, 560–567.
96. Nakanishi, S., Kita, T., Nakamura, M., Chang, C.Y., Cohen, S.N., and Numa, S. (1979) Nucleotide sequence of cloned cDNA, for bovine corticotropin–beta-lipotropin precursor. Nature (Lond.) 278, 423–427.
97. Nambi, P., and Sharma, R.K. (1981) Adrenocorticotropic hormone-responsive guanylate cyclase in the particulate fraction of rat adrenal glands. Endocrinology 108, 2025–2027.
98. Noble, N.L., and Papageorge, E. (1955) Loss of adrenal glycogen in the rat following stress or treatment with various hormones. Endocrinology 57, 492–497.
99. Pearlmutter, A.F., Rapino, E., and Saffran, M. (1973) Comparison of steroidogenic effects of cAMP and dbcAMP in the rat adrenal gland. Endocrinology 92, 679–686.
100. Pedersen, R.C., Brownie, A.C., and Ling, N. (1980) Pro-adrenocorticotropin/endorphin-derived peptides: Coordinate action on adrenal steroidogenesis. Science 208, 1044–1046.
101. Peron, F.F., and Koritz, S.B. (1958) On the exogenous requirements for the action of ACTH in vitro on rat adrenal glands. J. Biol. Chem. 233, 256–259.
102. Peron, F.G., Moncloa, F., and Dorfman, R.I. (1960) Studies on the possible inhibitory

effect of corticosterone on corticosteroidogenesis at the adrenal level in the rat. Endocrinology 67, 379–388.

103. Ramachandran, J., Hagman, J., and Muramoto, K. (1981) Persistent activation of steroidogenesis in adrenocortical cells by photoaffinity labeling of corticotropin receptors. J. Biol. Chem. 256, 11424–11427.

104. Ramwell, P.W., Shaw, J.E., Douglas, W.W., et al. (1964) Efflux of prostaglandins from adrenal glands stimulated with acetylcholine. Nature 210, 273–274.

105. Reiss, M., Brummel, E., Halkerston, I.D.K., Badrick, F.E., and Fenwick, M. (1953) The in vitro action of ACTH on the oxygen consumption of slices of cattle adrenal cortex. J. Endocrinol. 9, 379–390.

106. Reitherman, R., Chen, L., Wen, S., and Harding, B.W. (1981) Adenosine 3′,5′-monophosphate (cAMP)-binding proteins and cAMP-dependent protein kinases in bovine adrenal cortical cell plasma membrane. Endocrinology 109, 301–306.

107. Rivier, J., Spiess, J., and Vale, W. (1983) Characterization of rat hypothalamic corticotropin-releasing factor. Proc. Natl. Acad. Sci. U.S.A. 80, 4851–4855.

108. Robison, G.A., Butcher, R.W., and Sutherland, E.W. (1971) Cyclic AMP. Academic Press, New York, pp 317–337.

109. Rochefort, G.J., and Saffran, M. (1957) Distribution of adrenocorticotrophic hormone in the adrenal gland. Can. J. Biochem. Physiol. 35, 471–480.

110. Rose, J.C., and Conklin, P.M. (1978) TSH and ACTH secretion and cyclic adenosine 3′5′ monophosphate content following stimulation with TRH or lysine vasopressin in vitro: Suppression by thyroxine and dexamethasone. Proc. Soc. Exper. Biol. Med. 158, 524–529.

111. Rubin, R.P., Shen, J.C., and Laychock (1980) Evidence for the mobilization of cellular calcium by prostacyclin in cat adrenocortical cells: the effect of TMB-8. Cell Calcium 1, 391–400.

112. Saffran, M., and Bayliss, M.J. (1953) In vitro bioassay of corticotrophin. Endocrinology 52, 140–148.

113. Saffran, M., Bayliss, M.J., and Webb, J.L. (1951) In vitro studies on adrenal ascorbic acid. Fed. Proc. 10, 116 (Abs.).

114. Saffran, M., and Dokas, L.A. (1983) Sites of nonspecificity in the response of the adrenocortical system to stress. In: H. Selye (ed.) Selye's Guide to Stress Research, Vol. 3, Scientific and Academic Editions, New York, pp. 79–85.

115. Saffran, M., Grad, B., and Bayliss, M.J. (1952) Production of corticoids by rat adrenals in vitro. Endocrinology 50, 639–643.

116. Saffran, M., Matthews, E.K., and Pearlmutter, F. (1971) Analysis of the response to ACTH by rat adrenal in a flowing system. Rec. Progr. Horm. Res. 27, 607–630.

117. Saffran, M., and Schally, A.V. (1955) The release of corticotrophin by anterior pituitary tissue in vitro. Can. J. Biochem. Physiol. 33, 408–415.

118. Saffran, M., and Schally, A.V. (1977) The status of the corticotropin releasing factor (CRF). Neuroendocrinology 24, 359–375.

119. Saffran, M., Schally, A.V., and Benfey, B.G. (1955) Stimulation of the release of corticotropin from the adenohypophysis by a neurohypophysial factor. Endocrinology 57, 439–444.

120. Sala, G.B., Hayashi, K., Catt, K.J., and Dufau, M.L. (1979) Adrenocorticotropin action in isolated adrenal cells. The intermediate role of cyclic AMP in stimulation of corticosterone synthesis. J. Biol. Chem. 254, 3861–3865.

121. Sayers, G. (1951) The adrenal cortex and homeostasis. Physiol. Rev. 30, 241–320.

122. Sayers, G., Sayers, M.A., Fry, E.G., White, A., and Long, C.N.H. (1944) The effect of the adrenotrophic hormone of the anterior pituitary on the cholesterol content of the adrenals, with a review of the literature on adrenal cholesterol. Yale J. Biol. Med. 361–362.

123. Sayers, G., Sayers, M.A., Liang, T.Y., and Long, C.N.H. (1946) Effect of pituitary adrenotrophic hormone on the cholesterol and ascorbic acid content of the adrenal of the rat and guinea pig. Endocrinology 38, 1–9.

124. Sayers, G., White, A., and Long, C.N.H. (1943) Preparation and properties of pituitary adrenotropic hormone. J. Biol. Chem. 149, 425–436.
125. Sayers, M.A., Sayers, G., and Woodbury, L.A. (1948) The assay of adrenocorticotrophic hormone by the adrenal ascorbic acid-depletion method. Endocrinology 42, 379–393.
126. Schachter, S.S., Johnson, L.K., Baxter, J.D., and Roberts, J.L. (1982) Differential regulation by glucocorticoids of proopiomelanocortin mRNA levels in the anterior and intermediate lobes of the rat pituitary. Endocrinology 110, 1442–1444.
127. Schonbaum, E., Birmingham, M.K., and Saffran, M. (1953) Metabolism of glucose and steroid formation by rat adrenals in vitro. Can. J. Biochem. Physiol. 34, 527–533.
128. Schulster, D., Richardson, M.C., and Palfreyman, J.W. (1974) The role of protein synthesis in adrenocorticotrophin action: Effects of cycloheximide and puromycin on the steroidogenic response of isolated adrenocortical cells. Mol. Cell. Endocrinol. 2, 17–29.
129. Seltzman, T.P., Finn, F.M., Widnell, C.C., and Hofmann, K. (1975) Lipids of bovine adrenal plasma membranes. J. Biol. Chem. 250, 1193–1196.
130. Sharma, R.K., Ahmed, N.K., Sutliff, L.S., and Brush, J.S. (1974) Metabolic regulation of steroidogenesis in isolated adrenal cells of the rat. ACTH regulation of cGMP and cAMP levels and steroidogenesis. FEBS Lett. 45, 107–110.
131. Sharma, R.K., Hashimoto, K., and Kitabchi, A.E. (1972) Steroidogenesis in isolated adrenal cells of rat. III. Morphological and biochemical correlation of cholesterol and cholesterol ester content in ACTH and N^6-2′-0-dibutyryl-adenosine-3′,5′-monophosphate activated adrenal cells. Endocrinology 91, 994–1003.
132. Sharma, S.K., Johnstone, R.M., and Quastel, J.H. (1963) Active transport of ascorbic acid in adrenal cortex and brain cortex in vitro and the effects of ACTH and steroids. Can. J. Biochem. Physiol. 41, 597–604.
133. Sharma, S.K., Johnstone, R.M., and Quastel, J.H. (1964) Corticosteroids and ascorbic acid transport in adrenal cortex in vitro. Biochem. J. 92, 565–573.
134. Shepherd, R.G., Wilson, S.D., Howard, K.S., Bell, P.H., Davis, D.S., Davis, S.B., Eigner, E.A., and Shakespeare, N.E. (1956) Studies with corticotropin. III. Determination of the structure of B-corticotropin and its active degradation products. J. Am. Chem. Soc. 78, 5067–5076.
135. Shima, S., Kawashima, Y., Hirai, M., and Asakura, M. (1980) Studies on cyclic nucleotides in the adrenal gland. X. Effects of adrenocorticotropin and prostaglandin on adenyl cyclase activity in the adrenal cortex. Endocrinology 106, 948–951.
136. Slusher, M.A., and Roberts, S. (1954) Fractionation of hypothalamic tissue for pituitary-stimulating activity. Endocrinology 55, 245–254.
137. Sobel, H., Levy, R.S., Marmorston, J., Schapiro, S., and Rosenfeld, S. (1955) Increased excretion of urinary corticoids by guinea pigs following administration of pitressin. Proc. Soc. Exp. Biol. Med. 89, 10–13.
138. Spiess, J., Rivier, J., Rivier, C., and Vale, W. (1981) Primary structure of corticotropin-releasing factor from ovine hypothalamus. Proc. Natl. Acad. Sci. U.S.A. 78, 6517–6521.
139. Steiner, D.F., and Oyer, P.E. (1967) The biosynthesis of insulin and a probable precursor of insulin by a human islet cell adenoma. Proc. Natl. Acad. Sci. U.S.A. 57, 473–480.
140 Stone, D., and Hechter, O. (1954) Studies on ACTH action in perfused bovine adrenals. The site of action of ACTH in corticosteroidogenesis. Arch. Biochem. Biophys. 51, 457–469.
141. Sutherland, E.W., and Rall, T.W. (1957) Properties of an adenine ribonucleotide produced with cellular particles, ATP, Mg^{++}, and epinephrine or glucagon. J. Am. Chem. Soc. 79, 3608.
142. Swartz, S.L., and Williams, G.H. (1983) Role of prostaglandins in adrenal steroidogenesis. Endocrinology 113, 992–996.
143. Sydnor, K.L., and Sayers, G. (1954) Blood and pituitary ACTH in intact and adrenalectomized rats after stress. Endocrinology 55, 621–636.
144. Thomson, M.E., and Hedge, G.A. (1978) Inhibition of corticotropin secretion by hypothalamic administration of indomethacin. Neuroendocrinology 25, 212–220.

145. Vale, W., Vaughan, J., Smith, M., Yamamoto, G., Rivier, J., and Rivier, C. (1983) Effects of synthetic ovine corticotropin-releasing factor, glucocorticoids, catecholamines, neurohypophysial peptides, and other substances on cultured corticotropic cells. Endocrinology 113, 1121–1131.

146. Vale, W., Spiess, J., Rivier, C., and Rivier, J. (1981) Characterization of a 41-residue ovine hypothalamic peptide that stimulates secretion of corticotropin and beta-endorphin. Science 213, 1394–1397.

147. Vogt, M. (1944) Observations on some conditions affecting the rate of hormone output by the suprarenal cortex. J. Physiol. (Lond.) 103, 317–332.

148. Ways, D.K., Zimmerman, C.F., Ontjes, D.A. (1976) Inhibition of adrenocorticotropin effects on adrenal cell membranes by synthetic adrenocorticotropin analogues: Correlation of binding and adenylate cyclase activity. Mol. Pharmacol. 12, 789–799.

149. White, W. F. (1953) Studies on pituitary adrenocorticotropin-A. J. Am. Chem. Soc. 75, 4877–4878.

150. Wolfsen, A.R., McIntyre, H.D., and Odell, W.D. (1972) Adrenocorticotropin measurement by competitive binding receptor assay. Endocrinology 34, 684–689.

S.Y. TAN, M.D.

CONTROL OF ADRENAL SECRETION OF MINERALOCORTICOIDS

From the early studies of Deane et al. (37) emerged the concept that the major steroid secreted by the zona glomerulosa (i.e., aldosterone) was independent of the adenohypophysis but was affected by sodium and potassium intake. It is now recognized that the control of aldosterone secretion is far more complex, although the principal factors are known to include the renin–angiotensin system, K^+, and adrenocorticotrophic hormone (ACTH). Angiotensin II is believed to represent the most potent stimulus for aldosterone production in humans; in other species, however, it may play a less critical role. Alterations in plasma potassium levels constitute an important signal for aldosterone biosynthesis, and ACTH can profoundly affect aldosterone levels when administered acutely. Other factors (e.g., serum sodium), probably play a secondary role in the overall control of aldosterone (Figure 1).

THE RENIN–ANGIOTENSIN SYSTEM

A major physiological regulator of aldosterone secretion is the renin–angiotensin system (29,75,76). Renin is an enzyme synthesized in the

From the University of Hawaii, John A. Burns School of Medicine, Honolulu, Hawaii. Formerly of the Department of Medicine, Medical College of Ohio, Toledo, Ohio.

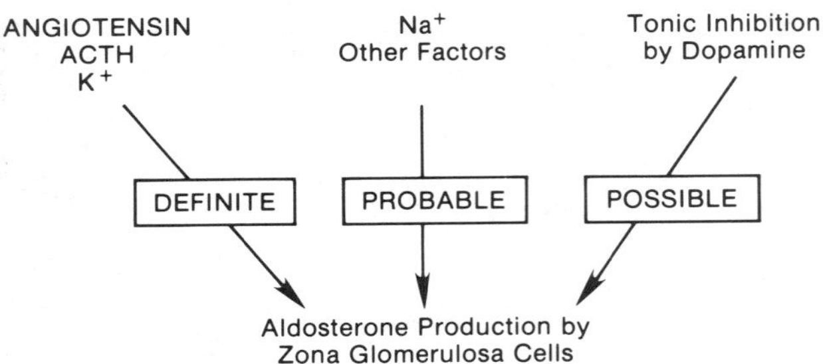

FIGURE 1. Control of aldosterone secretion.

kidney; it acts upon a substrate, angiotensinogen, which is made in the liver, to form angiotensin I. This decapeptide is then converted by an enzyme (converting enzyme) into an octapeptide, angiotensin II, the active principle in this system (Figure 2). Tonin, a recently described enzyme isolated from the rat submandibular salivary gland, directly forms angiotensin II from a natural protein substrate (toninogen), or the synthetic tetradecapeptide renin substrate. It can also act on angiotensin I to form angiotensin II (14). Its role in the human renin–angiotensin system is, however, unknown.

The main actions of angiotensin II are to stimulate aldosterone biosynthesis and to increase peripheral resistance, thus raising the blood pressure. A large percentage of the plasma angiotensin I is converted to angiotensin II in one passage through the lung, although other tissues can also effect this conversion (74). Recent developments point to the presence of a 7-amino-acid peptide (des-aspartyl angiotensin II) termed angiotensin III, which is also a potent stimulator of aldosterone secretion, though less active than angiotensin II as a vasopressor agent (47). Inactivation of the angiotensins occurs in many tissues via angiotensinases.

The juxtaglomerular cells are the site of renin formation in the kidney (49). They are located in the media of the afferent arterioles just before entering the glomeruli. Each renal tubule returns to a point near the glomerulus from which it starts and, in the angle between the arterioles, it comes into close contact with juxtaglomerular cells. At this point the epithelium of the distal convoluted tubule contains many tall, columnar cells with large nuclei and is called the macula densa, which, together with the juxtaglomerular cells, makes up the juxtaglomerular apparatus.

In 1960, Tobian proposed that the juxtaglomerular cells are baroreceptors and respond to changes in the pressure gradient between intraluminal arterial pressure and interstitial pressure (95). When this gradient is large, renin is inhibited; when it is small, renin is stimulated. It appears that the mean arterial pressure rather than the pulse pressure is the modulator. Decreases in effective blood volume or perfusion pressure as in hemorrhage, Na^+ depletion, or renovascular constriction thus result in an increase in renin and, secondarily, in aldosterone secretion. In addition to this baroreceptor mechanism, it is known that the sodium

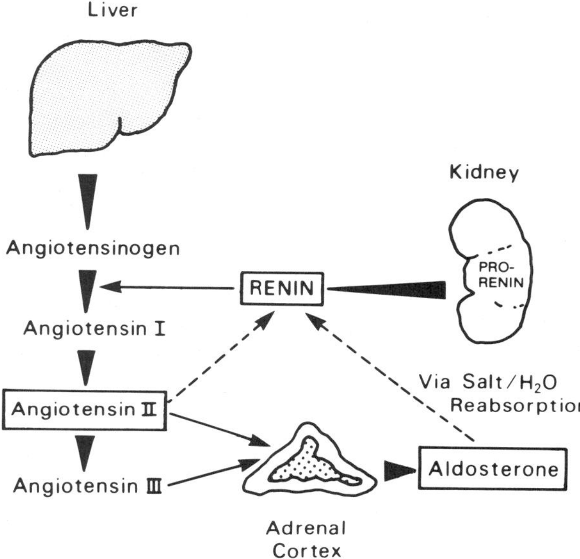

FIGURE 2. The renin–angiotensin–aldosterone system.

concentration of the renal tubular fluid at the macula densa also regulates renin release (97). It is controversial, however, whether increased or decreased Na^+ delivery signals the release of renin. The sympathetic nerves to the kidney modify renin secretion as well (3,45). In the absence of these nerves, the renin response to sodium depletion is blunted (22). A β-adrenergic receptor may be involved, because beta blockers (such as propranolol) inhibit renin release, whereas α-adrenergic blockers do not (3,45). Acute infusion of norepinephrine can increase renin secretion, but infusions of angiotensin decrease it (96). This latter effect represents the short-loop negative feedback (Figure 2). Direct infusion of aldosterone into the renal artery has no effect, although chronic administration of aldosterone reduces renin secretion by means of sodium retention and volume expansion (long-loop feedback). Potassium may also directly alter renin secretion quite independent of its effect on aldosterone. Potassium loading decreases while potassium depletion increases renin release (1,23).

Prostaglandins have recently been implicated as mediators of renin release. In the nonfiltering kidney model, inhibition of prostaglandin biosynthesis by indomethacin diminished the release of renin in response to pressure changes (28). In man, indomethacin inhibits renin release during sodium restriction (91). Indomethacin has also been reported to lower basal plasma renin activity, and the response of renin to posture and to furosemide has been shown (80,93). In a study of 12 human volunteers, indomethacin was shown to inhibit renal prostaglandin production as reflected by radioimmunoassay of urinary prostaglandin E_2. The increases in plasma renin activity and plasma and urinary aldosterone following acute furosemide challenge were reduced by 50%–75% in the presence of indomethacin, whereas cortisol levels were unchanged (93). These results have been interpreted as evidence of the pivotal role of renal prostaglandins in modulating the responsiveness for a renin–angiotensin–aldosterone axis. Direct stimulation of renin release by prostaglandins and by arachidonic acid, the substrate for prostaglandin biosynthesis, has also been demonstrated (59,100).

Inactive forms of renin can be found in plasma derived from both renal and extrarenal sources (35,60,85). Their clinical significance is under study. Various treatments can result in activation (e.g., acidification or exposure to cold or trypsin). Big renin is a larger molecular weight species (~50–60,000 vs ~43,000 for normal renin) found in various tissues including plasma and kidney (35). It is inactive at physiologic pH but is activated at pH 3.3. The possibility exists that inactive renin may be a zymogen (prorenin), being converted to active renin either within the kidney or upon release into the circulation.

The administration of renin or angiotensin increases the width of the zona glomerulosa and aldosterone secretion while nephrectomy lowers aldosterone secretion and prevents its increase following hemorrhage, salt depletion, and thoracic inferior vena caval constriction (30,31,72). In humans, angiotensin infusions increase aldosterone (10,57) and plasma renin levels are increased in those conditions associated with increased aldosterone secretion, such as sodium depletion, cirrhosis of the liver with ascites, nephrosis, and malignant hypertension (20). A high-salt intake plus a mineralocorticoid decrease both renin and aldosterone. Angiotensin II is believed to be the most potent stimulus for aldosterone production in man, and a close correlation exists between plasma renin activity and urinary aldosterone in normal subjects.

Since angiotensin II, and perhaps angiotensin III, are the active principles affecting aldosterone secretion, factors that influence angiotensin II generation in turn determine aldosterone levels. The concentrations of renin enzyme and of renin substrate (i.e., angiotensinogen) govern the rate of angiotensin I generation. Converting enzyme is widely available and is not believed to be a limiting factor. Stimuli for renin release (e.g., upright posture, diuretics, hemorrhage, etc.) lead to a secondary increase in aldosterone, whereas renin inhibition (e.g., following salt loading, propranolol, or indomethacin therapy) results in a decrease in aldosterone. Likewise, an increase in angiotensinogen leads to an increase in both renin and aldosterone. Such a situation occurs with estrogen or glucocorticoid administration (56,89).

Angiotensin II stimulates aldosterone biosynthesis both in vivo and in vitro and its effect can be blocked by the angiotensin II antagonist, saralasin (75). In most species, including humans, angiotensin II is believed to selectively stimulate aldosterone production but not cortisol production. However, this does not appear to be true in dogs (46). The renin–angiotensin system is also not felt to be an important modulator of deoxycorticosterone (DOC) or 18 hydroxy-deoxycorticosterone (18 OH-DOC) production. Human DOC production is under the primary control of ACTH and is not influenced by changes in salt intake. Under some circumstances, however, DOC production from the zona glomerulosa can be demonstrated (e.g., during concurrent dexamethasone suppression and sodium depletion) (92). In the case of 18 OH-DOC, studies in the rat provide no evidence for a regulatory role of angiotensin II (94); in humans the evidence is less clear (98). Like aldosterone, 18-hydroxycorticosterone is also a product of the zona glomerulosa under the primary control of the renin–angiotensin system (42). Most of the evidence indicates that angiotensin acts early in the biosynthetic pathway for aldosterone. In vitro, it stimulates the conversion of cholesterol, but not of pregnenolone, progesterone, deoxycorticosterone, or corticosterone to aldosterone (53,69) (Figure 3). In humans treated with dexamethasone and the 11-β-hydroxylase inhibitor, metyrapone, angiotensin II increases deoxycorticosterone indicating an effect at a step prior to the formation of deoxycorticosterone (21). Although it is clear that the acute effect of angiotensin II is at an early biosynthetic step, there is evidence that prolonged exposure to the peptide results in an enhanced conversion of corticosterone to aldosterone (i.e., the late or final steps in aldosterone biosynthesis) (2,34).

Angiotensin's stimulation of adrenal steroidogenesis is not accompanied by an increase in cAMP concentration (83). In this aspect, it differs from the action of ACTH. It can increase aldosterone secretion by bovine adrenals even in the presence of maximum doses of ACTH or cAMP (52). Like ACTH, angiotensin action requires Ca^{++} and is blocked by puromycin (52) and other inhibitors of protein synthesis.

The heptapeptide angiotensin III has the same affinity for adrenal receptor sites and stimulates aldosterone secretion to the same extent as angiotensin II. Its action can be blocked by its selective antagonist 7-Ile-angiotensin III.

FIGURE 3. Stimulation of aldosterone by angiotensin II, K^+, and ACTH.

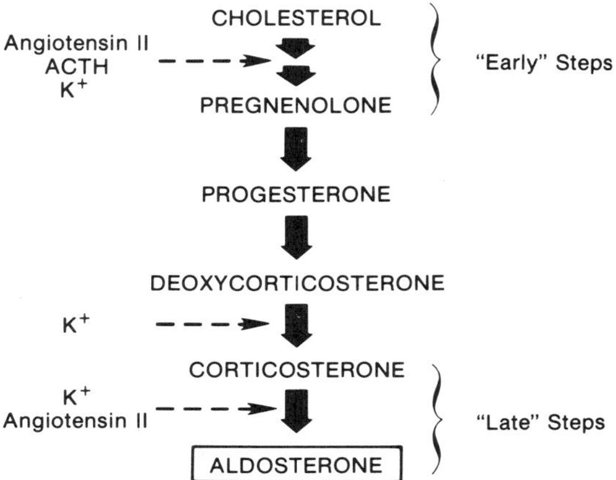

POTASSIUM

The K^+ ion has a marked influence on the secretion of aldosterone (24,44,51,58,88). Potassium loading increases while potassium depletion decreases aldosterone secretion; the latter circumstance also prevents the stimulation that ordinarily follows sodium depletion. It has been shown by both in vitro and in vivo studies (26,32,52,68) that potassium acts directly on the adrenal gland. This effect of potassium may be related to the serum concentration; changes in serum potassium concentration of less than 1 mEq/L can influence the aldosterone secretion rate (17,18, 43,50). It is possible that adrenal cell potassium concentration is the more important factor, because it is involved in the action of many stimuli that increase aldosterone production. Ouabain, an inhibitor of Mg^{++}-dependent, Na^+-K^+ activated ATPase, prevents K^+ uptake by adrenal cells in vitro, leading to intracellular potassium depletion. Ouabain diminishes the stimulation of aldosterone production by K^+, ACTH, and cAMP, yet ouabain has no effect on glucocorticoid production by the inner zone cells. Baumber et al. (6) have shown that intraadrenal K^+ is increased in a variety of conditions in which there is increased aldosterone biosynthesis e.g. administration of ACTH, or angiotensin II, sodium depletion, and hyperkalemia. The possibility therefore exists that increased adrenocortical potassium promotes increased aldosterone synthesis during sodium depletion independent of alterations in the renin–angiotensin system, ACTH, and plasma electrolytes. This suggestion would also help explain the increased aldosterone production seen in sodium depletion in the sheep without demonstrable changes in angiotensin II, ACTH, sodium, or potassium concentrations. However, Mendelsohn and Mackie have not detected uniform increases in intraadrenal K^+ concentrations during stimulation of adrenal steroidogenesis (66).

In humans, potassium loading or sodium depletion enhances the aldosterone response to a subsequent potassium infusion even though the preinfusion serum K^+ is normal (38). Early experiments tended to indicate that aldosterone biosynthesis is increased if K^+ levels are raised to unphysiologically high levels. There is now no question that minor K^+ changes within the physiologic range can affect aldosterone biosynthesis. In the dog, a rise in plasma K^+ of 1.3 mEq/L increases aldosterone secretion (32); in the sheep, 0.5 mEq/L would suffice (43), and in humans, effects are discernible at 0.1 mEq/L (50). The studies of Williams et al (38,39,50) in man indicate that an increase of 0.2 mEq/L or a reduction of 0.5 mEq/L in serum K^+ leads to a 46% change in plasma aldosterone levels. These findings are particularly pertinent to a number of clinical situations where the increase in aldosterone does not quite match the marked hyperreninemia. Hypokalemia is commonly present in these situations (e.g., Bartter's syndrome or diuretic use) and is responsible for the blunted aldosterone response: repletion of potassium results in a marked increase in aldosterone.

It appears that K^+ primarily stimulates an early step in the biosynthetic pathway, i.e., from cholesterol to pregnenolone (21,69). The last steps, conversion of corticosterone to aldosterone, are not increased by acute changes in K^+ concentration. However, prolonged K^+ loading can increase the rate of the last steps, increase the width of the zona glomerulosa and cause ultrastructural changes which are similar to those found during sodium depletion (4). Potassium has also been reported to stimulate the 11-β-hydroxylation step, i.e., conversion of deoxycorticosterone to corticosterone (5) (Figure 3).

In anephrics, K^+ appears to be the major regulator of aldosterone (7), although aldosterone levels are quite low in the absence of the renin–angiotensin system (86). A significant correlation between plasma aldosterone and K^+ in anephrics has been reported by Bayard et al. (7). In nephrectomized decapitated dogs, McCaa et al. (63) have shown that the rise in aldosterone with time as well as following hemorrhage is associated with increases in serum K^+; normalization of serum K^+ with hemodialysis abolished the aldosterone response. Others have invoked an as yet unknown mechanism for the aldosterone response to posture and hemodialysis (67,81) in anephrics since they were unable to detect changes in serum K+ or ACTH.

ACTH

Unlike other adrenal steroids, aldosterone is not under the primary control of the pituitary gland. It is well known that the zona glomerulosa of the adrenal does not undergo marked atrophy after hypophysectomy while the inner zones do (36). As early as 1948, Deane et al. (37) showed that a low sodium diet increased the width of the zona glomerulosa in hypophysectomized rats, indicating that another mechanism independent of the pituitary gland was stimulating the growth of the zona glomerulosa. However, more recent evidence indicates that despite the increased width of the zona glomerulosa, the adrenals of sodium-depleted hypophysectomized rats secrete very little aldosterone (79).

It has now become evident that the pituitary gland does play a very important role in maintaining the growth and biosynthetic ability of the zona glomerulosa cell. The extent of its role varies from species to species. In man, acute hypophysectomy does not lower the basal rate of aldosterone secretion or prevent the rise following sodium depletion. However, patients who have had hypopituitarism for several years show little or no increase in aldosterone secretion after sodium depletion (61,99). In the rat, hypophysectomy completely inhibits the rise following sodium depletion, and ACTH does not restore the response despite a return of adrenal size and corticosterone secretion to normal (77). Adrenocorticotrophic hormone plus growth hormone can maintain the adrenal gland's response, but the evidence suggests that another pituitary factor may be involved (77). In the dog, hypophysectomy markedly reduced the aldosterone response to sodium depletion. Indeed, the effects of hypophysectomy on secondary aldosteronism seem to be much greater than that of nephrectomy in the dog (33).

In humans, injections of ACTH acutely stimulate aldosterone secretion. Only small doses of ACTH are necessary; it has been estimated that plasma ACTH need only rise to stress levels, or even remain within the range normally present at 8 A.M. (54,73). An interesting aspect of the aldosterone response to ACTH is its transient nature; prolonged administration leads to a decline in aldosterone secretion, which may be secondary to sodium retention and renin suppression or to the kaliuretic effect of ACTH.

The response to ACTH is augmented during increased K+ intake and is diminished in K^+-deficient rats. Sodium deficiency sensitizes the adrenal to angiotensin II, K^+ as well as ACTH. In primary aldosteronism, there is a hyperresponse of aldosterone to ACTH (55). This is true for both the adenomatous and hyperplastic forms of the disease. In low-renin essential hypertension, however, the response is normal.

The mechanism of action of ACTH on aldosterone biosynthesis is the same as on glucocorticoid synthesis (48). The primary site of action is on the conversion of cholesterol to pregnenolone. Cyclic AMP is believed to mediate the action of ACTH since its increase precedes steroidogenesis, and exogenous cAMP also stimulates the conversion of cholesterol to pregnenolone (Figure 3).

OTHER FACTORS

Sodium

Perfusion studies of isolated adrenals have shown that low serum sodium concentration increases, whereas a high serum sodium concentration decreases aldosterone secretion (13,32). Local increases in adrenal arterial plasma Na^+ can transiently decrease aldosterone secretion by approximately 25% in the sheep. The response to angiotensin II was also reduced. A significant increase in aldosterone secretion was noted by Davis et al. in hypophysectomized nephrectomized dogs when plasma sodium concentration was reduced by 20 mEq/L. It is unlikely, however, that the serum sodium concentration is a major regulator of aldosterone secretion. Serum Na^+ remains normal during Na^+ depletion, which is a well-known stimulus for aldosterone production; moreover, when vasopressin and water are given to sodium-depleted subjects, aldosterone secretion drops despite a fall in serum sodium concentration. The dehydration of water deprivation increases aldosterone as well as the serum sodium concentration. Therefore, it is the extracellular fluid volume (via the renin–angiotensin system) rather than serum sodium concentration which influences aldosterone output in most circumstances.

Central Nervous System

The role of the central nervous system in regulating aldosterone secretion has been a controversial subject. There have been claims that the central nervous system can both inhibit and stimulate aldosterone secretion (40). Certainly, the neural mechanisms regulating ACTH release play a role.

The original studies suggesting that the pineal gland and surrounding tissue contained a stimulatory substance, adrenoglomerulotropin, later identified as a carboline derivative, have not been confirmed. The sympathetic nervous system, by modulating the secretion of renin, has an indirect effect on aldosterone secretion (96).

It has been proposed that the brain contains an intrinsic renin-angiotensin system which may be active in vivo. Renin substrate, converting enzyme, and a renin-like enzyme are known to be present in brain tissue. Some workers feel that this enzyme is Cathepsin D, a protease capable of forming angiotensin I from the synthetic tetradecapeptide substrate but not from the natural renin substrate angiotensinogen. Conflicting answers, related in part to methodology, surround the question as to whether angiotensin is present in the brain (82), but more recent evidence supports the presence of a separate brain renin-angiotensin system (46a).

Growth hormone is known to increase adrenal size, and in the hypophysectomized rat, growth hormone plus ACTH restore adrenal sensitivity towards normal. By itself, growth hormone does not acutely increase aldosterone secretion in the dog. In humans, exogenous growth hormone is said to increase plasma aldosterone (9). However, hypoaldosteronism has not been reported in growth-hormone deficient states, and a recent study indicates a little or no role for this hormone in aldosterone regulation in man (64). Aldosterone responded normally to sodium restriction and ACTH in subjects with isolated growth hormone deficiency but not in panhypopituitarism; despite growth hormone therapy for 12 months, the latter patients continued to display a subnormal aldosterone responsiveness. It appears that a pituitary factor other than growth hormone may be involved in the control of aldosterone. Other pituitary peptides such as α-MSH, β-lipotrophin, and β-MSH can stimulate aldosterone production in vitro or in vivo (41a,62a). Whether these peptides play a physiological role in the control of aldosterone remains to be determined.

Prolactin has been suggested as having a possible effect on adrenal steroidogenesis since the adrenal is rich in prolactin receptors. Most studies, however, do not support this. Changes in dietary sodium markedly affect renin and aldosterone; prolactin levels on the other hand are unchanged. Thyrotropin-releasing hormone, a potent stimulus for prolactin release, does not elevate plasma aldosterone levels (41). Of greater interest is the recent demonstration that metoclopramide, a dopamine antagonist, can acutely elevate plasma aldosterone when administered into human volunteers (25). Cortisol, potassium, and renin were unchanged. Angiotensin II increased aldosterone further. Bromocryptine, a dopamine agonist, did not diminish the response of aldosterone to angiotensin II infusion. These results have been interpreted to mean that aldosterone secretion may normally be under maximum tonic dopaminergic inhibition, which can be overridden with stimulation by angiotensin II. Dopamine has also been shown to inhibit the aldosterone response to angiotensin II by bovine adrenal cells although basal production was unaffected. This inhibition was believed to occur at the late steps of aldosterone biosynthesis (65).

Miscellaneous

Magnesium deficiency stimulates aldosterone secretion in the rat; corticosterone production is unaltered. In man, however, magnesium deficiency failed to change aldosterone secretion in two patients (27), and only a slight increase occurred following magnesium replenishment. Monovalent cations (e.g., ammonium, cesium, and rubidium) have also been shown to stimulate aldosterone formation by rat adrenal slice; the latter two compounds have also been shown to be effective in the perfused dog adrenal gland.

Acidosis has recently been reported to stimulate aldosterone secretion in humans (84).

A number of observations suggest the existence of an unidentified mechanism regulating aldosterone secretion (11,12,15,62,78,90). Data are especially impressive in sheep, in which significant discrepancies between renin and aldosterone levels exist (11,12). For example, continuous infusion of angiotensin II cannot maintain aldosterone secretion at high levels, and aldosterone secretion can be altered appropriately during sodium loading and depletion despite a continuous infusion of renin. Rabbits immunized against angiotensin II increased aldosterone production during sodium depletion yet do not respond to infusions of angiotensin II (62). In the rat, potassium appears to be more important in the aldosterone response to sodium depletion than the renin system (17,18). In man, infusions of angiotensin do not elevate plasma aldosterone concentrations to levels attained during sodium depletion, despite higher plasma angiotensin concentration (15). One group of investigators could not demonstrate an increase in plasma angiotensin II during a low sodium diet (8). The presence of bilateral adrenal hyperplasia in patients with primary aldosteronism and low plasma renin suggests that another trophic factor exists.

Recently, a protein fraction has been extracted from normal human urine which when injected into rats, stimulates aldosterone but not corticosterone secretion (87). It also causes sustained hypertension which is accompanied by volume expansion and Na^+ retention. This peptide appears to originate in the pituitary gland, has a molecular weight of 26,000 daltons, and is found in high concentrations in the plasma and urine of patients with ideopathic primary aldosteronism (25).

REFERENCES

1. Abbrecht, P.H., and Vander, A.J. (1970) Effects of chronic potassium deficiency on plasma renin activity. J. Clin. Invest. 49, 1510–1516.
2. Aguilera, G., and Marusic, E.T. (1971) Role of the renin–angiotensin system in the biosynthesis of aldosterone. Endocrinology 89, 1524–1529.
3. Assaykeen, T.A., and Ganong, W.F. (1971) The sympathetic nervous system and renin secretion. Front. Neuro Endocrinol, pp. 67–102.
4. Baumann, K., and Muller, J. (1972) Effect of potassium intake on the final steps of aldosterone biosynthesis in the rat. I. 18 hydroxylation and 18-hydroxydehydrogenation. Acta Endocrinol. 69, 701–717.

5. Baumann, K., and Muller, J. (1972) Effect of potassium on the final steps of aldosterone biosynthesis in the rat. II. 11-β hydroxylation. Acta Endocrinol. 69, 718–730.
6. Baumber, J.S., Davis, J.O., Johnson, J.A., et al. (1971) Increased adrenocortical potassium in association with increased biosynthesis of aldosterone. Am. J. Physiol. 220, 1094–1099.
7. Bayard, F., Cooke, R.C., Tiller, D.J., Beitins, I.Z., Kowarski, A., Walker, W.G., and Migeon, C.J. (1971) The regulation of aldosterone in anephric man. J. Clin. Invest. 50, 1585–1595.
8. Best, J.B., Coghlan, J.P., Bett, J.H.N., Cran, E.J., and Scoggins, B.A. (1971) Circulating angiotensin II and aldosterone levels during dietary sodium restriction. Lancet 2, 1353–1354.
9. Birkhauser, M., Gaillard, R., Riondel, A.M., and Zahnd, G.R. (1974) Influence of acute administration of human "growth" hormone and alpha-MSH on plasma concentration of aldosterone, cortisol, corticosterone, and growth hormone in man. Acta Endocrinol. 79, 16–24.
10. Biron, P., Koiw, E., Nowaczynski, W., Brouillet, J., and Genest, J. (1961) The effects of intravenous infusions of valine-5 angiotensin II and other pressor agents on urinary electrolytes and corticosteroids, including aldosterone. J. Clin. Invest. 40, 338–347.
11. Blair-West, J.R., Cain, M.D., Catt, K.J. et al. (1971) The dissociation of aldosterone secretion and systemic renin and angiotensin II levels during the correction of sodium deficiency. Acta Endocrinol. 66, 229–247.
12. Blair-West, J.R., Coghlan, J.P., Denton, D.A., Funder, J.W., and Scoggins, B.A. (1972) The role of the renin-angiotensin system in control of aldosterone secretion. Adv. Exp. Med. Biol. 17, 167–187.
13. Blair-West, J.R., Coghlan, J.P., Denton, D.A., Goding, J.R., Wintour, M., and Wright, R.D. (1963) The control of aldosterone secretion. Rec. Prog. Horm. Res. 19, 311–363.
14. Boucher, R., DeMassieux, S., Garcia, R., and Genest, J. (1977) Tonin–angiotensin II system. In: J. Genest, E. Koiw, and O. Kuchel (eds.), Hypertension. McGraw-Hill, New York, pp. 256–260.
15. Boyd, G.W., Adamson, A.R., James, V.H.T., and Peart, W.S. (1969) The role of the renin–angiotensin system in the control of aldosterone in man. Proc. Roy. Soc. Med. 62, 1253–1254.
16. Boyd, J.E., Manuelidis, L., and Mulrow, P.J. (1972) The importance of potassium in the regulation of aldosterone biosynthesis. In: Proceedings, 4th Int. Cong. Endocrinol. pp. 785–789.
17. Boyd, J.E., and Mulrow, P.J. (1972) Further studies of the influence of potassium upon aldosterone production in the rat. Endocrinology 90, 299–301.
18. Boyd, J.E., Palmore, W.P., and Mulrow, P.J. (1971) Role of potassium in the control of aldosterone secretion in the rat. Endocrinology 88, 556–565.
19. Brown, J.J., Davies, D.L. Lever, A.F., and Robertson, J.I.S. (1964) Variations in plasma renin concentration in several physiological and pathological states. Can. Med. Assoc. J. 90, 201–206.
20. Brown, R.D., Strott, C.A., and Liddle, G.W (1972) Site of stimulation of aldosterone biosynthesis by angiotensin and potassium. J. Clin. Invest. 51, 1413–1418.
21. Brubacher, F.S., and Vander, A.J. (1968) Sodium deprivation and renin secretion in unanesthetized dogs. Am. J. Physiol. 214, 15–21.
22. Brunner, H.R., Baer, L., Sealey, J.E., Ledingham, J.G.G., and Laragh, J.H. (1970) The influence of potassium administration and of potassium deprivation on plasma renin in normal and hypertensive subjects. J. Clin. Invest. 49, 2128–2138.
23. Cannon, P.J., Ames, R.P., and Laragh, J.H. (1966) Relation between potassium balance and aldosterone secretion in normal subjects and in patients with hypertensive or renal tubular disease. J. Clin. Invest. 45, 865–879.
24. Carey, R.M., Thorner, M.O., and Ortt, E.M. (1979) Effects of metoclopramide and bromocriptine on the renin–angiotensin–aldosterone system in man. J. Clin. Invest. 63, 727–735.

25. Carey, R. M., Sen, S., Dolan, L., Malchoff, C.D., and Bumpus, M.F. (1984) Ideopathic hyperaldosteronism: A possible role for aldosterone stimulating factor. N. Engl. J. Med. 311, 94–100.
26. Coghlan, J.P., Denton, D.A., Goding, J.R., and Wright, R.D. (1960) The control of aldosterone secretion. Postgrad. Med. J. 36, 76–102.
27. Cope, C.L., and Pearson, J. (1963) Aldosterone secretion in magnesium deficiency. Br. Med. J. 2, 1385–1386.
28. Data, J.L., Gerber, J.G., Crump, W.J., Frolich, J.C., and Nies, A.S. (1978) The prostaglandin system: A role in canine baroreceptor control of renin release. Circ. Res. 42, 454–458.
29. Davis, J.O. (1967) Regulation of aldosterone secretion. In: A.B. Eisenstein (ed.), The Adrenal Cortex. Little, Brown and Co., Boston, pp. 203–247.
30. Davis, J.O., Ayers, C.R., and Carpenter, C.C.J. (1961) Renal origin of aldosterone-stimulating hormone in dogs with thoracic caval constriction and in sodium depleted dogs. J. Clin. Invest. 40, 1466–1474.
31. Davis, J.O., Carpenter, C.C.J., Ayers, C.R., Holman, J.E., and Bahn, R.C. (1961) Evidence for secretion of an aldosterone-stimulating hormone by the kidney. J. Clin. Invest. 40, 684–696.
32. Davis, J.O., Urquhart, J., and Higgins, J.T., Jr. (1964) The effects of alterations of plasma sodium and potassium concentration on aldosterone secretion. J. Clin. Invest. 42, 597–609.
33. Davis, J.O., Urquhart, J., Higgins, J.T., Jr., Rubin, E.C., and Hartroft, P.M. (1964) Hypersecretion of aldosterone in dogs with a chronic aortic-caval fistula and high output heart failure, Circ. Res. 14, 471–485.
34. Davis, W.W., Berwell, L.R., Casper, A.G.T., and Bartter, F.C. (1968) Sites of action of sodium depletion on aldosterone biosynthesis in the dog. J. Clin. Invest. 47, 1425–1434.
35. Day, R.P., and Luetscher, J.A. (1974) Big-renin: A possible prohormone in kidney and plasma of a patient with Wilm's tumor. J. Clin. Endocrinol. Metab. 38, 923–926.
36. Deane, H.G. (1962) The anatomy, chemistry and physiology of adrenocortical tissue. Handbuch Exp. Pharmackol. 14, 1–185.
37. Deane, H.W., Shaw, J.H., and Greep, R.O. (1948) The effect of altered sodium or potassium intake on the width and cytochemistry of the zona glomerulosa of the rat's adrenal cortex. Endocrinology 43, 133–153.
38. Dluhy, R.G., Axelford, L., Underwood, R.H., and Williams, G.H. (1972) Studies of the control of plasma aldosterone concentration in normal man. J. Clin. Invest. 51, 1950–1957.
39. Dluhy, R.G., Cain, J.P., and Williams, G.H. (1974) The influence of dietary potassium on the renin and aldosterone response to diuretic-induced volume depletion. J. Lab. Clin. Med. 83, 249–255.
40. Farrell, G.L. (1964) Recent contributions to the study of the role of the central nervous system in aldosterone secretion. In: E.E. Baulieu and R. Robel (eds.), Aldosterone—A symposium. Blackwell Scientific Publications, Oxford, pp. 243–249.
41. Fernandez-Cruz, A., Jr., Noth, R.H., Tan, S.Y., Donabedian, R.K., and Mulrow, P.J. (1976) The role of prolactin in the control of aldosterone secretion in man. Endocrine Soc. 58th Ann. Meeting, (abst 540), 327.
41a. Franco-Saenz, R., Mulrow, P.J., and Kim, K. (1984) Ideopathic aldosteronism: A possible disease of the intermediate lobe of the pituitary. JAMA 251, 2555–2558.
42. Fraser, R., and Lantos, C.P. (1978) 18-hydroxycorticosterone: A review. J. Ster. Biochem. 9, 273–286.
43. Funder, J.W., Blair-West, J.R., Coghlan, J.P., Denton, D.A., Scoggins, B.A., and Wright, R.D. (1969) Effect of plasma K^+ on the secretion of aldosterone. Endocrinology 85, 381–384.
44. Gann, D.S., Delea, C.S., Gill, J.R., Jr., Thomas, J.P., and Bartter, F.C., (1964) Control of aldosterone secretion by change of body potassium in normal man. Am. J. Physiol. 202, 991–996.

45. Ganong, W.F. (1972) Sympathetic effects on renin secretion: Mechanisms and physiological role. Adv. Exp. Med. Biol. 17, 17–32.
46. Ganong, W.F. (1973) Review of medical physiology, 6th Ed. Lange, Los Altos, Calif.
46a. Ganten, D., Hermann, K., Unger, T., and Lang, R.E. (1983) The tissue renin-angiotensin systems: Focus on brain angiotensin, adrenal gland, and arterial wall. Clin. and Exp. Hyper.—Theory and Practice A5 (7 and 8), 1099–1118.
47. Goodfriend, T.L., and Peach, M.J. (1975) Angiotensin III (des-aspartic acid)-angiotensin II: Evidence and speculation for its role as an important agonist in the renin-angiotensin system. Circ. Res. 36 (Suppl I), 38–48.
48. Hall, P.F., and Young, D.G. (1968) Site of action of trophic hormones upon the biosynthetic pathways to steroid hormones. Endocrinology 82, 559–568.
49. Hartroft, P.M. (1966) The juxtaglomerular complex. Ann. Rev. Med. 17, 113–122.
50. Himathongkam, T., Dluhy, R.G., and Williams, G.H. (1975) Potassium–aldosterone–renin interrelationships. J. Clin. Endocrinol. Metab. 41, 153–159.
51. Johnson, B.B., Lieberman, A.H., and Mulrow, P.J. (1957) Aldosterone excretion in normal subjects depleted of sodium and potassium. J. Clin. Invest. 36, 757–766.
52. Kaplan, N.M. (1965) The biosynthesis of adrenal steroids: Effects of angiotensin II, adrenocorticotropin and potassium. J. Clin. Invest. 44, 2029–2039.
53. Kaplan, N.M., and Bartter, F.C. (1962) The effect of ACTH, renin, angiotensin II and precursors on biosynthesis of aldosterone by adrenal slices. J. Clin. Invest. 41, 715–724.
54. Kem, D.C., Gomez-Sanchez, C., Kramer, N.J., Holland, O.B., and Higgins, J.R. (1975) Plasma aldosterone and renin activity response to ACTH infusion in dexamethasone-suppressed normal and sodium-depleted man. J. Clin. Endocrinol. Metab. 40, 116–124.
55. Kem, D.C., Weinberger, M.H., Higgins, J.R., Kramer, N.J., Gomez-Sanchez, C., and Holland, O.B. (1978) Plasma aldosterone response to ACTH in primary aldosteronism and in patients with low renin hypertension. J. Clin. Endocrinol. Metab. 46, 552–560.
56. Krakoff, L.R. (1973) Measurement of plasma renin substrate by radioimmunoassay of angiotensin I: Concentration in syndromes associated with steroid excess. J. Clin. Endocrinol. Metab. 37, 110–117.
57. Laragh, J.H., Cannon, P.J., and Ames, R.P. (1964) Interaction between aldosterone secretion, sodium and potassium balance, and angiotensin activity in man. Studies in hypertension and cirrhosis. Can. Med. Assoc. J. 90, 248–256.
58. Laragh, J.H., and Stoerk, H.C. (1957) A study of the mechanism of secretion of the sodium-retaining hormone (aldosterone). J. Clin. Invest. 36, 383–392.
59. Larsson, C., Weber, P., and Anggard, E. (1974) Arachidonic acid increases and indomethacin decreases plasma renin activity in the rabbit. Eur. J. Pharmacol. 28, 391–394.
60. Leckie, B.J., McConnell, A., Grant, J., Morton, J.J., Tree, J., and Brown, J.J. (1977) An inactive renin in human plasma. Circ. Res. 40 (Suppl. I), 146–151.
61. Lieberman, A.H., and Leutscher, J.A., Jr. (1960) Some effects of abnormalities of pituitary, adrenal or thyroid function on excretion of aldosterone and the response to corticotropin or sodium deprivation. J. Clin. Endocrinol. 20, 1004–1016.
62. Lowenstein, J., Boyd, G.W., Rippon, A.E., James, V.H.T., and Peart, W.S. (1972) Increased aldosterone in response to sodium deficiency in the angiotensin II-immunized rabbit. In: J. Genest and E. Koiw (eds.), Hypertension. Springer-Verlag, Heidelberg, Berlin, New York, pp. 481–489.
62a. Matsuoka, H., Mulrow, P.J., Franco-Saenz, R., and Li, C.H. (1981) Effects of β-Lipotropin and β-Lipotropin derived peptides on aldosterone production in the rat adrenal gland. J. Clin. Invest. 68, 752–759.
63. McCaa, R.E., McCaa, C.S., Cowley, A.W., Olt, C.E., and Guyton, A.C. (1973) Stimulation of aldosterone secretion by hemorrhage by dogs after nephrectomy and decapitation. Circ. Res. 32, 356–362.
64. McCaa, R.E., Montalvo, J.M., and McCaa, C.S. (1978) Role of growth hormone in the regulation of aldosterone biosynthesis. J. Clin. Endocrinol. Metab. 46, 247–253.
65. McKenna, T.J., Island, D.P., Nicholson, W.E., and Liddle, G.W. (1979) Dopamine

inhibits angiotensin-stimulated aldosterone biosynthesis in bovine adrenal cells. J. Clin. Invest. 64, 287–291.

66. Mendelsohn, F.A., and Mackie, C. (1975) Relation of intracellular K^+ and steroidogenesis in isolated adrenal zona glomerulosa and fasciculata cells. Clin. Sci. Mol. Med. 49, 13–26.
67. Mitra, S., Genuth, S., Berman, L.B., and Vertes, V. (1972) Aldosterone secretion in anephric patients. N. Engl. J. Med. 286, 61–64.
68. Muller, J. (1965) Aldosterone stimulation in vitro. Acta Endocrinol. 50, 301–309.
69. Muller, J. (1971) Regulation of aldosterone biosynthesis. Springer-Verlag, New York.
70. Mulrow, P.J., and Ganong, W.F. (1964) The role of the renin-angiotensin system in the regulation of aldosterone secretion in the dog and man. In: E.D. Baulieu and P. Robel (eds.), Aldosterone—A Symposium. Blackwell Scientific Publications, Oxford, pp. 265–278.
71. Mulrow, P.J., Ganong. W.F., and Boryczka, A.T. (1963) Further evidence for a role of the renin-angiotensin system in regulation of aldosterone secretion. Proc. Soc. Exp. Biol. 112, 7–10.
72. Mulrow, P.J., Ganong, W.F., Cera, G., and Kuljian, A. (1962) The nature of the aldosterone-stimulating factor in dog kidneys. J. Clin. Invest. 41, 505–518.
73. Nicholls, M.G., Espiner, E.A., and Donald, R.A. (1975) Plasma aldosterone response to low dose ACTH stimulation. J. Clin. Endocrinol. Metab. 41, 186–188.
74. Ng, K.K.F., and Vane, J.R. (1967) Conversion of angiotensin I to angiotensin II. Nature 216, 762–766.
75. Oparil, S., and Haber, E. (1974) The renin-angiotensin system. N. Engl. J. Med. 291, 389–401 and 446–457.
76. Page, I.H., and Bumpus, F.M. (1961) Angiotensin. Physiol. Rev. 41, 331–390.
77. Palmore, W.P., Anderson, R., and Mulrow, P.J. (1970) Role of the pituitary in controlling aldosterone production in sodium-depleted rats. Endocrinology 86, 728–734.
78. Palmore, W.P., Marieb, N.J., and Mulrow, P.J. (1969) Stimulation of aldosterone secretion by sodium depletion in nephrectomized rats. Endocrinol. 84, 1342–1351.
79. Palmore, W.P., and Mulrow, P.J. (1967) Control of aldosterone secretion by the pituitary gland. Science 158, 1482–1484.
80. Patak, R.V., Mookerjee, B.K., Bentzal, C.J., Hysert, P.E., Babej, J., and Lee, J.B. (1975) Antagonism of the effect of furosemide by indomethacin in normal and hypertensive man. Prostaglandins 10, 649–659.
81. Read, V.H., McCaa, C.S., Bower, J.D., and McCaa, R.E. (1973) Effect of hemodialysis on the metabolic clearance rate, plasma concentration and blood production rate of aldosterone in anephric man. J. Clin. Endocrinol. Metab. 36, 773–778.
82. Reid, I.A. (1977) Is there a brain renin-angiotensin system? Circ. Res. 41, 147–153.
83. Saruta, T., Cook, R., and Kaplan, N.M. (1972) Adrenocortical steroidogenesis: Studies on the mechanism of action of angiotensin and electrolytes. J. Clin. Invest. 51, 2239–2245.
84. Schambelan, M., and Sebastian, A. (1977) Adrenocortical hormone response to metabolic acidosis in normal man. Clin. Res 25, 301A.
85. Sealey, J.E., Moon, C., Laragh, J.H., and Atlas, S.A. (1977) Plasma prorenin in normal, hypertensive and anephric subjects and its effect on renin measurements. Circ. Res. 40 (Suppl. I), 141–145.
86. Sealey, J.E., White, R.P., Laragh, J.H., Case, D.B., and Rubin, A.L. (1978) Studies of plasma aldosterone in anephric people: Evidence for the fundamental role of the renin system in maintaining aldosterone secretion. J. Clin. Endocrinol. Metab. 47, 52–60.
87. Sen, S., Bravo, E.L., and Bumpus, F.M. (1977) Isolation of a hypertension-producing compound from normal human urine. Circ. Res. 40 (Suppl. I), 15–110.
88. Singer, B., and Stack-Dunne, M.P. (1955) The secretion of aldosterone and corticosterone by the rat adrenal. J. Endocrinol. 12, 130–145.

89. Skinner, S.L., Lumbers, E.R., Symonds, E.M. (1969) Alterations by oral contraceptives of normal menstrual changes in plasma renin activity, concentration and substrate. Clin. Sci. 36, 67–76.
90. Slater, J.D.H. (1969) The role of the renin–angiotensin system in the control of aldosterone secretion. Proc. Roy. Soc. Med. 62, 1251–1252.
91. Speckart, P., Zia, P., Zipser, R., and Horton, R. (1977) Effect of sodium restriction and prostaglandin inhibition on the renin-angiotensin system in man. J. Clin. Endocrinol. Metab. 44, 832–837.
92. Tan, S.Y., and Mulrow, P.J. (1975) The contribution of the zona fasciculata and glomerulosa to plasma 11-deoxycorticosterone levels in man. J. Clin. Endocrinol. Metab. 41, 126–130.
93. Tan, S.Y., and Mulrow, P.J. (1977) Inhibition of the renin-aldosterone response to furosemide by indomethacin. J. Clin. Endocrinol. Metab. 45, 174–176.
94. Tan, S.Y., and Mulrow, P.J. (1978) Regulation of 18-hydroxydeoxycorticosterone in the rat. Endocrinology 102, 1113–1117.
95. Tobian, L. (1960) Physiology of juxtaglomerular cells. Ann. Intern. Med. 52, 395–410.
96. Vander, A.J. (1967) Control of renin release. Physiol. Rev. 47, 359–382.
97. Vander, A.J., and Miller, R. (1964) Control of renin secretion in the anesthetized dog. Am.J. Physiol. 207, 537–546.
98. Williams, G.H., Braley, L.M., and Underwood, R.H. (1976) The regulation of plasma 18-hydroxy 11-deoxycorticosterone in man. J. Clin. Invest. 58, 221–229.
99. Williams, G.H., Rose, L.I., Dluhy, R.G., Dingman, J.F., and Lauler, D.P. (1971) Aldosterone response to sodium restriction and ACTH stimulation in panhypopituitarism. J. Clin. Endocrinol. Metab. 32, 27–35.
100. Yun, J., Kelly, G., Bartter, F.C., and Smith, H. (1977) Role of prostaglandins in the control of renin secretion in the dog. Circ. Res. 40, 459–464.

JUDITH SAFFRAN, Ph.D

RECEPTORS FOR HORMONES OF THE ADRENAL CORTEX

INTRODUCTION

The adrenal cortex is composed of three different histologic zones, the zona glomerulosa, the zona fasciculata, and the zona reticularis. Each zone secretes a mixture of hormones, reflecting differences in the distribution of the enzymes that convert cholesterol to the adrenal cortical hormones.

The mineralocorticoid aldosterone is synthesized in the zona glomerulosa. The zona fasciculata and the zona reticularis are sources of the glucocorticoids cortisol and corticosterone, as well as of the adrenal androgens. Although the primary physiologic activities of mineralocorticoids, glucocorticoids, and androgens are very different, all the steroid hormones of the adrenal cortex share a common mechanism of action with the steroid hormones of the gonads and with vitamin D.

According to this unified theory, all steroid hormones diffuse into cells with ease, and bind with high affinity to protein receptors that are present only in the cytoplasm of target cells (Figure 1). The binding is specific for target tissues and for steroids with hormonal activity. Because the number of receptor molecules in a cell is limited, the binding is also saturable.

From the Departments of Biochemistry and Pathology, Medical College of Ohio, Toledo, Ohio.

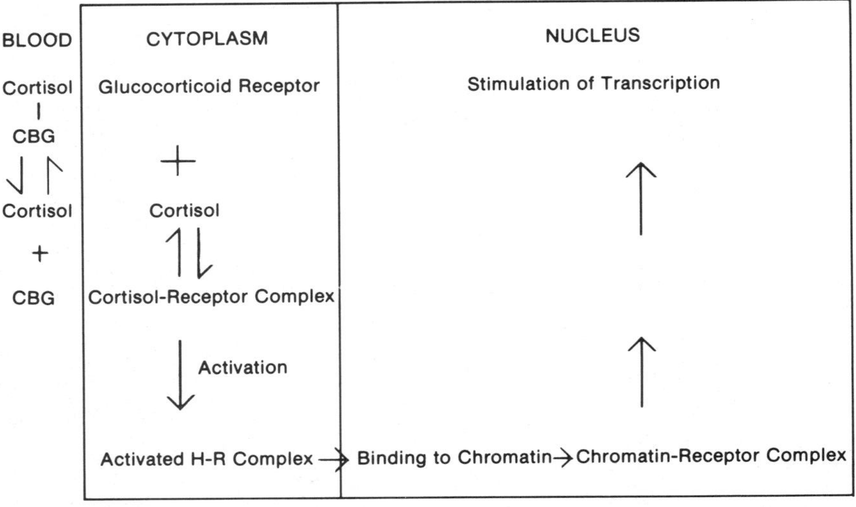

FIGURE 1. Model of steroid hormone action. Cortisol is used as an example. **CBG**, Corticosteroid-binding globulin; **R**, receptor; **H**, hormone.

Steroid hormones bind to other proteins in target cells, but this binding is neither specific nor saturable. The hormone-receptor complex undergoes an as yet unclear process of "activation" or "transformation" that enables it to enter the nucleus and bind to chromatin. This binding is essential for the activity of the hormone, and results in the stimulation of transcription and, ultimately, in increased protein synthesis.

The major target organ of the mineralocorticoids is the kidney; receptors for mineralocorticoids have been studied mainly in the kidney. Glucocorticoids affect the metabolic activity of nearly all cells of the body, and receptors for glucocorticoids have been identified throughout the body. Because of overlapping activities of mineralocorticoids and glucocorticoids, there is an overlap in the presence of receptors in target tissues.

DISTRIBUTION OF GLUCOCORTICOID RECEPTORS IN VARIOUS TISSUES

The physiologic effects of the glucocorticoid hormones vary in different target organs, and may be either anabolic or catabolic. Catabolic actions predominate in lymphoid tissue, and cell death and lympholysis result from hormone action. In the liver, glucocorticoids induce the synthesis of the enzymes that mediate the effects of the hormones. The liver is the major site of gluconeogenesis and the enzymes tyrosine aminotransferase, tryptophane oxygenase, and ornithine decarboxylase are synthesized here and switch the metabolism of the organism to carbohydrate-forming pathways. The ultimate effect is protein catabolism in the organism as a whole.

The liver was the subject of early investigations of the mechanism of action of glucocorticoids. Beato et al. (19) reported the presence of a glycoprotein in the liver of adrenalectomized rats, which bound [^{3}H]-cortisol and was involved in the transport of the hormone into the nucleus, resulting in increased transcription of liver chromatin.

The work of several groups of investigators showed that rat liver contains several proteins that bind glucocorticoids. However, only one binds both natural and synthetic glucocorticoids and has all the properties of a receptor. In spite of a confusing diversity of nomenclature, a protein designated G protein (90) and binder II (106) seems to represent the glucocorticoid receptor of liver. The liver also contains transcortin (corticosteroid-binding globulin) and other proteins that bind only natural glucocorticoids. Their properties and purification have been extensively studied by Litwack et al. (25,106), who isolated six fractions, designated as follows: IA (Ligandin, a GSH-S-alkyl transferase); IB (a binder present at 1/10 the concentration of binder II, binding both natural and synthetic glucocorticoids); II (the receptor); IIIA and IIIB, which bind metabolites of glucocorticoids and IV (transcortin). Binder IB may have a role in hormone action (107).

Studies of the binding of natural glucocorticoids in liver are complicated by the presence of protein binders other than the receptor, and also by the rapid metabolism of cortisol and corticosterone by liver enzymes. The use of synthetic glucocorticoids, such as dexamethasone, is advantageous because they are not metabolized and because they bind to the receptor, but not to transcortin.

Another approach to the study of glucocorticoid action in hepatic tissue was the use of tissue cultured from a rat hepatoma (hepatoma tissue culture or HTC cells). Glucocorticoids induce the synthesis of the enzyme tyrosine aminotransferase in these cells and the enzyme is a useful biochemical marker of hormone action. Binding to the glucocorticoid receptor is a prerequisite for enzyme induction, and there is a good correlation of the binding affinity of various steroids and their ability to stimulate enzyme induction (18). Some steroids (e.g., progesterone) are competitive inhibitors of enzyme synthesis and binding affinity and inhibitory action also are related.

As a result of this work. Rousseau et al. (150) postulated a model of hormone action and suggested that adrenal steroids act as allosteric effector molecules. They classified steroids into four groups, based on their ability to influence the induction of tyrosine aminotransferase in HTC cells. Steroids with high activity were optimal inducers and bound to the cytoplasmic receptor with high affinity. Suboptimal inducers had less potency and binding affinity, while inactive compounds had neither activity nor affinity. Antiinducers did not stimulate the enzyme, but they bound to the receptor and, thus, inhibited the activity of potent glucocorticoids. The cytoplasmic receptor seems to exist in two conformational forms in equilibrium with one another. One form is active and the other inactive. In the absence of hormone the receptor is in the inactive form. Binding by "inducer" steroids shifts the equilibrium toward the active form in proportion to hormonal activity (optimal inducers > suboptimal inducers). The complex can then be translocated to the nucleus and initiate hormonal effects. Antiinducer steroids also bind to the receptor, but do not increase the concentration of the active form and, hence, competitively inhibit the action of inducers. All steroids are thought to bind to the same receptor site, but only inducers are capable of effecting nuclear translocation of the steroid-receptor complex (152). An alternative model to explain the ability of some steroids to act as suboptimal inducers or antiinducers was proposed by Suthers et al. (188). They suggested that the receptor might have a second class of binding sites with a selective affinity for antagonist steroids. Occupation of the second site might reduce the affinity between the active site and the inducer steroid, causing a dissociation of the active hormone-receptor complex and resulting in a decrease in biologic activity. They thought that optimal inducers might have no affinity for the second site, but that suboptimal inducers might have partial affinity for both sites. Progesterone is an antagonist of both glucocorticoids and mineralocorticoids. Wambach and Higgins (196) found that progesterone increased the rate of dissociation of the dexamethasone-receptor complex of liver and of the aldosterone-receptor complex of kidney, supporting the alternative model.

The glucocorticoid receptor of HTC cells has properties that are similar to those of the rat liver receptor and may be the same protein. The human liver glucocorticoid receptor also is similar to that in rat liver (3) and to the receptor in an induced liver tumor (179).

The lymphatic system is another important target of glucocorticoid hormones and also was an early focus of studies on the mechanism of hormone action. Lymphatic tissue responds to glucocorticoids with inhibition of protein synthesis and involution.

Rat thymus cells bind [^{3}H]-cortisol in vitro. Specific sites are saturated at physiologic concentrations of the hormone and the hormone-receptor complex is translocated to the nucleus in a temperature-dependent process (203). Cortisol is not readily metabolized by isolated thymocytes, making it practical to use natural, as well as synthetic, glucocorticoids. In early studies of cortisol binding by thymocytes, it was found that there was a correlation between the levels of ATP in the cell and the magnitude of specific binding (128). It was then suggested that ATP exerts its effects in an energy-dependent cell cycle of receptor action. It was postulated that the hormone-receptor complex enters the nucleus to bind to chromatin and, thus, to exert its effects; the receptor is then released from the nucleus in a form that must be reactivated before it can function again. These early speculations were remarkably prophetic. This will be discussed more fully in the section on receptor properties.

The antiglucocorticoid cortexolone (11-deoxycortisol) is a competitive inhibitor of active glucocorticoids in rat thymocytes. Turnell et al. (194) suggested that the cortexolone-receptor complex was taken up by the nucleus but, because of altered conformation and decreased acceptor site affinity, was not active. In contrast, Rousseau et al. (152) found that antiglucocorticoid-receptor complexes in HTC cells were not translocated to the nucleus.

Both normal and neoplastic rat and mouse lymphatic tissue contained receptors for glucocorticoids (89,195). In human leukocytes, also, there was good correlation between binding activity and the physiologic effects of glucocorticoids (177,178).

The glucocorticoids themselves regulate the secretion of hormones from the zona fasciculata and reticularis of the adrenal cortex through the feedback inhibition of ACTH secretion from the anterior pituitary. This control may be exerted via the secretion of corticotropin-releasing factor from the hypothalamus, or by a direct effect on the pituitary, or both.

A search for glucocorticoid receptors in the hypothalamus and pituitary showed that specific binding sites were present in the hypothalamus of adrenalectomized rats (74,115,116,181), of pigs (184,185), of cattle (200), and in the anterior pituitary of rats (42,91). Rotsztejn et al. (149) demonstrated a relationship between ACTH inhibition by corticosterone and the saturation of pituitary binding sites for corticosterone.

The binder(s) are proteins with properties characteristic of receptors (high affinity, hormonal specificity, and saturability), and are distinguishable from transcortin (74,115,200). Specific binding has been found in both cytosol and nuclear fractions, as required for true receptor binding (42,91,116,149,184).

Mouse pituitary tumor cells in tissue culture (A_tT-20 cells) secrete ACTH, which is inhibited by glucocorticoids. These cells contain glucocorticoid receptors that can be translocated to the nucleus (75,190,198). Indeed, nuclear translocation showed a better correlation with the ability of a steroid to inhibit ACTH production than did the binding affinity in cytosol (190).

In addition to the regulation of ACTH secretion, glucocorticoids have an influence on the neuroendocrine activity of the brain, on mood and behavior. Receptors are not restricted to the hypothalamus and pituitary, but are more widely distributed in the brain (31), with the highest concentrations in the limbic system. There is fairly general agreement that localization is predominantly in the hippocampus, followed by septum and amygdala (74,116,117,181,183,185). There was a diurnal variation in the amount of corticosterone bound by proteins in the brain, which was dependent on the presence of the adrenal cortex and was inversely proportional to the concentration of circulating corticoids (182,183).

The localization of receptors by means of binding of glucocorticoids was confirmed by radioautographic studies after the administration of natural and synthetic glucocorticoids (63,187). Coutard et al. (40) compared the localization of [^{3}H]-dexamethasone in several tissues (heart, liver, kidney, and brain) of adrenalectomized mice by both autoradiography and the measurement of specific binding. Specific binding was seen in the cytosol and nuclei of all tissues, but autoradiography demonstrated displaceable binding only in cell nuclei. In brain tissue, autoradiography showed the highest concentration of dexamethasone in the medial basal hypothalamus.

A puzzling discrepancy was seen in the distribution of binding sites for natural and synthetic hormones in brain tissue (117). Dexamethasone was concentrated in cell nuclei of the anterior pituitary and was found in much lower concentration in the hippocampus and hypothalamus. Corticosterone binding was highest in the hippocampus and septum, and lower in the pituitary.(118,185). McEwen et al. (118) found the differences to be more pronounced in experiments in vivo than in vitro. The differences in the distribution of the different steroids also appeared in radioautograms (187).

It seemed possible that there were at least two different binding sites with different binding properties for natural and synthetic glucocorticoids. In support of this, dexamethasone and corticosterone had different binding properties in competitive binding experiments. Unlabeled dexamethasone and corticosterone both competed effectively with [^{3}H]-dexamethasone binding, but unlabeled dexamethasone did not compete with [^{3}H]-corticosterone (43,183). Maclusky et al. (109) were able to separate at least two binding components by isoelectric focusing, and DeKloet and Burbach (46) reported a 200-fold purification of one of the receptors by affinity chromatography.

Koch et al.(91) confirmed the presence of two classes of binding sites in the anterior pituitary. One of the binders resembled transcortin but was not of plasma origin. It was suggested that the transcortin-like protein might be bound to plasma membranes (92,93).

Glucocorticoid receptors have been identified in many other tissues whose metabolism is regulated by the hormones. Receptor instability has been a great problem in the detection and measurement of receptors in many of these tissues. In some cases, successful measurement of receptors has required the use of inhibitors of proteolysis, agents protective of sulfhydryl (SH), the presence of glycerol in buffers and, especially, the presence of the hormone itself. The unbound glucocorticoid receptor is very unstable, but its stability is increased when it is in bound form.

Some tissues are most markedly affected by glucocorticoids during development in utero. The properties of the receptors in these tissues will be discussed in a section on the ontogenesis of receptors.

Lung tissue, both in the fetus and in the adult, contains receptors for glucocorticoids (13,72,191). The adult lung is exceeded only by the liver and lymphatic tissue in its content of receptors.

Mammary tissue from virgin, pregnant, and lactating rodents, as well as cultured mammary cells and transplanted and carcinogen-induced mammary tumors, all contain glucocorticoid receptors. As with hepatic tissue, the receptors in the normal and neoplastic mammary glands are similar (30,70,192,194).

Muscle contains receptors (possibly different) for both natural (cortisol) and synthetic (dexamethasone, triamcinolone acetonide) glucocorticoids. (113,114).

Glucocorticoid receptors have been demonstrated in adipose tissue, both brown and white (55,57), bone (29,54,10), the gastrointestinal tract

(143), heart (60,172), arteries (95), and interstitial cells of the testis (52).

The presence of glucocorticoid receptors in so many different tissues (11) gives rise to the question, "Is the same receptor present in all of the tissues?" This is especially pertinent because glucocorticoids have different effects in different tissues and some tissues (e.g., testis) have receptors but their function is not yet certain. Feldman et al. (56) studied dexamethasone binding in tissues with diverse glucocorticoid actions. They chose kidney (anabolic effects), thymus (catabolic effects), and adipose tissue (permissive effects), and concluded that the binding sites in all tissues seemed to be the same. Acs et al. (1) independently reached the same conclusion.

MINERALOCORTICOID RECEPTORS

The main function of aldosterone is the regulation of sodium and potassium excretion by the kidney. Kidney cytosol contains receptors for aldosterone, which are translocated to the nucleus and bind to chromatin. The receptor protein is saturated at physiologic concentrations of aldosterone, and there is generally good correlation of the relative binding affinity of a variety of steroids and their potency as mineralocorticoids. Aldosterone also binds in kidney cytosol to sites that exhibit lower affinity of binding (58,111,151).

The two classes of aldosterone binding sites appear to represent mineralocorticoid receptors, which have been designated type I sites (higher affinity) and glucocorticoid receptors, which have been designated type II sites (lower affinity for aldosterone). The type II sites bind dexamethasone with high affinity. Coutard et al. (40) called into question the presence of type II sites in this tissue, because the autoradiographic localization of dexamethasone was not definite. In addition, there are corticosterone-binding sites resembling corticosteroid-binding globulin (CBG), which have been called type III sites (59). Type III sites have low affinity for dexamethasone and are similar, but not identical, to the CBG of blood plasma. They have different sedimentation properties (8S for type III sites of kidney; 4S for plasma CBG) and, unlike CBG, can undergo nuclear translocation. The type III sites are localized in the inner medulla-papilla of the kidney, rather than in the cortex (53) and this has been confirmed by autoradiography (186).

Doucet and Katz (48) measured [^{3}H]-aldosterone binding along microdissected nephron segments from rabbit kidney. Specific binding, in highest concentration, was present in branched collecting tubule, cortical collecting tubule, and outer medullary collecting tubule. This corresponds to the site of aldosterone action. There was negligible binding in proximal convoluted tubule, pars recta, medullary thick ascending limb, cortical thick ascending limb, and distal convoluted tubule.

Kidney receptors for aldosterone have been separated by ion exchange chromatography into four binding components, one of which may be the mineralocorticoid receptor (2).

Mineralocorticoid receptors also have been identified in parotid gland

(58), toad bladder (4) gut mucosa (143), and brain (5). Lung tissue from adult rats contains low levels of high affinity aldosterone binders, in addition to high concentrations of glucocorticoid receptors (98). Smooth muscle cells and fibroblasts cultured from rat aorta contain material binding both aldosterone and corticosterone with high affinity (119). However, the binding properties differ from those of classical glucocorticoid and mineralocorticoid receptors. Anterior pituitary, in contrast, contains authentic mineralocorticoid receptors, suggesting that the pituitary might be involved in the feedback regulation of aldosterone (99).

PROPERTIES OF GLUCOCORTICOID RECEPTORS

The glucocorticoid receptor has properties that are common to all steroid hormone receptors. Like other cytoplasmic receptors it is a protein, representing a very small percent (less than 0.01%) of the total protein in the cytoplasm. Binding is specific for hormonal activity and the binding affinity usually parallels the biologic activity. Furthermore, binding is saturated at a concentration of hormone that has physiologic activity. Equilibrium dissociation constants, calculated from Scatchard analysis of saturation curves, are in the neighborhood of 10^{-9}M. In cell-free binding studies, the cytoplasmic receptors must undergo a process of "activation" (or "transformation") to enable them to bind to nuclei. The receptor complex can be extracted from nuclei using buffers with a salt concentration (KCl or NaCl) greater than 0.15−0.2 M, but a portion of the receptor resists extraction and remains bound to chromatin.

On sucrose gradient centrifugation the sedimentation coefficient of the receptor complex in cytosol depends on the ionic strength and is 7-8S in buffers of low ionic strength and approximately 4S at higher salt concentrations (0.3−0.4 M KCl). The nuclear receptor, on the other hand, sediments at 3-4S, regardless of salt concentration.

Middlebrook and Aronow (121) made a systematic study of the physiochemical properties of unpurified glucocorticoid receptors in cytosol and nuclei of mouse fibroblasts. The isoelectric points and partial specific volumes were the same for receptors in cytosol and in nuclear fractions (extracted with 0.3 M KCl and resistant to extraction). Isoelectric focusing experiments gave three peaks of activity at pH 5.8−5.9 (75% of the total), pH 6.4 (20%), and pH 6.9 (5%).

On the other hand, sedimentation properties of cytoplasmic and nuclear receptors were different. The sedimentation coefficients in cytosol varied with the ionic strength of the buffer, and were approximately 6S at low ionic strength, decreasing to 4S when the concentration of KCl was 0.2 M or greater. The receptor extracted from nuclei had a sedimentation coefficient of 4S that was not dependent on ionic strength. The receptor resistant to extraction (nuclear residual form) aggregated on sucrose gradients.

Stokes radii also were different for different receptor forms and were 73Å, 59Å, and 32Å respectively, for cytosol at low and isotonic salt concentrations and for isotonic nuclear extract. These studies suggest that the cytoplasmic receptor probably is an asymmetric protein, while the nuclear form is globular. Calculated molecular weights were 172,000, 109,000, and 54,000 for cytosol in low salt and isotonic buffers and for nuclear extract, respectively. Molecular weights of cytoplasmic receptors determined by gel filtration are not reliable because of the asymmetric shape of the receptor molecule.

The receptors in cytosol and nuclear extracts were unstable at 30°C, but the nuclear residual form was much more stable.

Litwack et al. (108) also reported the results of a careful study of the physical properties of the glucocorticoid receptor of rat liver cytosol. On sucrose gradient centrifugation, two forms with sedimentation coefficients of 7-8S (unactivated) and 5.1S (activated by NaSCN) were seen. Activation at 25°C did not change the sedimentation coefficient of 8S. In addition, an aggregating form that disaggregated on dilution was seen. The Stokes radius (3.5 nm) and the molecular weight (78,000) were both somewhat lower than those reported for fibroblast cytosol by Middlebrook and Aronow (121).

In spite of generally similar physical properties, steroid hormone receptors have differing stabilities. The glucocorticoid receptor is rather less stable than the estrogen and androgen receptor, and conditions were devised to preserve the receptor for experimental studies (13,72,166). Empirical observations showed that instability was most marked when the receptor was not bound to its hormone. Oxidation of sulfhydryl groups led to a loss of binding capacity, especially when the receptor was unbound, and SH compounds, such as dithiothreitol, thioglycerol, and mercaptoethanol protected the receptor. Glycerol also had a protective effect. The ionic strength and pH of buffers were critical and, in rat liver, optimal conditions were pH 7.5 in the presence of 20 mM tris buffer, 50 mM KCl, and 20% glycerol (166).

More recently, the properties of glucocorticoid receptors in rat liver, mouse fibroblast L929 cells, and rat thymocytes have received a thorough study with results that now permit a rational choice of experimental conditions for studying the receptors (134,135,160−162). In addition, an understanding of the properties of the receptor should result in a better understanding of its mechanism of action.

Nielsen et al. (134) found that purified alkaline phosphatase (calf intestine) inactivated unbound glucocorticoid receptors in mouse fibroblast and rat liver cytosol. Arsenate, which inhibits the ability of alkaline phosphatase to cleave phosphate from chemically defined substrates, inhibited receptor inactivation by the purified enzyme preparation. This suggests that receptor inactivation involves the removal of phosphate. The loss of binding capacity was not caused by proteolysis, since inhibitors of proteolysis were not protective. Inhibitors of proteolysis, however, did stabilize the glucocorticoid receptors of adipose tissue (55).

An endogenous enzyme with similar inactivating properties was found in the particulate fraction of rat thymocytes, rat liver, and mouse fibroblasts (135). The activity of the enzyme and its exact distribution differ in thymocytes, liver, and fibroblasts, with the greatest activity present in thymocytes and the smallest in liver. This may account for the fact that the receptor in thymocytes is most unstable, followed in order of increasing stability by fibroblast and liver.

Indirect evidence indicates that the inactivation caused by the endogenous enzyme is the result of dephosphorylation and not proteolysis. Receptor inactivation was inhibited by known inhibitors of phosphatase. Molybdate was most effective, followed by fluoride and glucose-1-phosphate. However, glucose-1-phosphate was the only effective inhibitor of inactivation in thymocyte cytosol.

A factor in mouse fibroblast cytosol of molecular weight between 5,000 and 15,000 was able to reactivate the binding capacity of thymocyte cytosol, but the mechanism is not yet understood (160).

In further studies with mouse fibroblast cytosol, Sando et al. (161) showed that ATP reactivated binding capacity after it had been lost. Magnesium seemed to be required for this process. The logical conclusion was that activation involved an ATP-dependent phosphorylation process, possibly of the receptor itself, although there was no definite proof of this. The very labile thymocyte receptor required both SH-protective compounds (dithiothreitol) and ATP for reactivation (162).

On the basis of the studies just described and of empirical observations, it can be concluded that the unbound glucocorticoid receptor is active (able to bind hormones) when it is in the reduced (SH) form and phosphorylated state, and is inactivated by oxidation and removal of phosphate.

These studies confirm and extend the earlier observations of Munck et al. (128) and Ishii et al. (79) that the glucocorticoid receptor requires energy (ATP) to enable it to bind hormone and to function in the cell.

ACTIVATION OR TRANSFORMATION OF GLUCOCORTICOID RECEPTORS

Before the complex of glucocorticoid receptor and hormone can bind in the nucleus, it must first undergo a process of "activation" or "transformation," a property it shares with all steroid hormone receptor complexes. The terms "activation" and "transformation" refer to the same process, i.e., the change in the cytoplasmic hormone-receptor complex that enables it to bind to nuclei at O°C, in cell-free incubations.

It is generally agreed that activation involves changes only in the cytoplasmic receptor and does not affect the nucleus. Milgrom et al. (122) studied the glucocorticoid receptor of rat liver and dissected glucocorticoid action into three parts: 1) the association of hormone and receptor, which takes place at low temperature and low ionic strength; 2) the activation of the hormone-receptor complex; and 3) the binding of the activated complex by nuclei. Only the hormone-receptor complex, not the free receptor, is believed to be activated and to bind the nuclei. The activated and unactivated receptor complexes normally exist in equilibrium and, even under favorable circumstances, at least 40% of the receptor is not activated (7). However, in the presence of an excess of nuclear acceptor the equilibrium can be shifted in the direction of activation (8).

Under what conditions does activation take place? The cytoplasmic receptor and hormone associate fairly rapidly at 0°C, but the complex is not translocated to the nucleus at an appreciable rate at 0°C. Activation does take place slowly at 0°C, however, and after 24 hours equilibrium is reached (86). Warming the glucocorticoid-receptor complex greatly increased the rate of activation; but as the temperature increased, the possibility of receptor inactivation also increased. Activation is usually carried out at 20−25°C, a temperature at which activation is rapid, but the receptor is reasonably stable (65,66,69,86,124).

The rate of activation at 0°C is greatly increased when the ionic strength of the buffer is increased. Usually, 0.3−0.4 M KCl or NaCl is used. (66,86,122). The effect of divalent cations is not clear. Milgrom et al. (122) found that Ca^{++} inhibited activation, while Kalimi et al. (86) found activation to be facilitated by Ca^{++}, both in studies of the glucocorticoid receptor of rat liver. ATP also activated the glucocorticoid receptor of rat liver at 0°C (81). Thiocyanate (140) and theophylline (26) both increased activation. Theophylline acted directly on the hormone-receptor complex and not by a cyclic-AMP-dependent mechanism.

The hormone-receptor complex is very susceptible to activation and many treatments result in the formation of activated complex. Dilution of the cytosol and gel filtration on several types of gels cause activation (10,27,69,77,140).

Differences in the binding properties of activated and unactivated complexes have been used as the basis of separation. Phosphocellulose separates the activated glucocorticoid-receptor complex, which binds, from unactivated complex, which does not (7,37−39). In fact, exposure to phosphocellulose activates the complex. Separation of activated and unactivated complexes has been effected on DEAE Sephadex and carboxymethyl Sephadex (140), and on DEAE-cellulose, as well (157). Protamine sulfate precipitation can be used to separate unactivated and activated glucocorticoid receptors because only the activated receptor complex is precipitated (87).

The difference in binding properties of activated and unactivated receptors also has been used to purify receptor complexes by sequential chromatography; and upwards of a 1000-fold purification has been achieved in this way (7,37−39, 50). The glucocorticoid receptor of rat liver has been purified using protamine sulfate precipitation and chromatography (affinity chromatography on deoxycorticosterone-Sepharose, followed by DEAE-cellulose) (71). Two homogenous dexamethasone-binding components of molecular weight 45,000 and 90,000, respectively, were obtained. Antibodies to the two binders showed mutual cross-reactivity. The investigator suggested that the 90,000-dalton component was a dimer of the 45,000-dalton protein, and resulted from activation of the receptor during purification. Parchman and Litwack (140) also found that the rat liver glucocorticoid receptor was activated during the course of purification. Since binding ability decreases, or is lost after activation, detection of the receptor becomes difficult (140). However, receptor measurement by immunoassay overcomes this difficulty (71).

Sodium molybdate inhibits receptor activation and facilitates the separation of unactivated and activated receptor complexes (41). This should allow the preparation of the unactivated receptor complex in quantities that are adequate for a study of its properties.

What changes in receptor properties result from activation? It is generally agreed that activation increases the affinity of the glucocorticoid-receptor complex for nuclei. The affinity for DNA increases and a preparation of DNA cellulose has been used as a surrogate nucleus in many binding studies (86). The affinity of the receptor for a variety of polyanions (homologous and heterologous DNA and RNA, carboxymethyl and sulfopropyl Sephadex) increases as a result of activation (39,122). This suggests that activation causes an increase in the number of positive groups on the surface of the receptor molecule (122). In agreement, Parchman and Litwack (140) found that the activated receptor was more basic than the unactivated receptor. They suggested that the molecule was an acidic protein with localized basic regions. However, Kalimi et al. (86) reported that the isoelectric point decreased from 7.1 to 6.1 as a result of activation, suggesting that the molecule became not more basic, but more acidic. Pyridoxal phosphate reversibly inhibits the binding of activated glucocorticoid-receptor complex to DNA cellulose (28). Formation of covalent bonds by reduction with sodium borohydride results in irreversible inhibition. Cake et al. (28) suggested that pyridoxal phosphate acted by forming a Schiff base with ξ-amino group of lysine appearing at the surface of the complex as a result of activation.

There is no agreement as to the effects of activation on the sedimentation properties of the receptor. Kalimi et al. (86) found no change from a sedimentation coefficient of 7-8S after activation. Giannopoulos (65,66) found that heat activation did not change the sedimentation coefficient (7S) of the fetal lung glucocorticoid receptor, but the receptor activated with 0.4 M KCl at 0°C had a sedimentation coefficient of 5S. Litwack et al. (108) also found that the sedimentation coefficient of heat-activated receptor was not changed, but that thiocyanate activation decreased the sedimentation coefficient to approximately 5S.

What is the mechanism of activation? Beyond the statement that activation involves a conformational change in hormone-receptor complex (8,122), the mechanism is not known. The fact that dilution and gel filtration facilitate activation suggests that either the receptor dissociates into subunits or that an inhibitor of activation is removed. The latter theory is favored.

There is agreement that molybdate inhibits activation. Because molybdate is an inhibitor of phosphatases, it has been suggested that activation may involve dephosphorylation (16,81,102). There is a good deal of experimental support for this theory, but it remains speculative.

The effects of molybdate are concentration-dependent. At low concentrations (10−20 mM), activation is inhibited, but activated receptor complexes can still bind to the nucleus (132,136). At higher concentrations (50 mM), nuclear translocation is inhibited (132). Unfortunately, the way in which molybdate acts is not understood. Therefore, studies using molybdate have not really clarified the mechanism of activation.

Pyridoxal phosphate, a more physiologic substance, also affects activation and/or nuclear translocation (171). Like molybdate, it alters surface charge and binding of glucocorticoid receptors to polyanions. It changes the sedimentation coefficient of the receptor complex and protects against proteolysis (34,138). Its relation to molybdate, however, is not clear. Its possible role in glucocorticoid action will be discussed in the section "The Regulation of Receptor Concentrations In Vivo."

It can be argued that activation is an artifact of the in vitro conditions under which it is nearly always studied. Munck and Foley (131) have evidence that activation occurs in whole cells as a physiologic concomitant of glucocorticoid action.

NUCLEAR BINDING

It is generally accepted that the cytoplasmic hormone-receptor complex is translocated to the nucleus after it has been "activated" ("transformed"). In support of this concept, the concentration of cytoplasmic glucocorticoid receptor (in liver, HTC tissue culture cells, and cultured pituitary tumor cells) decreases while the concentration of nuclear receptor increases by an equivalent amount (21,22,152,199).

The evidence seems overwhelming that glucocorticoid and mineralocorticoid receptors are translocated to the nucleus only when they are complexed with their respective hormones. However, the dogma that steroid hormone receptors enter the nucleus only as hormone-receptor complexes may be susceptible to modification. Uterine estrogen receptors (24,163) and progesterone receptors (155,156) can be activated in the absence of hormone and bind to nuclei. Free estrogen receptors have been found in the nucleus of cultured MCF-7 cancer cells (204,205) and of the ovariectomized rat uterus (82).

The results of early investigations indicated that binding in the nucleus, like that in the cytoplasm, was to a small number of high affinity acceptor sites (K_d of approximately 10^{-10}M) (77,78,85,105,173). It later became evident, however, that the apparent saturation of nuclear binding was an artifact (124). Crude cytosol was found to contain macromolecular inhibitor(s) of nuclear binding. As the concentration of the receptor increased, so did the concentration of the inhibitor, leading to a deceptive appearance of saturation. The inhibitor interacted with the hormone-receptor complex in cytosol to prevent binding to the nucleus (9,175). Nuclear binding is now thought to be of high capacity and not saturable (125,153). However, Pfahl et al. (142) have evidence for the presence of both low and high affinity sites in the nuclei of a lymphoid cell line.

Although there is target cell specificity for cytoplasmic receptors, the evidence for such specificity of nuclear binding is controversial. Kalimi et al. (85) found that the glucocorticoid-receptor complex of liver bound preferentially to liver nuclei. Climent et al. (38) reported that liver chromatin bound more purified cytoplasmic receptor of liver than did chicken erythrocyte chromatin. Climent et al. (38) also measured receptor binding to chromatin subunits (nucleosomes) and found that the tissue specificity was not present in the nucleosomes, concluding that specificity resides in another part of the genome. Milgrom et al.(125) found no species specificity, and Higgins et al. (78) agreed that nuclear receptors were not restricted to target tissues.

In spite of considerable work, the composition of the acceptor site for the hormone-receptor complex and the precise nature of the binding also remain controversial. The hormone-receptor complex binds to chromatin, and there is little doubt that DNA is involved in the binding. The complex binds to purified DNA (153) and to DNA adsorbed to cellulose (21). The requirements for binding to DNA are the same as for nuclear binding. The hormone and the receptor must both be present and the resulting complex must be activated. Binding can then take place at 0°C (21,32,125,153). DNA of many sources (procaryotic and eucaryotic) binds the receptor complex (125,175), but denatured DNA binds less well than native DNA (153). The hormone-receptor complex does not bind to RNA (153).

Simons et al. (175) reported that the acceptor capacity of DNA was greater than that of nuclei but that the affinity of the hormone-receptor complex for nuclei was greater than the affinity for DNA. They concluded that the chromosomal proteins associated with DNA had an important influence on binding, reducing the number of acceptor sites, and increasing the affinity of binding to DNA. Milgrom et al. (125) found no difference in the binding capacity of native or denatured DNA, but in other respects agreed with Simons et al. (175) that binding to DNA was of higher capacity than binding to nuclei. The nature of the chromatin proteins that modify glucocorticoid receptor binding is not known.

The interaction of the receptor complex and DNA probably involves electrostatic interactions. In cell-free studies the amount of binding is critically dependent on the pH and ionic strength (77,85,142). Binding takes place at low ionic strength. At high ionic strength (0.15 M KCl and greater) binding is inhibited and the complex is extracted from nuclei (21,125,153,199). Digestion with DNAse, but not RNAse, also extracts the receptor complex from nuclei and DNA cellulose (21,199).

The receptor complexes bound to DNA cellulose and to nuclei are not equally susceptible to extraction with KCl solutions, or to digestion with DNAse. In general, binding to DNA cellulose is more easily disrupted (32). Cidlowski and Thanassi (33,34) found that pyridoxal phosphate extracted 75%−80% of the dexamethasone-receptor complex from nuclei.

The physiologic activity of all steroid hormones begins when the hormone and receptor bind to chromatin. Therefore, it is essential to understand the nature and the regulation of receptor binding in the nucleus. Our knowledge of this process and of the events subsequent to it is still incomplete. However, our general understanding is expanding, albeit at an uneven pace for different steroid hormones.

MULTIPLE RECEPTOR FORMS

Glucocorticoid receptors have been found in nearly all tissues of the body and do not seem to differ from tissue to tissue. Nevertheless, in many tissues there are several binding components for glucocorticoids. Liver contains proteins that bind synthetic glucocorticoids, and natural glucocorticoids and their metabolites with somewhat differing binding affinities. The "receptor" of rat liver has been separated by chromatographic means from transcortin-like material and from other binding proteins (20,90,108,166,167). Rat heart contains three glucocorticoid-binding proteins. One of these resembles the receptor of rat liver, one is similar to transcortin, and one may represent true transcortin contamination (172).

There is ample evidence, although indirect, that there are multiple glucocorticoid binders in rat brain: 1) There is a difference in the distribution of injected corticosterone and dexamethasone. Corticosterone is localized in the limbic system, predominantly in cell nuclei of the hippocampus, septum, and amygdala. Dexamethasone has a more diffuse distribution in brain cell nuclei and is localized in the anterior pituitary (42–44, 118). 2) There is a difference in the temperature stability of corticosterone and dexamethasone binding. Binders for dexamethasone are considerably less stable than those for corticosterone. 3) Competitive binding studies provide evidence for the presence of several binders (43–45). Unlabeled dexamethasone is not a very good competitor for [^{3}H]-corticosterone binding, in spite of its biologic activity as a glucocorticoid (74,183).

Transcortin-like material is present in the pituitary, in addition to the classical glucocorticoid receptor, but little transcortin is found in brain (43,92,93).

Maclusky et al. (109) used isoelectric focusing to separate components with different isoelectric points and binding properties. Hippocampus and hypothalamus cytosol separated into fractions with isoelectric points of 6.8, 5.9, and 4.3. The 4.3 pH fraction bound only corticosterone, a characteristic of transcortin-like material. The 6.8 pH fraction had a preference for corticosterone over dexamethasone, and the fraction with pH 5.9 preferred dexamethasone. Anterior pituitary cytosol contained two fractions with isoelectric points of 4.3 (corticosterone-binding) and 5.9 (dexamethasone-binding). Although chromatography did not initially successfully separate the binding proteins in brain, De Kloet and Burbach (46) succeeded in separating two binding proteins with differing affinities for corticosterone and dexamethasone in hippocampus cytosol by means of ion exchange chromatography.

An anatomical basis for the diversity of glucocorticoid binding in brain has been suggested (45). Autoradiography confirmed binding measurements of the distribution of corticosterone- and dexamethasone-binding sites in the brain. [^{3}H]-corticosterone was concentrated in cell nuclei of neurons in the hippocampus, septum, and amygdala. [^{3}H]-dexamethasone was found in neurons and glial cells throughout the brain (63,187,197).

Neurons and glial cells may contain different receptor proteins with characteristic binding properties.

This may also be the case in the kidney. The kidney has receptors for both mineralocorticoids and glucocorticoids (154). They have been designated binders, I, II, and III (53,59). Binder I is the mineralocorticoid receptor and binds aldosterone with high affinity. Binder II is the glucocorticoid receptor and binds synthetic and natural glucocorticoids with high affinity, but has lesser affinity for aldosterone. Binder III binds natural, but not synthetic glucocorticoids or aldosterone. It is similar, but not identical, to transcortin. The various binders may be localized in different anatomic parts of the kidney. Strum et al. (186) found both autoradiographic and binding evidence that type III sites were concentrated in the collecting tubules of the outer medulla of the kidney.

Other tissues that contain both glucocorticoid and mineralocorticoid receptors are aorta (95), gastrointestinal tract (143), and possibly even brain (5). The heart binds [^{3}H]-aldosterone, but the binding seems to be to glucocorticoid receptors (60).

Bovine tissues contain a receptor with unusual binding properties, in addition to the usual glucocorticoid receptor (47,96). The unique binder has greater temperature stability than the labile glucocorticoid receptor. It can survive a temperature of 37°C for 24 hrs. It binds dexamethasone with moderate affinity (K_d~14 nM), but has virtually no affinity for the even more potent glucocorticoid, triamcinolone acetonide. The function of this binder is not known.

MEMBRANE RECEPTORS

The strict separation of hormones into those that bind to receptors on the plasma membrane of target cells (peptide and catecholamines) and those that bind to receptors in the cytoplasm (steroid hormones) may not be entirely valid. Peptide hormones are increasingly found inside cells (94) and, from time to time, it is suggested that receptors on the plasma membrane play a role in steroid hormone action (17). There is evidence both for (123) and against (127,141) the participation of membrane receptors in the action of β-estradiol on the uterus, in particular on the entry of estradiol into the cell.

Rao et al. (144–146) obtained evidence for the presence of a protein receptor on the plasma membrane of liver cells, which acted to transport corticosterone into the cell. Uptake into hepatocytes was saturable and was inhibited by KCN. p-Chloromercuribenzoate depressed the binding. Suyemitsu and Terayama (189) also found that plasma membranes of liver cells had both high and low affinity binders for natural, but not for synthetic glucocorticoids.

The anterior pituitary contains transcortin-like material, which may be bound to the plasma membrane (92,93). Plasma membranes of rat kidney contain an aldosterone-binding protein that is saturable and of high affinity (139). The importance of this binder is suggested but has not yet been proven.

REGULATION OF RECEPTOR CONCENTRATIONS IN VIVO

The fate of the glucocorticoid hormone-receptor complex, after it has exerted its effects in the nucleus, is not known. Over a long span of time (e.g., days) degradation and resynthesis of receptors undoubtedly takes place. But over the shorter periods of time in which the hormone acts, there is evidence that "used" nuclear receptor returns to the cytoplasm, seemingly in an inactive form, and is then reactivated and used again. The reactivation and possibly also the release from the nucleus require energy (ATP), but not protein synthesis. Experiments with rat thymocytes, mouse fibroblasts, and hepatoma tissue culture cells all point to a cycle of receptor movement from cytoplasm to nucleus and back again.

Rousseau et al. (152) incubated active glucocorticoids (cortisol, dexamethasone) with HTC cells and found that the concentration of cytoplasmic receptor decreased, while the nuclear receptor increased by an equivalent amount. When the hormone was removed from the incubation, there was a rapid decrease of nuclear receptor and a return of cytoplasmic receptor to its original level.

Incubation of rat thymocytes in the absence of oxygen or glucose resulted in low levels of ATP and poor specific binding of cortisol (23,128). However, this was reversible and either oxygen or glucose restored both ATP levels and specific binding. Therefore there appeared to be a correlation between ATP and binding ability. Protein synthesis was not necessary, but a source of energy was essential. Metabolism of the hormone did not take place before the release of the receptor from thymocyte nucleus (129).

Experiments with cultures of mouse fibroblast L 929 cells gave similar results (79,120). As with thymocytes, incubation with metabolic inhibitors of protein synthesis resulted in low levels of cytoplasmic receptor and an apparent accumulation of receptor in the cell nucleus, especially the fraction of the nuclear receptor that was tightly bound to chromatin. It was suggested that the release of receptor from binding in the nucleus required energy as ATP (130).

The role of ATP in glucocorticoid action is now somewhat clearer, although by no means definitely understood (see the section "Properties of Glucocorticoid Receptors"). The ability of the receptor in fibroblasts, thymocytes, and liver to bind the hormone is lost after dephosphorylation and can be regained after ATP-dependent phosphorylation. Whether or not the receptor itself is phosphorylated and dephosphorylated is not yet certain. Sando et al. (162) have proposed that phosphorylation of the reduced receptor (SH form) may be needed for the initial binding of the hormone, but removal of phosphate may be essential for activation (transformation) of the receptor to the form that is translocated to the cell nucleus (Figure 2).

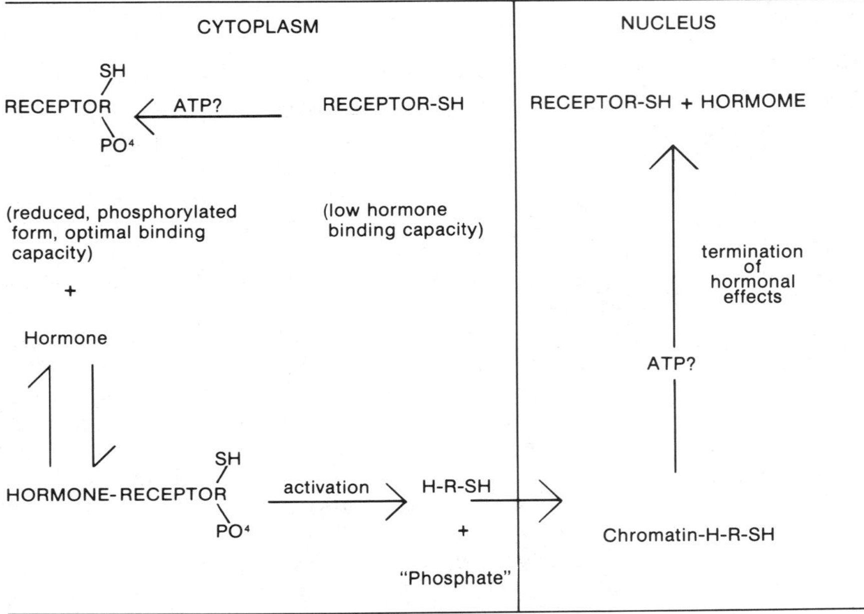

FIGURE 2. Hypothetical cycle of glucocorticoid receptors in target cells. **H**, hormone; **R**, receptor.

Cidlowski and Thanassi (34) have proposed a potential role for pyridoxal phosphate in recycling of used receptors from the nucleus to the cytoplasm. At physiologic concentrations, pyridoxal phosphate extracts glucocorticoid receptors from thymocyte nuclei and stabilizes the receptors against proteolysis. Pyridoxal phosphate might interfere with the interaction between receptor and nuclear acceptor and thus facilitate the release of the receptor. This is entirely speculative.

Little is known of the long-term regulation of glucocorticoid receptors. There is evidence that receptor levels are regulated, at least to some extent, by the hormones themselves. The concentration of receptors was increased in the liver of adrenalectomized rats (22) and suppressed by the administration of glucocorticoids (148).

The concentration of glucocorticoid receptors in HeLaS3 cells was reduced when the cells were grown in the presence of active glucocorticoids (35). Mineralocorticoid receptors also are subject to "self regulation." Receptor levels in the kidneys of adrenalectomized rats were higher than in normal rats, but decreased after the kidneys were perfused with aldosterone (36).

Other hormones also influence receptor levels. Hypophysectomy, as well as adrenalectomy, increases receptor levels, but to a greater extent in females than in males (51). Therefore, sex hormones exert an effect, but one not yet understood.

CORRELATION OF PHYSIOLOGIC ACTIVITY WITH RECEPTORS

A good deal of support for the hypothesis that cytoplasmic receptors mediate the action of steroid hormones has come from the fact that specific binding is restricted to target tissues and that there is a good correlation of binding affinity with biologic activity. With only a few exceptions (47,61,96) the binding affinity of a glucocorticoid parallels its activity (e.g., the ability to induce the enzyme tyrosine amino transferase in hepatoma tissue culture cells). Hormone-resistant mutants of cultured cells have much less receptor than do responsive cells (62,174). This also is true in whole animals. In a comparison of strains of mice with different sensitivity to glucocorticoid-induced cleft palate in the embryos, the insensitive strain had less receptor than the sensitive strain(159). As a species, the guinea pig is resistant to glucocorticoids, while the mouse is sensitive. The glucocorticoid receptor of guinea pig spleen cytosol had a lower affinity for dexamethasone ($K_d \sim 10^{-7}$M) than mouse spleen cytosol ($K_d \sim 10^{-9}$M) (97). Similarly, in Long–Evans rats resistant to deoxycorticosterone (DOC)-induced hypertension, there was a deficiency of DOC-binding protein in the hypothalamus (101).

Some steroids, such as progesterone or 11-deoxycortisol, have the ability to block the action of glucocorticoids by competing with active glucocorticoids for binding to the receptor. However, the antiglucocorticoid receptor complex is unable to complete the normal sequence of events that results in biologic activity (84,196). Progesterone also has antimineralocorticoid action in rats. An antimineralocorticoid, spironolactone (112) acts in the same way to inhibit the action of aldosterone and may be used therapeutically, e.g., in hypertension and liver disease with ascites.

ONTOGENY OF RECEPTORS

Glucocorticoids have an influence on development in many tissues, both pre- and postnatally. In particular, a number of enzymes and other biologically active substances are induced by glucocorticoids, and early maturation of these systems can be brought about by administration of the hormones. It is not surprising that many investigators tried to identify glucocorticoid receptors in developing tissues and to correlate their presence with the biochemical events.

The surfactant dipalmitoyl lecithin ensures the stability of lung alveoli after the transition of the fetus to an air-breathing neonate. The biosynthesis of surfactant increases as parturition approaches and is controlled by glucocorticoids, which may induce some of the responsible enzymes (reviewed by Ballard, 13).

Giannapoulos (64) identified glucocorticoid receptors in the lungs of fetal rats, rabbits, guinea pigs, and humans. In human lung the receptor level increased threefold from 9 to 17 weeks of gestation. Ballard and Ballard (12) also found receptors in human fetal lung, but the concentration was constant throughout fetal life. In rat lung the receptor concentration was highest around the time of birth (76). The receptor in rabbit fetal lung was translocated from cytoplasm to the nucleus, and had the physicochemical properties characteristic of all glucocorticoid receptors (65,66). Giannopoulos (64) was able to find receptors in adult lung only in the rabbit. Granberg and Ballard (72) made a careful study of the properties of glucocorticoid receptors in a variety of fetal and adult tissues and in cultured cells. They found that the unbound receptors were exceedingly unstable, but could be stabilized with SH-protective agents (e.g., dithiothreitol). In this way receptors could be demonstrated in adult lung and other tissues where previously they had not been seen. Glucocorticoid receptors were found in the cells that synthesized surfactant, i.e., in freshly isolated type II epithelial cells and in cell lines from these cells (14).

In the small intestine glucocorticoids influence the changing pattern of enzyme production as young animals develop, mature, and are weaned. In rats, during the 3rd week after birth, there is a decrease in lactase and an increase in peptidases, sucrase, and alkaline phosphatase. Henning et al. (76) found glucocorticoid receptors in the intestine of rats from late fetal life through adulthood, but the highest concentration was present during the first two weeks after birth. The presence of receptors preceded the presence of the enzymes that were induced by glucocorticoids, since the enzymes were first seen between days 16–20 after birth. Lee et al. (103), Lee and Solomon (104), and Solomon and Lee (180) found cytoplasmic and nuclear glucocorticoid receptors in rabbit intestine. The cytosol receptors were maximal at day 25 of gestation and then decreased. Nuclear receptors were detected at day 22 of gestation and were maximal at day 26, declining thereafter. The enzyme alkaline phosphatase was just detected at day 25 and then increased rapidly. Thus, during the development of the rabbit small intestine also, receptor development preceded the development of the enzymes that presumably were mediated by the complex of hormone and receptor. In fetal liver, receptors also were found before the ability of the liver to respond to glucocorticoids (67,68). The receptors in the liver of the fetal and adult animals seemed to have different properties.

Glucocorticoids influence function in developing brain and induce the enzyme glutamine synthetase, which converts glutamate to glutamine. Glucocorticoid receptors were present in the neural retina of chick embryos and, again, levels were high before those of the induced enzyme (126,202). Although such results have prompted most investigators to conclude that the ontogeny of glucocorticoid-induced phenomena was not dependent on the presence of receptors, this conclusion may not be warranted. If the response to the hormone requires the presence of its receptor, it is really not surprising that in the process of development the receptor is seen first.

STRUCTURE–ACTIVITY RELATIONSHIPS

Glucocorticoid activity is not the property of one unique hormone. The adrenal cortex secretes two potent glucocorticoids, cortisol and corticosterone, and a number of still more potent glucocorticoids have been made synthetically. There also is an overlap of glucocorticoid and mineralocorticoid activity; aldosterone has some glucocorticoid activity (suboptimal glucocorticoid). What structural features are responsible for glucocorticoid action? The C4-C5 double bond and C3 ketone group in ring A, and 11 β hydroxyl group in ring C, and a sidechain having a C20-ketone and a C21-hydroxyl are all essential. The addition of other functional groups to the steroid nucleus (OH, CH_3, F, double bonds) modifies the activity, in some cases yielding very potent compounds (e.g., dexamethasone), in others decreasing activity.

Binding to a glucocorticoid receptor is thought to precede physiologic activity. In order to determine which molecular structures are responsible for binding and for biologic activity, it is necessary to correlate binding affinity with physiologic activity, and molecular structure with both. In a series of four papers, G.G. Rousseau and J.P. Schmit reported the results of such a study and also determined the effects of changes in the chemical structure on the exact geometry of a series of steroids with differing glucocorticoid activities (154,168–170).

The binding affinity of the compounds was measured by competition for the binding of [^{3}H]-dexamethasone to the cytosol receptor of cultured HTC cells (154). The index of biologic activity was the ability to induce the enzyme tyrosine amino transferase (TAT) in these cells. This is a good model system, because the induction of TAT correlates well with other effects of glucocorticoids (thymolysis, antiinflammatory action), and HTC cells do not (or very rarely) metabolize the steroids being tested. In addition, problems of drug absorption and transport are avoided.

Correlation of molecular structure with binding and activity requires a precise knowledge of the geometry of the compounds studied. This can be acquired by x-ray crystallography, but x-ray crystallographic measurements are available for only a limited number of steroids. In addition, there are difficulties in comparing structural data obtained on crystals with those of steroids in solution in the cell. There also are inaccuracies when molecular dimensions are calculated from bond lengths and angles (Dreiding model). Schmit and Rousseau (168) chose to determine molecular structure using a computerized method of geometry optimization based on minimization of molecular energy (calculation according to a Westheimer model). The results agreed in general with crystallographic data and were used to describe in depth a series of 15 compounds (169,170). This method describes the molecules in their lowest energy state, in a form where different compounds are comparable with one another.

Schmit and Rousseau (169) studied molecules (pregnanes) with substitutions that produced definite effects on biologic activity. The positions altered were C11 (α- and β-OH), C16 (α- and β-CH_3), and substituents on C17 and C21, which affected the position of the sidechain relative to the D ring. The studies enabled the investigators to determine how functional groups affected the overall shape of the molecule (molecular volume, surface area), as well as effects in specific regions of the molecule (on rings A, B, C, D, and the sidechain) resulting from variations in structure (169). They concluded that binding of the hormone and receptor probably affected the conformation of both the steroid and the receptor. The most mobile parts of the steroid are the A ring, which is deformable, and the sidechain, which is free to rotate about the C17−C20 bond. The D ring also is susceptible to some conformational modification.

Factors of probable importance in binding were thought to be the conformation of the sidechain and ring A. The A ring is responsible for initiating and maintaining binding, while the D ring controls the expression of activity (49). The optimized structure of the A ring seemed to be a 1α, 2β half-chair in which C3, C4, C5, and C10 are in the same plane, while C1 is below the plane and C2 is above the plane of the ring. In interacting with the receptor, the sidechain may adopt a conformation which is specific, and similar for all steroids. Rings B and C are rather rigid and little affected by substitution.

RECEPTORS AND DISEASE STATES

There is increasing evidence that some endocrine disorders may be the result of receptor dysfunction, rather than of hormonal insufficiency or excess. Disorders of peptide hormones have received the greatest amount of attention; e.g., insulin resistance has been associated with a decrease in the number of insulin receptors on cell membranes (reviewed by Jacobs and Cuatrecasas, 80, and Kahn 83). However, some steroid receptor deficiencies are already well established. Androgen insensitivity in the testicular feminization syndrome can be caused by a lack of androgen receptors in target tissues of both mice (15) and humans (88). Recently, Oberfield et al. (137) reported a case of pseudohypoaldosteronism, in which there was defective responsiveness to both endogenous and exogenous mineralocorticoids. A receptor defect was suggested as an explanation for the problem.

An interesting use of glucocorticoid receptors has been described by Lan and Baxter (100). They used competition for [^{3}H]-dexamethasone binding in cultured pituitary tumors cells to measure unbound glucocorticoids in plasma. This replaces a cumbersome and difficult procedure with one that is easy to carry out. In addition, the method measures total glucocorticoid activity in the plasma of patients receiving steroid medication.

SUMMARY

Glucocorticoids affect the metabolism of nearly all tissues, and receptors for glucocorticoids are present throughout the body, as well as in cell lines that respond to glucocorticoids. Mineralocorticoid receptors are present mainly in the kidney, where aldosterone exerts its major effects. However, there is overlap of both hormonal activity and receptor binding affinity between glucocorticoids and mineralocorticoids.

Glucocorticoid and mineralocorticoid receptors have physicochemical properties that are characteristic of all steroid hormone receptors. In the absence of hormone(s), they are found in the cytosol. In the presence of hormone(s) saturable binding of high affinity ($K_d \sim 10^{-9}$M) is seen, and the complex of hormone and receptor is then activated (transformed) and translocated to the nucleus, where binding to chromatin takes place.

The unbound glucocorticoid receptor is very unstable, but stability is increased when the receptor is bound to the hormone, and in the presence of SH-protecting reagents. The receptor is inactivated by removal of phosphate but can be reactivated with ATP. It is suggested that the receptor must be in the reduced (SH) and phosphorylated form in order to bind hormone. After the receptor complex has acted in the nucleus it may return to the cytoplasm and its ability to bind glucocorticoids may be restored. ATP may be needed for both processes.

REFERENCES

1. Acs, Z., Stark, E., and Folly, G. (1975) Steroid-binding properties of corticosteroid receptors in different target tissues of the rat. J. Steroid Biochem. 6, 1127–1130.
2. Agarwal, M.K., (1976) Identification and properties of renal mineralocorticoid receptors in relation to glucocorticoid binders in rat liver and kidney. Biochem. J. 154, 567–575.
3. Agarwal, M.K. (1976) Human liver glucocorticoid receptors are similar to those in rat liver. Naturwissenschaft 63, 50.
4. Alberti, K.G.M.M., and Sharp, G.W.G. (1969) Macromolecular binding of aldosterone in the toad bladder. Biochim. Biophys. Acta 192, 335–346.
5. Anderson, N.S., and Fanestil, D.D. (1976) Corticoid receptors in rat brain: Evidence for an aldosterone receptor. Endocrinology 98, 676–684.
6. Aronow, L. (1978) The glucocorticoid receptor of mouse fibroblasts. Fed. Proc. 37, 162–166.
7. Atger, M., and Milgrom, E. (1976) Chromatographic separation on phosphocellulose of activated and nonactivated forms of steroid-receptor complex. Purification of the activated complex. Biochem 15, 4298–4304.
8. Atger, M., and Milgrom, E. (1976) Mechanism and kinetics of the thermal activation of glucocorticoid hormone receptor complex. J. Biol. Chem. 251, 4758–4762.
9. Atger, M., and Milgrom, E. (1978) Interaction of glucocorticoid receptor complexes with rat liver nuclei. Biochim. Biophys. Acta 539, 41–53.
10. Bailly, A., Sallas, N., and Milgrom, E. (1977) A low molecular weight inhibitor of steroid receptor activation. J. Biol. Chem. 252, 858–863.
11. Ballard, P.L., Baxter, J.D., Higgins, S.J., Rousseau, G.G., and Tomkins, H. G.M. (1974) General presence of glucocorticoid receptors in mammalian tissues. Endocrinology 94, 998–1002.
12. Ballard, P.L., and Ballard R.A. (1974) Cytoplasmic receptor for glucocorticoids in lung of the human fetus and neonate. J. Clin. Invest. 53, 477–486.
13. Ballard, P.L. (1977) Glucocorticoid receptors in the lung. Fed. Proc. 36, 2660–2665.
14. Ballard, P.L., Mason, R.J., and Douglas, W.H.J. (1978) Glucocorticoid binding by isolated lung cells. Endocrinology 102, 1570–1575.

15. Bardin, C.W., Bullock, L.P., Janne, O., and Jacob, S.T. (1975) Genetic regulation of the androgen receptor—A study of testicular feminization in the mouse. J. Steroid Biochem. 6, 515–520.
16. Barnett, C.A., Schmidt, T.J., and Litwack, G. (1980) Effect of calf intestinal alkaline phosphatase, phosphatase inhibitors and phosphorylated compounds on the rate of activation of glucocorticoids-receptor complexes. Biochemistry 12, 5446–5455.
17. Baulieu, E.E. (1979) Aspects of steroid hormone target-cell interactions. In: W.W. Leavitt and J.H. Clark (eds.), Steroid Hormone Receptor Systems, Plenum Press, New York, pp. 377–399.
18. Baxter, J.D., and Tomkins, G.M. (1971) Specific cytoplasmic glucocorticoid hormone receptors in hepatoma tissue culture cells. Proc. Nat. Acad. Sci. U.S.A. 68, 932–937.
19. Beato, M., Brandle, W., Biesewig, D., and Sekeris, C.E. (1970) On the mechanism of hormone action XVI. Transfer of [1,2 ^{3}H] cortisol from the cytoplasm to the nucleus of rat liver cells. Biochim. Biophys. Acta 208, 125–136.
20. Beato, M., and Feigelson, P., (1972) Glucocorticoid-binding proteins of rat liver cytosol. I. Separation and identification of the binding proteins. J. Biol. Chem. 247, 7890–7896.
21. Beato, M., Kalimi, M., Konstam, M., and Feigelson, P. (1973) Interaction of glucocorticoids with rat liver nuclei. II. Studies on the nature of the cytosol transfer factor and the nuclear acceptor site. Biochemistry 12, 3372–3379.
22. Beato, M. Kalimi, M., Beato, W., and Feigelson, P. (1974) Interaction of glucocorticoids with rat liver nuclei: Effect of adrenalectomy and cortisol administration. Endocrinology 94, 377–387.
23. Bell, P.P., and Munck, A. (1973) Steroid-binding properties and stabilizations of cytoplasmic glucocorticoid receptors from rat thymus cells. Biochem. J. 136, 97–107.
24. Buchi, K., and Villee, C.A. (1976) Influence of heating and estradiol on the activation and transformation of the estradiol receptor of the rat uterus. J. Steroid Biochem. 7, 539–544.
25. Cake, M.H., and Litwack, G. (1975) The glucocorticoid receptor. In: Biochemical Actions of Hormones, Academic Press, New York, pp. 317–390.
26. Cake, M.H., and Litwack, G., (1975) Effects of theophylline on the activation and nuclear translocation of the hepatic glucocorticoid receptor at low temperature. Biochem. Biophys. Res. Comm. 66, 828–835.
27. Cake, M.H., Goidl, J.A., Parchman, L.G., and Litwack, G. (1976) Involvement of a low molecular weight component(s) in the mechanism of action of the glucocorticoid receptor. Biochem. Biophys. Res. Comm. 71; 43–52.
28. Cake, M.H., DiSorbo, D.M., and Litwack, G. (1978) Effect of pyridoxal phosphate on the DNA binding site of activated hepatic glucocorticoid receptor. J. Biol. Chem. 253, 4886–4891.
29. Chen, T.L., Aronow, L., and Feldman, D. (1977) Glucocorticoid receptors and inhibition of bone cell growth in primary culture. Endocrinology 100, 619–628.
30. Chomczynski, P., and Zwierczchowski, L. (1976) Mammary glucocorticoid receptor of mice in pregnancy and lactation. Biochem. J. 158, 481–483.
31. Chytil, F., and Toft, D. (1972) Corticoid binding component in rat brain. J. Neurochem. 19, 2877–2880.
32. Cidlowski, J.A., and Munck, A. (1978) Comparison of glucocorticoid-receptor complex binding to nuclei and DNA cellulose. Evidence for different forms of interaction. Biochim. Biophys. Acta 543, 545–555.
33. Cidlowski, J.A., and Thanassi, J.W. (1978) Extraction of nuclear glucocorticoid receptor complexes with pyridoxal phosphate. Biochem. Biophys. Res. Comm. 82, 1140–1146.
34. Cidlowski, J.A., and Thanassi, J.W. (1981) Pyridoxal phosphate: A possible cofactor in steroid hormone action. J. Steroid Biochem. 15, 11–16.
35. Cidlowski, J.A., and Cidlowski, N.B. (1981) Regulation of glucocorticoid receptors by glucocorticoids in cultured He.La S_3 cells. Endocrinology 109, 1975–1982.

36. Claire, M., Oblin, M-E., Steimer, J-L., Nakane, H., Misumi, J., Michaud, A., and Corvol, P. (1981) Effect of adrenalectomy and aldosterone on the modulation of mineralocorticoid receptors in rat kidney. J. Biol. Chem. 256, 142–147.
37. Climent, F., Bugany, H., and Beato, M. (1976) Partial purification of the activated glucocorticoid receptor of rat liver. FEBS Lett. 66, 317–321.
38. Climent, F., Doenecke, D., and Beato, M. (1977) Properties of the partially purified activated glucocorticoid receptor of rat liver. Binding to chromatin subunits. Biochemistry 16, 4694–4703.
39. Colman, P.D., and Feigelson, P. (1976) Partial purification of the activated hepatic glucocorticoid receptor complex. Molec. Cell. Endocrinol. 5, 33–40.
40. Coutard, M., Osborne-Pellegrin, M.J., and Funder, J.W. (1978) Tissue distribution and specific binding of tritiated dexamethasone in vivo: Autoradiographic and cell fractionation studies. Endocrinology 103; 1144–1152.
41. Dahmer, M.K., Quasney, M.W., Bissen, S.T., and Pratt, W.B. (1981) Molybdate permits resolution of untransformed glucocorticoid receptors from the transformed state. J. Biol. Chem. 256, 9401–9405.
42. DeKloet, R., Wallach, G., and McEwen, B.S. (1975) Differences in corticosterone and dexamethasone binding to rat brain and pituitary. Endocrinology 96, 598–609.
43. DeKloet, R., and McEwen, B.S. (1976) Differences between cytosol receptor complexes with corticosterone and dexamethasone in hippocampal tissue from rat brain. Biochim. Biophys. Acta 421, 124–132.
44. DeKloet, R., and McEwen, B.S. (1976) Glucocorticoid interactions with brain and pituitary. In: Gispen, W.H. (ed.), Molecular and functional neurobiology, Elsevier Scientific Publishing Co., New York pp. 257–307.
45. DeKloet, E.R., Dam, C.W., and Bobus, F. (1977) In: Agarwal, M.K. (ed.), Multiple molecular forms of steroid hormone receptors. Elsevier/North Holland, Amsterdam, pp. 65–79.
46. DeKloet, E.R., and Burbach, P. (1978) Selective purification of a single population of glucocorticoid receptors from rat brain. J. Neurochem. 30, 1505–1507.
47. Do, Y.S., Loose, D.S., and Feldman, D. (1979) Heterogeneity of glucocorticoid binders: A unique and a classical dexamethasone-binding site in bovine tissues. Endocrinology 105, 1055–1063.
48. Doucet, A., and Katz, A. (1981) Mineralocorticoid receptors along the nephron: [^{3}H] aldosterone binding in rabbit tubules. Am. J. Physiol. 241, F-605–611.
49. Duax, W., Griffin, J.F., Rohrer, D.C., Swenson, D.C., and Weeks, C.M. (1981) Molecular details of receptor binding and hormonal action of steroids derived from x-ray crystallographic investigations. J. Steroid Biochem. 15, 41–47.
50. Eisen, H.J., and Glinsmann, W.H. (1978) Maximizing the purification of the activated glucocorticoid receptor by DNA-cellulose chromatography. Biochem. J. 171, 177–183.
51. Endres, D.B., Milholland, R.J., and Rosen, F. Sex differences in the concentration of glucocorticoid receptors in rat liver and thymus. J. Endocrinol. 80, 21–26.
52. Evain, D., Morera, A.M., and Saez, J.M. (1976) Glucocorticoid receptors in interstitial cells of the rat testis. J. Steroid Biochem. 7, 1135–1139.
53. Feldman, D., Funder, J.W., and Edelman, I.S. (1973) Evidence for a new class of corticosterone receptors in the rat kidney. Endocrinology 92, 1429–1441.
54. Feldman, D., Dziak, R., Koehler, R., and Stern, P. (1975) Cytoplasmic glucocorticoid binding proteins in bone cells. Endocrinology 96, 29–36.
55. Feldman, D., and Loose, D., (1977) Glucocorticoid receptors in adipose tissue. Endocrinology 100, 398–405.
56. Feldman, D., Funder, J., and Loose, D. (1978) Is the glucocorticoid receptor identical in various target organs? J. Steroid Biochem. 9, 141–145.
57. Feldman, D. (1978) Evidence that brown adipose tissue is a glucocorticoid target organ. Endocrinology 103, 2091–2097.

58. Funder, J.W., Feldman, D., and Edelman, I.S., (1972) Specific aldosterone binding in rat kidney and parotid. J. Ster. Biochem. 3, 209–218.
59. Funder, J.W., Feldman, D., Edelman, I.S. (1973) Glucocorticoid receptors in rat kidney: The binding of tritiated dexamethasone. Endocrinology 92, 1005–1013.
60. Funder, J.W., Duval, D., and Meyer, P. (1973) Cardiac glucocorticoid receptors—The binding of tritiated dexamethasone in rat and dog heart. Endocrinology 93, 1300–1308.
61. Funder, J.W., Mercer, J., Ingram, B., Feldman, D., Wynne, K., and Adam, W.R. (1978) 19-nor Deoxycorticosterone (19-nor DOC): Mineralocorticoid receptor affinity higher than aldosterone, electrolyte activity lower. Endocrinology 103, 1514–1517.
62. Garroway, N.W., Orth, D.N., and Harrison, R.W. (1976) Binding of cytosol receptor-glucocorticoid complexes by isolated nuclei of glucocorticoid responsive and non-responsive cultured cells. Endocrinology 98, 1092–1100.
63. Gerlach, J.L., and McEwen, B.S. (1972) Rat brain binds adrenal steroid hormone: Radioautography of hippocampus with corticosterone. Science 175, 1133–1136.
64. Giannopoulos, G. (1974) Variations in the levels of cytoplasmic glucocorticoid receptors in lungs of various species at different developmental stages. Endocrinology 94, 450–458.
65. Giannopoulos, G. (1975) Glucocorticoid receptors in lung. Mechanism of specific glucocorticoid uptake by fetal rabbit lung nuclei. J. Biol. Chem. 250, 2896–2903.
66. Giannopoulos, G. (1975) Glucocorticoid receptors in lung. Comparison between non-activated and activated forms of the cytoplasmic glucocorticoid binding protein and their relationship to the nuclear binding protein of fetal rabbit lung. J. Biol. Chem. 250, 2904–2910.
67. Giannopoulos, G. (1975) Ontogeny of glucocorticoid receptors in rat liver. J. Biol. Chem. 250, 5847–5851.
68. Giannopoulos, G. (1975) Early events in the action of glucocorticoids in developing tissues. J. Steroid Biochem. 6, 623–631.
69. Goidl, J.A., Cake, M.H., Dolan, K.P., Parchman, L.G., and Litwak, G. (1977) Activation of the rat liver glucocorticoid-receptor complex. Biochemistry 16, 2125–2130.
70. Goral, J.E., and Wittliff, J.L. (1975) Comparison of glucocorticoid-binding proteins in normal and neoplastic mammary tissues of the rat. Biochemistry 14, 2944–2952.
71. Govindan, M.V. (1979) Purification of glucocorticoid receptors from rat liver cytosol. Preparation of antibodies against major receptor proteins and application of immunological techniques to study activation and translocation. J. Steroid Biochem. 11, 323–332.
72. Granberg, J.P., and Ballard, P.L. (1977) The role of sulfhydryl groups in the binding of glucocorticoids by cytoplasmic receptors of lung and other mammalian tissues. Endocrinology 100, 1160–1168.
73. Grekin, R.J., and Sider, R.S (1978) Aldosterone receptor assay in rat kidney cytosol. Abstracts of the 60th Annual Meeting of the Endocrine Society, (abst. 468), pp. 309.
74. Grosser, B.F., Stevens, W., and Reed, D.J. (1973) Properties of corticosterone-binding macromolecules from rat brain cytosol. Brain Res. 57, 387–395.
75. Harrison, R.W., Fairfield, S., and Orth, D.N. (1976) Multiple glucocorticoid binding components of intact AtT-20/D-1 mouse pituitary tumor cells. Biochim. Biophys. Acta 444, 487–496.
76. Henning, S.J., Ballard, P.L., and Kretchmer, N. (1975) A study of cytoplasmic receptors for glucocorticoids in intestine of pre and post weaning rats. J. Biol. Chem. 250, 2073–2079.
77. Higgins, S.J., Rousseau, G.G., Baxter, J.D., and Tomkins, G.M. (1973) Early events in glucocorticoid action. Activation of the steroid receptor and its subsequent specific nuclear binding studied in a cell-free system. J. Biol. Chem. 248, 5866–5872.
78. Higgins, S.J., Rousseau, G.G., Baxter, J.D., and Tomkins, G.M. (1973) Nature of nuclear acceptor sites for glucocorticoids and estrogen-receptor complexes. J. Biol. Chem. 248, 5873–5879.

79. Ishii, D.N., Pratt, W.B., and Aronow, L. (1972) Steady-state level of the specific glucocorticoid binding component in mouse fibroblasts. Biochemistry 11, 3896–3904.
80. Jacobs, S., and Cuatrecasas, P. (1977) Cell receptors in disease, N. Engl. J. Med. 297, 1383–1386.
81. John, J.K., Moudgil, V.K. (1979) Activation of glucocorticoid receptor by ATP. Biochem. Biophys. Res. Comm. 90, 1242–1248.
82. Jungblut, P.W., Gaues, J., Hughes, A., Kallweit, E., Sierratta, W., Szendro, P., and Wagner, R.K (1976) Activation of transcription-regulating proteins by steroids. J. Steroid Biochem. 7, 1109–1116.
83. Kahn, C.R. (1977) Receptors for peptide hormones—New insights into pathophysiology of disease states in man. Ann. Int. Med. 86, 205–219.
84. Kaiser, N., Mayer, M., Milholland, R.J., and Rosen, F. (1979) Studies on the antiglucocorticoid action of progesterone in rat thymocytes: Early in vitro effects. J. Steroid Biochem. 10, 379–386.
85. Kalimi, M., Beato, M., and Feigelson, P. (1973) Interaction of glucocorticoids with rat liver nuclei. I. Role of the cytosol proteins. Biochemistry 12, 3365–3371.
86. Kalimi, M., Colman, P., and Feigelson, P. (1975) The activated hepatic glucocorticoid-receptor complex. Its generation and properties. J. Biol. Chem. 250, 1080–1086.
87. Kalimi, M. (1978) The activated hepatic glucocorticoid-receptor complex: A simple one-step method for its separation from nonactivated complex. Anal. Biochem. 86, 166–174.
88. Kaufman, M.C., Straisfeld, C., and Pinsky, L. (1976) Male pseudohermaphroditism presumably due to target unresponsiveness to androgens. Deficient 5α dihydrotestosterone binding in cultured skin fibroblasts. J. Clin. Invest. 58, 345–350.
89. Kirkpatrick, A.F., Kaiser, N., Milholland, R.J., and Rosen, F. (1972) Glucocorticoid-binding macromolecules in normal tissues and tumors. Stabilization of the specific binding component. J. Biol. Chem. 247, 70–74.
90. Koblinsky, M., Beato, M., Kalimi, M., and Feigelson, P. (1972) Glucocorticoid-binding proteins of rat liver cytosol. II. Physical characterization and properties of the binding proteins. J. Biol. Chem. 247, 7897–7904.
91. Koch, B., Lutz, B., Briaud, B., and Mialhe, C. (1975) Glucocorticoid binding to adenohypophysis receptors and its physiological role. Neuroendocrinology 18, 299–310.
92. Koch, B., Lutz, B., Briaud, B., and Mialhe, C. (1976) Heterogeneity of pituitary glucocorticoid binding. Evidence for a transcortin-like compound. Biochim. Biophys. Acta 444, 497–507.
93. Koch, B., Lutz-Bucher, B., Briaud, B., and Mialhe, C. (1978) Specific interaction of corticosteroids with binding sites in the plasma membranes of rat anterior pituitary gland. J. Endocrinol. 79, 215–222.
94. Kolata, G.B. (1978) Polypeptide hormones: What are they doing in cells? Science 201, 895–897.
95. Kornel, L., Kanamarla Pudi, N., Patel, N., and Travers, T. (1978) Further studies on mineralocorticoid and glucocorticoid intracellular receptors in arterial blood vessels. J. Steroid Biochem 9, 839 (abst. 124).
96. Kraft, N., Barlow, J., and Funder, J.W. (1978) Predominant high affinity [^{3}H]-dexamethasone binding in bovine tissues is not to classical glucocorticoid receptors. J. Steroid Biochem. 9, 836 (abst. 113).
97. Kraft, N., Hodgson, A.J., and Funder, J.W. (1979) Glucocorticoid receptor and effector mechanisms: A comparison of the corticosensitive mouse with the corticoresistant guinea pig. Endocrinology 104, 344–349.
98. Krozowski, Z., and Funder, J.W. (1981) Mineralocorticoid receptors in rat lung. Endo crinology 109, 1811–1813.
99. Krozowski, Z., and Funder, J.W. (1981) Mineralocorticoid receptors in rat anterior pituitary: Toward a redefinition of "mineralocorticoid hormone." Endocrinology 109, 1221–1224.

100. Lan, N.C., and Baxter, J.K. (1982) A radioreceptor assay for direct measurement of plasma free glucocorticoid activity. J. Clin. Endocrinol. Metab. 55, 516–523.

101. Lassman, M.D., and Mulrow, P.J. (1974) Deficiency of deoxycorticosterone-binding protein in the hypothalamus of rats resistant to deoxycorticosterone-induced hypertension. Endocrinology 94, 1541–1546.

102. Leach, K.L., Stratford, C.A., Dahmer, M.K., Hammond, N.D., and Pratt, W.B. (1979) Multiple effects of molybdate on glucocorticoid receptors. Eleventh International Congress of Biochemistry, abstract 11-6-S9, p. 613.

103. Lee, D.K.H., Stern, M., and Solomon, S. (1976) Cytoplasmic glucocorticoid receptors in the developing small intestine of the rabbit fetus. Endocrinology 99, 379–388.

104. Lee, D.K.H., and Solomon, S. (1978) Characteristics and ontogeny of nuclear receptor for glucocorticoids in the rabbit fetal small intestine. Endocrinology 102, 312–320.

105. Lippman, M.E., and Thompson, E.B. (1973) Differences between cytoplasmic glucocorticoid-binding proteins shown by heterogeneity of nuclear acceptor sites. Nature 246, 352–355.

106. Litwack, G., Filler, R., Rosenfield, S.A., Lichtash, N., Wishman, C.A., and Singer, S. (1973) Liver cytosol corticosteroid binder II, a hormone receptor. J. Biol. Chem. 248, 7481–7486.

107. Litwack, G. and Rosenfield, S.A. (1975) Liver cytosol corticosteroid binder IB, a new binding protein. J. Biol. Chem. 250, 6799–6805.

108. Litwack, G., Cake, M.H., Filler, R., and Taylor, K. (1978) Physical measurements of the liver glucocorticoid receptor. Biochem. J. 169, 445–448.

109. Maclusky, N.J., Turner, B.B., and McEwen, B.S. (1977) Corticosteroid binding in rat brain and pituitary cytosols: Resolution of multiple binding components by polyacrylamide gel based isoelectric focusing. Brain. Res. 130, 564–571.

110. Managolas, S.C. and Anderson, D.C. (1978) Detection of high affinity glucocorticoid binding in rat bone. J. Endocrin. 76, 379–380.

111. Marver, D., Goodman, D., and Edelman, I.S. (1972) Relationships between renal cytoplasmic and nuclear aldosterone receptors. Kidney Int. 1, 210–223.

112. Marver, D., Stewart, J., Funder, J.W., Feldman, D., and Edelman, I.S. (1974) Renal aldosterone receptors: Studies with [^{3}H] aldosterone and the antimineralocorticoid [^{3}H] spirolactone (SC-26304). Proc. Natl. Acad. Sci. USA 71, 1431–1435.

113. Mayer, M., Kaiser, N., Milholland, R.J., and Rosen, F. (1974) The binding of dexamethasone and triamcinolone acetonide to glucocorticoid receptors in rat skeletal muscle. J. Biol. Chem. 249, 5236–5240.

114. Mayer, M., Kaiser, N., Milholland, R.J., and Rosen, F. (1975) Cortisol binding in rat skeletal muscle. J. Biol. Chem. 250, 1207–1211.

115. McEwen, B.S., Magnus, C., and Wallach, G. (1972) Soluble corticosterone-binding macromolecules extracted from rat brain. Endocrinology 90, 217–226.

116. McEwen, B.S., and Wallach, G. (1973) Corticosterone binding to hippocampus: Nuclear and cytosol binding in vitro. Brain Res. 57, 373–386.

117. McEwen, B.S., Luine, V.N., Plapinger, L., and DeKloet, E.R. (1975) Putative estrogen and glucocorticoid receptors in limbic brain. J. Steroid Biochem. 6, 971–977.

118. McEwen, B.S., DeKloet, R., and Wallach, G. (1976) Interactions in vivo and in vitro of corticoids and progesterone with cell nuclei and soluble macromolecules from rat brain regions and pituitary. Brain Res. 105, 129–136.

119. Meyer, W.J., and Nichols, N.R. (1981) Mineralocorticoid binding in cultured smooth muscle cells and fibroblasts from rat aorta. J. Steroid Biochem. 14, 1157–1168.

120. Middlebrook, J.L., Wong, M.D., Ishii, D.N., and Aronow, L. (1975) Subcellular distribution of glucocorticoid receptors in mouse fibroblasts. Biochemistry 14, 180–186.

121. Middlebrook, J.L., and Aronow, L. (1977) Physiochemical properties of glucocorticoid receptors from mouse fibroblasts. Endocrinology 100, 271–282.

122. Milgrom, E., Atger, M., and Baulieu, E.-E. (1973) Acidophilic activation of steroid hormone receptors. Biochemistry 12, 5198–5205.

123. Milgrom, E., Atger, M., and Baulieu, E.-E., (1973) Studies on estrogen entry into uterine cells and on estradiol receptor complex attachment to nucleus—Is the entry of estrogen into uterine cells a protein mediated process? Biochim. Biophys. Acta 320, 267–283.
124. Milgrom, E., and Atger, M. (1975) Receptor translocation inhibitor and apparent saturability of the nucleus acceptor. J. Steroid Biochem. 6, 487–492.
125. Milgrom, E., Atger, M., and Bailly, A. (1976) Interaction of rat-liver glucocorticoid receptor with DNA. Eur. J. Biochem. 70, 1–6.
126. Moscona, A.A. (1975) Hydrocortisone-mediated regulation of gene expression in embyronic neural retina: Induction of glutamine synthetase. J. Steroid Biochem. 6, 633–638.
127. Muller, R.E., Johnston, T.C., Traish, A.M., and Wotiz, H.H. (1979) Studies on the mechanism of estradiol uptake by rat uterine cells and on estradiol binding to uterine plasma membranes. In: Steroid Hormone Receptor Systems, W.W. Leavitt, J.H. Clark (eds.), Plenum Press, New York, pp. 401–421.
128. Munck, A., Wira, C., Young, D.A., Mosher, K.M., Hallahan, C., and Bell, P.A. (1972) Glucocorticoid-receptor complexes and the earliest steps in the action of glucocorticoids on thymus cells. J. Steroid Biochem. 3, 567–578.
129. Munck, A., and Brinck-Johnson, T. (1974) Is cortisol metabolized as it dissociates from glucocorticoid receptors in thymus cells? J. Steroid Biochem. 5, 203–205.
130. Munck, A., and Foley, R., (1976) Kinetics of glucocorticoid-receptor complexes in rat thymus cells. J. Steroid Biochem. 7, 1117–1122.
131. Munck, A., and Foley, R. (1979) Activation of steroid hormone-receptor complexes in intact target cells in physiological conditions. Nature 278, 752–754.
132. Murakami, N., and Moudgil, V.K. (1981) Inactivation of rat liver glucocorticoid receptor by molybdate. Biochem. J. 198, 447–455.
133. Nielsen, C.J., Vogel, W.M., and Pratt, W.B. (1977) Inactivation of glucocorticoid receptors in cell-free preparations of rat liver. Cancer Res. 37, 3420–3426.
134. Nielson, C.J., Sando, J.J., and Pratt, W.B. (1977) Evidence that dephosphorylation inactivates glucocorticoid receptors. Proc. Natl. Acad. Sci. U.S.A. 74, 1398–1402.
135. Nielson, C.J., Sando, J.J., Vogel, W.M., and Pratt, W.B. (1977) Glucocorticoid receptor inactivation under cell-free conditions. J. Biol. Chem. 252, 7568–7578.
136. Noma, K., Nakao, K., Sato, B. Nishigawa, Y., Matsumoto, K., and Yamamura, Y. (1980) Effect of molybdate on activation or stabilization of steroid receptors. Endocrinology 107, 1205–1211.
137. Oberfield, S., Levine, L.S., Carey, R.M., Bejar, R., and New, M.I. (1979) Pseudohypoaldosteronism: Multiple target organ unresponsiveness to mineralocorticoid hormones. J. Clin. Endocrinol. Metab. 48, 228–234.
138. O'Brien, M.J., and Cidlowski, J. (1981) Interaction of pyridoxal phosphate with glucocorticoid receptors from $HeLaS_3$ cells. J. Steroid Biochem. 14, 9–18.
139. Ozegović, B., Schon, E., and Milković, S. (1977) Interaction of [^{3}H]-aldosterone with rat kidney plasma membranes. J. Steroid Biochem. 8, 815–819.
140. Parchman, L.G., and Litwack, G. (1977) Resolution of activated and unactivated forms of the glucocorticoid receptor from rat liver. Arch. Biochem. Biophys. 183, 374–382.
141. Peck, E.J., Burgner, J., and Clark, J.H. (1973) Estrophilic binding sites of the uterus. Relation to uptake and retention of estradiol in vitro. Biochemistry 12, 4596–4603.
142. Pfahl, M., Sandros, T., and Bourgeois, S. (1978) Interaction of glucocorticoid receptors from lymphoid cell lines with their nuclear acceptor sites. Mol. Cell. Endocrinol. 10, 175–191.
143. Pressley, L., and Funder, J.W. (1975) Glucocorticoid and mineralocorticoid receptors in gut mucosa. Endocrinology 97, 588–596.
144. Rao, G.S., Schulze-Hagen, K., Rao, M.L., and Breuer, H. (1976) Kinetics of steroid transport through cell membranes: Comparison of the uptake of cortisol with binding of cortisol to rat liver cytosol. J. Steroid Biochem. 7, 1123–1129.

145. Rao, M.L., Rao, G.S., Holler, M., Breuer, H., Schattenberg, P.J., and Stein, W.D. (1976) Uptake of cortisol by isolated rat liver cells. A phenomenon indicative of carrier-mediation and simple diffusion. HoppeSeyler's Z. Physiol. Chem. 357, 573–584.

146. Rao, G.S., Rao, M.L., Eckel, J., and Allera, A. (1978) Mode of entry of corticosterone into the liver cell. J. Steroid Biochem. 9, 834 (abst. 102).

147. Rees, A.M., and Bell, P.A. (1975) The involvement of receptor sulphydryl groups in the binding of steroids to the cytoplasmic glucocorticoid receptor from rat thymus. Biochim. Biophys. Acta 411, 121–132.

148. Rosner, W., and Polimeni, S.T. (1978) An exchange assay for the cytoplasmic glucocorticoid receptor in the liver of the rat. Steroids 31, 427–438.

149. Rotsztejn, W.H., Normand, M., Lalonde, J., and Fortier, C. (1975) Relationship between ACTH release and corticosterone binding by the receptor sites of the adenohypophysis and dorsal hippocampus following infusion of corticosterone at a constant rate in the adrenalectomized rat. Endocrinology 97, 223–230.

150. Rousseau, G.G., Baxter, J.D., and Tomkins, G.M. (1972) Glucocorticoid receptors: Relations between steroid binding and biological effects. J. Mol. Biol. 67, 99–115.

151. Rousseau, G.G., Baxter, J.D., Funder, J.W., Edelman, I.S., and Tomkins, G.M. (1972) Glucocorticoid and mineralocorticoid receptors for aldosterone. J. Ster. Biochem. 3, 219–227.

152. Rousseau, G.G., Baxter, J.D., Higgins, S.J., and Tomkins, G.M. (1973) Steroid-induced nuclear binding of glucocorticoid receptors in intact hepatoma cells. J. Mol. Biol. 79, 539–554.

153. Rousseau, G.G. Higgins, S.J., Baxter, J.D., Gelfand, D., and Tomkins, G.M. (1975) Binding of glucocorticoid receptors to DNA. J. Biol. Chem. 250, 6015–6021.

154. Rousseau, G.G., and Schmit, J-P. (1977) Structure-activity relationships for glucocorticoids. I. Determination of receptor binding and biological activity. J. Steroid Biochem. 8, 911–919.

155. Saffran, J., Loeser, B.K., Bohnett, S.A., and Faber, L.E. (1976) Binding of progesterone receptor by nuclear preparations of rabbit and guinea pig uterus. J. Biol. Chem, 251, 5607–5613.

156. Saffran, J., and Loeser, B.K. (1979) Nuclear binding of guinea pig uterine progesterone receptor in cell-free preparations. J. Steroid Biochem. 10, 43–51.

157. Sakau, Y., and Thompson, E.B. (1977) Characterization of two forms of glucocorticoid hormone-receptor complex separated by DEAE-cellulose column chromatography. Biochem. Biophys. Res. Comm. 77, 533–541.

158. Salomon, D.S., and Pratt, R.M. (1976) Glucocorticoid receptors in murine embryonic facial mesenchymal cells. Nature 264, 174–177.

159. Salomon, D.S., Zubairi, Y., and Thompson, E.R. (1978) Ontogeny and biochemical properties of glucocorticoid receptors in mid-gestation embryos. J. Steroid Biochem. 9, 95–107.

160. Sando, J.J., Nielsen, C.J., and Pratt, W.B. (1977) Reactivation of thymocyte glucocorticoid receptors in a cell-free system. J. Biol. Chem. 252, 7579–7582.

161. Sando, J.J., LaForest, A.C., and Pratt, W.B. (1979) ATP-dependent activation of L cell glucocorticoid receptors to the steroid binding form. J. Biol. Chem. 254, 4772–4778.

162. Sando, J.J., Hammond, N.D., Stratford, C.A., and Pratt, W.B. (1979) Activation of thymocyte glucocorticoid receptors to the steroid binding form. The roles of reducing agents, ATP and heat-stable factors. J. Biol. Chem. 254, 4779–4789.

163. Sato, B., Nishizawa, Y., Noma, K., Matsumoto, K., and Yamamura, Y. (1979) Estrogen-independent nuclear binding of receptor protein of rat uterine cystol by removal of low molecular weight inhibitor. Endocrinology 104, 1474–1479.

164. Sato, B., Yoma, K., Nishizawa, Y., Nakao, K., Matsumoto, K., and Yamamura, Y. (1980) Mechanism of activation of steroid receptors: Involvement of low molecular weight inhibitor in activation of androgen, glucocorticoid and estrogen receptor systems. Endocrinology 106, 1142–1148.

165. Schaumburg, B.P. (1972) Investigations on the glucocorticoid binding protein from rat thymocytes. II Stability, kinetics and specificity of binding steroids. Biochim. Biophys. Acta 261, 219–235.
166. Schmid, W., Grote, H., and Sekeris, C.E. (1976) Stabilization and characterization of the dexamethasone-binding proteins in rat liver cytosol. Mol. Cell. Endocrinol. 5, 223–241.
167. Schmid, W., and Grote, H. (1977) Multiple forms of glucocorticoid binding proteins in glucocorticoid target cells. In: Multiple Molecular Forms of Steroid Hormone Receptors. Agarwal, M.K. (ed.), Elsevier/North Holland, New York, pp. 35–48.
168. Schmit, J.P., and Rousseau, G.G. (1977) Structure-activity relationships for glucocorticoids—II. Theoretical approach of molecular structures based on energy optimization of a Westheimer model. J. Steroid Biochem. 8, 921–928.
169. Schmit, J.P., and Rousseau, G.G. (1978) Structure-activity relationships for glucocorticoids—III. Structural and conformational study of the rings and side-chain of steroids which bind to the glucocorticoid receptor. J. Steroid Biochem. 9, 909–920.
170. Schmit, J.P., and Rousseau, G.G. (1978) Structure-activity relationships for glucocorticoids—IV. Effects of subtituents on the overall shape of steroids which bind to the glucocorticoid receptor. J. Steroid Biochem. 9, 921–927.
171. Sekula, B.C., Schlmit, T.S., and Litwack, G. (1981) Redefinition of modulator as an inhibitor of glucocorticoid receptor activation. J. Steroid Biochem. 14, 161–166.
172. Seleznev, Y.M., Danilov, S.M., and Smernov, V.N. (1979) Separation of three glucocorticoid-binding fractions from cytosol of rat heart. J. Steroid Biochem. 10, 215–220.
173. Shyamala, G. (1975) Glucocorticoid receptors in mouse mammary tumors. Specific binding to nuclear components. Biochemistry 14, 437–444.
174. Sibley, C.H., and Tomkins, G.M. (1974) Mechanisms of steroid resistance. Cell 2, 221–227.
175. Simons, S.S., Martinez, H.M., Garcea, R.L., Baxter, J.D., and Tomkins, G.M. (1976) Interactions of glucocorticoid receptor steroid complexes with acceptor sites. J. Biol. Chem. 251, 334–343.
176. Simons, S.S (1977) Glucocorticoid receptor-steroid complex binding to DNA. Competition between DNA and DNA-cellulose. Biochim. Biophys. Acta 496, 349–358.
177. Simonsson, B. (1975) Evidence for a glucocorticoid receptor in human leukocytes. Acta Phys. Scand. 98, 131–135.
178. Smith, K.A., Crabtree, G.R., Kennedy, S.J., and Munck, A.U. (1977) Glucocorticoid receptors and glucocorticoid sensitivity of mitogen stimulated and unstimulated human lymphocytes. Nature 267, 523–526.
179. Snart, R.S., and Thorne, J. (1978) Glucocorticoid binding and response in rat liver and diethylnitrosamine (DENA)-induced hepatomas. J. Steroid Biochem. 9, 709–715.
180. Solomon, S., and Lee, D.K.H. (1977) Binding of glucocorticoids in fetal tissues. J. Steroid Biochem. 8, 453–461.
181. Stevens, W., Grosser, G.I., and Reed, D.J. (1971) Corticosterone-binding molecules in rat brain cytosols. Regional distribution. Brain Res. 35, 602–607.
182. Stevens, W., Reed, D.J., Erickson, S., and Grosser, B.I. (1973) The binding of corticosterone to brain proteins: diurnal variation. Endocrinology 93, 1152–1156.
183. Stevens, W., Reed, D.J., and Grosser, B.I. (1975) Binding of natural and synthetic glucocorticoids in rat brain. J. Steroid Biochem. 6, 521–527.
184. Stith, R.D., and Bottoms, G.D. (1972) Intracellular binding of [^{3}H]-cortisol and its effect on RNA polymerase activity in hypothalamus of the pig. Brain Res. 41, 423–434.
185. Stith, R.D., Person, R.J., and Dana, R.C. (1976) Uptake and binding of [^{3}H]-hydrocortisone by various pig brain regions. Brain Res. 117, 115–124.
186. Strum, J.M., Feldman, D., Taggart, B., Marver, D., and Edelman, I.S. (1975) Autoradiographic localization of corticosterone receptors (type III) to the collecting tubule of the rat kidney. Endocrinology 97, 505–516.
187. Stumpf, E.W., and Sar, M. (1976) Steroid hormone target sites in the brain: The

differential distribution of estrogen, progestin, androgen and glucocorticosteroid. J. Steroid Biochem. 7, 1163–1170.

188. Suthers, M.B., Pressley, L.A., and Funder, J.W. (1976) Glucocorticoid receptors: Evidence for a second, non-glucocorticoid binding site. Endocrinology 99, 260–269.
189. Suyemitsu, T., and Terayama, H. (1975) Specific binding sites for natural glucocorticoids in plasma membranes of rat liver. Endocrinology 96, 1499–1508.
190. Svec, F., and Harrison, R.W. (1979) The intracellular distribution of natural and synthetic glucocorticoids in the At T-20 cell. Endocrinology 104, 1563–1568.
191. Toft, D., and Chytil, F. (1973) Receptors for glucocorticoids in lung tissue. Arch. Biochem. Biophys. 157, 464–469.
192. Tucker, H.A., Larson, G.L., Gorski, J. (1971) Cortisol binding in cultured bovine mammary cells. Endocrinology 89, 152–160.
193. Turnell, R.W., Beers, P.C., and Wittliff, J.W. (1974) Glucocorticoid-binding macromolecules in the lactating mammary gland of the vole. Endocrinology 95, 1770–1773.
194. Turnell, R.W., Kaiser, N., Milholland, R.J., and Rosen, F. (1974) Glucocorticoid receptors in rat thymocytes. Interactions with the antiglucocorticoid cortexolone and mechanism of its action. J. Biol. Chem. 249, 1133–1138.
195. Turnell, R.W., and Burton, A.F. (1975) Glucocorticoid receptors and lymphocytolysis in normal and neoplastic lymphocytes. Mol. Cell. Biochem. 9, 175–189.
196. Wambach, G., and Higgins, J.R. (1978) Antimineralocorticoid action of progesterone in the rat: Correlation of the effect on electrolyte excretion and interaction with renal mineralocorticoid receptors. Endocrinology 102, 1686–1693.
197. Warembourg, M. (1975) Radiographic study of the rat brain after injection of [1,2-^{3}H] corticosterone. Brain Res. 89, 61–70.
198. Watanabe, H., Orth, D.N., and Toft, D.O. (1973) Glucocorticoid receptors in pituitary tumor cells, cytosol receptors. J. Biol. Chem. 248, 7625–7630.
199. Watanabe, H., Orth, D.N., and Toft, D.O. (1974) Glucocorticoid receptors in mouse pituitary tumor cells. II Nuclear binding. Biochemistry 13, 332–336.
200. Watanabe, H. (1975) Dexamethasone-binding receptor in bovine pituitary cytosol. J. Ster. Biochem. 6, 27–33.
201. Watanabe, H. (1975) Binding of glucocorticoid hormones in bovine hypothalamic and pituitary cytosol. J. Ster. Biochem. 6, 1113–1119.
202. Wiggert, B., and Chader, G.J. (1975) A glucocorticoid and progesterone receptor in the chick optic tectum. J. Neurochem. 24, 585–586.
203. Wira, C., and Munck, A. (1970) Specific glucocorticoid receptors in thymus cells. J. Biol. Chem. 245, 3436–3438.
204. Zava, D.T., Chamness, G.C., Horwitz, K.B., and McGuire, W.L. (1977) Human breast cancer: Biologically active estrogen receptor in the absence of estrogen. Science 196, 663–664.
205. Zava, D.T., and McGuire, W.L. (1977) Estrogen-receptor-unoccupied sites in nuclei of a breast tumor-cell line. J. Biol. Chem. 252, 3703–3708.

PAUL H. BRAND, Ph.D
JAMES T. HIGGINS, JR., M.D.

EFFECT OF ADRENAL HORMONES ON WATER AND ELECTROLYTE METABOLISM

INTRODUCTION

In this chapter we will consider the important role of adrenocortical hormones in the regulation of water, acid–base, and electrolyte metabolism, as well as some of the clinical manifestations that result from abnormalities of adrenocortical hormone secretion or tissue responsiveness. The adrenal hormone that is most important in mineral metabolism is aldosterone, although other endogenous (e.g., deoxycorticosterone) and exogenous (e.g., 9-α fluorohydrocortisone) steroids have similar physiologic effects, though with lower potencies. These steroids are collectively regarded as "mineralocorticoids." The primary role of aldosterone appears to be conservation of sodium and excretion of potassium and, perhaps, hydrogen ion as well. To accomplish these processes, aldosterone stimulates various epithelia to absorb sodium and to secrete potassium and hydrogen ion (or reabsorb bicarbonate, in either case, to achieve net secretion of acid). The mineralocorticoid hormones act on a variety of epithelia, such as the renal tubule, colon, salivary ducts, sweat ducts, urothelium, and on tissues in nonmammalian vertebrates, such as amphibian skin and urinary bladder. Since the mechanism of action of the

From the Departments of Physiology and Medicine, Medical College of Ohio, Toledo, Ohio.

hormone appears to be similar in all of these tissues, we will concentrate our discussion on the best studied mechanisms: mammalian renal tubule and amphibian urinary bladder. By necessity, the discussion of cellular action of these hormones will deal mostly with their effect on sodium transport, which has been extensively investigated in the past 20 years. In contrast, the mechanism by which these hormones stimulate potassium and acid secretion remains largely unexplained. An effect of mineralocorticoid hormones on nonepithelial tissues to cause redistribution of potassium across cell membranes has also been observed and may have important clinical implications. Since the cellular mechanisms for this effect have not been extensively investigated, this aspect of mineralocorticoid action is discussed only in the section on systemic effects.

Cortisol and other endogenous and exogenous glucocorticoid hormones have important effects on water metabolism, which also will be considered. At very high concentrations these hormones can cause mineralocorticoid-like responses in aldosterone-sensitive tissues, due to the fact that the specificity lies in the cellular receptor for the hormones and probably in the cellular response to the hormone–receptor complex as well. Some aspects of this specificity will be discussed.

CELLULAR ACTION OF MINERALOCORTICOID HORMONES

Aldosterone Binding and Cell Response

Although the very existence of aldosterone was deduced from its effect to reduce urinary sodium excretion in man (34), much of our understanding of the cellular response to the mineralocorticoid hormones has come about from the study of amphibian epithelia. Most attention has been directed to the urinary bladder of the toad, because this large bilobed structure transports sodium actively, responds to aldosterone by increasing sodium transport, and its single-cell–thick epithelium contains only four cell types of which more than 80% are of one type, the granular cell. The next most abundant is the mitochondria-rich cell, and probably less than 5% of cells are mucus-secreting goblet cells and basilar precursor cells. When the toad bladder is mounted as a sheet in a chamber separating two identical physiologic salt solutions, it generates a serosa-positive electrical potential (Figure 1). If an external current source is applied to the chamber in sufficient magnitude to nullify the spontaneous transepithelial potential generated by the bladder, it can be shown that the current applied is equivalent to the mucosa-to-serosa active transport of sodium (97). This method of determining transepithelial ion currents is referred to as the short-circuit current (SCC), and was developed by Ussing and Zerahn (166) using frog skin. The lag time between exposure of the toad bladder to aldosterone and the first observation of increased SCC suggested to investigators that intermediate steps were involved. The fact that the aldosterone effect was blocked by both actinomycin D and puromycin indicated that both RNA synthesis and protein synthesis participated (Figure 2) (27,39,125). The elegant studies from the laboratory of

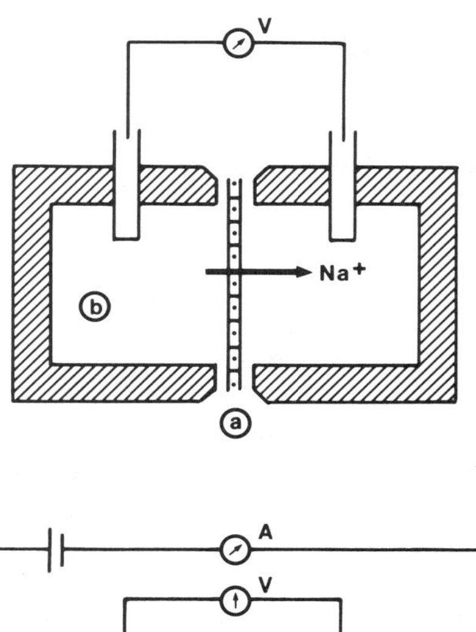

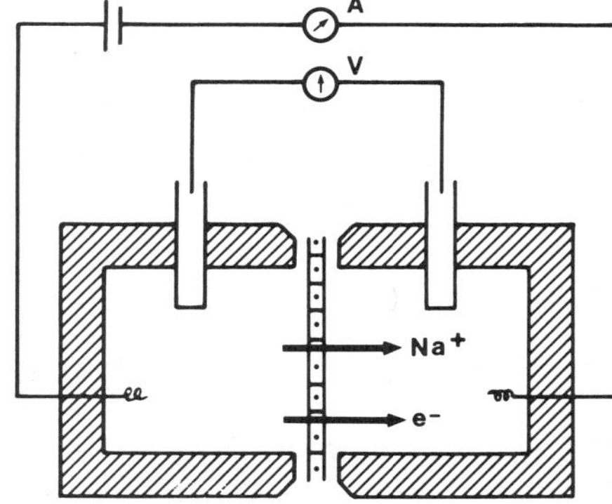

FIGURE 1. The Ussing apparatus for determination of SCC. In the upper diagram, a sheet of isolated epithelium (**a**) is seen mounted in a plastic chamber so that the tissue separates similar electrolyte solutions (**b**). The electrical potential generated by transport of an electrolyte, here indicated by Na^+, is read from a voltmeter (**V**) attached to appropriate electrodes in the baths. As shown in the lower diagram, an external current source can be applied through the chamber, in a polarity opposite to that of the spontaneous potential. When the transport rate through the tissue, and the external current (**e**) are exactly opposite, the voltage measured at the meter (**V**) is 0. Under these conditions, the current measured at the ammeter (**A**) indicates the transport rate of ions by the tissue and is referred to as the SCC.

Edelman et al. (39, 125) also demonstrated that (a) cellular uptake of aldosterone preceded the biologic effect, (b) radiolabeled aldosterone bound preferentially to cell nuclei, (c) uptake of radiolabeled uridine into epithelial cell RNA was increased by aldosterone and preceded biologic action, and (d) the increase in SCC in response to aldosterone required energy.

Three key points in this sequence are: The nature of the cellular receptor, the nature of the newly synthesized RNA, and the role of the new protein in the biologic response to aldosterone.

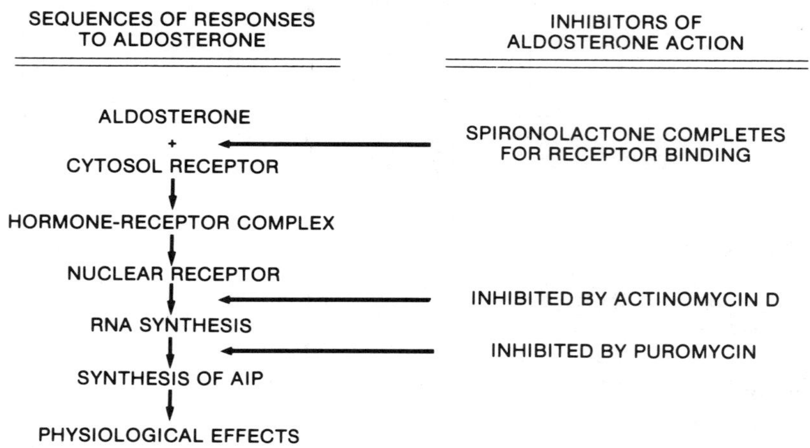

FIGURE 2. Sequence of events in cells responding to aldosterone. The corticosteroid binds to specific cytosolic receptors, and the hormone-receptor is translocated to nuclear receptors where new RNA synthesis is initiated. The new RNA leads to synthesis of new proteins, referred to as aldosterone-induced proteins (AIP), which are responsible for the biologic response to the hormone. Specific inhibitors for various steps in the sequence are indicated.

The Aldosterone Receptor. The cytosol of disrupted kidney cells contains proteins to which aldosterone binds, as do the nuclei. It has been found that the steroid binds first to the cytosolic receptor, following which the steroid–receptor complex is translocated to a soluble nuclear receptor and, subsequently, to a chromatin-bound complex (49,111). More recent studies using kidney have shown that the cytosol contains several distinct receptors to which steroid hormones bind, and the affinity of these receptors for different steroids has led to the identification of four distinct receptor types. The receptor with the highest affinity for aldosterone has been termed type I receptor and shows the following selectivity sequence: aldosterone > deoxycorticosterone > corticosterone > progesterone > dexamethasone. This affinity sequence, obtained by sophisticated kinetic analysis of radioligand binding, correlates very well with the ability to stimulate Na^+ in toad bladder: aldosterone > deoxycorticosterone > cortisol > corticosterone > progesterone (126). Matulich et al. (113) related renal receptor affinities to biologic responses and found them comparable. Type II receptor has been termed the glucocorticoid receptor because the sequence of affinities shows: dexamethasone > corticosterone > deoxycorticosterone > aldosterone > cortisol > progesterone > estradiol and dihydrotestosterone. Type III or corticosterone receptor shows these affinities: corticosterone > cortisol > deoxycorticosterone > progesterone > aldosterone > dexamethasone. The physiologic role of the type III receptor, as well as that of a fourth renal cytosolic receptor with highest affinity for deoxycorticosterone (109) is unknown. The specificities and putative roles of these receptors have been reviewed by

Fanestil and Park (43). The precise nature of the mineralocorticoid receptor remains obscure, but Feldman et al. (49) have proposed an allosteric behavior with active and inactive forms of the receptor existing in the cytosol. Later studies from this same group (112) showed that both aldosterone and the aldosterone antagonist spironolactone compete for the same cytosolic receptor. The aldosterone-receptor complex was found to condense to form aggregates of larger molecular size in gradients of low salt concentration, and to transfer to nuclear chromatin acceptor sites. The spironolactone-receptor complex showed neither of these properties, and it was proposed that the receptor remained in the inactive form if combined with spironolactone.

The technique of tubular microdissection has recently allowed the identification of aldosterone-binding sites in the mammalian renal tubule. Strum et al. (158) used autoradiographic methods to demonstrate type III binding sites in cells of cortical collecting tubules and outer medullary collecting tubules of rat kidney. Bonvalet et al. (11) showed binding sites in microdissected rabbit distal convoluted tubules. It is now recognized that the distal convoluted tubule is actually composed of three morphologically and functionally distinct segments (see below, "Distal Tubule and Cortical Collecting Tubule," for further discussion of this distinction). Doucet and Katz (37) have recently localized this "distal tubule" binding of aldosterone to the branched collecting tubule, also known as the cortical connecting tubule, and confirmed specific binding in the medullary collecting tubule. These investigators found negligible binding of [^{3}H]-aldosterone to other tubular segments. The binding sites in the branched and medullary collecting tubule segments showed a dissociation constant, K_D, of 2.2×10^{-9}M, a value within the physiologic range for plasma aldosterone concentration, and had the specificity: aldosterone > DOC > spironolactone > dexamethasone > 5α-dihydrotestosterone = progesterone = 17β-estradiol.

We should emphasize that steroid binding should not be equated with a specific physiologic response, such as increased sodium transport. It was pointed out above that spironolactone binds to the aldosterone receptor with relatively high affinity, yet the spironolactone-receptor complex fails to bind to nuclear sites or to have a direct effect on transport. On the other hand, another chemically similar aldosterone-antagonist steroid, which also has no direct effect on sodium transport, is capable of stimulating acidification by the turtle urinary bladder to the same extent as aldosterone (119). Finally, in vitro protein binding does not necessarily correlate with in vivo activity, because of the differences in nonspecific binding of the steroids to plasma proteins. For instance, Funder et al. (56) showed that 19-nordeoxycorticosterone, a putative mineralocorticoid found in urine of rats with adrenal-regeneration hypertension, had 140% of the affinity of aldosterone for renal receptors in kidney slices in protein-free solution. However, the affinity, compared to that of aldosterone, was only 40% when plasma was added in vitro, and 33% in vivo. In the in vivo Kagawa rat assay, 19-nordeoxycorticosterone had only 10–30% of the agonist potency of aldosterone and did not antagonize the effect of aldosterone on urinary electrolyte excretion.

Aldosterone Effect on RNA Synthesis. Even before the identification of specific cytosolic receptors for aldosterone, it had been shown that [^{3}H]-aldosterone accumulated preferentially in the nuclei of epithelial cells of the toad bladder (39) and that the sodium-transport effect of aldosterone both in rat kidney (175) and in toad bladder (27,39) was blocked by actinomycin D, an inhibitor of RNA synthesis. Marver et al. (111) suggested from time-course studies that the cytoplasmic receptor−hormone complex binds first to tris-soluble nuclear receptors and then to a chromatin-bound site. Recent studies (135) of specific RNAs have shown that aldosterone increases synthesis of polyadenylated messenger RNA (poly A(+) mRNA) after a latent period of 30−60 minutes. After 90−240 minutes new 18S and 28S cytoplasmic ribosomal RNAs (rRNA) are induced. Actinomycin D, which blocks aldosterone-stimulated sodium transport by intact epithelia, blocks synthesis of both poly A(+) mRNA and non-polyadenylated RNA (poly A(−) mRNA). 3′-deoxyadenosine, which inhibits synthesis of poly A(+) RNA, but not that of poly A(−) RNA, blocks only ~ 50% of the aldosterone effect of SCC, suggesting that poly A(−) RNA also plays a role in the aldosterone stimulation of SCC. The long delay in synthesis of rRNA after exposure of the tissue to aldosterone, as well as the lack of effect on SCC of 3′-deoxycytidine, which blocks synthesis of rRNA but not mRNA, suggests that the early phase of the response of SCC to aldosterone is not dependent on new rRNA synthesis.

Aldosterone Induction of Protein Synthesis. Inhibition of the effect of aldosterone on SCC by puromycin (27,39) indicated that synthesis of new protein was necessary for the increased sodium transport stimulated by the hormone. Using radionuclide-labeled protein precursors, such as ^{35}S-methionine, with subsequent identification of label after protein separation techniques, in toad bladder it was shown that aldosterone stimulates synthesis of new proteins with molecular weights given variously as 12,000 (9), 17,000−38,000 (147), 70,000 (in cytosolic fraction), and 15,000 (in microsomal fraction) (60).

Recent studies of mitochondria-rich cells of toad bladder by Scott et al. (145,147) have shown that aldosterone induces synthesis of proteins of 170,000, 85,000, and 12,000 mol. wt. in plasma membrane, and cytosolic proteins of 36,000, 12,000, and 6,000 mol. wt. Furthermore, these investigators were able to extract aldosterone-induced RNA with properties of polyadenylated messenger RNA and use it in a cell-free system to induce synthesis of two proteins, one of which had the same molecular weight as an aldosterone-induced plasma membrane protein from the intact cell system (145).

Note should be made here that Scott et al. have carried out their studies on toad bladder epithelial cells separated by density-gradient technique into granular cell and mitochondria-rich cell fractions. These investigators have shown that radiolabeled aldosterone accumulates in nuclei of mitochondria-rich cells but not in granular cell nuclei where it can be displaced by DOC but not by cortisol. By contrast, labeled corticosterone was bound equally by mitochondria-rich and granular cells suggesting that the mitochondria-rich cell is a target for aldosterone (136). Using double-labeling techniques, these same investigators found that aldosterone induced new protein synthesis in the mitochondria-rich cells. Corticosterone induced new protein synthesis in granular cells, but this protein had different physical properties from the new protein induced by aldosterone in the mitochondria-rich cells (147). Since most investigators consider the granular cells to be the site of active transport, the relationship between induction of protein by aldosterone in mitochondria-rich cells and increased sodium transport in granular cells remains to be explained.

Physiologic Role of the Aldosterone-Induced Proteins

The physiologic role(s) of the aldosterone-induced protein(s) have not been conclusively identified. Before addressing this question we should briefly consider the generally accepted mechanisms for sodium uptake across epithelia, such as renal tubule, colon, and amphibian bladder and skin (Figure 3). All of these epithelia are composed of asymmetrical cells

FIGURE 3. A generalized schema for transport of sodium across epithelium. A single cell is indicated, bound by tight-junctions near the luminal surface to neighboring cells. Sodium ions diffuse passively along an electrochemical gradient through the luminal membrane (**a**), probably through the aegis of protein molecules within the lipids of the membrane. Sodium ions are carried against their electrochemical gradient out of the cell at the serosal or basolateral membrane, in exchange for potassium ions moving into the cell, by Na-K-ATPase (**c**). Energy for this active transport step in the form of ATP is generated by consumption of substrate (**b**).

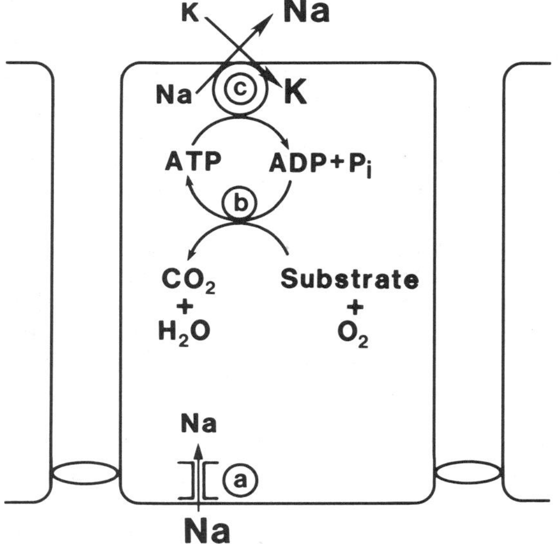

with the luminal or mucosal surface of the cell dissimilar in structure and function from the serosal or basolateral membrane. Sodium diffuses down its electrochemical gradient across the luminal cell membrane into the cell. Although no specific transport protein for sodium is known to exist in this membrane, it appears likely that proteins would be required to allow passage of the highly hydrophilic sodium ion through the lipid membrane. Maintenance of a low intracellular sodium concentration and, hence, maintenance of the electrochemical gradient for sodium diffusion across the luminal membrane, is achieved by active transport of sodium across the basolateral membrane against its electrochemical gradient. This transport step, by virtue of its being against an electrochemical gradient, requires an energy source such as ATP and is associated with simultaneous transport of potassium ions against their electrochemical gradient into the cell. The "sodium pump" involved here would appear to be the ubiquitous sodium- and potassium-activated adenosine triphosphate or Na-K-ATPase as described by Skou (153).

Returning to the role(s) of the aldosterone-induced proteins, it is evident that they might be involved (a) by serving as the luminal membrane sodium-conducting pathway or involved with the synthesis of such protein, (b) by contributing to synthesis of new Na-K-ATPase or activating Na-K-ATPase already present, or (c) by furnishing the energy to the sodium pump as component of any of several ATP-generating systems. An increase in sodium transport across an epithelium will necessarily involve increased movement of sodium across both cell membranes and, thus, it becomes difficult to tell which process is initiated by aldosterone-induced protein and which process follows secondarily.

One of the earliest mechanisms proposed for the action of aldosterone was that of increased entry of sodium into epithelial cells across the outer or luminal cell membrane (26,105,150). Electrophysiologic studies of amphibian urinary bladder have shown that most of the resistance to transepithelial movement of ions resides in the luminal cell membrane (55,72) and that the transepithelial conductance is directly related to SCC, a measure of sodium transport as discussed earlier (71). Similar observations have been made in rabbit urinary bladder (99,100). While not localizing the specific cellular site of sodium conductance changes, studies of transepithelial electrical parameters have demonstrated that aldosterone simultaneously increases conductance while it is increasing SCC in both toad bladder (20,152) and rabbit urinary bladder (99). Thus, it has been proposed that aldosterone-induced proteins could be involved in creating low resistance channels in the hydrophobic lipid cell membrane through which sodium ions might pass. Support for this hypothesis has come from studies with amiloride, a pyrazine diuretic that binds reversibly with the luminal cell membrane to block sodium entry. Cuthbert and Shum (29) used ^{14}C-amiloride to demonstrate saturable binding sites for this compound on toad bladder epithelial cells. The number of amiloride binding sites fell after prolonged in vitro incubation of the cells (a technique known to sensitize amphibian bladder to the SCC-stimulating effect of mineralocorticoid hormones) and rose after pretreatment of the bladders with aldosterone. The effect of aldosterone to increase amiloride binding sites, like its effect to increase SCC, was blocked by actinomycin D or cycloheximide. The conclusion from these studies is that aldosterone increases the number of sites, probably proteins, in the luminal membrane through which sodium passes and at which amiloride binds to block the passage of sodium.

The foregoing discussion suggests that an aldosterone-induced protein might lead directly to increased permeation of sodium ions through the luminal membrane of epithelial cells, either by acting as conducting channels or by inducing information of sodium conducting channels. Alternatively, increased extrusion of sodium from the cell across the basolateral membrane by Na-K-ATPase would lower cytoplasmic sodium concentration and increase the driving force for sodium entry into the cell across the luminal membrane. This possibility has led investigators to examine Na-K-ATPase activity in aldosterone-sensitive tissues. Early studies by Landon et al. (94) and Chignell and Titus (18) showed that adrenalectomy resulted in lower Na-K-ATPase activity in rat kidney, and Chignell and Titus found the K_m for ATP, Na, and K to be unchanged. This led to the conclusion that the amount of enzyme present might be lowered by adrenalectomy. Landon et al. found that enzyme activity was not restored by physiologic amounts of aldosterone but could be restored by larger amounts. Jørgensen's studies (83) showed that aldosterone increased the Na-K-ATPase activity in a rat kidney microsomal preparation. The greatest effect was seen in microsomes from the outer renal medulla but this response required six or more hours to become evident, whereas, the effect of aldosterone on sodium conservation is seen much earlier. It was suggested on the basis of these and later studies (84) that the early effect of aldosterone was to increase sodium entry into cells, after which the higher intracellular sodium concentration led to an increase in the number of binding sites for ATP on Na-K-ATPase, thus, increasing the velocity of the enzymatic reaction as seen after 14 hours. Longer exposure to the hormone, it was proposed, might lead to an increase in the amount of enzyme through new protein synthesis. This latter hypothesis was supported by the work of Knox and Sen (91), who found that after 5 days of aldosterone treatment in adrenalectomized rats, Na-K-ATPase activity was restored in the heavy microsomal fraction of the kidney. In addition, isotope labeling showed synthesis of new protein that had in vitro physical properties similar to Na-K-ATPase. Westenfelder et al. (173) reported studies indicating that the effect of aldosterone on renal Na-K-ATPase might be secondary to a more immediate effect on sodium metabolism. These investigators found that providing a high salt intake to adrenalectomized rats restored renal tissue Na-K-ATPase activity even without hormonal replacement. The work of Hendler et al. (70) showed that restoration of Na-K-ATPase activity in kidneys of adrenalectomized rats did not depend upon replacement of mineralocorticoid hormone, but could be accomplished by the glucocorticoid methylprednisolone. The effect appeared to be due to synthesis of new enzyme, for the number of ouabain-binding sites was increased after treatment with the hormone.

Rodriguez et al. (132) also examined the effects of mineralocorticoid and glucocorticoid hormones on renal ATPase of adrenalectomized rats. Dexamethasone elevated both Na-K-ATPase activity and gluconeogenesis in a dose-dependent fashion but had a minimal effect on electrolyte excretion and no effect on inulin clearance. Acute administration of aldosterone failed to stimulate Na-K-ATPase activity but had the expected effect on electrolyte excretion, whereas at high doses aldosterone stimulated gluconeogenesis as well. Daily administration of aldosterone at a dose that optimally affected electrolyte excretion (1–4 μg/100 g body weight) similarly failed to increase either Na-K-ATPase activity or gluconeogenesis. Daily administration of aldosterone at doses 100–200 times greater increased both Na-K-ATPase activity and gluconeogenesis. These investigators proposed that stimulation of Na-K-ATPase activity was a glucocorticoid response rather than a mineralocorticoid response to steroid hormone administration. Studies in toad bladder also failed to provide evidence for a direct effect of aldosterone on Na-K-ATPase. Electron microscopic studies by Laird and Yates (93) had demonstrated increased precipitation of lead phosphate at the basolateral membranes of aldosterone-stimulated tissues suggesting increased ATPase activity in response to aldosterone. Hill et al. (73), however found no effect of aldosterone at 10^{-6}M on Na-K-ATPase of toad bladder in vitro. These latter studies examined not only total enzyme activity but also the dependence of enzyme activity on sodium and ATP concentrations and the dissociation constant of the enzyme–sodium complex.

Since the number of aldosterone-sensitive cells may be a small percentage of the total cell mass of the kidney, and even of the toad bladder, it seemed desirable to examine Na-K-ATPase activity only in those cell populations known to respond to aldosterone. The technical difficulties of isolating aldosterone-sensitive segments of the renal tubule and performing enzyme assays on so little tissue are obvious and it is not surprising that results have been conflicting. Schmidt et al. (141) microdissected renal tubules from rats and found that adrenalectomy lowered Na-K-ATPase activity in the proximal convoluted tubule, the thick ascending limb of the loop of Henle, and the distal convoluted tubule. Administration of aldosterone, 5 μg/100 g body weight 1 hour before sacrifice, was found to restore enzyme activity to normal. The restoration of enzyme activity by aldosterone could be blocked by concurrent administration of cycloheximide or actinomycin D. This same group later showed decreased Na-K-ATPase activity in cortical thick ascending limb and cortical collecting tubule of adrenalectomized animals (74). As in their previous studies, enzyme activity was restored within 1 hr by aldosterone, this time administered in vitro, and a dose–response curve showed that maximum enzyme activity could be achieved by aldosterone at a concentration of 10^{-6}M. The effect of aldosterone was blocked by spironolactone and was not induced by dexamethasone. This short time-course for the observed effect of aldosterone is in sharp contrast to the long time reported by Jørgensen (83), Hendler et al., (70) and Landon et al. (94). Garg et al. (59) used an indirect coupled fluorometric method to assess Na-K-ATPase activity in 11 different segments of isolated rabbit tubules, and found the enzyme activity levels to correlate with rates of sodium transport reported in other studies. Enzyme activity in the cortical collecting duct was increased by administration of either deoxycorticosterone acetate (DOCA) or a low sodium diet to the rabbits. Doucet and Katz (37) were careful to document the sensitivity of their Na-K-ATPase assay and found it capable of discriminating 20% changes in enzyme activity. Using this assay method to study isolated mouse and rabbit proximal convoluted tubule, medullary ascending limb of Henle's loop, distal convoluted tubule, and cortical collecting tubule, these investigators found that adrenalectomy resulted in decreased Na-K-ATPase activity in all four tubule segments. Enzyme activity was not restored by aldosterone administered in vivo. Aldosterone receptors probably exist in only two of these tubule segments, the distal convoluted tubule and the cortical collecting tubule, and Doucet and Katz concluded that the effects of adrenalectomy were nonspecific. Katz (85) found that another known stimulus of renal Na-K-ATPase, potassium loading, stimulated enzyme activity both in adrenalectomized rats and in rats given spironolactone to block the effect of endogenous aldosterone secreted in response to the potassium administration. Katz calculated that intracellular ATP and extracellular potassium concentrations are normally close to the optimal levels for maximal Na-K-ATPase activity, whereas intracellular sodium concentration is below enzyme-saturating level, and concluded that changes in intracellular sodium concentration could be sufficient to determine enzyme activity. This conclusion is supported by the observations of Petty et al. (124), using the technique of microperfusion of the isolated rabbit collecting tubule. It was found that adrenalectomy lowered and aldosterone replacement restored tubule Na-K-ATPase activity. However, the restoration of enzyme activity by aldosterone was blocked by addition of amiloride to the luminal perfusate to block entry of sodium into the cells across the luminal membrane. Thus, the evidence seems to support an effect of aldosterone to increase sodium entry into cells across the luminal membrane and a secondary effect of intracellular sodium to determine Na-K-ATPase activity.

Aldosterone Effect on Energy Generation

Active transport of sodium by Na-K-ATPase requires energy in the form of ATP and another role postulated for the aldosterone-induced proteins has been the generation of ATP via any of several metabolic pathways. Early studies of the toad bladder showed a stoichiometric relationship between sodium transport and oxygen consumption and the effect of aldosterone on sodium transport was shown to be dependent upon the presence of metabolizable substrate (98,151). Aldosterone was found to stimulate activity of the oxidative enzymes succinic dehydrogenase and cytochrome oxidase (50) and later it was shown to stimulate activity of several other enzymes in the citric acid cycle (86,87,89,107). Law and Edelman (95) have shown that aldosterone not only increases the activity of citrate synthase but also leads to synthesis of new enzyme. Kirsten et al. (89) observed that the increase in activity of citric acid cycle enzymes induced by aldosterone takes place even if sodium is absent from the solution bathing the mucosal surface of the bladder tissue. Therefore, the change in enzyme activity is not a secondary response to increased cell sodium concentration induced by aldosterone. An interesting related observation by Kirsten et al. (88) is the reduced cytochrome-a activity of renal mitochondria from adrenalectomized rats and its restoration to normal by aldosterone treatment. These investigators point out that increased nicotinamide adenine dinucleotide (NADH) production by the aldosterone-stimulated citric acid cycle might stimulate cytochrome oxidase activity or, alternatively, a fall in NADH due to increased cytochrome oxidase activity might stimulate the citric acid cycle, thus illustrating the difficulty faced in trying to unravel the primary and secondary events arising from the action of aldosterone.

Because aldosterone had been shown to stimulate succinic dehydrogenase, Tan and Trachewsky (160) and Fazekas and Sandor (48) examined the synthesis of flavin nucleotides, which are linked to succinic dehydrogenase. Fazekas and Sandor found that adrenalectomy lowered, and aldosterone treatment partially restored synthesis of flavin–adenine dinucleotide (FAD) from radiolabeled riboflavin in rat liver. There was no effect on flavin mononucleotide (FMN) levels and treatment with corticosterone or cortisol decreased both FAD and FMN synthesis from riboflavin. These investigators found no change in synthesis of renal FMN or FAD by any of the manipulations. However, others have demonstrated increased synthesis of FAD in the kidney in response to aldosterone if synthesis of the nucleotide was first suppressed by giving the rats dexamethasone (160). The aldosterone effect could be reproduced by 9α-fluorohydrocortisone, but not by progesterone or corticosterone, and it was blocked by spironolactone or actinomycin D but not by cycloheximide. Trachewsky (163) later showed increased synthesis of both FMN and FAD in rat kidneys after aldosterone administration. Either of two riboflavin analogs, which act as competitive inhibitors of flavokinase, reduced the formation of FMN from labeled riboflavin and blocked the antinatriuretic but not the kaliuretic effect of aldosterone on the kidney. This latter finding again demonstrates the dissociation of the effects of aldosterone on excretion of sodium and potassium by the intact kidney.

Another mechanism by which aldosterone might increase Na-K-ATPase activity has been proposed by Goodman et al. (62,63). These investigators found that within 20 minutes after exposure of the toad bladder to aldosterone there was increased decarboxylation of 1-^{14}C-glucose to produce $^{14}CO_2$, indicating increased activity of the hexose monophosphate (HMP) shunt. By comparison, production of labeled CO_2 from 6-^{14}C-glucose required 40 minutes. Increased HMP shunt activity in response to aldosterone suggests that there might be an effect on lipid synthesis and incorporation of 2-^{14}C-pyruvate into phospholipid was examined. It was observed that 6 hours after exposure to aldosterone, both weight percentage and specific activity of label in several long-chain fatty acids was increased (63,64). The effects of aldosterone on lipid synthesis could be blocked by cordycepin, an inhibitor of RNA synthesis, as well as by cycloheximide, an inhibitor of protein synthesis (102). Further evidence for the importance of aldosterone's effect on cell membrane lipid was provided using an inhibitor of acetyl-coenzyme A carboxylase, TPIA (2-methyl-2-[p-(1,2,3,4-tetrahydro-1-naphthyl) phenoxyl] proprionic acid) (102,146). When TPIA was applied to the toad bladder, it inhibited sodium transport as well as lipid synthesis. Amiloride limits sodium entry into the epithethial cell layer but had no effect on lipid synthesis, suggesting that the effects of aldosterone on lipid synthesis are not mediated via effects of increased intracellular sodium concentration. On the basis of all these observations it has been proposed that aldosterone may exert an effect on sodium transport via an effect on cell membrane lipids to cause a change in the environment of membrane-bound Na-K-ATPase.

The foregoing discussion centers on the mechanisms by which aldosterone might stimulate epithelial absorption of sodium. Less well understood are the mechanisms by which aldosterone stimulates secretion of potassium and hydrogen ion. Study of the effects of aldosterone on sodium transport has been greatly facilitated by use of the amphibian skin and urinary bladder but these tissues have not been shown to secrete potassium. Barger et al. (4) examined the effects of acute mineralocorticoid treatment on renal sodium and potassium excretion in the intact dog. They observed that direct infusion of aldosterone or 9-α fluorohydrocortisone into the renal artery over a 1.5–2-hour period stimulated kaliuresis but not antinatriuresis. The animals studied were moderately saline loaded and the relatively large natriuretic effect of the saline load might have masked the effect of the mineralocorticoid to stimulate sodium reabsorption. Adrenalectomized dogs treated in the same fashion showed both antinatriuretic and kaliuretic responses to mineralocorticoid hormone. Similar findings in intact and adrenalectomized rats were reported by Morris et al. (117). Divergence of the effects of aldosterone on sodium and potassium excretion by the kidneys of the rat (53,175) and dog (103) was shown by the use of actinomycin D, which blocked the antinatriuretic effect but not the kaliuretic effect of aldosterone. The effects of corticosteroids on the kidney are discussed in more detail below.

The toad bladder is capable of acidifying its luminal bathing solution. The acidification process is stimulated by physiologic concentrations of aldosterone with a time course similar to that of the stimulation of sodium transport (108). Unlike sodium transport, acidification is also stimulated by dexamethasone (108). The effect of aldosterone on acidification is not blocked by actinomycin D, puromycin, or cycloheximide, all of which stimulate acidification (103,109).

ADRENOCORTICOID ACTION AT THE ORGAN LEVEL

Na^+ and K^+ Transport in the Urinary Tract

Proximal Tubule. While most recent work has continued to focus on the effects of mineralocorticoids on the distal nephron, Gutsche and Hegel (68) have demonstrated that the time constant for leakage of electrolytes from peritubular plasma to proximal tubular luminal fluid is doubled by adrenalectomy in rats. Aldosterone replacement reverses this effect, suggesting that endogenous aldosterone has a role in maintaining the normal permeability of the proximal tubule to electrolytes.

Distal Tubule and Cortical Collecting Tubule. Recent interest has centered around new information on the site of action of aldosterone in the distal nephron. The renal distal tubule as usually defined in micropuncture experiments, i.e., that segment of the distal nephron extending from the macula densa to the point of union with another distal tubule to form a collecting duct, recently has been shown to be both functionally and morphologically heterogeneous. The so-called distal tubule, in fact, consists of at least two (66) and perhaps three (82) structurally and functionally distinct segments. What previously had been considered distal tubule actually consists of an initial convoluted distal tubular portion and a cortical collecting tubular portion. Adding to the complexity, Imai has described a functionally distinct third portion in the middle of this distal segment, the granular connecting tubule (82) (Figure 4).

Differences in mineralocorticoid responsiveness between the initial distal tubule and the cortical collecting tubule were described by Gross et al. (66) in 1975. They found that initial distal tubules dissected from kidneys of rabbits fed a standard laboratory chow, when perfused in vitro, always exhibited a lumen negative potential (mean value, −40 mV). In contrast, cortical collecting tubules showed a slightly positive electrical potential (mean value, +3.7 mV). However, if the rabbits were fed a low Na^+, high K^+ diet and given DOCA, the potential in the cortical collecting tubule was found to be −30 mV lumen negative, and the plasma aldosterone concentration increased 50-fold. The low Na^+, high K^+ diet plus DOCA had no effect on the electrical potential of the early distal tubule. The negative potential in both early distal tubule and collecting tubule (high aldosterone animals) was inhibited by ouabain and by amiloride. Gross et al. interpreted these results as indicating that the potential is secondary to active sodium transport in both segments, although no explanation is yet available as to why the potential of the cortical collecting tubule is affected by aldosterone and that of the early distal tubule is not.

The effect of DOCA or a high K^+−low Na^+ diet to shift the electrical potential of the isolated perfused rabbit cortical collecting tubule in a lumen-negative direction has been confirmed by O'Neil and Helman (120) and by Imai (82). O'Neil and Helman also found that when DOCA was administered to rabbits for a prolonged period, the maximal effect on the electrical potential occurred at 11−18 days, when the potential had changed from a control level of −6.6 mV to −53.8 mV. By 21−23 days of

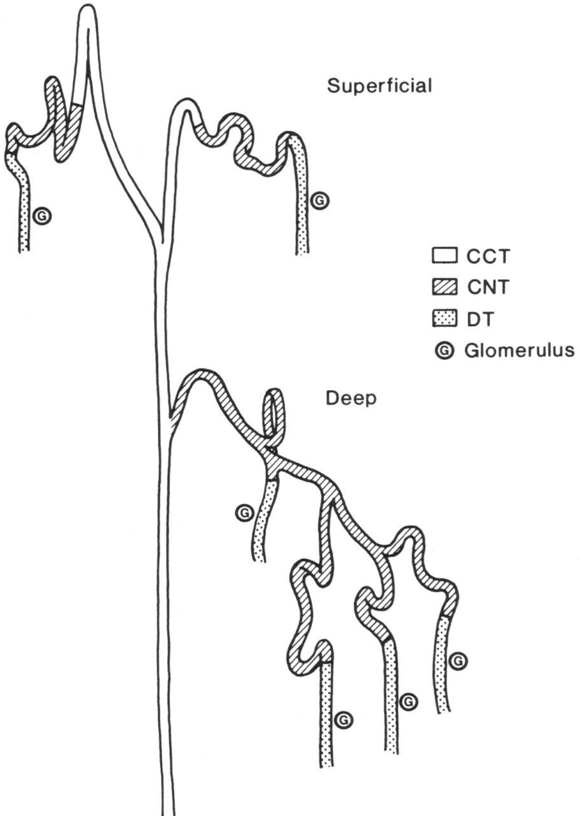

FIGURE 4. Segments of superficial and deep distal nephrons of rabbit. **CCT**, cortical collecting tubule; **CNT**, connecting tubule; **DT**, distal convoluted tubule; **G**, glomerulus for each nephron, adjacent to the macula densa region of the distal convoluted tubule. (Adapted from ref. 82 with permission).

DOCA administration, the potential had declined to −32.5 mV, a level still considerably more negative than the control value. The time of the peak negative luminal potential in these experiments (11−18 days) also corresponded to the time of maximal increase in net Na^+ reabsorption and net K^+ secretion (Figure 5). The observed increase in K^+ secretion was greater than would be expected from the more negative potential alone, so that DOCA must have increased either K^+ conductance or the electromotive force of the K^+ "pump." Amiloride inhibited the effect of DOCA on the transepithelial potential and also eliminated most of the effect of DOCA on net fluxes of Na^+ and K^+. These data indicate that in the cortical collecting tubule, mineralocorticoids stimulate Na^+ reabsorption and K^+ secretion, that the time required for the maximal effect of a mineralocorticoid at the tubular level is longer than previously detected

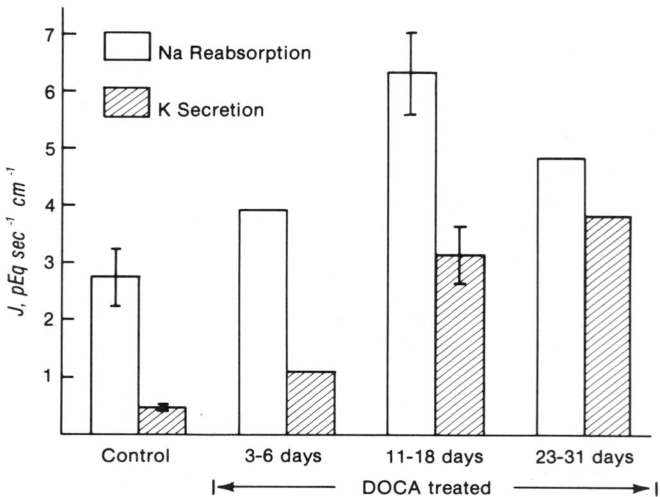

FIGURE 5. Effects of DOCA administration of sodium reabsorption and potassium secretion in isolated perfused rabbit cortical collecting tubules. The net transport rate (J) of sodium and potassium is indicated on the ordinate. Sodium reabsorption is maximal in tubules of animals treated 11–18 days, when transepithelial potential is greatest, but peak potassium excretion does not coincide with peak sodium reabsorption or potential (see text). (From ref. 120 with permission).

with clearance techniques, and that the increased luminal negativity corresponds to an amiloride-sensitive increase in net Na^+ absorption.

Gross and Kokko (67) also observed that isolated, perfused cortical collecting tubules dissected from rabbits on a regular chow diet or a diet supplemented with NaCl exhibit a low transtubular potential (mean value, +1 mV), which changed to −19 mV lumen negative after addition of d-aldosterone to the perfusate and bath. The latent period before the effect of aldosterone was detected was 10–40 minutes. Initial distal tubules, in contrast, showed a lumen negative potential that was not affected by either prior adrenalectomy or by administration of aldosterone in vitro. Spironolactone and triamterene in vitro inhibited the aldosterone-dependent potential in the cortical collecting tubule but had no effect on the potential of the initial distal tubule.

Schwartz and Burg (143) extended the observations on the effects of diet and DOCA on rabbit cortical collecting tubule function examined both by in vitro perfusion and by measurement of urinary electrolyte excretion. In their control animals, receiving standard rabbit chow, a mean transtubular electrical potential of 16 mV lumen negative was found that was not correlated with the lumen to bath Na^+ flux (i.e., Na^+ transport in the absorptive direction) in the same tubules. However, in tubules from rabbits receiving DOCA for 10–15 days, the lumen to bath Na^+ flux was doubled and the lumen became more negative (−46 mV). Additionally, net K^+ secretion increased fourfold. Although there were large changes in the rate of Na^+ and K^+ transport in cortical collecting tubules perfused in vitro, there was no change in the urine Na^+/K^+ ratio in the DOCA-treated animals, compared with control. Thus, DOCA stimulated ion transport in the cortical collecting tubule, but this stimulation did not alter the pattern of the electrolyte excretion, presumably due to the action of the collecting duct in vivo.

Other combinations of low and high Na^+ and K^+ diets were administered to produce large changes in plasma aldosterone concentration and the effect on cortical collecting tubule function was examined in vitro. The lumen to bath Na^+ flux, net K^+ secretion and the transtubular potential were all directly and closely correlated with the plasma aldosterone concentration. The persistence of an effect of diet on tubular function in vitro suggests that the action of aldosterone is via synthesis of enzymes or membrane components as has often been postulated. Wade et al. (168) used morphometric techniques to assess changes in membrane area in electron micrographs of sections of cortical collecting tubules from rabbits treated with DOCA for 11−18 days. Treatment with DOCA increased the basolateral membrane area (per millimeter of tubule) in the principal cells but had no effect on the luminal membrane, and no effect on either membrane of the intercalated cells. This study relates the long-term effects of DOCA on epithelial transport to underlying morphologic adaptations, and suggests that the hormonal effects on ion transport are mediated through synthesis of elements of the sodium pump in the basolateral membrane.

Stokes et al. (156) examined the transepithelial electrical potential of collecting tubules dissected from different regions of the rabbit kidney. When collecting tubules from the outer medulla of rabbits receiving DOCA were perfused in vitro they exhibited potentials ranging from −92 to +40 mV, in contrast to collecting tubules from the cortex of DOCA-treated rabbits, which always show a lumen negative potential in vitro. In DOCA-treated rabbits, however, the potential of the collecting tubule reversed from negative in the cortex to positive within the first millimeter of the outer medulla in association with a marked decrease in the number of the intercalated cells of the collecting tubule. The correlation between greater population density of intercalated cells and the aldosterone-stimulated lumen negative potential in cortical collecting tubules, and a positive potential and fewer intercalated cells in the outer medullary tubule led to the speculation that these cells may be responsible for the active Na^+ transport, which is thought to be the basis for the luminal negativity. Such speculation is not borne out by the morphometric studies of Wade et al. (168) (see above), which demonstrated that DOCA treatment of rabbits increase the basolateral membrane area of principal cells but has no effect on the intercalated cells. If the increase in basolateral membrane area with DOCA reflects the increased transport capacity for ions that occurs in cortical collecting tubules (143), then this increased capacity is not occurring in the intercalated cells and the change in cell population between cortical and outer medullary collecting tubules is not the basis for the change in sign of the transepithelial potential difference (PD). No evidence is yet available providing an explanation of the origin of the positive potential seen in the outer medullary collecting tubules.

In summary, the segment of the distal nephron between the macula densa and the collecting duct consists of at least two functionally distinct parts. The first part, the early distal convoluted tubule, exhibits a lumen negative transtubular potential that appears to be independent of the mineralocorticoid status of the animal. The second part, the collecting tubule, exhibits a transtubular potential whose sign and magnitude depend on the level of circulating aldosterone. However, even in DOCA-treated rabbits, the magnitude of the negative potential decrease as tubules closer to the medulla are examined, and collecting tubules dissected from the outer medulla show a reversal in sign, i.e., a lumen-positive potential.

Medullary Collecting Duct. In contrast to the clear evidence for an aldosterone effect in the cortical collecting tubule, the situation in the medullary collecting duct is somewhat obscured by the contradictory results obtained with different experimental approaches. Examination of net Na^+ reabsorption by the medullary collecting duct and the effect of volume expansion thereon has provided different results, depending on whether measurements were made with a microcatheterization method or by micropuncture. Sonnenberg (154), using microcatheterization, has shown that adrenalectomy, while producing the expected defects in urinary electrolyte excretion, did not affect net Na^+ reabsorption by the inner medullary collecting duct. Furthermore, infusion of blood inhibited medullary collecting duct sodium reabsorption in both adrenalectomized and sham-operated rats, implying that aldosterone does not mediate the acute natriuresis of volume expansion in this nephron segment. In response to Sonnenberg's report, Ullrich and Papavassiliou (165) repeated an earlier observation supporting the concept that mineralocorticoids, in fact, do influence medullary collecting duct function. In rats, using the split drop method, they found that net Na^+ absorption increased in animals on a low Na^+ diet and was inhibited in adrenalectomized animals. Administration of aldosterone to adrenalectomized animals resulted in an increase in Na^+ absorption. In comparing their results to those of Sonnenberg et al. (154, Table 2), Ullrich and Papavassiliou pointed out (165) that in Sonnenberg's study the final urine Na^+ concentration was higher in the adrenalectomized than in the control rats, conceivably reflecting the mineralocorticoid deficit. There is strong evidence for a role for mineralocorticoid in supporting medullary collecting duct Na^+ reabsorption in euvolemia, although a final conclusion will have to await clarification of the differences between micropuncture and microcatheterization experiments.

Mammalian Urinary Bladder. Although the mammalian urinary bladder has not been considered to play a significant role in electrolyte homeostasis, the bladder is the final site where urine is stored and is well vascularized. If the bladder epithelium exhibited a high permeability to water and electrolytes, the concentration and osmolar gradients between urine and plasma established by the distal nephron and collecting duct would be dissipated in the bladder. Recent reinvestigation of the transporting characteristics of the urinary bladder epithelium has shown that the tissue has a high electrical resistance (99), indicating a low permeability to electrolytes. Beyond that, this epithelium is capable of actively transporting Na^+ from urine to blood. Rabbit urinary bladder, examined in an Ussing chamber, showed a spontaneous potential in which the blood side was 24–70 mV positive to the urinary side (100). The SCC was stimulated by aldosterone and inhibited by replacement of Na^+ by choline, or by addition of amiloride to the mucosal solution. Studies with radioactive Na^+ and Cl^- confirmed that the SCC was due to net Na^+ absorption. Bladder epithelium taken from rabbits maintained on low Na^+ diets showed increased SCC (active Na^+ absorption), while tissue from rabbits on a high Na^+ diet showed a decreased SCC. While it is likely that the quantitative contribution of the urinary bladder to net Na^+ absorption by the urinary tract is small, the presence of high-resistance and aldosterone-stimulated Na^+ transport gives the bladder an adaptive role in Na^+ conservation, particularly during low Na^+ intake.

Renal H^+ Secretion

Recent studies have provided new evidence, both for a role of aldosterone in determining the rate of renal H^+ secretion, and for an effect of K^+ on mineralocorticoid-stimulated renal H^+ secretion.

K^+ Depletion. Evidence for a physiologic role of aldosterone in stimulating renal H^+ secretion has come from a reinvestigation of the effect of K^+ depletion on acid–base balance. Older studies had been interpreted as indicating that K^+ restriction leads to metabolic alkalosis. Burnell et al (15) reexamined the effect of K^+ depletion on acid–base balance in dogs. The animals were depleted of K^+ solely by restriction of dietary K^+ intake without the administration of exogenous mineralocorticoid. Under these conditions, a mild metabolic acidosis developed concomitant with decreases in urinary $NH_4{}^+$ and titratable acid excretion, and an increase in urine pH. The decreases in renal H^+ secretion occurred on the first day of dietary K^+ depletion, when plasma K^+ concentration had decreased but before a large decrease in body K^+ content could have occurred. Restoring K^+ to the diet promptly reversed the metabolic acidosis and renal H^+ secreting deficit (Figure 6).

A causative role for decreased aldosterone activity in the development of metabolic acidosis in dietary K^+ depletion has been postulated (79), since the metabolic acidosis and the decreased renal net acid excretion produced solely by K^+ restriction can be prevented by administration of physiologic doses of aldosterone. Additionally, in K^+ depletion, urinary

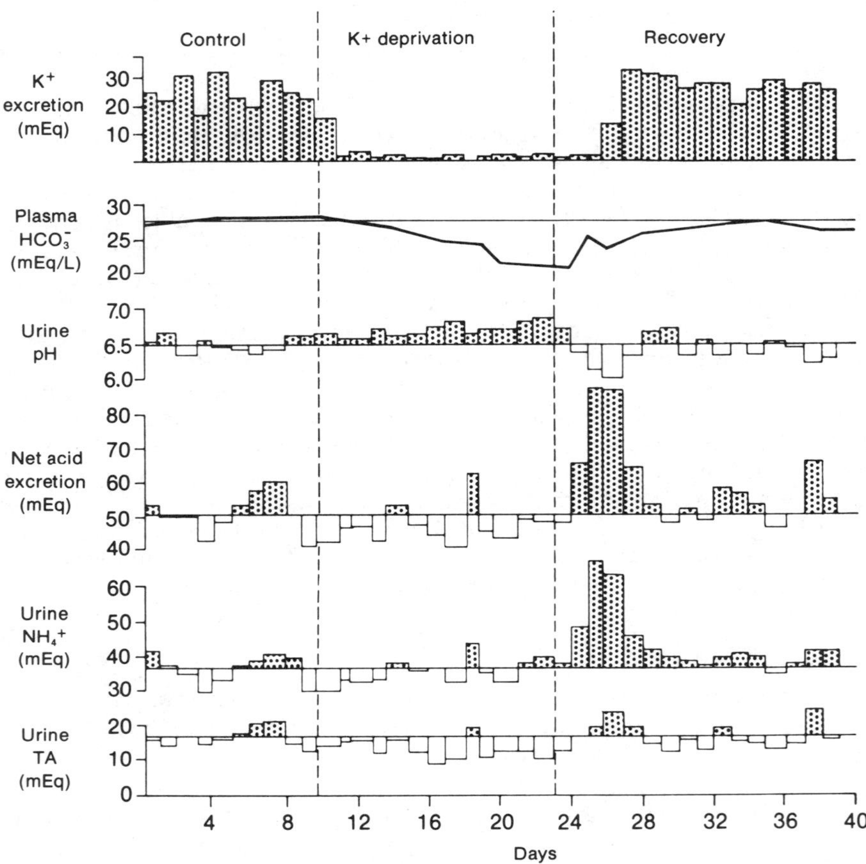

FIGURE 6. Induction of metabolic acidosis in conscious dogs deprived of dietary potassium. Dogs given low potassium diet, without exogenous mineralocorticoid hormone, developed metabolic acidosis with decreased urinary titratable acid and ammonium excretion. Restoration of dietary potassium restored acid excretion to normal. (From ref. 15 with permission).

aldosterone excretion rate is decreased as would be expected, since K^+ depletion depresses aldosterone secretion in dogs (79) and in humans (16). From these experiments, it is clear that restricting K^+ intake in dogs causes development of metabolic acidosis of renal origin, which can be prevented by injecting aldosterone. Burnell et al. (15) attributed previous data linking K^+ depletion and metabolic alkalosis to the effect on renal H^+ secretion produced by the simultaneous administration of exogenous mineralocorticoid in these earlier studies.

In a related study, Van Ypersele de Strihou and Dieu (167) examined the effect on renal acidifying capacity of restoring K^+ to the diet of K^+ depleted dogs that had been made chronically acidotic with acidifying salts. When K^+ was restored to the diet of these dogs there was an increase in plasma HCO_3^- concentration and in renal net acid excretion, and a decrease in urine pH.* These changes, indicating an increased rate of renal tubular H^+ secretion, occurred despite continued administration of the acidifying salts. The increase in net acid excretion was entirely due to increased NH_4^+ excretion. The effect on net acid excretion was specific for K^+; these dogs had also been Na^+ depleted, but restoring Na^+ to the diet had no effect on the state of H^+ balance. Thus, potassium depletion limits renal net acid excretion in both normal and acidotic dogs, independent of Na^+ balance.

The observation that K^+ depletion in dogs leads to hypoaldosteronism, which, in turn produces metabolic acidosis, suggests that aldosterone plays a significant role in maintaining the normal day-to-day rate of renal H^+ secretion. The well-known development of metabolic alkalosis with mineralocorticoid excess is an exaggeration of the physiologic role of the hormone in maintaining normal renal H^+ secretion.

Another recent study bearing on the mechanism of development of acid–base imbalances in K^+ depletion, by Garella et al. (58), consisted of observations of the changes in electrolyte and acid–base balance occurring during recovery from prolonged dietary K^+ depletion in dogs and rats. The results in dogs were quite similar to those of Burnell et al. (15) and Hulter et al. (79), i.e., with K^+ depletion the dogs develop metabolic acidosis with decreased renal net acid excretion. However, in rats under similar experimental conditions, again without administration of any exogenous mineralocorticoid, a severe metabolic alkalosis developed. Since this metabolic alkalosis developed in the rat without large changes in renal net acid excretion, the alkalosis must have been due to a shift of H^+ from the extracellular to the intracellular compartment. Metabolic alkalosis persisted in these rats as long as they were K^+ depleted. Garella et al. (58) suggested that metabolic acidosis developed in dogs because the kidney was unable to reabsorb the increased filtered load of HCO_3^- brought about by the increased plasma HCO_3^- concentration. The inability to reabsorb the large HCO_3^- load may have been due to a defect in H^+ secreting capacity brought about by the K^+ deficiency. This defect in H^+ secretion in the dog kidney is sufficient to overcome the alkalinizing effect of an intracellular shift of H^+ and to produce metabolic acidosis. In fact, the H^+ secreting defect in K^+ depleted dogs could well be due to the hypoaldosteronism of K^+ depletion as described above. These data imply that the ability of the dog kidney to secrete H^+ is more critically dependent on aldosterone than is that of the rat kidney.

Exogenous Mineralocorticoids. The studies discussed above have shown a role for aldosterone in the maintenance of normal levels of renal

*Net acid excretion is calculated as: Ammonium excretion plus titratable acid excretion minus bicarbonate excretion. Since NH_4^+ plus titratable acid excretion is equivalent to the amount of HCO_3^- generated by the kidneys, net acid excretion indicates the net addition or loss of HCO_3^- from body fluids as a result of renal H^+ secretion.

H^+ secretion. Related studies have investigated the mechanism of potentiation by K^+ depletion of the alkalosis that develops with mineralocorticoid excess. Hulter et al. (80) found that pharmacologic doses of DOCA produced a greater increase in net acid excretion in dogs that had been K^+ depleted (by ingestion of a K^+ free diet) than in K^+ replete dogs. The augmentation in net acid excretion began before there was any change in urinary K^+ excretion and was largely due to an increase in renal NH_4^+ excretion with no change in urine pH. Amiloride prevented the potentiating effect of mineralocorticoid on net acid excretion in K^+ depleted dogs (78). The effects of amiloride could not be ascribed to the acidosis that accompanies amiloride administration, since DOCA exhibited the same potentiating effects on plasma HCO_3^- concentration and net acid excretion in dogs made acidotic with HCl, and amiloride blocked the DOCA effect in these acidotic animals. Hulter et al. suggested that, since amiloride acts in the distal nephron in vivo at the doses used, it is at this nephron site that amiloride interferes with net H^+ secretion in the K^+ depleted, DOCA-stimulated animals. The effect of amiloride might be to diminish Na^+ reabsorption, thereby, decreasing the lumen-negative transepithelial potential, hence, reducing the electrochemical gradient favoring H^+ secretion. Reduced H^+ secretion would limit both net acid excretion and the increase in plasma HCO_3^- concentration.

Turning to the other side of the coin, the origin of the metabolic acidosis that develops with mineralocorticoid deficiency has been investigated in two recent studies. Hulter et al. (77) showed that metabolic acidosis in adrenalectomized dogs could be accounted for largely by a decrease in NH_4^+ excretion. In this study, NaCl was infused to maintain extracellular fluid volume, and K^+ intake was minimized to prevent hyperkalemia. The development of acidosis, despite these maneuvers, indicated that the effect of mineralocorticoid deficiency was directly on the renal tubule and was not mediated by ECF volume depletion or hyperkalemia. These investigators proposed a tonic effect of aldosterone to maintain normal renal acid excretion.

Contradictory results were obtained in a study by DiTella et al. (35), who stated that the impaired ammonium excretion of mineralocorticoid deficient rats was corrected by NaCl loading or by feeding a K^+ free diet. In their experiments, however, NaCl loading was accompanied by NH_4Cl, so that the resulting acidosis was due to both mineralocorticoid deficiency and acid loading, making intepretation of the results more difficult. Furthermore, the NH_4^+ excretion rate after NaCl (and NH_4Cl) loading when factored by glomerular filtration rate (GFR) and body weight, was actually slightly less than the NH_4^+ excretion rate in adrenalectomized rats, which had not received NaCl (35, Table 5 vs Table 2). This last observation contradicts their conclusion that NaCl loading corrected the defect in NH_4^+ excretion. In contrast, the adrenalectomized rats with restricted K^+ intake had a higher rate of NH_4^+ excretion than adrenalectomized rats on normal rat chow. Interestingly, however, there was no difference in the net acid excretion rate between these two groups of rats (recalculated from Tables 2 and 6, ref. 35, data factored by body weight and GFR).

These two studies suggest that the acidosis of mineralocorticoid deficiency is due to a primary defect in renal tubular H^+ secretion, and cannot be explained by secondary effects due to changes in Na^+ or K^+ balance. This conclusion lends further support to the role of mineralocorticoids in maintaining renal H^+ secretion.

Direct evidence for an effect of aldosterone on renal ammonia production comes from Welbourne and Francoeur (172), who demonstrated that administration of aldosterone to rats stimulated renal NH_4^+ excretion, an effect that could not be explained by changes in K^+ balance. These investigators also demonstrated that aldosterone administration stimulated renal glutamine uptake and glucose and CO_2 production by the isolated perfused rat kidney. The results were interpreted to suggest that aldosterone increases the flux of glutamine through the mitochondrial metabolic pathway, resulting in stimulation of renal ammonia production.

In a related study Hughey et al. (75) investigated the effect of adrenalectomy on renal glutamine extraction (A-V concentration difference) in response to metabolic acidosis induced by NH_4Cl feeding to rats. They observed that the extraction of glutamine was less in adrenalectomized acidotic rats than in intact acidotic rats, and concluded that adrenal hormones may facilitate the renal metabolic adaptation to acidosis. However, Hughey et al. did not consider the effects that changes in blood flow or urine flow accompanying NH_4Cl acidosis might have on the measurement of renal glutamine metabolism (19). Consequently, their results must be interpreted with caution.

Glucocorticoids. Hulter et al. (76) were prompted to look for an effect of glucocorticoids on acid–base balance, since metabolic alkalosis occurs in hyperglucocorticoid states, such as Cushing's syndrome. Hulter et al. observed that administration of triamcinolone (a synthetic glucocorticoid with minimal mineralocorticoid activity) to dogs at a low dosage (0.1 mg/kg/day), after 3–4 days resulted in a small increase in plasma HCO_3^- concentration, a decrease in urine pH, and increases in both net acid excretion and urinary unmeasured anion excretion. (Urinary unmeasured anion excretion is an estimate of urine organic anion content.) A tenfold larger dose of triamcinolone resulted initially in a decrease in plasma HCO_3^- concentration, along with greater decreases in urine pH and greater increases in net acid excretion and urinary unmeasured anion excretion than with the lower dose. However, after 4–6 days, plasma HCO_3^- concentration returned to control levels, while net acid excretion remained elevated. These results are consistent with two effects of triamcinolone. The increased organic anion excretion indicates increased organic acid production and reflects the catabolic activity of the glucocorticoid. The increased net acid excretion reflects primarily increased renal NH_4^+ excretion. Hulter et al. proposed that triamcinolone has a direct stimulatory effect on renal H^+ secretion and, hence, on net acid excretion. Such an increase in net acid excretion is consistent with the development of metabolic alkalosis in hyperglucocorticoid states, but even in the dogs receiving the higher dosage of triamcinolone metabolic alkalosis did not develop. Therefore, Hulter et al. suggested that the metabolic alkalosis of hyperglucocorticoidism might be due to the mineralocorticoid effect of cortisol, especially since the severity of the alkalosis is related to the degree of hypokalemia.

Glucocorticoids and Glomerular Filtration Rate

The well-known effect of glucocorticoids to increase GFR has been investigated by Baylis and Brenner (7). These investigators performed micropuncture experiments using the Munich–Wistar rat, which has many glomeruli accessible for puncture on the surface of the kidney. They found that animals that received methylprednisolone for 4 days had a 25% higher single nephron GFR, proportionately higher glomerular blood flow and, therefore, no change in single nephron filtration fraction. The increased flow rates could be explained by observed decreases in both afferent and efferent arteriolar resistance. The mechanism by which glucocorticoid decreases renal arteriolar resistance is not known, but Baylis and Brenner speculated that methylprednisolone might have an effect on the vascular smooth muscle rather than an effect secondary to changes in body fluid volumes.

Adrenocorticoids and Water Balance

Adrenocortical insufficiency has been associated with both inability to dilute the urine and excrete a water load at a normal rate, and inability to produce a maximally concentrated urine [for references to previous literature, see the excellent brief review by Schrier and Linas (142) and the paper by Schwartz and Kokko (144)]. In the last few years, the development of an accurate radioimmunoassay for plasma antidiuretic hormone (ADH) concentration and utilization of the isolated perfused tubule technique have provided a better understanding of the mechanisms underlying the abnormalities in water balance in adrenocortical insufficiency.

The inability of patients with adrenocortical insufficiency to excrete a water load has been alternatively attributed to increased plasma ADH concentration, and to increased distal nephron permeability to water due to a deficit of glucocorticoid hormone, even when plasma ADH concentration is very low. These contradictory hypotheses have been proposed since plasma ADH concentration had previously been reported by different laboratories to be either high or low in adrenocortical insufficiency when measured by bioassay. Use of the more accurate radioimmunoassay for ADH has recently shown increased plasma ADH concentration in adrenalectomized rats (142) and dogs (12). Moreover, in these recent studies careful experimental design has allowed the effects of mineralocorticoid and glucocorticoid deficiency to be separated (13).

Boykin et al. (12) examined the effect on water excretion of prolonged glucocorticoid deficiency in conscious adrenalectomized dogs receiving mineralocorticoid replacement by DOCA injection. After 5–9 days of glucocorticoid deficiency, these dogs were challenged with an intravenous water load and renal water excretion was measured. The animals failed to produce urine more dilute than plasma and, thus, to excrete excess water. Minimal urine osmolality was 425 mOsm/kg H_2O; free water clearance changed from −0.72 to −0.05 ml/min. Furthermore, in these glucocorticoid-deficient animals, despite a significant decrease in plasma osmolality, plasma ADH concentration doubled. Glucocorticoid deficiency had no effect on body weight, extracellular fluid volume, or cardiac output. There was a greater pulse rate, however, and consequently a smaller stroke volume in the glucocorticoid-deficient animals and these animals had a greater increase in pulse rate after water loading than did the control animals. These results were interpreted as showing that pure glucocorticoid deficiency of 5–9 days duration results in an elevated plasma ADH concentration and, therefore, a major defect in the ability to dilute the urine and to excrete a water load. The increased ADH secretion probably is occurring in response to the decreased stroke volume and is presumably mediated via cardiovascular mechanoreceptors.

In the adrenalectomized dogs studied by Boykin et al. (12), the possibility remained that some of the effects of adrenalectomy on water excretion may have been mediated via a deficiency of epinephrine. For this reason, and because pituitary insufficiency is the most common cause of glucocorticoid deficiency, Mandell et al. (110) used the radioimmunoassay for ADH to study the effects of anterior hypophysectomy and corticosterone replacement on water balance in rats. Fourteen days after surgery the response to an oral water load was examined. Hypophysectomized rats excreted only 34% of a water load within 3 hours, compared with 100% for controls. Some of the rats were then treated for 7 days with corticosterone and again given an oral water load. In rats receiving corticosterone replacement, both the percentage of the water load excreted in 3 hours and the minimal urine osmolality were restored almost to control levels. In the glucocorticoid deficient hypophysectomized rats, during water diuresis, plasma ADH concentration was three times higher than in the controls, despite a lower plasma osmolality. Corticosterone replacement decreased plasma ADH concentration during water diuresis. These results support the studies in dogs demonstrating that prolonged glucocorticoid deficiency produces a reversible defect in urinary diluting ability with elevated plasma ADH concentration despite plasma hypoosmolality. The excess ADH secretion is probably stimulated by changes in cardiovascular function produced by the glucocorticoid deficiency.

These two studies reveal an important role of pure glucocorticoid deficiency in the defect in water excretion that occurs in adrenal insufficiency. However, the earlier studies had suggested that mineralocorticoid deficiency might be involved as well. This question was examined (13) by studying plasma ADH concentration (measured by radioimmunoassay) in adrenalectomized dogs receiving both dexamethasone and DOCA replacement (controls), compared with adrenalectomized dogs that received only dexamethasone. The mineralocorticoid deficient dogs suffered a loss of body weight, a 50% decrease in GFR, and an increase in BUN, suggesting a large decrease in ECF volume. In addition, they showed both a profound decrease in plasma osmolality (largely due to decreased plasma Na^+ concentration), from 301 to 266 mOsm/kg H_2O, and an increased plasma ADH concentration. Thus, mineralocorticoid deficiency, like glucocorticoid deficiency, produces a nonosmolar stimulation of ADH release. The effects of mineralocorticoid deficiency on ADH secretion probably are mediated via severe volume depletion and cardiovascular receptors. The volume-contracted state produced by mineralocorticoid insufficiency also would be expected to enhance fluid reabsorption in the proximal convoluted tubule, reducing delivery of filtrate to the cortical diluting segment, also limiting the ability of the kidney to excrete a water load.

These in vivo studies have implicated nonosmolar (cardiovascular) stimulation of ADH secretion as the primary mechanism for the inability of the kidney to dilute the urine in adrenal insufficiency. It also has been suggested that glucocorticoids are necessary for maintenance of low water permeability in the distal nephron when antidiuretic hormone level is low (157). Green et al. (65) found that both mineralocorticoid and glucocorticoid replacement was necessary to restore renal diluting ability in the adrenalectomized rat with hereditary diabetes insipidus. However, neither Rayson et al. (129), studying the isolated collecting duct, nor Schwartz and Kokko, (144), using the isolated perfused cortical collecting tubule, were able to demonstrate any effect of adrenalectomy on water permeability of these structures. The results indicate that there is no direct effect of adrenal steroid deficiency on basal distal tubular water permeability, and the role of corticosteroids in maintenance of renal diluting capacity in intact animals appears to be indirect.

Schwartz and Kokko (144) also considered the ability of the kidney to produce maximally concentrated urine, which as noted above, is diminished in adrenocortical insufficiency. They found that adrenalectomized rabbits responded to injections of vasopressin with an increase in urine osmolality to 1327 mOsm/kg H_2O, whereas in control animals, urine osmolality increased to 1901 mOsm/kg H_2O. Replacement therapy with either dexamethasone or DOCA restored the ability of the adrenalectomized animals to concentrate the urine maximally. The inability of adrenalectomized animals to concentrate the urine maximally was reflected in diminished responsiveness to ADH in the isolated perfused cortical collecting tubule. Both net water absorption after addition of ADH and the calculated hydraulic conductivity coefficient (which is the rate of water absorption divided by the osmotic gradient) were almost five times lower in tubules from adrenalectomized rabbits than in tubules from controls. When the tubules from adrenalectomized rabbits were pretreated in vitro with either aldosterone or dexamethasone and ADH then added, net water absorption and the hydraulic conductivity coefficient were restored to near control levels. In contrast, progesterone was ineffective in restoring water permeability. Addition of a permeable analog of cAMP or a phosphodiesterase inhibitor also resulted in increased water permeability in collecting tubules from adrenalectomized rabbits. These results indicate that the concentrating defect of adrenal insufficiency is due to decreased responsiveness of the collecting tubules to ADH. This lack of responsiveness might be related to changes in intracellular cAMP concentration in the absence of adrenal hormones.

Adrenocorticoids and the Colon

Aldosterone administration or feeding of a low Na^+ diet will result in decreased fecal excretion of Na^+, due to increased Na^+ absorption by the colon. Recent studies of the effects of mineralocorticoids on electrolyte transport by mammalian colon in vitro have added significantly to our understanding of how aldosterone produces this increase in Na^+ absorption.

Frizzell and Schultz (54) examined the effects of aldosterone and amphotericin B on ion fluxes and SCC in a preparation of rabbit descending colon mucosa from which the muscular layer had been dissected away. When this stripped mucosa is mounted in an Ussing chamber it exhibits a spontaneous transepithelial potential difference, mucosal surface negative, as well as net active Na^+ transport from mucosa to serosa. The rabbits used for these experiments were given a high Na^+, low K^+ diet for 5 days, a regimen that was necessary to provide segments of colon that responded reproducibly with changes in electrolyte transport when exposed to aldosterone in vitro. Addition of aldosterone to these colon segments in vitro, after a 1-hour delay, resulted in an increased net Na^+ absorption due entirely to an increase in the mucosal to serosal Na^+ flux, with no change in the backflux. There also was an increase in the transepithelial electrical potential but aldosterone had no effect on the statistically not significant rate of K^+ secretion. Treatment with aldosterone was shown in tissue uptake experiments to increase the influx of Na^+ from lumen to mucosal cell. The magnitude of this increase was equal to the increase in net Na^+ absorption occurring after aldosterone stimulation. In fact, there was a close agreement between the influx of Na^+ at the mucosal membrane and the rate of net Na^+ absorption under both control conditions and after stimulation by aldosterone, so that the backflux of Na^+ from the cell across the mucosal membrane must be undetectably small.

Amphotericin B added to the mucosal solution in control tissues produced increases in SCC, net Na^+ absorption, and the unidirectional flux of Na^+ from mucosa to serosa. In aldosterone treated tissues, however, when amphotericin B was added, both the mucosal to serosal and the backfluxes of Na^+ increased to the same extent so that there was no increase in net Na^+ absorption. In fact, treatment of control tissues with amphotericin B increased the SCC and net Na^+ absorption up to the rates seen in aldosterone-stimulated tissue. This last observation indicates that the rate of Na^+ transport in aldosterone-stimulated tissue is the maximal rate of which the tissue is capable. Furthermore, the entire effect of aldosterone in these experiments was to increase Na^+ absorption by increasing the rate of passive entry of Na^+ into the cell at the mucosal membrane. Frizzell and Schultz (54) suggested that the mechanism of action of aldosterone on Na^+ absorption is to increase the permeability of the mucosal membrane to Na^+ sufficiently to saturate the active transport mechanism at the basolateral membrane. The maximal rate of Na^+ transport is then limited by the rate of activity of this basolateral "pump." No evidence was adduced to suggest that aldosterone might also affect the basolateral pump directly.

As noted above, in this study there was no significant net K^+ secretion. Previous experiments with mammalian colon have been interpreted as indicating either active or passive net K^+ secretion in this tissue (see Frizzell and Schultz for references). Although Frizzell and Schultz did not find a net K^+ secretion significantly different from zero, even after treatment with aldosterone, they suggested that the net K^+ secretion observed in vivo after aldosterone administration may be due to passive diffusion of K^+ into the lumen subsequent to the stimulatory effect of aldosterone on the transepithelial electrical potential.

Another aspect of the mechanism of action of aldosterone on colonic transport was examined by Will et al. (174) using rat colon mounted in an Ussing chamber. These investigators noted that the colon of the rat differs from that of other mammals in that the transepithelial potential is low (5 mV, lumen negative), the transepithelial Na^+ flux is electroneutral, i.e., this flux is two to six times greater than the SCC, and also is not inhibited by amiloride. However, descending colon taken from rats fed a Na^+ deficient diet for 2–3 days exhibits an increase in SCC, which is inhibited by amiloride added to the mucosal surface. If rats were maintained on a Na^+ deficient diet for 28–57 days, both the transmural potential and the SCC increased more than fourfold, compared with colon from control animals. After this prolonged period of Na^+ deficiency, amiloride inhibited the SCC by 95%. It was concluded that Na^+ deficiency induces a new mode of Na^+ absorption, presumably mediated via increased endogenous aldosterone, which is amiloride-sensitive. The role of aldosterone was confirmed by administration of the hormone to rats for 5 days, after which the SCC was inhibited 87% by amiloride. The effect of exogenous aldosterone could be blocked by simultaneous administration of spironolactone. Administration of DOCA, furosemide, or a high K^+ diet, all of which increase endogenous mineralocorticoid activity, results in induction of amiloride sensitivity of the increased SCC of isolated colon. Continuation of the Na^+ deficient diet also resulted in an increase in the scillaren-sensitive Na-K-ATPase activity of the colonic mucosa.

In summary, short-term Na^+ deficiency, acting via aldosterone, induces an increase in Na^+ absorption and SCC in rat colon. While control SCC is insensitive to amiloride, the increased current after aldosterone is inhibited by amiloride. These data suggest that aldosterone induces increased Na^+ transport, at least in part, by increasing mucosal membrane permeability to Na^+, as postulated for rabbit colon by Frizzell and Schultz (54) (see above). More prolonged Na^+ deficiency leads to a further increase in SCC as well as increased activity of Na-K-ATPase and a more negative luminal potential, all effects that are similar to the effect of prolonged Na^+ deficiency in the renal tubule (see above). Thus, the conclusion of Frizzell and Schultz that aldosterone's action on rabbit colonic mucosa can be explained entirely as being due to increased permeability of the luminal membrane to Na^+, may apply only to acute situations. Prolonged increases in plasma aldosterone concentration also may induce increased "pumping" capacity, i.e., Na-K-ATPase activity, both in the colon and in the distal nephron.

Similar results with respect to amiloride sensitivity of colonic Na^+ transport have been reported by Ferguson et al (51), studying the pattern of development of Na^+ transport in the neonatal pig colon in vitro. In distal colon taken from pigs at varying ages after birth, the net Na^+ absorption measured isotopically, or the SCC, both increase to a higher level within the 1st day postpartum. This increase corresponds to a sudden increase in plasma aldosterone concentration at birth. The increase in net Na^+ absorption can be prevented by administration of an aldosterone antagonist, canrenoate. Amiloride will also inhibit the increased Na^+ transport occurring postpartum in control animals, but has no effect on the colon of canrenoate-injected pigs. It appears that the postpartum increase in net Na^+ absorption in pig colon is aldosterone-dependent and it is only this aldosterone induced transport that can be inhibited by amiloride. Aldosterone or a Na^+ deficient diet also induce amiloride-sensitive Na^+ absorption in the lower intestine of the domestic fowl (162).

While all these studies support the role of aldosterone in mediating increased Na^+ absorption by the colon of animals on a Na^+ deficient diet, a somewhat different conclusion has been reached by Bastl et al. (6). They examined the effect of either aldosterone or dexamethasone injections on net ion and fluid transport of in situ perfused colon of adrenalectomized rats. Adrenalectomy itself resulted in inhibition of colonic Na^+ and water absorption and K^+ secretion, as well as in a decrease in the transmural PD. Injection of a physiologic replacement dose of dexamethasone restored all these parameters to the levels observed in control (nonadrenalectomized) rats. On the other hand, injection of aldosterone had much less effect. With a low dose of aldosterone, net K^+ secretion was partially restored but none of the other parameters was different from the values in the adrenalectomized, noninjected rats. With a higher dose of aldosterone (equivalent to the aldosterone secretion rate in Na^+ deficient rats), Na^+ and water absorption and K^+ secretion were returned almost to the level in control or dexamethasone-treated rats, while the transmural PD was entirely restored to the control level.

Two aspects of this study are of special interest. First, it appeared that a glucocorticoid, dexamethasone, was more effective than aldosterone in supporting colonic ion and fluid transport. Second, the observed changes in K^+ secretion and transmural PD do not support the hypothesis of Frizzell and Schultz (54) that K^+ secretion is passive and dependent on the PD. For example, the low dose of aldosterone restored K^+ secretion to

71% of the control value with no effect on the transmural PD. The high dose of aldosterone had no further effect on net K^+ secretion but restored the transmural PD to the control level.

While it is difficult to reconcile these results with previous work, the relatively unimportant effect of aldosterone in the experiments of Bastl et al. may reflect, in part, the method of measurement. Bastl et al. (6) perfused the colon from cecal junction to rectum in situ, thus, their results represent the average transport capacity of this entire organ. Will et al. compared the effect of aldosterone or of Na^+ deficiency on amiloride sensitivity of the ascending versus the descending colon. In fact, Bastl et al. noted that the transmural PD of the rat colon measured during in situ perfusion was greatest at 4 cm proximal to the rectum, i.e., probably somewhere in the descending colon. Thus, a part of the difference in results between Bastl et al. and others may reflect the fact that in situ perfusion gives results that represent averages of portions of the colon that respond differently to aldosterone. Nonetheless, their data support an important role for glucocorticoids in maintaining colonic fluid and electrolyte transport.

CLINICAL DISORDERS OF WATER AND ELECTROLYTE METABOLISM CAUSED BY ADRENOCORTICOID HORMONE ABNORMALITIES

Disorders of water and electrolyte metabolism can occur because of insufficient secretion or excess hormone secretion by the adrenal cortex. There are important differences in the clinical manifestations, depending on whether or not the abnormality in secretion involves mineralocorticoids or glucocorticoids, or both, and whether or not the abnormality resides within the adrenal cortex itself, or is due to abnormalities in the trophic hormones ACTH and the renin-angiotensin system. Moreover, the clinical presentation will depend on whether or not the abnormal adrenocortical secretion is chronic or acute and upon the needs of the organism. For example, a patient with chronic partial loss of adrenocortical function may exhibit little abnormality if unstressed and allowed adequate salt intake, but this same person would be in danger if subjected to trauma, surgical stress, or sodium restriction. We will consider first adrenocortical insufficiency, including the rare state of hormone resistance, and then adrenocortical hormone excess.

Adrenocortical Hormone Insufficiency

Secondary Adrenocorticoid Insufficiency. Secondary adrenocortical insufficiency occurs because of failure of the trophic hormones, ACTH, or angiotensin, to drive the adrenal cortex to produce sufficient amounts of glucocorticoid or mineralocorticoid hormone. Although isolated deficiency of ACTH may occur, more commonly there is insufficient secretion of most or all of the trophic hormones produced by the anterior pituitary. Anterior pituitary failure may result from surgical or other intentional ablation, from nonsecretory pituitary tumors, from metastatic tumor, from infarction, or from a wide variety of infectious, infiltrative, or granulomatous diseases. Supracellar tumors, trauma, infection, hydrocephalus, or infiltrative diseases may lead to a loss of hypothalamic releasing factors and secondarily cause adrenocortical insufficiency. Since the primary effect of ACTH is on control of cortisol synthesis and release, ACTH insufficiency is characterized primarily by the manifestations of glucocorticoid deficiency, and patients with hypopituitarism may not show signs of mineralocorticoid deficiency. With severe prolonged pituitary insufficiency, however, the adrenal cortex may undergo atrophy to the point where the zona glomerulosa is no longer able to respond to angiotensin or to elevated serum potassium concentration with increased aldosterone secretion, and the patient may develop signs and symptoms of aldosterone deficiency, as well as those of glucocorticoid deficiency.

Secondary aldosterone deficiency may result from loss of renal renin secretion due to nephrectomy (23) or insufficient renal renin secretion, usually from diseased kidneys, so called hyporeninemic hypoaldosteronism. Hyporeninemic hypoaldosteronism occurs most commonly in older individuals with mild to moderate renal insufficiency, is characterized by varying degrees of hyperkalemia, and appears to be due to an inability of the diseased kidneys to secrete renin in adequate amounts and in response to the usual stimuli (31,139,169,170). Schambelan et al. (138) studied 31 patients with hyperkalemia and moderate to severe renal insufficiency (creatinine clearance less than 31 ml/min). Although urinary aldosterone metabolite excretion indicated normal aldosterone secretion in a number of these subjects, it was abnormal in 23 of the 31 patients when expressed in relation to the elevated serum potassium concentration. In 19 of these 23 patients, plasma renin activity was low and responded poorly to sodium depletion. In contrast, only one subject with a normal urinary aldosterone to serum potassium ratio had low plasma renin activity. Thus, although in most of these subjects the hyperkalemia was associated with hyporeninemic hypoaldosteronism, some other unidentified cause occurred in a significant number of subjects (138). Diabetes mellitus also is common in patients with hyporeninemic hypoaldosteronism, (61,121) and it has been found in such patients that replacement of both insulin and mineralocorticoid is necessary to correct the hyperkalemia. Goldfarb et al. (61) suggested an effect of these hormones on uptake of potassium by the cells, and DeFronzo showed that either lack of insulin or adrenal insufficiency led to a greater than normal rise in serum potassium in rats given intravenous potassium chloride despite normal urinary potassium excretion. Thus, the hyperkalemia of hypoaldosteronism may be due to abnormal distribution of potassium, as well as to inadequate renal excretion and the abnormal distribution may be more severe in diabetes mellitus. The reduction in renin secretion that follows inhibition of prostaglandin production by nonsteroidal antiinflammatory agents also has been reported to cause hypoaldosteronism and hyperkalemia in patients with renal disease (161).

Glucocorticoid hormones produce a wide variety of effects on metabolism (reviewed elsewhere in this volume), but their major effects on water and salt metabolism appear to be exerted by effects on glomerular filtration and the ability of the kidney to dilute the urine (see above). Glucocorticoid insufficiency has long been recognized as a cause of reduction in glomerular filtration rate, and hormone replacement rapidly restores GFR to normal. The role of glucocorticoid hormones in water metabolism is evidenced by the inability of patients with pituitary or adrenal insufficiency to excrete a water load normally (118). In combined gluco- and mineralocorticoid deficiency, the extracellular fluid volume contraction caused by sodium wasting appears to function as a nonosmotic stimulus to vasopressin secretion so that renal water reabsorption and production of relatively concentrated urine occur despite extracellular hypotonicity. Administration of either saline or mineralocorticoid hormone causes the extracellular fluid to expand, thereby inhibiting vasopressin secretion and allowing appropriate dilution of the urine. An individual with secondary adrenal insufficiency would not be expected to manifest renal sodium wasting, due to preservation of control of aldosterone secretion by the renin-angiotensin system, but glucocorticoid deficiency would be expected to cause dilutional hyponatremia due to renal water retention for the reasons described.

Primary Adrenocorticoid Insufficiency. Primary adrenal insufficiency usually involves failure of secretion of all three steroid-producing layers of the cortex. Primary adrenal insufficiency may occur suddenly and totally with surgical adrenalectomy, infection, or hemorrhage, or it may occur gradually and insidiously due to infection, amyloid infiltration, replacement by malignant tumor, or destruction by autoimmune processes. Because of the simultaneous loss of all the adrenal cortical layers, both glucocorticoid and mineralocorticoid insufficiency result and the clinical presentation depends on the rapidity of loss of adrenal function and on the needs of the individual. As with secondary adrenocortical insufficiency, partial primary adrenocortical insufficiency may be fairly well tolerated in the unstressed individual with adequate salt intake. Mineralocorticoid deficiency results in decreased distal tubular sodium reabsorption and in decreased potassium and hydrogen ion secretion. The renal sodium wasting leads to extracellular fluid volume contraction with reduced cardiac output and lower blood pressure. Reduced potassium and hydrogen ion excretion result in hyperkalemia and metabolic acidosis. Glucocorticoid hormone deficiency results in decreased glomerular filtration, which is aggravated by the extracellular fluid volume contraction caused by renal sodium wasting. Due to the decreased glomerular filtration rate and increased proximal tubular reabsorption induced by the contracted extracellular fluid volume, there is decreased delivery of sodium to the distal tubule, which, on the one hand, allows sodium conservation but on the other hand limits the excretion of potassium and hydrogen ion that normally accompany sodium reabsorption in the distal segments of the renal tubule. The obvious clinical results of primary adrenal insufficiency are renal sodium wasting with hyponatremia, volume contraction, hypotension, renal insufficiency and vascular collapse, potassium retention with hyperkalemia and the risk of cardiac arrest, and metabolic acidosis.

The occurrence of metabolic acidosis in adrenal insufficiency has been recognized in humans for many decades. Sartorius et al. (137) reviewed this older literature and showed that within hours after adrenalectomy of rats there was a reduction in renal ammonia excretion that could be corrected by administration of deoxycorticosterone or by adrenocortical extract. Since renal excretion of ammonia as NH_4^+ is a major determinant of renal net acid excretion, defective renal ammoniagenesis may contribute importantly to the metabolic acidosis of adrenal insufficiency (see above). Mills et al. (115) reviewed early publications concerned with the effects of steroid hormones on renal function and showed that in normal human subjects aldosterone caused an increase in both potassium and acid excretion, whereas cortisol increased potassium excretion but caused either no change or a reduction in acid excretion. Similar results in human subjects were obtained by Bartter and Fourman (5), who also showed an effect of aldosterone to increase urinary excretion of ammonium and decrease urinary pH. The role of mineralocorticoids in the metabolic acidosis of adrenal insufficiency was questioned by Perez et al. (123), who withdrew mineralocorticoid replacement of adrenalectomized subjects and found that they did not develop acidosis or hyperchloremia. Information on the potassium balance of these subjects was not given and would be important for assessing the interplay of potassium and renal ammoniagenesis, as discussed below. More recently, Sebastian et al. (149) studied adrenalectomized patients maintained on glucocorticoid replacement. Addition of mineralocorticoid hormone at doses thought to be equivalent to basal aldosterone secretion rate resulted in excretion of urine with lower pH and higher ammonium and titratable acid content. It was observed that net acid excretion correlated positively with changes in sodium balance and negatively with changes in potassium balance. These investigators suggest that renal acidification is under "tonic" stimulation by mineralocorticoid hormones, but the relationships to sodium and potassium balance suggest important roles for extracellular fluid volume and potassium concentration as well.

The role of serum potassium concentration in control of renal ammoniagenesis in experimental animals has been discussed above. This effect is also seen in humans. Sebastian et al. (148) administered α-fluorohydrocortisone to four patients with renal insufficiency, hyporeninemic hypoaldosteronism, hyperkalemia, and metabolic acidosis. They observed a rise in renal net acid and potassium excretion, and serum bicarbonate concentration rose to near normal. Most of the increase in net acid excretion was accounted for by an increase in urinary ammonium excretion, which appeared to correlate closely with the degree of improvement in the serum potassium concentration. Szylman et al. (159) also observed correction of acidosis and increased urinary ammonium excretion in a hypoaldosteronemic patient when the hyperkalemia was corrected by administration of the cation exchange resin sodium polystyrene sulfonate. Mineralocorticoid replacement with up to 5 mg/day of fluorohydrocortisone only partially corrected the hyperkalemia and abnormal urinary ammonium excretion. On the other hand, Perez (122) studied a patient with hypoaldosteronism in whom deoxycorticosterone replacement for 8 days corrected the hyperkalemia but failed to correct the low urinary ammonium excretion. This patient also showed reduced renal bicarbonate conservation. Thus, the bulk of evidence suggests that aldosterone acts to maintain serum potassium concentration at normal levels, both by controlling renal potassium excretion and by determining distribution of potassium across cell membranes. Serum potassium concentration, in turn, exerts an important controlling effect of renal ammoniagenesis and renal ammonium excretion; thus, in hypoaldosteronism, hyperkalemia results in reduced urinary ammonium excretion and secondary metabolic acidosis.

Isolated aldosterone deficiency also occurs as a result of a defect in the terminal steps of adrenal biosynthesis (164). This inborn error has been shown to be the cause of renal salt-wasting in a group of Iranian Jews by Rösler et al. (133,134).

Hormone Resistance. Renal sodium wasting and hyperkalemia, findings expected in states of aldosterone deficiency, have been recognized in individuals who show renal unresponsiveness to mineralocorticoid hormones. This condition was first reported in 1958 by Cheek and Perry (17), who described a male infant with hypotension, renal sodium wasting, and hyperkalemia that did not respond to administration of DOCA. Because the child's perspiration showed low sodium concentration, it was postulated that endogenous mineralocorticoid secretion was normal; however, this was not documented. The electrolyte abnormalities could be corrected by high salt intake. This condition has been labeled pseudohypoaldosteronism. The disease may remit with maturity as shown in a child in whom pseudohypoaldosteronism had been diagnosed in infancy. The child was restudied at age 9 years and showed normal urinary and fecal electrolyte responses to extremes of salt intake and to spironolactone and 9α-fluorohydrocortisone administration (127). The cellular defect responsible for the failure of the kidney to respond to mineralocorticoids is unknown. Biopsy material from the colon of the child while in remission showed normal binding of ^{3}H-aldosterone to a nuclear fraction of mucosal cells. Additional cases have been described by Donnel et al. (36), Proesmans et al. (128), and Degli-Esposti et al. (33); the latter two reports contain reviews of the literature.

Acquired resistance to the renal effects of aldosterone has also been observed. Daughaday and Rendleman (30) reported a woman with chronic pyelonephritis and mild azotemia who had undergone adrenalectomy and subsequently required very large doses of fluorohydrocortisone to prevent hyperkalemia. Renal resistance to the kaliuretic effect of mineralocorticoid hormones has now been recognized to be relatively common in patients with various degrees of renal insufficiency (2,138,148) and has led to the practice of describing "relative" aldosterone deficiency as a condition characterized by a higher than normal ratio of urinary aldosterone excretion or plasma aldosterone concentration versus serum potassium concentration (138,148).

A number of case reports have appeared describing spontaneous, probably congenital, renal mineralocorticoid resistance, manifested not by sodium wasting but by hyperkalemia and metabolic acidosis. Arnold and Healey (1) reported a man with hypertension, hyperkalemia, and acidosis in whom kaliuresis could not be induced by sodium sulfate infusion, but who responded when given fluorohydrocortisone along with a low sodium diet and in whom both the hyperkalemia and acidosis could be corrected by combined chlorthiazide and sodium polystyrene sulfonate administration (this cation exchange resin exchanges sodium for potassium within the intestine). This patient had relatively low serum aldosterone concentration and low plasma renin activity, which increased after sodium depletion. These investigators postulated a defect in renal tubular secretion of potassium. Spitzer et al. (155) reported a child with normal blood pressure, acidosis, growth retardation, and hyperkalemia in whom aldosterone production was normal. Correction of the acidosis did not correct the hyperkalemia, but administration of chlorthiazide corrected both the acidosis and the hyperkalemia. It was proposed that the hyperkalemia was due to a defect in tubular secretion and that the hyperkalemia secondarily inhibited proximal tubular bicarbonate reabsorption. A child with similar findings was described by Weinstein et al. (171) and, subsequently, a family in Israel has been reported in whom three generations have shown hyperkalemia, systemic acidosis, hypertension, normal plasma aldosterone concentration, and low but stimulatable plasma renin activity (14,46,47). In this family, the acidosis was shown to be due to abnormally low proximal renal tubular bicarbonate reabsorption. Correction of the hyperkalemia with ion exchange resin corrected the bicarbonate reabsorption abnormality, thus, supporting the suggestion of Spitzer et al. that a primary tubular defect in potassium excretion leads to hyperkalemia, which in turn leads to proximal tubular bicarbonate wasting and a resulting acidosis. The nature of the renal tubular defect in potassium excretion and its failure to respond to aldosterone remain to be explained.

Adrenocortical Hormone Excess

Glucocorticoid Excess. States of excessive glucocorticoid hormone activity can be brought about by exogenous hormone administration, by secretion from the adrenal cortex in response to ACTH stimulation, and by secretion from autonomous adrenocortical adenomas or carcinomas. The end result on mineral metabolism of all three may be the same and reflects the relative effects on intermediary metabolism and the weak mineralocorticoid effects of these hormones. Although the glucocorticoid hormones are weak mineralocorticoids, in large excess they may cause renal sodium retention and potassium and acid wasting, producing hypertension, edema, hypokalemia, and systemic alkalosis. The catabolic action of the glucocorticoids causes loss of cellular potassium and can greatly accelerate the depletion of the body's potassium stores. The presence of hypokalemia and alkalosis in Cushing's syndrome is considered an ominous sign for it indicates secretion of very large amounts of glucocorticoid hormone and may indicate the presence of an adrenocortical carcinoma or ectopic ACTH production by a nonendocrine tumor (3). Another feature of adrenocortical carcinoma that may contribute to the development of electrolyte disturbance is altered steroid synthesis. Inadequate 11β-hydroxylation is common in adrenal tumors and may result in excessive secretion of deoxycorticosterone with its strong mineralocorticoid activity (28,106).

Electrolyte disturbances also may be brought about indirectly by excess glucocorticoid hormones. Hypertension is common in Cushing's syndrome and may lead to heart failure, edema formation, and renal failure with their attendant effects on electrolytes. The demineralizing effect on bone of the glucocorticoid hormones results in hypercalciuria, which may ultimately lead to nephrocalcinosis and nephrolithiasis. This process, as well as hypokalemia, if present, may lead to interstitial nephropathy, loss of urinary concentrating ability, renal salt wasting, and ultimately may result in renal failure. Other aspects of Cushing's syndrome are considered elsewhere in this volume.

Mineralocorticoid Excess. Disease states of mineralocorticoid excess are characterized by disturbances of electrolyte homeostasis and the circulatory system whose manifestations depend greatly on whether or not the endocrine abnormality is primary or secondary. Primary aldosteronism, as originally described by Conn (22), is caused by excessive secretion of aldosterone by an autonomous aldosterone-producing adrenal adenoma. The clinical hallmarks of this syndrome, hypokalemia and hypertension, are due to the effect of aldosterone on the kidney to cause sodium retention and potassium excretion. Aldosterone also produces the expected effects on epithelia of sweat glands (114), salivary glands (176), and colon (8,40,130), but those do not appear to be of clinical significance. The subject of primary aldosteronism is covered in detail elsewhere in the volume but some comments about the electrolyte disturbance are indicated here. Primary aldosteronism is notable for the absence of edema due to the ability of the kidney to escape from the sodium retaining properties of the hormone (90). During the first few days of exposure to excess mineralocorticoid, the normal subject retains sodium and excretes excessive amounts of potassium. Following this, even if the hormone exposure continues, the kidney begins to excrete an amount of sodium equal to the intake and a new state of sodium balance ensues, albeit, with an excess total body sodium content. Renal potassium wasting may continue and lead to potassium depletion and hypokalemia. Renal excretion of both sodium and potassium are responsive to sodium intake. When sodium intake is limited, urinary sodium excretion is reduced appropriately and potassium wasting is minimized. If a sodium load is administered to an individual in the state of mineralocorticoid escape, both urinary sodium and potassium excretion rise rapidly. This phenomenon was found useful as a diagnostic test (41). The mechanism allowing the kidney to escape from the sodium-retaining effects of the mineralocorticoids remains unexplained. This is a condition in which a putative natriuretic hormone has been proposed, but such a hormone remains to be identified and characterized. Other possible explanations are changes in filtration fraction and peritubular oncotic and hydrostatic pressures in the proximal tubule and shifts in fractional reabsorption of filtrate among the renal tubular segments.

Secondary aldosteronism occurs in patients with such clinical conditions as congestive heart failure, nephrotic syndrome, cirrhosis, or dehydration, in all of which the effective blood volume or cardiac output are reduced. The reduction in renal perfusion that results leads to increased renin secretion and secondarily to stimulation of aldosterone secretion via angiotensin stimulation of the adrenal cortex. Adrenergic stimulation of renin secretion also may play a role in these conditions. Patients with these conditions are usually edematous (with the obvious exception of dehydration) and there is no renal escape from the effect of aldosterone. Potassium wasting usually does not occur, probably because the avid reabsorption of sodium by the proximal renal tubule in these clinical states allows little delivery of sodium to distal tubule potassium-secreting sites.

SUMMARY AND CONCLUSIONS

Many of the very early clinical observations of electrolyte disorders in states of corticosteroid excess and deficiency can now be explained at the organ, cell, and even subcellular level. Studies of amphibian skin and urinary bladder, as well as mammalian kidney, have shown that corticosteroids bind to specific receptors to stimulate synthesis of new proteins that mediate transport of sodium through such diverse tissues as renal tubule, sweat gland ducts, colon, and salivary gland ducts. Refinements of laboratory techniques, such as binding kinetics of isotopically labeled hormone, microperfusion of isolated renal tubules, and radioimmunoassay have allowed identification of the major sites of aldosterone action and better understanding of the pathophysiology of water balance. Chemical and pharmacologic agents have been useful as biologic probes to understand the cellular actions of the corticosteroids, and increasing knowledge of these processes aids in development of clinically useful drugs. The effects of the corticosteroids on potassium and acid–base homeostasis are less well understood than those on sodium metabolism, and appear to be intimately interrelated. In the future, important new information can be expected to explain how the corticosteroids stimulate the cell to synthesize new proteins, and how these proteins act to increase sodium absorption and potassium and hydrogen ion secretion across epithelia.

REFERENCES

1. Arnold, J.E., and Healey, J.K. (1969) Hyperkalemia, hypertension and systemic acidosis without renal failure associated with a tubular defect in potassium excretion. Am. J. Med. 47, 461–472.
2. Arruda, J.A.L., Batlle, D.C., Sehy, J.T., Roseman, M.K., Baronowski, R.L., and Kurtzman, N.A. (1981) Hyperkalemia and renal insufficiency: Role of selective aldosterone deficiency and tubular unresponsiveness to aldosterone. Am. J. Nephrol. 1, 160–167.
3. Bagshawe, K.D. (1960) Hypokalemia, carcinoma and Cushing's syndrome. Lancet ii, 284–287.
4. Barger, A.C., Berlin, R.D., and Tulenko, J.F. (1958) Infusion of aldosterone, 9-α-fluorohydrocortisone and antidiuretic hormone into the renal artery of normal and adrenalectomized, unanesthesized dogs: Effect on electrolyte and water excretion. Endocrinology 62, 804–815.
5. Bartter, F.C., and Fourman, P. (1962) The different effects of aldosterone-like steroids and hydrocortisone-like steroids on urinary excretion of potassium and acid. Metabolism 11, 6–20.
6. Bastl, P.B., Binder, H.J., and Hayslett, J.P. (1980) Role of glucocorticoids and aldosterone in maintenance of colonic cation transport. Am. J. Physiol. 238, F181–F186.
7. Baylis, C., and Brenner, B.M. (1978) Mechanism of the glucocorticoid-induced increase in glomerular filtration rate. Am. J. Physiol. 234, F166–F170.
8. Beevers, D.G., Morton, J.J., Tree, M., and Young, J. (1975) Rectal potential difference in the diagnosis of aldosterone excess. Gut 16, 36–41.
9. Benjamin, W.B., and Singer, I. (1974) Aldosterone-induced protein in toad urinary bladder. Science 186, 269–272.
10. Binder, H.J. (1978) Effect of dexamethasone on electrolyte transport in the large intestine of the rat. Gastroenterology 75, 212–217.
11. Bonvalet, J.P., Farman, N., and Vandewalle (1979) Binding sites of aldosterone along the nephron: An attempt of localization by autoradiographic and binding studies on isolated tubules. Les colloques de l'INSERM: Controlé hormonal des transports epitheliaux 85, 113–120.
12. Boykin, J., de Torrenté, A., Erickson, A., Robertson, G., and Schrier, R. (1978) Role of plasma vasopressin in impaired water excretion of glucocorticoid deficiency. J. Clin Invest. 62, 738–744.
13. Boykin, J., de Torrenté, A., Robertson, G.L., Erickson, A., and Schrier, R.W. (1979) Persistent plasma vasopressin levels in the hyposmolar state associated with mineralocorticoid deficiency. Mineral Electrolyte Metabolism 2, 310–315.
14. Brautbar, N., Levi, J., Rosler, A., Leitesdorf, E., Djaldeti, M., Epstein, M., and Kleeman, C.R. (1978) Familial hyperkalemia, hypertension and hyporeninemia with normal aldosterone levels. A tubular defect in potassium handling. Arch. Int. Med. 138, 607–610.
15. Burnell, J.M., Teubner, E.J., and Simpson, D.P. (1974) Metabolic acidosis accompanying potassium deprivation. Am. J. Physiol. 227, 329–333.
16. Canon, P.J., Ames, R.P., and Laragh, J.H. (1966) Relation between potassium balance and aldosterone secretion in normal subjects and in patients with hypertensive or renal tubular disease. J. Clin. Invest. 45, 865–879.
17. Cheek, D.B., and Perry, J.W. (1958) A salt-wasting syndrome in infancy. Arch. Dis. Child. 33, 252–256.
18. Chignell, C.F., and Titus, E. (1966) Effect of adrenal steroids on a Na^+- and K^+-requiring adenosine triphosphatase from rat kidney. J. Biol. Chem. 241, 5083–5089.
19. Christy, N.P., and Laragh, J.H. (1961) Pathogenesis of hypokalemic alkalosis in Cushing's Syndrome. N. Engl. J. Med. 265, 1083–1088.
20. Civan, M.M., and Hoffman, R.E., (1971) Effect of aldosterone on electrical resistance of toad bladder. Am. J. Physiol. 220, 324–328.

21. Cohen, J.J., and Barac-Nieto, M. (1973) Renal metabolism of substrates in relation to renal function. I. Gaseous and substrate metabolism as related to the energy production and energy requirements of the kidney. In: Handbook of Physiology, Section 8, Renal Physiology. J. Orloff, and R. W. Berliner (eds.) American Physiological Society, Washington, D.C., pp. 909–927.
22. Conn, J.W. (1955) Primary aldosteronism: New clinical syndrome. J. Lab. Clin. Med. 45, 3–17.
23. Cook, C.R., Welton, P.K., and Moore, M.A. (1979) Dissociation of the diurnal variation of aldosterone and cortisol in anephric subjects. Kid. Int. 16, 669–675.
24. Cox, M., Guzzo, J., Shook, A., Huber, G., and Singer, I. (1979) Effects of tetracyclines on aldosterone-and-insulin mediated Na^+ transport in the toad urinary bladder. Biochim. Biophys. Acta 552, 162–168.
25. Cox, M., and Singer, I. (1977) Insulin-mediated Na^+ transport in the toad urinary bladder. Am. J. Physiol. 232, F270–F277.
26. Crabbé, J. (1961) Site of action of aldosterone on the bladder of the toad. Nature 200, 787–788.
27. Crabbé, J., and de Weer, P. (1964) Action of aldosterone on the bladder and skin of the toad. Nature 202, 298–299.
28. Crane, M.G., and Harris, J.J. (1966) Desoxycorticosterone secretion rates in hyperadrenocorticism. J. Clin. Endocrinol. Metab. 26, 1135–1143.
29. Cuthbert, A.W., and Shum, W.K. (1975) The effects of aldosterone on amiloride binding sites in toad bladder epithelial cells. J. Physiol. 245, 96P–97P.
30. Daughaday, W.H., and Rendleman, D. (1967) Severe symptomatic hyperkalemia in an adrenalectomized woman due to enhanced mineralocorticoid requirement. Ann. Int. Med. 66, 1197–1203.
31. DeFronzo, R.A. (1980) Hyperkalemia and hyporeninemic hypoaldosteronism. Kid. Int. 17, 118–134.
32. DeFronzo, R.A., Lee, R., Jones, A., and Bia, M. (1980) Effect of insulinopenia and adrenal hormone deficiency on acute potassium tolerance. Kid. Int. 17, 586–594.
33. Degli Esposti, A., Ambrosioni, G., and Zaniboni, M.G. (1977) Physiopathogenic, clinical and therapeutic considerations on pseudohypoaldosteronism, apropos 3 personal cases, compared with the world-wide cases. Minerva Pediatr. 29, 1853–1869.
34. Deming, Q.B., and Leutscher, J.A., Jr. (1950) Bioassay of desoxycorticosterone-like material in urine. Proc. Soc. Exp. Biol. Med. 73, 171–175.
35. DiTella, P.J., Sodhi, B., McCreary, J., Arruda, J.A.L., and Kurtzman, N.A. (1978) Mechanism of the metabolic acidosis of selective mineralocorticoid deficiency. Kid. Int. 14, 466–477.
36. Donnel, G.N., Litman, N., and Roldan, M. (1959) Pseudohypo-adrenalocorticism. Am. J. Dis. Child. 97, 813–828.
37. Doucet, A., and Katz, A.I. (1981) Short-term effect of aldosterone on Na-K-ATPase in single nephron segments. Am. J. Physiol. 241, F273–F278.
38. Doucet, A., and Katz, A.I. (1981) Mineralocorticoid receptors along the nephron: [^{3}H] Aldosterone binding in rabbit tubules. Am. J. Physiol. 241, F605–F611.
39. Edelman, I.S., Bogoroch, R., and Porter, G.A. (1963) On the mechanism of action of aldosterone on sodium transport: The role of protein synthesis. Proc. Natl. Acad. Sci., USA 50, 1169–1177.
40. Edmonds, C.J., and Godfrey, R.C. (1970) Measurement of electrical potentials of the human rectum and pelvic colon in normal and aldosterone-treated patients. Gut 11, 330–337.
41. Espiner, E.A., Tucci, J.R., Jagger, P.I., and Lauler, D.P. (1967) Effect of saline infusions on aldosterone secretion and electrolyte excretion in normal subjects and patients with primary aldosteronism. N. Engl. J. Med. 277, 1–7.
42. Fanestil, D.D., and Edelman, I.S. (1966) Characteristics of the renal nuclear receptors for aldosterone. Proc. Natl. Acad. Sci (USA) 56, 872–879.

43. Fanestil, D.D., and Park, C.S. (1981) Steroid hormones and the kidney. Ann. Rev. Physiol. 43, 637–649.

44. Fanestil, D.D., Porter, G.A., and Edelman, I.S. (1967) Aldosterone stimulation of sodium transport. Biochim. Biophys. Acta 135; 74–88.

45. Farah, A., Yamodis, N.D., and Pessah, N. (1969) The relation of changes in sodium transport to protein-bound disulfide and sulfhydryl groups in the toad bladder epithelium. J. Pharmacol. Exp. Ther. 170, 132–144.

46. Farfel, Z., Iaina, A., Levi, J., and Gafni, J. (1978) Proximal renal tubular acidosis. Association with familial normaldosteronemic hyperpotassemia and hypertension. Arch. Int. Med. 138, 1837–1840.

47. Farfel, Z., Iaina, A., Rosenthal, T., Waks, U., Shibolet, S., and Gafni, J. (1978) Familial hyperpotassemia and hypertension accompanied by normal plasma aldosterone levels. Possible hereditary cell membrane defect. Arch. Int. Med. 138, 1828–1832.

48. Fazekas, A.G., and Sandor, T. (1976) The influence of corticosteroids on flavin nucleotide biosynthesis in rat liver and kidney. J. Steroid Biochem. 7, 29–32.

49. Feldman, D., Funder, J.W., and Edelman, I. (1972) Subcellular mechanisms in the action of adrenal steroids. Am. J. Med. 53, 545–560.

50. Feldman, D., VanderWende, C., and Kessler, E. (1961) The effect of aldosterone on oxidative enzymes of the rat kidney. Biochim. Biophys. Acta 51, 401–403.

51. Ferguson, D.R., James, P.S., Paterson, J.Y.F., Saunders, J.C., and Smith, M.W. (1979) Aldosterone induced changes in colonic sodium transport occurring naturally during development in the neonatal pig. J. Physiol. 292, 495–504.

52. Field, M., (1978) Corticosteroids, Na, K-ATPase and intestinal water and electrolyte transport. Gastroenterology 75, 317–325.

53. Fimognari, G.M., Fanestil, D.D., and Edelman, I.S. (1967) Induction of RNA and protein synthesis in the action of aldosterone in the rat. Am. J. Physiol. 213, 954–962.

54. Frizzell, R.A., and Schultz, S.G. (1978) Effect of aldosterone on ion transport by rabbit colon in vitro. J. Membrane Biol. 39, 1–26.

55. Frömter, E., and Gebler, B. (1977) Electrical properties of amphibian urinary bladder epithelia. III. The cell membrane resistances and the effect of amiloride. Pflügers Arch. 371, 99–108.

56. Funder, J.W., Mercer, J., Ingram, B., Feldman, D., Wynne, K., and Adam, W.R. (1978) 19 nor-deoxycorticosterone (19 nor-DOC): Mineralocorticoid receptor affinity higher than aldosterone, electrolyte activity lower. Endocrinology 103, 1514–1517.

57. Funder, J.W., Robinson, J.A., Feldman, D., Wynne, K.N., and Adam, W.R. (1976) 16 β-hydroxy dehydroepiandrosterone: The dichotomy between renal receptor binding and urinary electrolyte activity. Endocrinology 99, 619–628.

58. Garella, S., Chang, B., and Kahn, S.I. (1979) Alterations of hydrogen ion homeostasis in pure potassium depletion: Studies in rats and dogs during the recovery phase. J. Lab. Clin. Med. 93, 321–331.

59. Garg, L.C., Krepper, M.A., and Burg, M.B. (1981) Mineralocorticoid effects on Na-K-ATPase in individual nephron segments. Am. J. Physiol. 240, F536–F544.

60. Geheb, M., Hercker, E., Singer, I., and Cox, M. (1981) Subcellular localization of aldosterone-induced proteins in toad urinary bladders. Biochim. Biophys. Acta 641, 422–426.

61. Goldfarb, S., Cox, M., Singer, I., and Goldberg, M. (1976) Acute hyperkalemia induced by hyperglycemia: Hormonal mechanisms. Ann. Int. Med. 84, 426–432.

62. Goodman, D.B.P., Allen, J.E., and Rasmussen, H. (1969) On the mechanism of action of aldosterone. Proc. Natl. Acad. Sci., USA 64, 330–337.

63. Goodman, D.B.P., Allen, J.E., and Rasmussen, H. (1971) Studies on the mechanism of action of aldosterone: Hormone-induced changes in lipid metabolism. Biochemistry 10, 3825–3831.

64. Goodman, D.B.P., Wong, M., and Rasmussen, H. (1975) Aldosterone-induced membrane phospholipid fatty acid metabolism in the toad urinary bladder. Biochemistry 14, 2803–2809.

65. Green, H.H., Harrington, A.R., and Valtin, H. (1970) On the role of antidiuretic hormone in the inhibition of acute water diuresis in adrenal insufficiency and the effects of gluco- and mineralocorticoids in reversing the inhibition. J. Clin. Invest. 49, 1724–1736.

66. Gross, J.B., Imai, M., and Kokko, J.P. (1975) A functional comparison of the cortical collecting tubule and the distal convoluted tubule. J. Clin. Invest. 55, 1284–1294.

67. Gross, J.B., and Kokko, J.P. (1977) Effects of aldosterone and potassium-sparing diuretics on electrical potential differences across the distal nephron. J. Clin. Invest. 59, 82–89.

68. Gutsche, H.U., and Hegel, U. (1980) Influence of aldosterone on epithelial leakiness of rat proximal tubules. Pflügers Arch. 385, 29–36.

69. Hawker, P.C., Mashiter, K.E., and Turnberg, L.A. (1978) Mechanisms of transport of Na, Cl, and K in the human colon. Gastroenterology 74, 1241–1247.

70. Hendler, E.D., Torretti, J., Kupor, L., and Epstein, F.H. (1972) Effects of adrenalectomy and hormone replacement on Na-K-ATPase in renal tissue. Am. J. Physiol. 222, 754–760.

71. Higgins, J.T., Jr., Cesaro, L., Gebler, B., and Frömter, E. (1975) Electrical properties of amphibian urinary bladder epithelia, I. Inverse relationship between potential difference and resistance in tightly mounted preparations. Pflügers Arch. 358, 41–56.

72. Higgins, J.T., Jr., Gebler, B., and Frömter, E. (1977) Electrical properties of amphibian urinary bladder epithelia, II. The cell potential profile in Necturus maculosus. Pflügers Arch. 371, 87–97.

73. Hill, J.H., Cortas, N., and Walser, M. (1973) Aldosterone action and sodium-and potassium-activated adenosine triphosphatase in toad bladder. J. Clin. Invest. 52, 185–189.

74. Horster, M., Schmid, H., and Schmid, U. (1980) Aldosterone in vitro restores nephron Na-K-ATPase of distal segments from adrenalectomized rats. Pflügers Arch. 384, 203–206.

75. Hughey, R.P., Rankin, B.R., and Curthoys, N.P. (1980) Acute acidosis and renal arteriovenous differences of glutamine in normal and adrenalectomized rats. Am. J.Physiol. 238, F199–F204.

76. Hulter, H.N., Licht, J.H., Bonner, E.L. Jr., Glynn, R.D., and Sebastian, A. (1980) Effects of glucocorticoid steroids on renal and systemic acid–base metabolism. Am. J. Physiol. 239, F30–F43.

77. Hulter, H.N., Licht, J.H., Glynn, R.D., and Sebastian, A. (1979) Renal acidosis in mineralocorticoid deficiency is not dependent on NaCl depletion or hyperkalemia. Am. J. Physiol. 236, F283–F294.

78. Hulter, H.N., Licht, J.H., and Sebastian, A. (1979) K^+ deprivation potentiates the renal excretory effect of mineralocorticoid: Obliteration by amiloride. Am. J. Physiol. 236, F48–F57.

79. Hulter, H.N., Sebastian, A., Sigala, J.F., Licht, J.H., Glynn, R.D., Schambelan, M., and Biglieri, E.G. (1980) Pathogenesis of renal hyperchloremic acidosis resulting from dietary potassium restriction in the dog: Role of aldosterone. Am. J. Physiol. 238, F79–F91.

80. Hulter, H.N. Sigala, J.F., and Sebastian, A. (1978) K^+ deprivation potentiates the renal alkalosis-producing effect of mineralocorticoid. Am. J. Physiol. 235, F298–F309.

81. Hutchinson, J.H., and Porter, G.A. (1975) Accelerated RNA turnover in toad urinary bladder epithelial cells during early aldosterone action. Physiol. Chem. Physics 7, 453–464.

82. Imai, M. (1979) The connecting tubule: A functional subdivision of the rabbit distal nephron segments. Kid. Int. 15, 346–356.

83. Jørgensen, P.L. (1969) Regulation of the (Na^+ + K^+)-activated ATP hydrolyzing enzyme system in rat kidney. Biochim. Biophys. Acta 192, 326–334.

84. Jørgensen, P.L. (1972) The role of aldosterone in the regulation of (Na^+ + K^+)-ATPase in the rat kidney. J. Steroid Biochem. 3, 181–191.

85. Katz, A.I. (1982) Renal Na-K-ATPase: Its role in tubular sodium and potassium transport. Am. J. Physiol. 242, F207–F219.
86. Kinne, R., and Kirsten, R. (1967) Enzymaktivitäten in der Niere normaler und adrenalektomierter Ratten vor und nach Aldosterongabe. Pflügers Arch. 294, 31.
87. Kinne, R., and Kirsten, R. (1968) Der Einfluss von Aldosteron auf die Aktivität mitochondrialer und cytoplasmatischer Enzyme in der Rattenniere. Pflügers Arch. 300, 244–254.
88. Kirsten, R., Brinkhoff, B., and Kinne, R. (1970) Increase in cytochromes a and a_3 in rat kidney mitochondria in response to administration of aldosterone in vivo. Pflügers Arch. 314, 231–239.
89. Kirsten, E., Kirsten, R., Leaf, A., and Sharp, G.W.G. (1968) Increased activity of enzymes of the tricarboxylic acid cycle in response to aldosterone in the toad bladder. Pflügers Arch. 300, 213–225.
90. Knox, F.G., Burnette, J.C., Jr., Kohan, D.E., Spielman, W.S., and Strand, J.C. (1980) Escape from the sodium-retaining effects of mineralocorticoids. Kid. Int. 17, 263–276.
91. Knox, W.H., and Sen, A.K. (1974) Mechanism of action of aldosterone with particular reference to (Na + K)-ATPase. Ann. N.Y. Acad. Sci. 242, 471–488.
92. Kurokawa, K., Aznar, E., Descoeudres, C., Zulueta, A., and Massry, S.G. (1978) Effects of glucocorticoid deficiency on renal medullary cyclic adenosine monophosphate of rats. Clin. Sci. Mol. Med. 54, 573–577.
93. Laird, R., and Yates, R. (1973) Ultrastructural observations on the aldosterone-stimulated toad urinary bladder epithelium-ATPase activity. J. Ultrastruct. Res. 44, 339–346.
94. Landon, E.J., Jazab, N., and Forte, L. (1966) Aldosterone and sodium-potassium-dependent ATPase activity of rat urinary membranes. Am. J. Physiol. 211, 1050–1056.
95. Law, P.Y., and Edelman, I.S. (1978) Induction of citrate synthase by aldosterone in the rat kidney. J. Membrane Biol. 41, 41–64.
96. Leaf, A. (1965) Transepithelial transport and its hormonal control in toad bladder. Ergeb. Physiol. Biol. Chem. Exp. Pharmacol. 56, 216–263.
97. Leaf, A., Anderson, J., and Page, L.B. (1958) Active sodium transport by the isolated toad bladder. J. Gen. Physiol. 41, 657–668.
98. Leaf, A., Page, L.B., and Anderson, J. (1959) Respiration and active sodium transport of isolated toad bladder. J. Biol. Chem. 234, 1625–1629.
99. Lewis, S.A., and Diamond, J.M. (1976) Na^+ transport by rabbit urinary bladder, a tight epithelium. J. Membr. Biol. 28, 1–40.
100. Lewis, S.A., and Diamond, J.M. (1975) Active sodium transport by mammary urinary bladder. Nature 253, 747–748.
101. Lien, E.L., Goodman, D.B.P., and Rasmussen, H. (1975) Effects of an acetylcoenzyme A carboxylase inhibitor and a sodium-sparing diuretic on aldosterone-stimulated sodium transport, lipid synthesis and phospholipid fatty acid composition in the toad urinary bladder. Biochemistry 14, 2749–2754.
102. Lien, E.L., Goodman, D.B.P., and Rasmussen, H. (1976) Effects of inhibitors of protein and RNA synthesis on aldosterone-stimulated changes in phospholipid fatty acid metabolism in the toad urinary bladder. Biochim. Biophys. Acta 421, 210–217.
103. Lifschitz, M.D., Schrier, R.W., and Edelman, I.S. (1973) Effect of actinomycin D on aldosterone-mediated changes in electrolyte excretion. Am. J. Physiol. 224, 376–380.
104. Linas, S.L., Peterson, L.N., Anderson, R.J., Aisenbrey, G.A., Simon, F.R., and Berl, T. (1979) Mechanism of renal potassium conservation in the rat. Kid. Int. 15, 601–611.
105. Lipton, P., and Edelman, I.S. (1971) Effects of aldosterone and vasopressin on electrolytes of toad bladder epithelial cells. Am. J. Physiol. 221, 733–741.
106. Lipsett, M.B., and Wilson, H. (1962) Adrenocortical cancer: Steroid biosynthesis and metabolism evaluated by urinary metabolites. J. Clin. Endocrinol. Metab. 22, 906–915.
107. Losert, W., Sitt, R., Senft, G., von Bergmann, K., and Schultz, G. (1967) Untersuchungen zum Wirkungsmechanismus des Aldosterons. Naunyn—Schmiedebergs Arch. Pharmak. Exp. Path. 257, 309–311.

108. Ludens, J.H., and Fanestil, D.D. (1974) Aldosterone stimulation of acidification of urine by isolated urinary bladder of the Colombian toad. Am. J. Physiol. 226, 1321–1326.

109. Ludens, J.H., Vaughn, D.A., and Fanestil, D.D. (1978) Stimulation of urinary acidification by aldosterone and inhibitors of RNA and protein synthesis. J. Membrane Biol. 40, 199–211.

110. Mandell, I.N., DeFronzo, R.A., Robertson, G.L., and Forrest, J.N., Jr. (1980) Role of plasma arginine vasopressin in the impaired water diuresis of isolated glucocorticoid deficiency in the rat. Kid. Int. 17, 186–195.

111. Marver, D., Goodman, D., and Edelman, I.S. (1972) Relationships between renal cytoplasmic and nuclear aldosterone receptors. Kid. Int. 1, 210–223.

112. Marver, D., Stewart, J., Funder, J.W., Feldman, D., and Edelman, I.S. (1974) Renal aldosterone receptors: Studies with [^{3}H] aldosterone and the antimineralocorticoid [^{3}H]spirolactone (SC-26304). Proc. Natl. Acad. Sci., USA 71, 1431–1435.

113. Matulich, D.T., Spindler, B.J., Schambelan, M., and Baxter, J.D. (1976) Mineralocorticoid receptors in human kidney. J. Clin. Endocrinol. Metab. 43, 1170–1174.

114. McConahay, T.P., Robinson, S., and Newton, J.L. (1964) d-Aldosterone and sweat electrolytes. J. Appl. Physiol. 19, 575–579.

115. Mills, J.N., Thomas, S., and Williamson, K.S. (1960) The acute effect of hydrocortisone, deoxycorticosterone and aldosterone upon the excretion of sodium, potassium and acid by the human kidney. J. Physiol. 151, 312–331.

116. Mimran, A., Banden, G., Casellas, D., and Soulas, D. (1977) Urinary kallikrein and changes in endogenous aldosterone in the rat. Eur. J. Clin. Invest. 7, 497–502.

117. Morris, D.J., Berek, J.S., and Davis, R.P. (1973) The physiological respone to aldosterone in adrenalectomized and intact rats and its sex dependence. Endocrinology 92, 989–993.

118. Moses, A.M., Gabrilove, J.L., and Soffer, L.J. (1958) Simplified water loading test in hypoadrenocorticism and hypothyroidism. J. Clin. Endocrinol. Metab. 18, 1413–1417.

119. Mueller, A., and Steinmetz, P.R. (1978) Spironolactone. An aldosterone agonist in the stimulation of H^+ secretion by turtle urinary bladder. J. Clin. Invest. 61, 1666–1670.

120. O'Neal, R.G., and Helman, S.I. (1977) Transport characteristics of renal collecting tubules: Influences of DOCA and diet. Am. J. Physiol. 233, F544–F558.

121. Perez, G.O., and Lespier, L., Jacobi, J., Oster, J.R., Katz, F.H., Vaamonde, C.A., and Fishman, L.M. (1977) Hyporeninemia and hypoaldosteronism in diabetes mellitus. Arch. Int. Med. 137, 852–855.

122. Perez, G.O., Oster, J.R., and Vaamonde, C.A. (1974) Renal acidosis and renal potassium handling in selective hypoaldosteronism. Am. J. Med. 57, 809–816.

123. Perez, G.O., Oster, J.R., and Vaamonde, C.A. (1976) Renal acidification in patients with mineralocorticoid deficiency. Nephron 17, 461–473.

124. Petty, K.J., Kokko, J.P., and Marver, D. (1981) Secondary effect of aldosterone on Na-K-ATPase activity in the rabbit cortical collecting tubule. J. Clin. Invest. 68, 1514–1521.

125. Porter, G.A., Bogoroch, R., and Edelman, I.S. (1964) On the mechanism of action of aldosterone on sodium transport: The role of RNA synthesis. Proc. Natl. Acad. Sci., USA 52, 1326–1333.

126. Porter, G.A., and Edelman, I.S. (1964) The action of aldosterone and related corticosteroids on sodium transport across the toad bladder. J. Clin. Invest. 43, 611–620.

127. Postel-Vinay, M.-C., Alberti, G.M., Ricour, C., Limal, J.-M., Rappaport, R., and Royer, P. (1974) Pseudohypoaldosteronism: Persistence of hyperaldosteronism and evidence for renal tubular and intestinal responsiveness to endogenous aldosterone. J. Clin. Endocrinol. Metab. 39, 1038–1044.

128. Proesmans, W., Geussens, H., Corbeel, L., and Eckels, R. (1973) Pseudohypoaldosteronism. Am. J. Dis. Child. 126, 510–516.

129. Rayson, B.M.R., Ray, C., and Morgan, T. (1978) The effect of adrenocortical hormones on water permeability of the collecting duct of the rat. Pflügers Arch. 373, 105–112.

130. Richards, P. (1973) Mineralocorticoids and rectal potential difference. Lancet ii, 798–799.

131. Rick, R., Dörge, A., Macknight, A.D.C., Leaf, A., and Thurau, K. (1978) Electron microprobe analysis of the different epithelial cells of toad urinary bladder. Electrolyte concentrations at different functional states of transepithelial sodium transport. J. Membrane Biol. 39, 257–271.

132. Rodriguez, H.J., Sinha, S.K., Starling, J., and Klahr, S. (1981) Regulation of renal Na^+-K^+-ATPase in the rat by adrenal steroids. Am. J. Physiol. 241, F186–F195.

133. Rösler, A., Rabinowitz, D., Theodor, R., Ramirez, L.C., and Ulick, S. (1977) The nature of the defect in a salt-wasting disorder in Jews of Iran. J. Clin. Endocrinol. Metab. 44, 279–291.

134. Rösler, A., Theodor, R., Boichis, H., Gerty, R., Ulick, S., Alagem, M., Tabachnik, E., Cohen, B., and Rabinowitz, D. (1977) Metabolic responses to the administration of angiotensin II, K and ACTH in two salt-wasting syndromes. J. Clin. Endocrinol. Metab. 44, 292–301.

135. Rossier, B.C. (1978) Role of RNA in the action of aldosterone on Na^+ transport. J. Membrane Biol. 40 (special issue), 187–197.

136. Sapirstein, V.S., and Scott, W.N. (1975) Binding of aldosterone by mitochondria-rich cells of the toad urinary bladder. Nature 257, 241–243.

137. Sartorius, O.W., Calhoon, D., and Pitts, R.F. (1953) Studies on the interrelationships of the adrenal cortex and renal ammonia excretion by the rat. Endocrinology 52, 256–265.

138. Schambelan, M., Sebastian, A., and Biglieri, E.G. (1980) Prevalence, pathogenesis and functional significance of aldosterone deficiency in hyperkalemic patients with chronic renal insufficiency. Kid. Int. 17, 89–101.

139. Schambelan, M., Stockigt, J.R., and Biglieri, E.G. (1972) Isolated hypoaldosteronism in adults: A renin-deficiency syndrome. N. Engl. J. Med. 287, 573–578.

140. Schmidt, U., and Dubach, U.C. (1971) Sensitivity of Na-K-adenosine triphosphatase activity in various structures of the rat nephron: Studies with adrenalectomy. Eur. J. Clin. Invest. 1, 307–312.

141. Schmidt, U., Schmid, J., Schmid, H., and Dubach, U.C. (1975) Sodium- and potassium-activated ATPase: A possible target of aldosterone. J. Clin. Invest. 55, 655–660.

142. Schrier, R.W., and Linas S.L. (1980) Mechanisms of the defect in water excretion in adrenal insufficiency. Min. Electr. Metab. 4, 1–7.

143. Schwartz, G.J., and Burg, M.B. (1978) Mineralocorticoid effects on cation transport by cortical collecting tubules in vitro. Am. J. Physiol. 235, F576–F585.

144. Schwartz, M.J., and Kokko, J.P. (1980) Urinary concentrating defect of adrenal insufficiency: Permissive role of adrenal steroids on the hydroosmotic response across the rabbit cortical collecting tubule. J. Clin. Invest. 66, 234–242.

145. Scott, W.N., Reich, I.M., Brown, J.A., Jr., and Yang, C.-P.H. (1978) Comparison of toad bladder aldosterone-induced proteins and proteins synthesized in vitro using aldosterone-induced messenger RNA as template. J. Membrane Bio. 40 (special issue), 213–230.

146. Scott, W.N., Reich, I.M., and Goodman, D.B.P. (1979) Inhibition of fatty acid synthesis prevents the incorporation of aldosterone-induced proteins into membranes. J. Biol. Chem. 254, 4957–4959.

147. Scott, W.N., and Sapirstein, V.S. (1975) Identification of aldosterone-induced proteins in the toad's urinary bladder. Proc. Natl. Acad. Sci, USA 72, 4056–4060.

148. Sebastian, A., Schambelan, M., Lindenfield, S., and Morris, R.C., Jr. (1977) Amelioration of metabolic acidosis with fluorocortisone therapy in hyporeninemic hypoaldosteronism. N. Engl. J. Med. 297, 576–583.

149. Sebastian, A., Sutton, J.M., Hutler, H.N., Schambelan, M., and Poler, S.M. (1980) Effect of mineralocorticoid replacement therapy on renal acid–base homeostasis in adrenalectomized patients. Kid. Int. 18, 762–773.

150. Sharp, G.W.G., and Leaf, A. (1964) Biological action of aldosterone in vitro. Nature 202, 1185–1188.
151. Sharp, G.W.G., and Leaf, A. (1966) Studies on the mode of action of aldosterone. Recent Prog. Horm. Res. 22, 431–471.
152. Siegel, B., and Civan, M.M. (1976) Aldosterone and insulin effects on driving force of Na^+ pump in toad bladder. Am. J. Physiol. 230, 1603–1608.
153. Skou, J.C. (1965) Enzymatic basis for active transport of Na^+ and K^+ across cell membrane. Physiol. Rev. 45, 596–617.
154. Sonnenberg, H. (1977) Effect of adrenalectomy on medullary collecting duct function in rats before and during blood volume expansion. Pflügers Arch. 368, 55–62.
155. Spitzer, A., Edelman, C.M., Jr., Goldberg, L.D., and Henneman, P.H. (1973) Short stature, hyperkalemia and acidosis: A defect in renal transport of potassium. Kid. Int. 3, 251–257.
156. Stokes, J.B., Tisher, C.C., and Kokko, J.P. (1978) Structural-functional heterogeneity along the rabbit collecting tubule. Kid. Int. 14, 585–593.
157. Stolte, H., Brecht, J.P., Wiederholt, M., and Hierholzer, K. (1968) Einfluss von Adrenalektomie und Glucocorticoiden auf die Wasserpermeabilität Corticaler Nephronabschnitte der Rattenniere. Pflügers Arch. 299, 99–127.
158. Strum, J.M., Feldman, D., Taggart, B., Marver, D., and Edelman, I. (1975) Autoradiographic localization of corticosterone receptors (type III) to the collecting tubule of the rat kidney. Endocrinology 97, 505–516.
159. Szylman, P., Better, O.S., Chaimowitz, C., and Rosler, A. (1976) Role of hyperkalemia in the metabolic acidosis of isolated hypoaldosteronism. N. Engl. J. Med. 294, 361–365.
160. Tan, E.L., and Trachewsky, D. (1975) Effect of aldosterone on flavin coenzyme biosynthesis in the kidney. J. Steroid Biochem. 6, 1471–1475.
161. Tan, S.Y., Shapiro, R., Franco, R., Stockard, H., and Mulrow, P.J. (1979) Indomethacin-induced prostaglandin inhibition with hyperkalemia. A reversible cause of hyporeninemic hypoaldosteronism. Ann. Int. Med. 90, 783–785.
162. Thomas, D.H., Jallageas, M., Munck, B.G., and Skadhauge, E. (1980) Aldosterone effects on electrolyte transport of the lower intestine (coprodeum and colon) of the fowl (*Gallus domesticus*) in vitro. Gen. Comp. Endocrinol. 40, 44–51.
163. Trachewsky, D. (1978) Aldosterone stimulation of riboflavin incorporation into rat renal flavin coenzymes and the effect of inhibition by riboflavin analogues on sodium reabsorption. J. Clin. Invest. 62, 1325–1333.
164. Ulick, S. (1976) Diagnosis and nomenclature of the disorders of the terminal portion of the aldosterone biosynthesis pathway. J. Clin. Endocrinol. Metab. 43, 92–96.
165. Ullrich, K.J., and Papavassiliou. (1979) Sodium reabsorption in the papillary collecting duct of rats. Effect of adrenalectomy, low Na^+ diet, acetazolamide, HCO_3^- free solutions and of amiloride. Pflügers Archiv. 379, 49–52.
166. Ussing, H.H., and Zerahn, K. (1951) Active transport of sodium as the source of electric current in the short-circuited isolated frog skin. Acta Physiol. Scand. 23, 110–127.
167. Van Ypersele de Strihou, C., and Dieu, J.P. (1977) Potassium deficiency acidosis in the dog: Effect of sodium and potassium balance on renal response to a chronic acid load. Kidney Int. 11, 335–347.
168. Wade, J.B., O'Neal, R.G., Pryor, J.L., and Boulpaep, E.L. (1979) Modulation of cell membrane area in renal collecting tubules by corticosteroid hormones. J. Cell. Biol. 81, 439–445.
169. Weidmann, P., Maxwell, M.H., Rowe, P., Winer, R., and Massry, S.G. (1975) Role of the renin-angiotensin-aldosterone system in the regulation of plasma potassium in chronic renal disease. Nephron 15, 34–39.
170. Weidmann, P., Reinhart, R., Maxwell, M.H., Rowe, P., Coburn, J.W., and Massry,

S.G. (1973) Syndrome of hyporeninemic hypoaldosteronism and hyperkalemia in renal disease. J. Clin. Endocrinol. Metab. 36, 965–977.

171. Weinstein, S.F., Allan, D.M.E., and Mendosa, S.A. (1974) Hyperkalemia, acidosis, and short-stature associated with a defect in renal potassium excretion. J. Pediatr. 85, 355–358.

172. Welbourne, T.C., and Francoeur, D. (1977) Influence of aldosterone on renal NH_3 production. Am. J. Physiol. 233, E56–E60.

173. Westenfelder, C., Arevalo, G.J., Baranowski, R.L., Kurtzman, N.A., and Katz, A.I. (1977) Relationship between mineralocorticoids and renal Na^+-K^+-ATPase: Sodium reabsorption. Am. J. Physiol. 233, F593–F599.

174. Will, P.C., Lebowitz, J.L., and Hopfer, U. (1980) Induction of amiloride-sensitive sodium transport in the rat colon by mineralocorticoids. Am. J. Physiol. 238, F261–F268.

175. Williamson, H.E. (1963) Mechanism of the antinatriuretic action of aldosterone. Biochem. Pharmacol. 12, 1449–1450.

176. Wotman, S., Goodwin, F.J., Mandel, I.D., and Laragh, J.H. (1969) Changes in salivary electrolytes following treatment of primary aldosteronism. Arch. Int. Med. 124, 477–480.

ROBERTO FRANCO-SAENZ, M.D.

DISEASES OF THE ADRENAL CORTEX

CUSHING'S SYNDROME

Definition and Historical Perspective

Cushing's syndrome is a term referring to the multiple symptoms and signs resulting from chronic exposure of the tissues to larger than physiological amounts of glucocorticoid.

In 1912 Harvey Cushing first described the cardinal symptoms and signs of the syndrome in a 23-year-old white female (77) with what Cushing called a "polyglandular syndrome" characterized by obesity, hypertrichosis, and amenorrhea with overdevelopment of secondary sexual characteristics (78). Although the origin of the syndrome was not established in the initial description, the possibility of pituitary or adrenal origin was suggested. In the same publication (78), Cushing refers to a symptom complex described in association with "certified adrenal lesions" and briefly reviews the clinical findings of Launois et al. (210) regarding a patient with an adrenal carcinoma. Also, he acknowledges five previously reported cases (with precisely the same syndrome) associated with adenomatous or hyperplastic adrenals, and makes the remark

From the Division of Endocrinology and Metabolism, Medical College of Ohio, Toledo, Ohio.

that "we may, per chance, be on the way toward recognition of consequences of hyperadrenalism." The association of the syndrome with basophilic adenomas of the pituitary body was also described by Cushing in 1932 in a monograph in which he expands the clinical observations on the original patient and reviews the history and findings of 11 similar cases reported in the literature between 1913 and 1928. Of the patients reported, five had pituitary tumors, three basophilic and two undifferentiated (78).

In 1938 Anderson et al. demonstrated that extracts of blood and urine from patients with Cushing's syndrome prolonged the life of adrenalectomized rats beyond the survivals of rats treated with extracts from normal subjects; they proposed that the cause of Cushing's syndrome was an excess of the hormone, cortin (10). Subsequently, Albright presented supporting evidence for this hypothesis and suggested that Cushing's syndrome was due to an excess of the carbohydrate regulating, or sugar, hormone (7). With the development of specific chemical methods to identify and measure the secretory products of the adrenal glands, it was soon confirmed that Cushing's syndrome was caused by an excess of cortisol (83,258,298,316).

The association of nonendocrine tumors with adrenal hyperplasia was first observed by Gabcke in 1896 in a patient with sarcoma of the thymus, skin pigmentation, and adrenal hyperplasia (109). Also, in 1928 Brown reported a case of adrenal hyperplasia associated with an oat cell carcinoma of the lung (48). However, the relationship between the nonendocrine tumor and adrenal hyperplasia was definitely established in 1962 by Meador et al., who first demonstrated the presence of an ACTH-like substance in nonendocrine tumors and introduced the term "ectopic ACTH syndrome" (243).

Classification and Pathogenesis

The term Cushing's *syndrome* is used to refer to the clinical manifestations of hypercortisolism independent of its cause. Cushing's *disease*, on the other hand, is a term reserved for pituitary-dependent hypercortisolism.

Cushing's syndrome can be classified according to its origin as: 1) pituitary Cushing's, with and without demonstrable tumor; 2) adrenal Cushing's, adenoma, carcinoma, nodular hyperplasia; 3) ectopic Cushing's—ectopic ACTH production by nonendocrine tumors; or 4) iatrogenic Cushing's, due to administration of glucocorticoids or ACTH. Cushing's syndrome can also be classified according to the pathogenesis of the hypercortisolism as ACTH-dependent and ACTH-independent (Table 1).

Cushing's Disease: Bilateral Adrenal Hyperplasia. Hypercortisolism due to pituitary excess of ACTH and adrenal-hyperplasia is the most common cause of Cushing's syndrome and accounts for over two-thirds of patients (50,155,297,387) (Table 1). The syndrome was originally as-

TABLE 1. Classification of Cushing's Syndrome

I. ACTH Dependent
  A. Adrenal hyperplasia
    1. Excess pituitary ACTH—with tumor
       —without tumor
    2. Ectopic ACTH
    3. Prolonged use of ACTH

II. ACTH Independent
  A. Adrenal neoplasia
    1. Adenoma
    2. Carcinoma
    3. Nodular hyperplasia (?)
  B. Prolonged use of glucocorticoids

cribed to basophilic adenomas of the pituitary gland. However, in a review of the histological findings of eight patients described up to 1932, Cushing found basophilic adenomas in only six of them (78). Since then, the frequency at which pituitary tumors have been reported has varied. In the early series, pituitary tumors were found in as many as 86% of the cases (94). In more recent series the incidence ranges between 3%–80% of the cases (50,134,280,305). This discrepancy in the incidence of pituitary tumors may partly be explained by the presence of microadenomas which may not cause distortion of the sella turcica and, therefore, may escape detection by currently available diagnostic techniques. Radiological evaluation of the sella turcica by conventional skull x-rays or "coned down views" of the sella reveals abnormalities suggestive of a tumor in only 10%–15% of patients with Cushing's disease (326). However, with the recent development of hypocycloidal or triaxial spiral tomograms of the sella the percentage of patients shown normal studies has dramatically changed. Of 33 patients with Cushing's disease seen at the Mayo Clinic between 1974 and 1977, only one had an abnormal sella on a plain skull film; in 12 of the remaining 32 patients, however, axial polytomography disclosed abnormalities suggestive of the presence of microadenoma (327).

Of 65 patients undergoing transsphenoidal microneurosurgery for Cushing's disease, 20 (33%) had normal sella turcica by polytomography and 59 of the 65 had microadenomas (tumors less than 10 mm in diameter), ranging in size between 1 and 9 mm in diameter (327,339,384). More recently, in a series of 37 patients with ACTH-producing pituitary tumors, Wilson et al. (399) found 31 microadenomas, 20 of which measured 5 mm or less. In Hardy's experience of 75 operated cases, tumors were found in 60 (52 microadenomas, four large adenomas, and four invasive tumors). In 15 cases no tumor was found at surgery; however, in four of these patients a total hypophysectomy was performed and three additional microadenomas were found at pathology. Forty-nine of these patients (65%) had no radiological anomalies of the sella turcica (134).

Tumors less than 2 mm in diameter are often missed during transsphenoidal exploration but have been identified in serial sections of totally excised glands (134,399).

Although Cushing's original description suggested that the syndrome was caused by a basophilic tumor, recent evidence indicates that the tumor may be basophilic, chromophobic, or mixed. In fact, chromophobe adenomas appear to be the most common type of ACTH-secreting pituitary adenomas causing Cushing's disease.

Of 15 tumors stained by conventional histological techniques, 10 were chromophobic, three were mixed basophilic/chromophobic, and two were basophilic adenomas (384). Microadenomas are more often intraglandular and may be distributed almost equally in the lateral lobes and middle of the anterior lobe (399), although in Hardy's experience the majority of the microadenomas were located in the center of the gland, most often near or within the neural lobe (134). Occasionally, the tumor may occupy or derive from the pars intermedia. One of the original cases compiled by Cushing (the Raab–Krause case) was a pars intermedia tumor (79).

The anterior and the intermediate lobe of the pituitary gland share the capacity to synthesize the common ACTH precursor, 31-K ACTH or proopiomelanocortin (POMC). This peptide is a precursor for ACTH, β-lipotropin (β-LPH), the endorphins, and the melanotropins (237) (Figure 1). However, a number of differences in the neurotransmitter regulation, negative feedback suppression by glucocorticoids, and processing of the precursor peptide exist between the POMC system of the anterior and that of the intermediate lobe of the pituitary. Corticotropin-releasing factor appears to be a major stimulus for the release of POMC from both lobes. Catecholamines have a stimulatory effect in the anterior lobe system and prostaglandins suppress the release of POMC products from the anterior lobe. Dopamine, on the other hand, is the most potent inhibitor of POMC products from the intermediate lobe and has little or no effect on the anterior lobe corticotrophins. Also, whereas the POMC system of the anterior lobe of the rat and the horse is exquisitely sensitive to glucocorticoid inhibition, the system from the intermediate lobe is relatively resistant to feedback suppression by glucocorticoids (283,301, 320). A difference in the processing of POMC has also been demonstrated in these two species (236,283). The major products of secretion of the POMC system from the anterior lobe are ACTH, β-LPH and β-endorphin (Figure 1). In contrast, the intermediate lobe releases little or no ACTH and the major products of secretion are α-melanotropin stimulating hormone (α-MSH), corticotropin-like intermediate lobe peptide (CLIP), β-LPH, γ-LPH, β-MSH, and β-endorphin.

Equine Cushing's disease is always associated with adenomas or adenomatous hyperplasia of the intermediate lobe of the pituitary (285). A variant of Cushing's disease with distinct clinical and laboratory characteristics has recently been described in association with tumors derived from the intermediate lobe of the pituitary gland (206). These tumors may be found in the intermediate or anterior lobe of the pituitary but are

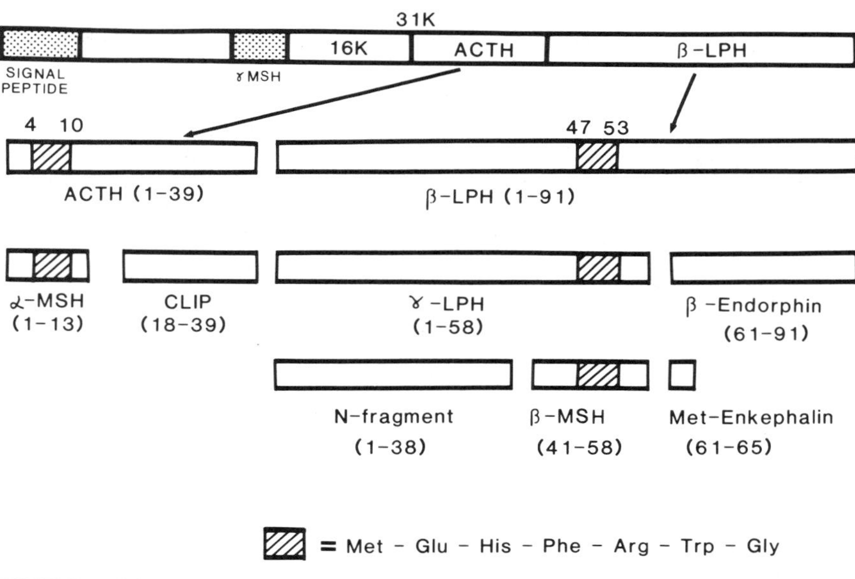

FIGURE 1. Schematic diagram of the ACTH precursor, proopiomelanocortin (POMC), and the peptides derived from it. The hatched portion represents the heptapeptide sequence common to ACTH and β-LPH and some of the peptides derived from them.

characterized by the presence of nerve fibers surrounding the cells. Patients with tumors arising from the intermediate lobe have a tendency to recur after hypophysectomy and are relatively resistant to dexamethasone suppression. In addition, pars intermedia tumors may have high prolactin levels and the elevated levels of ACTH and cortisol are significantly suppressed by bromocriptine and other dopaminergic agonists.

The majority of pituitary tumors causing Cushing's syndrome are benign, but in rare occasions these tumors may become locally invasive and may spread intracranially (393). This is more common with large adenomas. Also, in rare occasions the tumors may be malignant and have extracranial metastasis. In a review of 55 patients with large adenomas, Rovit and Berry (321) found five with hepatic metastasis. Corticotropic adenomas are usually PAS and lead hematoxylin positive. Immunocytochemical studies of pituitary tumors causing Cushing's disease may show variable staining for POMC-derived peptides, but all tumors stain with ACTH antibody (138,314). β-LPH and β-endorphin have been demonstrated in some and as many as 20% of the cells may stain for α-MSH. Using immunocytochemical stains for POMC peptides, a number of "silent" corticotropic pituitary adenomas have been described in patients with no clinical or laboratory evidence of hypercortisolism (137,150). It has been estimated that 4%−10% of endocrinologically normal people may harbor POMC producing adenomas (196). Abnormalities of secretion, processing, or a biologically inactive crossreacting material may explain the endocrinological silence of these tumors.

The ultrastructural features of ACTH adenomas are characteristic (351). A prominent feature is the presence of bundles of 70 nm microfilaments surrounding the nucleus and lying randomly within the cytoplasm. Larger than normal (approximately 700 μm) secretory granules, which tend to align beneath the cell membrane, are common in these tumors. An additional feature identifiable in the cytoplasm of extratumoral ACTH-producing cells is Crooke's hyalin changes. This abnormality occurs with hypercortisolism of any cause. Crooke's changes result in cellular enlargement with a ring-like pattern of cytoplasmic hyalinization with marked reduction in the number of secretory granules. It has been suggested that Crooke's changes represent a "physiological brake" in the mechanism of granule secretion (335). Basophilic hyperplasia with or without tumor has been noticed in several cases (114,196,340). The extent of basophilic hyperplasia has been variable. The presence of hyperplasia is suggestive of excessive hypothalamic drive by corticotropin releasing factor (CRF). Corticotroph hyperplasia often accompanies ACTH-producing adenomas (335).

The pathogenesis of the pituitary tumor causing Cushing's is not known. That the primary defect is at the level of the pituitary and not at the hypothalamic level is suggested by the sequence of events that follows successful removal of the tumor. After removal of the microadenoma, there is usually a period of ACTH and cortisol deficiency followed by recovery of normal ACTH and cortisol secretion over a period of months. Also, there is return of the diurnal rhythm and normal suppression by glucocorticoids (327,339,384). On the other hand, a cyproheptadine reversible defect in the cortisol feedback suppression of ACTH was found in four patients who had undergone adrenalectomy for Cushing's disease and in five patients with Nelson's syndrome studied 2 years after transsphenoidal removal of the pituitary tumor. These findings have been interpreted as suggesting that higher centers, such as the hypothalamus, may be involved in the pathogenesis of the pituitary adenoma (209). The role of CRF in the pathogenesis of tumors is a matter of controversy. The injection of CRF stimulated ACTH release in vivo in two patients with pituitary microadenomas, causing Cushing's disease studied by Orth et al. (282). Pieters et al. (294) reported a normal ACTH and cortisol response to CRF in three patients, hyperresponse in two patients with classical pituitary-dependent Cushing's disease, and in another patient with Cushing's disease due to bilateral micro- and macronodular hyperplasia, unresponsiveness to CRF was shown. Nakahara et al. (257) reported a lower than normal ACTH response to CRF in four patients with Cushing's disease, but an exaggerated response in a patient with Nelson's syndrome. Recently, the same group of investigators found that the level of immunoreactive CRF in the spinal fluid of 13 of 14 patients with Cushing's disease was lower than normal and returned to normal 2–9 months after adrenalectomy. These results suggest that spinal fluid CRF in Cushing's disease is suppressed by the increased corticosteroid levels. If the levels of CRF are representative of the concentrations in the portal system, it may indicate that CRF is not involved in the pathogenesis of microadenomas (382). Furthermore, in an in vitro study of three microadenomas, Shibasaki et al. (355) showed that these tumors responded to arginine vasopressin but did not respond to CRF.

Patients with Cushing's disease and Nelson's syndrome respond normally to vasopressin and metyrapone and to higher than normal doses of dexamethasone (197,198,275,305). In contrast to normal subjects, patients with Cushing's and Nelson's syndrome respond with an increase in ACTH after the injection of TRH (198,292,293). This abnormal response is probably due to a receptor abnormality of the pituitary corticotroph. This possibility has been substantiated by the in vitro release of ACTH by the AtT-20 ACTH-secreting mouse pituitary tumor in response to thyrotropin releasing hormone (TRH) (116). An increase in β-endorphin has also been observed after injection of TRH in Nelson's syndrome (275). Similarly, increase in plasma cortisol and ACTH have been reported in patients with Cushing's disease after the injection of luteinizing hormone releasing factor (LHRH) (292,293) and in contrast to the response of normal subjects, somatostatin suppresses ACTH and β-endorphin levels in patients with Nelson's syndrome (174,385). Therefore, it appears that in patients with Cushing's disease the pituitary ACTH receptor may have a loss of specificity similar to the one described in some adrenal carcinomas (341). In reference to the increased resistance to the negative feedback suppression by glucocorticoids observed in pituitary Cushing's, it appears that in these patients there is a defect in the fast (rate-sensitive) feedback response to cortisol administration (99) and that cyproheptadine corrects these abnormalities (208). Recent evidence suggests that 6-hydroxy-dopamine decreases glucocorticoid binding in the hypothalamus (370). Further suggestive evidence for the role of dopamine in glucocorticoid receptors is the fact that the POMC system of the intermediate lobe of the pituitary is suppressed by dopamine and it is known to be resistant to negative feedback by glucocorticoids. Other possibilities that have been suggested to explain the resistance to glucocorticoid suppression include: defective translocation of the glucocorticoid receptor to the nucleus; modifications in the DNA with decreased nuclear receptor binding sites (69); and chemical or structural modifications in the glucocorticoid receptors (76).

In spite of the evidence suggesting a tumoral origin for Cushing's disease there remain some cases in which there is no histological evidence of tumor in the pituitary gland, suggesting the possibility that there may be at least two types of Cushing's disease, one dependent on abnormal hypothalamic function and the other of primary pituitary origin. The possibility of dysfunction of the neurotransmitters involved in the regulation of CRF secretion has been suggested to explain those cases of Cushing's syndrome associated with basophilic hyperplasia without a tumor (199). Abnormalities in the periodicity of other pituitary hormones, as well as in the stages of sleep, have been described in patients with Cushing's disease and have been interpreted as evidence of hypothalamic dysfunction (194). Another line of evidence suggestive of hypothalamic dysfunction has been the report that cyproheptadine, a drug that interferes with serotoninergic neurotransmission in the hypothalamus, causes remission in some patients with Cushing's disease (194); also, cyproheptadine lowers plasma ACTH and cortisol levels in patients with documented tumors of the pars intermedia (206). Moreover, Asa et al. (14a) recently reported a case of Cushing's disease and pituitary corticotropic hyperplasia associated with an intrasellar gangliocytoma producing CRF. This case supports the theory that some cases of Cushing's disease may be of hypothalamic origin. Therefore, it appears that Cushing's disease may be of heterogeneous etiology and that it may be of primary pituitary origin, as in the case of anterior lobe microadenomas, or secondary to central nervous system or hypothalamic dysfunction, as in the case of patients with pars intermedia adenomas or basophilic hyperplasia.

The adrenal glands in Cushing's disease show simple bilateral hyperplasia in the majority of cases. In simple hyperplasia the adrenals may show mild to moderate increase in weight (6–12 g per adrenal as compared to 2–6 g per normal adrenals) (375). Histologically, these glands show widening of the zona fasciculata and a compact broad zona reticularis. In approximately 15%–20% (12) the adrenals may contain nodules in addition to hyperplasia. This condition has been called nodular or adenomatous hyperplasia. The nodules are multiple and bilateral and, in contrast with single functional adrenal adenomas in which the surrounding tissue and the contralateral adrenals are atrophic, in nodular hyperplasia the surrounding tissue is hyperplastic and the contralateral adrenal may also be hyperplastic and contain nodules. Of 69 cases of bilateral adrenal hyperplasia causing Cushing's syndrome reviewed by Neville and Symington (268), 50 had simple bilateral adrenal hyperplasia, 10 had nodular hyperplasia, and nine had hyperplasia secondary to ectopic ACTH syndrome. This form of hyperplasia is particularly common in children (267).

Adrenal Cushing's, Cushing's Syndrome, Adrenal Adenoma, and Adrenal Carcinoma. Adrenal adenomas are responsible for the development of Cushing's in approximately 10% of the cases. In a series of 195 patients with Cushing's syndrome, adrenal adenomas accounted for 11% of the cases and carcinomas accounted for 7% (24). Whereas adrenal adenomas occurred more frequently on the left side than on the right (2:1), adrenal carcinomas occurred with equal frequency on either side (24). Adenomas and carcinomas are 4–6 times more common in females than in males. Adrenal adenomas are well encapsulated and may range in size from a few centimeters to 5–7 cm in diameter. Adrenal carcinomas, on the other hand, are usually much larger. The mean weight of 22 adenomas reported by Bertagna was 36 g, whereas that of 14 adrenal carcinomas was 508 g. It is not unusual for adrenal carcinomas to have metastases at the time of diagnosis. In the absence of metastases or local invasion, pathological differentiation of adenomas from carcinomas may be difficult (342). Large tumor weight has been thought to be a reliable indicator of malignancy (200). A disproportionately high excretion of 17-ketosteroids as compared to 17-hydroxycorticosteroids may also be an indicator of malignancy. In a mathematic analysis of clinical and pathologic data in 41 patients with adrenocortical tumors, Hough et al. (151) found that the most significant indicators of malignancy were evidence of weight loss, broad fibrous bands traversing the tumor, a diffuse growth pattern, vascular invasion, tumor cell necrosis, and tumor mass. Nevertheless, none of these criteria are absolute and in clinical practice a long-term follow-up is necessary to establish recurrence of an occult metastatic lesion.

Adrenal adenomas may have fluctuating activity (125) and occasionally undergo spontaneous remission (34). Because of inefficient steroidogenesis adrenal carcinomas may attain a large size before clinical detection and are often associated with massive elevation of the urinary 17-ketosteroids. Also, carcinomas frequently have a relative deficiency of 11-β-hydroxylase and excrete large quantities of 11-deoxycortisol (Compound S) (228,229) urinary-free deoxycorticosterone (DOC) (181) and other steroid precursors. Adrenal carcinomas are usually unresponsive to exogenous ACTH, which may be an indication of an abnormality of the cell plasma membrane at the site of interaction of ACTH with its receptor or a postreceptor defect (324). Defect in steroidogenesis in steps beyond the generation of cyclic AMP has been described in a mouse adrenocortical carcinoma (341). In addition, this tumor had the abnormal presence of receptors for epinephrine and luteinizing hormone (LH). Adrenal carcinomas are the commonest cause of Cushing's syndrome in children (156,366). Functional adrenal adenomas are usually spherical and compress the atrophic adrenal tissues surrounding it. The cut surface is usually yellow with brown or red areas. Occasionally, the tumor may appear black due to accumulation of lipofucsin. Pathological differentiation of benign from malignant is often difficult by histologic examination alone. Conventional evidence of malignancy is absent. Mitoses are rare and cell pleomorphism is uncommon. However, some tumors have gross evidence of malignancy, such as invasion to the capsule or blood vessel, or evidence of metastasis. Nevertheless, in tumors of over 70 g, regardless of the benign histological appearance, only a long-term follow-up will secure the benign nature of the tumor.

Ectopic ACTH Syndrome. Ectopic production of ACTH by nonendocrine tumors causing Cushing's syndrome account for approximately 15%–20% of cases of Cushing's (50,278,297). The molecular basis by which these tumors produce ACTH are not known. It is postulated that these tumors arise from a single progenitor cell embryologically derived from the neural crest and capable of producing peptide hormones (APUD cells) (290). However, in a study of 51 cases of ectopic ACTH-β-LPH-producing tumors, only 84% were categorized as APUD tumors (159). Another possibility is that portions of DNA that are inactive during normal cell differentiation become activated or derepressed during neoplastic transformation, leading to ectopic production of hormones. A third explanation is that neoplastic tissue undergoes a process of dedifferentiation by which the tissue regresses to a more primitive cell expression than that of the parent cell (19). ACTH-producing tumors have been shown to synthesize the common precursor for ACTH, proopiomelanocortin. Synthesis of this precursor is directed by a single m-RNA transcribed from one gene. Evidence for a similar synthetic sequence has now been obtained in human lung cancer cells in culture (25). Release of several POMC-derived peptides has been shown in a variety of tumors. All tumors have been found to elaborate and release β-LPH, γ-LPH, and β-endorphin (161,284). In addition, some, but not all, tumors have been found to contain α-MSH and CLIP, which derives from cleavage of ACTH (1,304). The most common tumors associated with ectopic Cushing's are listed in Table 2.

An estimated 2% of patients with bronchogenic carcinoma develop the clinical syndrome (319), and plasma immunoreactive levels of ACTH are markedly elevated. This is in contrast to pituitary Cushing's in which nearly half of the patients have ACTH levels in the normal range; these levels, however, are inappropriately high relative to the levels of plasma cortisol (27). Approximately 50% of patients with lung cancer without the syndrome may have elevated plasma levels of ACTH without hypercortisolism (27,303) and virtually all lung tumor extracts contain ACTH (117). The absence of symptoms and signs in patients with high plasma levels of immunoreactive ACTH has been attributed to release of biological inactive fragments of ACTH that crossreact in the immunoassay (303). Therefore, it appears that the clinical expression of the syndrome depends on the capability of the tumor to synthesize the precursor molecule, process it, and release the biologically active form of ACTH. In addition to ACTH some tumor extracts have been found to contain corticotropin-releasing factor, CRF (160,386). The adrenal glands in the ectopic ACTH syndrome are symmetrically enlarged and usually weigh more than 15 g each, and sometimes as much as 40 g each (379).

TABLE 2. Tumors Most Commonly Associated with Ectopic ACTH Production

1. Small cell anaplastic (oat cell) carcinoma of the lung
2. Thymoma
3. Carcinoid tumors—lung
—gastrointestinal tract
4. Pancreatic carcinoma
5. Neural crest neoplasm—pheochromocytoma
—neuroblastoma
—ganglioma
—paraganglioma
6. Medullary carcinoma of the thyroid
7. Melanoma
8. Prostatic carcinoma

Clinical Manifestations

Cushing's syndrome occurs in all races and is more frequent in people between the ages of 20 and 60 years. However, it can also occur in children, although less frequently. Pituitary Cushing's and Cushing's associated with adrenal tumors is approximately four times more frequent in females than in males. On the other hand, Cushing's secondary to the ectopic ACTH syndrome is more common in males and has a higher frequency in patients over 50 years of age. This is probably because of oat cell carcinoma of the lung is the most common cause of the syndrome, and this tumor is 10 times more common in males of this age group. The frequency of symptoms and signs of Cushing's syndrome is shown in Table 3. The pathophysiological basis for many of the symptoms of Cushing's syndrome remains unknown. Obesity is the most common feature of Cushing's. Central redistribution of fat-pads leads to the typical accumulation of fat in the face, trunk, and cervicodorsal regions leading to the classical "moon facies," "buffalo hump," and fullness of the supraclavicular fossa. The abdomen is often protuberant and pendulous and the extremities are thin, owing to muscle wasting. Obesity may also be general without centripetal distribution, but extreme obesity is rare. Patients with ectopic ACTH syndrome secondary to malignant tumors may not be obese and may lack the typical cushingoid habitus; in fact, patients with ectopic Cushing's may present with a history of weight loss owing to the catabolic effects of the tumor and the sudden and rapidly deteriorating clinical course. Body composition studies in patients with Cushing's show that there is an increase in total body fat (202). The increased body fat has been attributed to increased caloric intake caused by the excess of glucocorticoid-decreased turnover of fatty acids with sparing of fat (33) and to increased lipogenesis secondary to hyperinsulinism (139). The factors that determine the typical cushingoid habitus are not known.

The face is frequently plethoric. The skin is atrophic with thinning of

TABLE 3. Frequency of Clinical Manifestations of Cushing's Syndrome in 601 Cases

	Percent
Obesity	88
Plethora	75
Hypertension	74
Hirsutism	64
Muscle weakness	61
Menstrual disorders	60
Acne	45
Easy bruising	42
Back pain	40

Source: Modified from Ross, E.J., Marshall-Jones, P., Friedman, M. (1966), Q. J. Med. 35:149.

the stratum corneum and increased transparency permitting the underlying capillary plexus to be seen (353). Loss of connective tissue and atrophy of the skin lead to easy bruising and minor trauma causes skin breaks and ulcerations. This is particularly apparent in the lower extremities, forearms, and dorsum of the hands. Ecchymosis and purpuric lesions are common at venopuncture site. Broad purple striae are often seen around the abdomen, hips, upper thigh, and axillary region. Fungal infections and tinea versicolor are common.

Muscle weakness and atrophy are frequent, especially involving the proximal muscles of the pelvic and shoulder girdle. Muscle weakness may be due to hypokalemia which, on occasion, may be severe. Wasting and atrophy of muscles may be related to muscle protein breakdown resulting from the excess glucocorticoids that make increased levels of amino acids available to the liver to increase gluconeogenesis (401). In addition, changes in ribosomal and mitochondrial function of muscles have been described in experimental animals receiving glucocorticoids (49). Back pain is a common complaint and usually results from osteoporosis and fractures of the spine. Osteoporosis can be generalized, but the most vulnerable places are the spinal column and rib cage. In some patients the major presenting symptom may be bone pain from osteoporosis (152,322). The mechanism by which excess glucocorticoids cause osteoporosis is multifactorial. In glucocorticoid-induced osteoporosis, bone formation is decreased and bone reabsorption is increased. This bone loss preferentially affects the axial skeleton, rich in trabecular bone, and, to a lesser degree, affects the appendicular skeleton as well. Excess glucocorticoids cause a direct inhibition of osteoblastic function with a decreased collagen synthesis (54) and inhibition of the conversion of progenitor cells to functioning osteoblasts (43,107,172). The mechanism whereby glucocorticoids increase bone reabsorption is probably indirect and thought to be mediated by parathyroid hormone. In experimental animals glucocorticoid-induced bone reabsorption is prevented by parathyroidectomy (166). In patients treated with glucocorticoids the levels of parathyroid hormone are frequently elevated (132). This secondary hyperparathyroidism is likely to be caused by the negative calcium balance resulting from the inhibitory effects of corticosteroids on calcium absorption (185) and decrease renal conservation of calcium leading to hypercalciuria (377). The secondary hyperparathyroidism of glucocorticoid excess can be corrected by calcium infusions (231), pharmacological doses of vitamin D or 1-25 dihydroxy vitamin D (132), and correction of hypercalciuria by hydrochlorothiazide (377).

Mild to moderate hypertension occurs in approximately 75%–80% of patients and evidence of left ventricular hypertrophy is common. Paradoxically, patients with ectopic Cushing's syndrome have a lower prevalence of hypertension, occurring in approximately 30%–50% of patients (160,220). This is despite very high levels of ACTH and cortisol (220,308). Patients with Cushing's syndrome have different patterns of steroid hypersecretion. A mixture of cortisol and mineralocorticoid excess may occur in some patients. Plasma renin activity (PRA) may be normal or high in patients with isolated hypersecretion of cortisol or in patients receiving large doses of synthetic glucocorticoids (190). Low PRA can also be seen, especially in patients with adrenal carcinoma or ectopic Cushing's, and indicates concurrent hypersecretion of mineralocorticoids (31). Mineralocorticoid-induced hypertension requires a high sodium intake and depends upon a positive sodium balance (191), whereas experimental glucocorticoid-induced hypertension develops in spite of low sodium intake (95). In contrast to PRA, plasma renin substrate is uniformly elevated (190) as a consequence of the glucocorticoid action upon the liver to increase synthesis and release of renin substrate (105). Administration of the angiotensin II antagonist, saralasin, reduced the blood pressure of five patients with Cushings's syndrome and with high PRA, suggested that the hypertension of these patients was mediated in part by angiotensin II (81). However, in patients with Cushing's syndrome with normal or low PRA, saralasin does not lower the blood pressure. Patients with Cushing's syndrome have been shown to have an increased vascular sensitivity to pressor agents (249).

Glycosuria and impaired glucose tolerance occurs in approximately 80% of patients, but fasting blood glucose is frequently normal. In 20% of patients, overt diabetes may be present. It is likely that patients who develop frank diabetes are those with a genetic predisposition to the disease. Hyperglycemia in Cushing's usually coexists with hyperinsulinemia which suggests an insulin-resistant state. Glucocorticoids have widespread effects on carbohydrate metabolism. The carbohydrate intolerance of patients with Cushing's syndrome may be due to a combination of increased gluconeogenesis and decreased glucose uptake by cells. It has been reported that glucocorticoids influence intracellular metabolic pathways of glucose metabolism (53) and decrease glucose transport (276). The effects of glucocorticoids on the insulin receptor are controversial. Cortisol has been shown to increase (20), decrease (86,177), or not affect (97) receptor binding of insulin. A postreceptor defect in insulin action has been shown after acute glucocorticoid administration (313); in a study of five patients with Cushing's syndrome, Nosadini et al. (272) showed an impaired maximal glucose disposal with normal insulin receptor binding indicating that insulin resistance in Cushing's syndrome is due to an impairment of peripheral insulin action located beyond the hormone-receptor binding step (272).

Menstrual disorders, hirsutism, and acne are equally prevalent, but true virilization, such as temporal balding, deepening of the voice, and clitoral enlargement are rare. When present, they should alert the physician to the possibility of adrenal carcinoma because carcinomas frequently have coexistent excess of adrenal androgens. However, plasma testosterone levels are significantly elevated in female patients with pituitary Cushing's and this may account for the hirsutism and acne (361). In contrast to females, male patients with Cushing's have significant reduction in plasma testosterone levels which is associated with low follicle stimulating hormone (FSH) and LH (233). Unresponsiveness of the pituitary to LHRH has been shown in male and female patients with Cushing's syndrome and is thought to be caused by inhibition of release of pituitary gonadotropins by the excess cortisol (38,233). This abnormality is reversible and is thought to be responsible for the menstrual irregularities in females and for the impotence, loss of libido, and oligospermia seen in male patients with Cushing's syndrome (111).

Hyperpigmentation similar to that seen in Addison's disease occurs in approximately 25% of patients with the ectopic ACTH syndrome (160). It may also be present in patients with pituitary tumors (78) and may become very prominent after adrenalectomy for Cushing's syndrome (Nelson's syndrome). Increased pigmentation does not occur in patients with Cushing's syndrome due to adrenal tumors nor in iatrogenic Cushing's. The increased pigmentation was initially thought to be due to an increase in the production and release of β-MSH by the pituitary and by tumors causing ectopic Cushing's (2). However, it appears that β-MSH does not circulate in the blood and that previous measurements of this peptide were the result of an artifact of plasma and tissue extraction (37,349). It is now believed that the hyperpigmentation results from the markedly elevated levels of ACTH and other POMC-derived peptides with melanotropic activity, such as β-LPH, γ-LPH, and α-MSH (159).

Mental symptoms occur in approximately one-half of the patients (120) and may include a wide spectrum of psychiatric illness, ranging from personality changes, irritability, severe depression, leading in some cases to suicide or even frank psychosis. On the other hand, emotional and psychiatric difficulties are often demonstrable before the onset of illness (118). It is noteworthy that some patients with primary severe depression may show many of the biochemical abnormalities associated with Cushing's syndrome and differentiation from primary Cushing's syndrome may be difficult (27). Nephrolithiasis owing to hypercalciuria is seen in about 20% of cases and exophthalmos may be found in some patients. In patients with pituitary tumors, headaches, and signs of compression of the optic chiasma with bitemporal hemianopsia and progressive loss of vision may be present, but are rare in the untreated patient.

In a comparison of the electrolyte abnormalities of patients with pituitary Cushing's syndrome with those of patients with ectopic Cushing's, Prunty et al. (300) found that the serum potassium of patients with pituitary Cushing's ranged from 2.9−4.5 mEq/L and serum bicarbonate from 24−39 mEq/L whereas in patients with ectopic ACTH, the serum potassium ranged from 1.3−3.8 mEq/L and serum bicarbonate from 28−52 mEq/L.

Hypersecretion of cortisol has been suggested as one of the causes of the hypokalemic alkalosis (40). However, marked elevations of the mineralocorticoid DOC and corticosterone have been found in patients with adrenal carcinoma (73,103) and in the ectopic ACTH syndrome (45,334). The clinical manifestations of iatrogenic Cushing's are similar to the ones of endogenous Cushing's with the exception that benign intracranial hypertension, glaucoma, cataracts, pancreatitis, "avascular necrosis" of bone, and panniculitis occur in iatrogenic Cushing's but do not occur in the endogenous type (68).

Diagnosis

Laboratory Findings. Routine laboratory examinations may show a number of findings that are consistent, but not diagnostic of Cushing's syndrome. Mild to moderate leukocytosis with neutrophilia and reduction of lymphocytes to below 20% is a common finding. Eosinophils are usually absent from the differential count. The hematocrit is normal in the majority of patients, although in approximately 10% of the patients mild erythrocytosis may be present. Hyperglycemia and glycosuria are seen in 20% of patients, but the glucose tolerance test may be abnormal in approximately 80% of patients. Serum electrolytes are usually normal, but hypokalemia and metabolic alkalosis occur in some patients. Severe hypokalemia and alkalosis in the absence of diuretic use may be an important clue to the presence of the ectopic ACTH.

Specific Laboratory Tests. A major problem in the diagnosis of Cushing's syndrome is the lack of any specific manifestations unique to Cushing's syndrome. This is complicated by the fact that the most common clinical features of the syndrome are highly prevalent in the general population (e.g., obesity, hypertension, carbohydrate intolerance) and even the association of more than one feature is not uncommon (e.g., obesity, hypertension, and diabetes). Therefore, in patients in whom the history and physical findings are highly suggestive, a sequential diagnostic approach is to be followed (Figure 2). The initial diagnostic evaluation of patients suspected of having Cushing's syndrome should be directed at identifying patients with nonsuppressible cortisol output by using a screening test such as the overnight dexamethasone suppression. As an important preliminary step all drugs should be stopped, if possible, during the diagnostic period. This is important in view of the fact that a large number of analgesics, tranquilizers, diuretics, and antimicrobial agents are known to interfere with the technique for determination of the 17-hydroxycorticosteroid (17-OHCS or Porter–Silber chromogen) and 17-ketosteroids. Furthermore, some drugs may induce changes in cortisol secretion, metabolism, or excretion or may interfere with drugs used for diagnostic purposes, such as dexamethasone or metapyrone, leading to unreliable results.

Screening Tests

Overnight Dexamethasone Suppression Test. As an outpatient screening test, the overnight dexamethasone suppression test is the simplest, most reliable test (273,289). Test results have been found to be abnormal in approximately 98% of patients with Cushing's syndrome. In a review of 154 patients with Cushing's syndrome from 13 series only three patients (1.9%) showed normal suppression (74). False positive results were seen in 1.1% of 466 normal control subjects. However, 13% of 173 obese control subjects and 23% of 320 hospitalized, chronically ill controls gave false positive results (74). Furthermore, patients taking Dilantin or potent

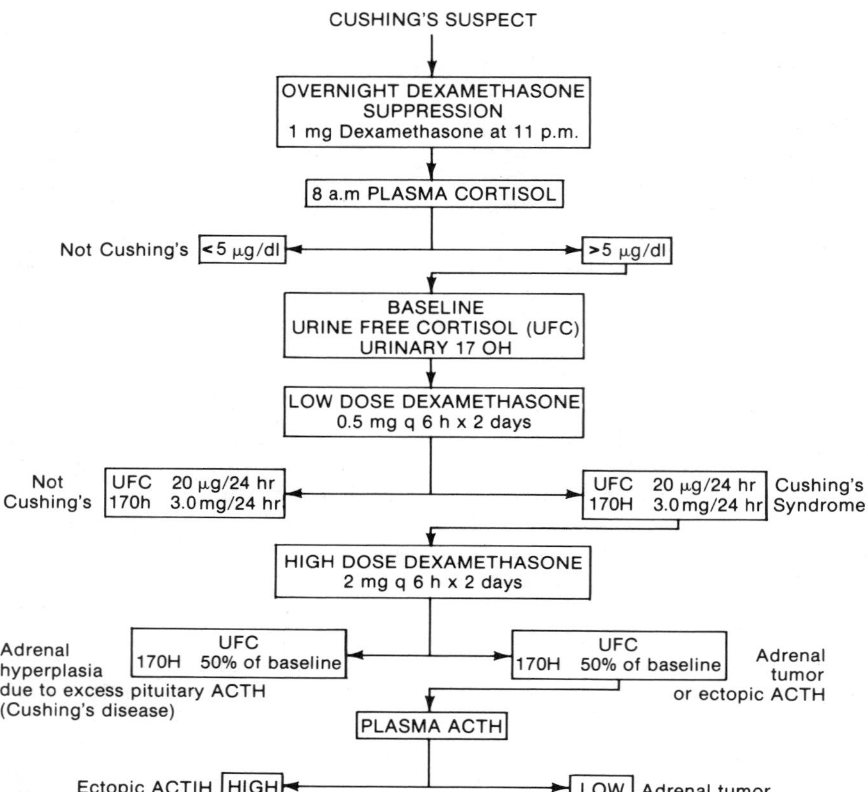

FIGURE 2. Diagnostic flowchart for patients suspected of having Cushing's syndrome.

estrogens may show false positive results (15,273). The test is performed by administering 1 mg of dexamethasone orally at 11:00 P.M. and then obtaining a plasma cortisol between 8:00 and 9:00 A.M. the following morning. In normal persons the early morning surge of ACTH is suppressed by this dose of dexamethasone and the 8:00 A.M. plasma cortisol is generally 5 μg/dl or less. In patients with Cushing's syndrome, cortisol secretion is not suppressed and the 8:00 A.M. plasma cortisol usually exceeds 10 μg/dL. Although there was marked variation among the different studies in the upper limit of normal of the 8:00 A.M. plasma cortisol after the overnight dexamethasone suppression, (range 3.5–10 μg/dL), recently the test has become more standardized and most authors accept 5 μg/dL as the upper normal range (87,332,395). Because of the high reliability of this test, normal suppression of the 8:00 A.M. plasma cortisol virtually excludes patients with Cushing's syndrome. On the other hand, any patient showing lack of suppression should undergo further confirmatory tests.

Plasma Cortisol. Plasma cortisol can be measured by a variety of techniques, including colorimetric assays using the Porter–Silber reaction (298,356), fluorimetrically (85,242), double-isotope derivative assays (188), competitive protein binding (255), or radioimmunoassay. Because of the high sensitivity, specificity, and reliability, the radioimmunoassay of plasma cortisol is now the method of choice in the majority of clinical and research laboratories. Several studies have shown that the plasma cortisol level is characterized by a series of peaks and troughs resulting from episodic secretion of cortisol. Combined studies of plasma cortisol in normal subjects and patients with Cushing's syndrome indicate that it is very difficult to make the diagnosis of Cushing's syndrome with basal plasma cortisol measurements (74).

Diurnal Variation. Although patients with Cushing's syndrome often lack the normal diurnal variation of plasma cortisol it has been shown that this test is not reliable for the definitive diagnosis of Cushing's. By use of the criteria of Krieger et al. (193) which defines a normal diurnal variation as a pattern where all plasma cortisol levels from 4:00 P.M. to midnight should be less than 75% of the 8:00 A.M. plasma cortisol, 77% of patients with Cushing's syndrome reported by Nichols et al. (269) had evening plasma cortisol levels less than 75% of the 8:00 A.M. level (74). Even changing the definition of normal diurnal variation from 75%–50% of the 8:00 A.M. cortisol level, the distinction between Cushing's patients and normal control subjects remained poor (74).

Urinary Free Cortisol. Determination of urinary free cortisol is an excellent screening test for the diagnosis of Cushing's syndrome. Urinary free cortisol represents cortisol that is excreted in the urine in an unconjugated and unaltered form. The sensitivity of this method is based on the fact that all of the "free cortisol" in the plasma (not bound to cortisol-binding globulin, CBG) is filterable at the glomerulus. In hypercortisolism when plasma cortisol exceeds 20 μg/dL, CBG is saturated and the concentration of free plasma cortisol rises with a proportional increase in the filtered load at the glomerulus resulting in high urinary free cortisol excretion. Urinary free cortisol is measured by organic solvent extraction of urine followed by a colorimetric method (318), competitive protein binding assay (256), or radioimmunoassay. Similar to plasma cortisol, the preferred method widely used in clinical laboratories is the radioimmunoassay. In a review of 479 lean, obese, and chronically ill subjects from 15 separate studies, 3.3% had elevated 24-hour urinary free cortisol (74) and only 5.6% of 248 patients with Cushing's syndrome had normal urinary free cortisol excretion. Normal nonstressed persons excrete less than 100 μg/24 hours as measured by radioimmunoassay.

Urinary 17-hydroxycorticosteroids (17-OHCS). The 24-hour urinary excretion of 17-OHCS can be used as another measure of the cortisol production rate. The 17-OHCS are measured by the Porter–Silber reaction between phenylhydrazine and corticosteroids containing 17,21 dihydroxy -20 ketosteroids side chain (298). This reaction measures about 50% of the metabolites of cortisol appearing in the urine (108). The Porter–Silber reaction does not measure all of the 17-OHCS. Total 17-OHCS can be measured by conversion of the 17-OHCS to 17-ketosteroids followed by assay by the Zimmerman reaction (271). These compounds are called 17-ketogenic steroids (17-KGS). Normal urinary excretion of 17-OHCS was found in 11% of 354 patients with Cushing's syndrome (74) and false positive results occurred in 27% of 173 obese control subjects. The urinary excretion of 17-ketogenic steroids is even less specific or reliable as shown by normal urinary excretion in 24% of 235 patients with Cushing's syndrome (74). A better discrimination between obese subjects and normal subjects is obtained by expressing the urinary excretion of 17-OHCS as per gram of creatinine per day (373). Normal urinary excretion rate of 17-OHCS is 3–7 mg/g of creatinine/24 hours, whereas patients with Cushing's have excretion rates greater than 9 mg/g of creatinine/day (220).

Determination of urinary creatinine is of critical importance to assess the completeness of collection when several 24-hour urines are obtained. Creatinine excretion in an individual subject is relatively constant and day-to-day variations should not exceed 20%. In spite of the shortcomings, the determination of 17-OHCS has been a valuable asset for the study of adrenocortical function.

17-Ketosteroids. Measurement of the 17-ketosteroids has no diagnostic value in Cushing's syndrome. Urinary 17-ketosteroids can be normal, subnormal, or supernormal (220). However, great elevations of the 17-ketosteroids are seen in over half of the patients with adrenal carcinoma.

Diagnostic Tests

Low-Dose Dexamethasone Suppression. The low-dose dexamethasone suppression was first introduced by Liddle in 1960 (219). This test is the most reliable and discriminating diagnostic test for Cushing's syndrome. After collecting two baseline samples for determinations of urinary free cortisol and 17-OHCS, 0.5 mg of dexamethasone are given orally every 6 hours for 2 consecutive days. On the second day of administration of dexamethasone, another 24-hour urine is obtained for determination of urinary free cortisol and 17-OHCS. In normal subjects the urinary excretion of 17-OHCS is suppressed to less than 3 mg/24 hours or 2.5 mg/g of creatinine/day (383,395) or the free urinary cortisol below 20 μg/24 hours (50,92). Only 3.1% of 225 separate patients with Cushing's syndrome had normal suppression of the 17-OHCS or 17-KGS (74) and two of 45 patients (4.2%) showed normal suppression of the urinary free cortisol. In spite of the reliability of the test, there have been several reports of patients with Cushing's syndrome that showed normal suppression and some that showed paradoxical responses to dexamethasone. The normal suppressibility of Cushing's patients has been attributed to abnormalities of dexamethasone metabolism (56,59,247,337) or periodic hormonogenesis (18, 46,62,216,319). On the other hand, some patients without Cushing's syndrome show lack of suppressibility after dexamethasone. This is particularly common in patients with severe mental depression (27,52), patients taking dilantin (173), or in chronic alcoholics (204,309,360).

In order to avoid the inconvenience associated with 24-hour urine collection, such as mistakes during the collection of the specimen which may lead to erroneous results, several investigators have attempted to measure the plasma cortisol values at different times of the day following two days of dexamethasone administration. Besser and Liddle proposed that the values in plasma cortisol should be less than 5 μg/dl after 2 days of 0.5 mg of dexamethasone (27,222). However, there is not enough published data to establish the validity and reliability of this criteria. In a prospective study, Aschraft et al. (16), recently tried to establish the cut-off point of serum cortisol during the second day of low- and high-dose dexamethasone suppression test. In their study a level of 5 μg/dL, or less, at 4:00 P.M. during the second day of the low-dose dexamethasone test was selected as the cut-off point and it provided a sensitivity of 86% and a specificity of 92%. Also, they established a cut-off point of 10 μg/dL at 4:00 P.M. (1600 hours) during the second day of high-dose dexamethasone. With these levels the sensitivity of the test was 100% and the specificity 92%. These values compared favorably with the 17-OHCS using a cut-off point of 4 mg/24 hours which had a sensitivity of 78% and a specificity of 93%. This test offers many advantages, but, in view of the relatively small number of patients studied in this fashion, further clinical experience is necessary to establish the validity and reliability of this criterion.

Differential Diagnosis of Cushing's Syndrome

High-Dose Dexamethasone Suppression. This test was also described by Liddle in 1960 (219). The test is performed by administering 2 mg of dexamethasone orally every 6 hours for 2 consecutive days and then determining the 24-hour urinary excretion of 17-hydroxycorticosteroids and urinary free cortisol during the second day of administration of dexamethasone. Failure to suppress with the low-dose dexamethasone, but suppression to less than 50% of the baseline values of urinary free cortisol or 17-OHCS, is highly suggestive of pituitary Cushing's, that is, bilateral adrenal hyperplasia caused by an excess of pituitary ACTH. A reduction of 40%–50% of the baseline values was found in 87% of 165 patients with Cushing's disease (74). Patients with Cushing's disease associated with nodular adrenal hyperplasia may or may not show suppression. Approximately 60% of them do not suppress. In a recent review of 43 patients with nodular adrenal hyperplasia, Aron et al. (12) found no suppression with the high dexamethasone dose in 67% of the cases.

Approximately one-quarter of the patients with the ectopic ACTH syndrome, especially those patients with bronchial carcinoids, show suppression with the high dexamethasone dose.

The majority of the unexpected responses to dexamethasone are probably the result of spontaneous, cyclic, endogenous changes in cortisol production. Careful studies in four patients with Cushing's syndrome indicate that in some patients there are cyclic episodes of high endogenous cortisol production which alternate with periods of normal or low cortisol production. In two patients with Cushing's disease and pituitary tumors, there were spontaneous, cyclic periods of 11 (46) and 85 days (216). Furthermore, two patients with ectopic ACTH caused by ACTH-secreting bronchial adenoma showed cyclic periods of 7 days (62) and 18 days (18). This phenomenon could explain some of the "paradoxical responses" to dexamethasone in patients in whom an endogenous high cycle starts between the collection of the baseline sample and the dexamethasone suppression test (317). Similarly, lack of suppression with the high dexamethasone dose in patients with pituitary Cushing's, and suppression of patients with the ectopic ACTH, can also be explained by this phenomenon. Therefore, it is often important to repeat the dexamethasone testing at several intervals for an accurate differential diagnosis of the cause of Cushing's syndrome. Resistance to dexamethasone suppression can also be found in patients with Cushing's disease due to tumors or hyperplasia of the intermediate lobe of the pituitary (206) which, in contrast to the anterior lobe tumors, are relatively resistant to dexamethasone.

The mechanism by which dexamethasone causes a reduction in ACTH and cortisol output in Cushing's disease is not known. An abnormally high "set point" for negative feedback by plasma cortisol at the level of the hypothalamus or at the pituitary level could explain the pathophysiological basis of this syndrome and the response to the high-dose dexamethasone. Whether a deficiency or abnormality of glucocorticoid receptors of the pituitary corticotrophs or the CRF-producing cells of the median eminence is responsible for this phenomenon has not been ascertained.

Plasma ACTH. With the development of sensitive and specific techniques for measurement of ACTH in plasma, the assay of ACTH has become important in the differential diagnosis of Cushing's syndrome. Plasma ACTH can be measured by bioassay measuring the corticosterone levels in the adrenal vein of hypophysectomized rats in response to injections of ACTH (226,227). Although this assay is reliable, it is relatively insensitive. A more sensitive bioassay is that described by Sawyer and Beall (333), using the corticosterone response of isolated rat adrenal cells to ACTH extracted from plasma. This assay can detect plasma ACTH concentrations in the order of 5 pg/mL. Another sensitive bioassay is the radioreceptor assay (215,400). This assay is based on competitive binding of ACTH to the ACTH-receptors isolated from rat adrenal cells. The sensitivity of this assay is also approximately 5 pg/mL. The most sensitive assay for ACTH is the cytochemical redox bioassay of Chayen et al. (64,306). This assay employs the change in redox state of guinea pig adrenal cells induced by ACTH which leads to a change in the prussian blue staining which is detected by a scanning differential microdensitometer. This assay is capable of detecting ACTH quantities in the femtogram range (10^{-15}g/mL). This assay can detect plasma ACTH levels which may be undetectable by any other technique. In a patient with adrenal adenoma causing Cushing's syndrome, the circulating level of ACTH measured by cytochemical redox technique was 80 fg/mL. Unfortunately, all of the bioassay techniques for ACTH are technically difficult and because only a relatively small number of samples can be processed every day; these assays are not practical and, therefore, are not available for clinical use (82,146).

ACTH Radioimmunoassay. The radioimmunoassay of ACTH is highly specific and sensitive for ACTH (23,281,307). With recent improvements this assay is now available in many clinical laboratories and is one of the most reliable procedures for the differential diagnosis of Cushing's syndrome. Similar to plasma cortisol, plasma ACTH levels demonstrate frequent, large fluctuations in normal subjects, as well as in patients with Cushing's disease (74). All 45 patients with adrenal adenomas reviewed by Crapo (74) had undetectable ACTH levels. Patients with Cushing's disease (189 patients) had either normal or elevated ACTH levels and patients with ectopic ACTH had markedly elevated levels of ACTH (150 patients), although there was significant overlap in the levels of these two groups of patients. Patients with nodular adrenal hyperplasia may have low, normal, or high levels of ACTH (67,305,322). On occasions, differentiation between pituitary Cushing's and ectopic Cushing's may be difficult after standard testing. In these rare cases, selective venous catheterization of the pituitary venous drainage for measurements of ACTH may help to establish a cranial to peripheral gradient in ACTH concentration which helps in the localization of the tumor (72,308). Selective catheterization of other vascular beds has also helped to identify ectopic sources of ACTH (344). Another recent approach to differentiate pituitary from ectopic Cushing's has been the measurement of other peptides derived from the common precursor, POMC. Plasma concentrations of ACTH and β-LPH are equimolar under basal conditions and after several stimuli (129,195,380).

In patients with Cushing's disease and Nelson's syndrome the blood levels of several POMC-derived peptides are elevated. Elevations of plasma ACTH, β-LPH, β-endorphin, γ-LPH, and the 16K N-terminal fragment of POMC have been reported (26,63,119,147,148,195,376). In patients with Cushing's disease the molar ratio of ACTH/β-LPH has been reported to be lower than in normal subjects, whereas the ratio of β-endorphin/β-LPH is higher than in normal subjects (196). However, other investigators have reported higher than normal ACTH/β-LPH ratio in patients with Cushing's disease (119) and low ACTH/β-LPH ratio in patients with ectopic Cushing's. Unfortunately, because of the presence of common sequences in several of the POMC-derived peptides, and the different degrees of crossreactivity and specificity of the antibodies employed for these studies, as well as differences in the metabolic clearance rates of these peptides, the reliability of this approach is questionable and therefore of limited value for the differential diagnosis of Cushing's disease.

Other Tests

The Metyrapone Test. The metyrapone test was introduced by Liddle et al. (217,218). Metyrapone is a powerful inhibitor of 11-β-hydroxylase and, therefore, blocks the synthesis of cortisol at the level of 11-deoxycortisol. As a consequence in normal subjects and patients with Cushing's disease (pituitary Cushing's) there is a compensatory increase in ACTH which, in turn, increases adrenal synthesis of steroids to the step of 11-deoxycortisol (compound S). The increased levels of compound S can be measured in plasma or urine and can cause a concomitant increase in the levels of 17-OHCS. The test consists of the administration of 750 mg of metyrapone orally every 4 hours for a total of six doses. Daily 24-hour urines are collected for determination of 17-OHCS on the day before, the day of administration of metyrapone, and the day after. Normal subjects show a two- to fourfold increase in the 24-hour urine excretion of 17-OHCS on the day of administration of metyrapone or the day after. Patients with pituitary Cushing's show a significant increase in the urinary excretion of 17-OHCS and often an exaggerated response to metyrapone. Patients with adrenal tumors show either no change or fall in the excretion of 17-OHCS. Approximately 50% of the patients with nodular adrenal hyperplasia and ectopic ACTH may show a response to metyrapone (74). Dilantin or estrogen treatment may cause a false-negative test by increasing the metabolism of metyrapone (245,246). This problem can be overcome by doubling the dose of metyrapone. In a recent study comparing the accuracy of the metyrapone test against the high dexamethasone test for differentiation of pituitary Cushing's from adrenal Cushing's, Sindler et al. (359) reported the metyrapone test as superior (100%) to the high dexamethasone test (81%) for this purpose in a series of 25 consecutive patients with Cushing's syndrome.

Corticotropin-Releasing Factor Stimulation Test. Recently, Chrousos et al. (68a) reported that injection of corticotropin-releasing factor was helpful in differentiating patients with Cushing's disease from those with the ectopic ACTH syndrome. In 13 patients with pituitary Cushing's, injections of ovine corticotropin-releasing hormone (1 μg/kg) caused a further increase in the already high levels of plasma ACTH and cortisol. On the other hand, six patients with the ectopic ACTH syndrome with high basal levels of plasma ACTH and cortisol did not respond to the injections of

CRF. Unfortunately, others have found that the plasma ACTH and cortisol responses to CRF in patients with Cushing's disease are quite variable (285a). Furthermore, Lytras et al. (234a) reported a patient with ectopic ACTH syndrome that responded to CRF. Therefore, it appears that although the CRF stimulation test may provide a more rapid test, it is unlikely that it will replace the dexamethasone suppression test in the differential diagnosis of Cushing's syndrome.

ACTH-stimulation Test. The ACTH-stimulation test has been used by several investigators for the differential diagnosis of Cushing's syndrome (74). However, there is considerable overlap, and in our experience it does not add any significant information to the diagnosis of the cause of Cushing's syndrome. Most patients with pituitary Cushing's show an exaggerated response to ACTH. The majority of patients with adrenal carcinoma do not respond to ACTH and approximately 50% of patients with adrenal adenoma may respond to ACTH.

The cortisol production rate (70,291) has also been used for the diagnosis of Cushing's syndrome. Unfortunately, although it may be a useful measurement, it is not clinically available and is used primarily for research purposes. The excretion of 6-β-hydroxycortisol is higher than normal in patients with Cushing's syndrome and has been suggested as a good test for the diagnosis of Cushing's syndrome(390).

Insulin Tolerance Test. This test consists of the administration of 0.05−0.1 units of regular insulin/kg of body weight and determinations of the plasma cortisol before and at 30-minute intervals for 1½ hours (28, 207). Lowering of the plasma glucose below 40 mg/dL causes an increase of 5−8 μg/dL in the plasma cortisol level to a level usually greater than 15−25 μg/dL in normal subjects. Patients with Cushing's syndrome often do not respond to insulin-induced hypoglycemia. In a review by Crapo (74) approximately 18% of 74 patients with primary Cushing's syndrome had a normal cortisol response rendering this test of questionable value for the diagnosis. It is claimed, however, that this test is useful in the differentiation of severely depressed patients with nonsuppressible levels of cortisol from patients with Cushing's syndrome. In contrast to Cushing's patients, depressed patients usually have a plasma cortisol response to insulin-induced hypoglycemia (27,52).

The administration of lysine vasopressin by the intravenous or intramuscular route has been used by some investigators for the differential diagnosis of Cushing's syndrome (131,207). Normal subjects and patients with Cushing's disease show an increment in cortisol after the injection of LVP, whereas patients with adrenal adenomas do not respond (29). In a recent study Raux et al. (305) reported that in patients with pituitary tumors causing radiological destruction of the sella turcica, LVP caused a more than threefold higher increment in ACTH as compared to those without a demonstrable pituitary tumor. Table 4 shows the most commonly used test in the differential diagnosis of Cushing's syndrome.

Radiological Examinations. A variety of radiological examinations, including skull x-rays with cone down views of the sella turcica, polytomograms, computerized tomography (CT), pneumoencephalography, venography, and angiography, are used for the diagnosis of Cushing's syndrome. Gross enlargement of the sella turcica by conventional skull or sella turcica roentgenograms is found in only 15% of cases (235,321,326). However, with the use of multidirectional polytomography (hypocycloid or triaxial) approximately 40%–60% of microadenomas produce sufficient alterations in the bony walls of the sella turcica to suggest the presence of an intrasellar tumor (134,153,327,339,385). With the advent of CT and the remarkable improvements of the third- and fourth-generation scanners, evaluation of the pituitary fossa by CT has become a very important tool for the detection of pituitary microadenomas. Axial and coronal sections with and without contrast infusion permit sagittal and coronal reconstructions without further scanning. The sensitivity and specificity of CT in the evaluation of pituitary tumors vary in relation to the degree of sellar enlargement and the presence of extrasellar extensions (153). The CT examination of pituitary fossa is remarkably sensitive in detection of suprasellar extension and is now the procedure of choice for this purpose. Furthermore, CT scan after intrathecal injection of metrizamide provides similar information to that obtained by pneumoencephalogram and has recently become the preferred test for the visualization of an empty sella. Although highly sensitive, the specificity of CT in the evaluation of suprasellar masses is lower. Very large suprasellar extensions of pituitary tumors, especially those located anteriorly in the suprasellar cistern, may be difficult to differentiate from other kinds of tumors. Small anterior extensions may be confused with aneurysms and meningiomas. Para-

TABLE 4. Laboratory Tests in the Differential Diagnosis of Cushing's Syndrome

	Plasma Cortisol			Baseline urinary Steroids	
	Overnight dexamethasone suppression	Diurnal rhythm	Plasma ACTH	Urinary free cortisol μg/24 hr	17-OHCS mg/g creatinine
Normal	<5 μg/dl	N	N	<100	3-7
Pituitary-dependent adrenal hyperplasia	↑	A	N° or ↑	↑	↑
Autonomous adrenal tumor	↑	A	↓ or U	↑	↑
Ectopic ACTH	↑	A	↑↑	↑↑	↑↑

Abbreviations: A = absent; N = normal; NC = no change; U = undetectable; ° = "inappropriately" high for levels of plasma cortisol.

sellar extensions, on the other hand, are easier to differentiate from other lesions. In a preliminary evaluation of the experience at the Mayo Clinic, Houser et al. (153) reported that approximately 70% of surgically proven microadenomas could be detected by CT scan. Distortions of the sellar wall was the most common finding, being present in approximately 50% of the cases.

Pneumoencephalography was widely used in the past for evaluation of suprasellar extensions and for exclusion of an empty sella. However, the combined use of CT scan and the intrathecal injection of metrizamide has replaced pneumoencephalography as the procedure of choice for these purposes.

Angiography. Bilateral common or internal carotid angiograms are performed with magnification ×2 and single-order substraction (153). Kricheff and Schotland (192) were the first to report a tumor "stain" in a pituitary tumor. However, it was not until Powel et al. (299) identified abnormalities of the cavernous branches of the internal carotid that the potential of this technique for the evaluation of pituitary tumors was recognized. A localized intrasellar stain on the magnified lateral view was present in 70% of patients with microadenomas of all types and in over 80% of patients with ACTH-secreting tumors (153). Angiography is also useful in ruling out the possibility of aneurysms and meningiomas. With the continuing improvement and high resolution in the CT scanners, it is likely that angiography may not be necessary in the future. Moreover, preliminary experience with the nuclear magnetic resonance scanning appears to be a very promising technique for the evaluation of the pituitary.

TABLE 4. *(continued)*

Low-dose dexamethasone test		**High-dose dexamethasone test**		
Urinary free cortisol μg/24 hr	**17-)CHS mb/24 hr**	**Urinary free cortisol μg/24 hr**	**17-OCHS mg/24 hr creatinine**	**Metyrapone test (17-OHCS)**
<20	<3.0	<20	<3.0	2–4 X baseline
↑	↑	<50% baseline	<50% baseline	3–6 X baseline
↑	↑	↑	↑	NC or ↓
↑	↑	↑	↑	NC or ↑

For the diagnosis of adrenal Cushing's, computerized axial tomography is the most useful tool for the detection of adrenal tumors and for bilateral hyperplasia of the adrenals (Figure 3) (91). Occasionally, adrenal masses may be discovered incidentally during the course of an examination for other purposes (71). Ultrasound has also been useful in the evaluation of adrenal tumors (328,403,404). Selective adrenal arteriography is of value in demonstrating small adrenal tumors (176). Retrograde venography has also been used in the past but should only be done in selected cases and by an experienced radiologist. Venography offers the advantage of being able to obtain cortisol measurements from the venous affluents of both adrenals in addition to outlining the adrenal pathology (312). However, the incidence of complications is relatively high. Hemorrhage of the adrenal develops in approximately 5% (61,270) of the cases and failure to visualize the right adrenal occurs in approximately 15% of the cases.

A number of isotopic procedures have recently been developed for the evaluation of the adrenal glands. Adrenal scanning using ^{131}I-19-iodocholesterol was first introduced by Beierwaltes et al. in 1971 (21,223). A significant improvement in the technique was accomplished with the use of ^{131}I-6β-iodomethyl-19-norcholesterol (NP-59) (331,381) which, in their hands, had a diagnostic accuracy of 90% or greater for Cushing's syndrome. The patterns of imaging in Cushing's syndrome depend upon the etiology of the process involved. In Cushing's syndrome, caused by pituitary-dependent ACTH excess, or ectopic ACTH syndrome, the scans

FIGURE 3. CAT scan of the abdomen demonstrating a large left adrenal adenoma in a patient with Cushing's syndrome.

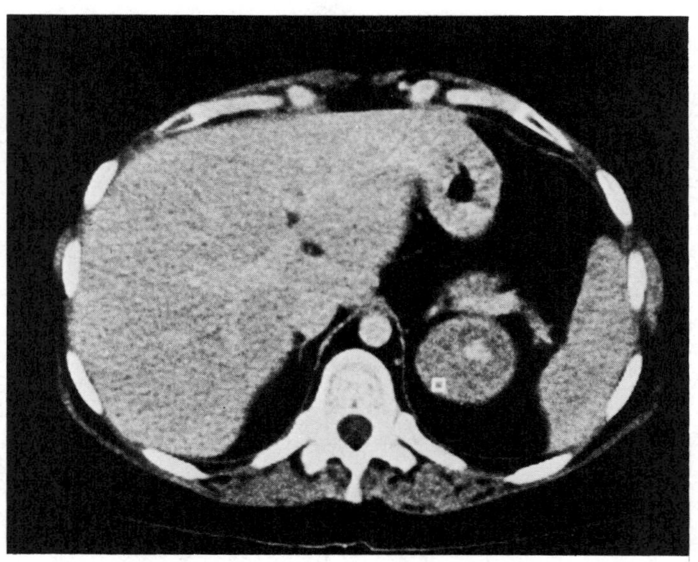

demonstrate excessive bilateral adrenal cortical uptake of the tracer (331, 343,381). Autonomous adrenal function from either nodular hyperplasia or a solitary adenoma shows either marked asymmetry or unilateral visualization and functioning adrenal carcinoma provides a pattern of bilateral nonvisualization (350,381). Also, Gross et al. (127) showed that in patients with ACTH-dependent Cushing's syndrome, there was a significant correlation between the urinary free cortisol excretion and the level of NP-59 adrenal uptake suggesting that the quantitative uptake of iodocholesterol may be another parameter to estimate adrenal disease activity in Cushing's (127). Recently, Shapiro et al. (351) reported their experience using a new adrenal imaging agent, ^{75}SE-seleno-methylcholesterol. Overall predictability of the type of adrenal disorder was 90.6% in 12 cases of Cushing's disease, seven cases of ectopic ACTH, five cases of unilateral adenoma, three cases of adrenal carcinoma, and three cases of postadrenalectomy regrowths. This isotope offers the advantage of a longer adrenal retention time permitting scanning 14 days or longer after the administration of the isotope, a time when the nonadrenal background activity has fallen to a low level. However, the total radiation dose is similar to that of iodocholesterol.

The diagnosis of ectopic Cushing's may require several specialized radiographic and endoscopic techniques. However, since bronchogenic carcinoma is the most frequent cause of ectopic ACTH, chest roentgenograms localized the tumor in 50% of the cases (17,221). Establishment of ACTH gradients by selective venous sampling may be helpful in some cases (308,344). The CT scanning of the chest and abdomen have recently become the most useful test for localization of the tumor. Among other procedures used in Cushing's syndrome, x-rays of the spine show variable degrees of osteoporosis and in some patients, isolated skeletal involvement secondary to Cushing's syndrome has been the only clinical expression of the disease (152). Visual field examinations and perimetry are sensitive indicators of compression of the optic chiasma.

Differential Diagnosis. Patients with Cushing's syndrome must be differentiated from patients with cushingoid habitus, which may be hypertensive, diabetic with hirsutism and menstrual irregularities. The overnight dexamethasone test is especially helpful for this purpose. Some patients with severe mental depression may show several of the biochemical abnormalities of Cushing's syndrome; however, depressed patients often lack the clinical manifestations of the syndrome. According to Besser and Edwards (27), insulin-induced hypoglycemia causes a release of cortisol in depressed patients whereas it does not in patients with Cushing's syndrome (27). Some chronic alcoholic patients develop a cushingoid habitus and hypersecretion of cortisol. The biochemical abnormalities of alcohol-induced pseudo-Cushing's syndrome revert to normal on ethanol withdrawal (101,171,204,309,360). Therefore, if diagnostic errors are to be avoided, a history of alcohol intake should always be sought in a patient in whom the diagnosis of Cushing's syndrome is suspected.

Treatment

The treatment of Cushing's syndrome should be directed toward the primary abnormality causing hypersecretion of cortisol. Therefore, differentiation between pituitary Cushing's, adrenal Cushing's, and ectopic ACTH is of fundamental importance for proper treatment.

Treatment of Cushing's Disease (Pituitary Cushing's). Several treatments have been used for the therapy of pituitary Cushing's, including pituitary surgery, adrenalectomy, pituitary radiation, and pharmacologic therapy. With the refinement of transsphenoidal microsurgery and the high incidence of microadenomas, transsphenoidal microsurgery is presently the treatment of choice for Cushing's disease, even in patients in whom there is no detectable abnormality of the sella turcica. In Hardy's experience of 75 operations, initial cure was obtained in 63 cases (84%) and two of these patients had recurrences 10 and 30 months later. The initial cure was greater in patients with noninvasive tumors, 50 of 59 patients (88%). Also, in 10 of 12 patients without evidence of tumor, in whom a partial or total hypophysectomy was performed, correction of the hypercortisolism was accomplished in 83% of the cases (134). All patients who had successful correction of the hypercortisolism developed transient adrenal insufficiency and required maintenance doses of cortisol for periods of 3–12 months after the operation (134). Similarly, in the Mayo Clinic series of 66 operations, clincial remission and correction of hypercortisolism was accomplished in 53 patients (80%). In 51 of the 53 patients remission was associated with very low postoperative plasma cortisol level and restoration of the normal hypothalamic pituitary adrenal axis required several months. Recurrences have occurred in two of the 53 patients with an average follow-up period of 20 months (214). In the third largest series, reported by Wilson et al. (399), of 37 patients undergoing transsphenoidal microsurgery (31 microadenomas and six macroadenomas) initial cure was accomplished in 28 of the 31 microadenomas (90%) and three of the six macroadenomas (50%), for an overall initial cure rate of 84% (399). In most instances successful correction of hypercortisolism was followed by resumption of normal hypothalamic pituitary function.

Similar experiences have been reported from Europe. In the British series of Carmalt, 11 of the 12 patients with Cushing's disease were in complete remission 2–11 years after the operation (55).

In most instances successful correction of hypercortisolism is followed by transient secondary adrenal insufficiency (100) although few successfully treated patients have not experienced hypoadrenalism or required supplemental therapy with glucocorticoids in the postoperative period (32). In most successfully treated patients there is restoration of normal hypothalamic–pituitary–adrenal function after surgery. In Fitzgerald's experience, dexamethasone suppressibility returned to normal 8–18 months postoperatively and the majority of patients had a normal cortisol response to ACTH stimulation and insulin hypoglycemia (100); also, the abnormalities of other pituitary hormones are usually corrected postoperatively. On the other hand circadian periodicity of cortisol remains abnormal in approximately half of the patients for periods of up to 18 months after surgery (41,201,399).

Recently Lambert et al. (205) reported failure of clinical remission after transsphenoidal removal of a microadenoma surrounded by hyperplastic adenomatous cells (205). In a subsequent report the same group of investigators describe the clinical and biochemical characteristics of six patients thought to have tumors or hyperplasia of cells derived from the intermediate lobe of the pituitary. In this group of patients transsphenoidal microsurgery is less successful and recurrence rates appear to be high. If confirmed by other investigators, these observations may be important for the selection of patients with Cushing's disease to undergo transsphenoidal resection, since in patients with intermediate lobe tumors dopamine agonist and cyproheptadine may be the treatment of choice (206).

Adrenalectomy. Prior to the refinement in the technique for transphenoidal hypophysectomy and up to the late 1960s and early 1970s bilateral adrenalectomy was considered to be the treatment of choice for Cushing's disease (142,248,280,347,348,367). Bilateral adrenalectomy has the advantage of rapid correction of hypercortisolism. However, it carries a significant operative mortality ranging from 4% to 10% of the cases in different series (96,393). Furthermore, it requires lifelong dependency on replacement therapy with glucocorticoids and mineralocorticoids. Recurrent hypercortisolism from hyperplastic adrenal remnants or ectopic adrenal tissue occurs in approximately 10% of the cases (96,287). Rapid growth of pituitary tumors and hyperpigmentation occurs postoperatively in 8%–20% of the cases (Nelson's syndrome) (259,326). To avoid lifelong dependency on replacement with adrenocortical hormones, total adrenalectomy followed by adrenal autotransplantation has been attempted with limited success (179). Today, total bilateral adrenalectomy is the treatment of choice for patients with micro- or macronodular hyperplasia of both adrenals and in selected patients in whom recurrences after transsphenoidal hypophysectomy or radiation to the pituitary have occurred.

Pituitary Irradiation. Pituitary irradiation has been used as an alternative and as an adjunct to surgery in Cushing's disease. Conventional cobalt 60 (high-voltage radiotherapy, dosage of 4,000–5,000 rads delivered over a period of one month is generally safe). A major shortcoming of this type of therapy is the considerable lag period necessary for correction of the hypercortisolism which in some patients may take 12–18 months after completion of radiotherapy. In the experience of Vanderbilt University Hospital, pituitary radiation cured 10 of 51 patients (20%) and improvement was observed in 13 additional patients (25%) (280). In other series the success rate of pituitary radiation varies from 40% to 83% of cases (88,143,362).

Pituitary radiation appears to be more effective in children than in adults. In a recent report 12 of 15 children with Cushing's disease treated by pituitary radiation were cured (169). This type of pituitary radiation does not affect linear growth, fertility, or other functions of the pituitary gland. However, in a small number of patients malignant cranial neoplasms have been reported following radiation (121,363,391).

Photon beam irradiation delivering 10,000−15,000 rads to the pituitary over five days has been employed by two groups of investigators (186,224) with a reported cure rate of 60% of cases and improvement in an additional 30% (212). Unfortunately, the incidence of cranial nerve paralysis and permanent pituitary failure is higher, approaching approximately 8% of cases (42,186). It appears that with the recent improvements in the linear accelerator delivery systems the morbidity may be reduced (225).

Pituitary implantation of yttrium 90 or gold 198 has been reported to be effective for the treatment of Cushing's disease and Nelson's syndrome, with improvement in 81% of patients (51,58); however, radiation implants require transsphenoidal surgery and have been associated with pituitary necrosis and permanent hypopituitarism in some cases.

Pharmacologic Therapy. Pharmacologic therapy for Cushing's disease can be divided into two major groups of agents: 1) drugs that may interfere with the neurotransmitter regulation of CRF and/or ACTH; and 2) drugs that inhibit one or more enzymatic steps in the biosynthesis of cortisol. In addition to the inhibition of steroid biosynthesis some drugs such as *o,p'*-DDD (mitotane) have a direct adrenolytic effect. Experimental evidence indicates that ACTH secretion is regulated by a number of neurotransmitters. Serotonin is thought to stimulate the release of CRF and dopamine is an inhibitor of ACTH secretion. This experimental evidence led several groups of investigators to the use of serotonin antagonist and dopamine agonist for the treatment of Cushing's disease and Nelson's syndrome. Cyproheptadine is a drug with peripheral as well as central antiserotoninergic actions. In normal subjects cyproheptadine appears to block ACTH release, acting at the level of the hypothalamus. Cyproheptadine blocks the ACTH response to metyrapone (296), and the nocturnal rise in plasma ACTH concentration (65). On the other hand, cyproheptadine does not affect the adrenal response to ACTH (296). Metergoline, a more specific antiserotoninergic agent, inhibits the ACTH response to insulin-hypoglycemia (60); however, neither cyproheptadine nor metergoline block the ACTH and cortisol response to vasopressin (60,115). Krieger et al. first reported clinical improvement and reduction of ACTH and cortisol levels in a small number of patients with Cushing's disease treated with cyproheptadine. Of approximately 100 patients treated with cyproheptadine to date, the remission rate varies from 30% to 50% (196). In responsive cases, clinical and laboratory evidence of remission appears within 2−3 months after reaching a daily dose of 24 mg/day. The remission rate in children is significantly lower. The longest successful treatment period has been five years (154). Usually, relapses occurred soon after discontinuation of therapy and in some patients even while still under treatment. Major side effects are increased appetite, weight gain, and somnolence. Metergoline has been reported to be more successful in children than in adults (196).

Bromocriptine, a dopaminergic agonist, has been used in patients with Cushing's disease. In the experience of Lambert et al., six of 13 patients with Cushing's disease showed a decrease in plasma ACTH concentrations after the acute administration of bromocriptine (203). Initial clinical and laboratory improvement was reported in four of five patients who underwent chronic treatment with bromocriptine, although in two patients, escape from therapy occurred within 2–6 weeks. More recently the same group of investigators have reported that patients with anterior lobe tumors do not respond whereas patients with intermedial lobe tumors do respond to bromocriptine therapy (206). There are a number of conflicting reports in the literature, however, regarding the efficacy of bromocriptine in the treatment of Cushing's disease and Nelson's syndrome (9,174,178,183,277).

Another neurotransmitter that appears to inhibit CRF release and may play a role in glucocorticoid feedback at the hypothalamic level is gamma amino butyric acid (GABA) (4,170). Based on this evidence, the GABA agonist, sodium valproate, has been used in patients with Cushing's and Nelson's syndrome. However, Allolio et al. (8) were unable to demonstrate any effect on plasma ACTH or cortisol levels in five patients with Cushing's disease, and Dornhorst et al. (90) reported lowering of the plasma ACTH levels and restoration of circadian rhythm in only two of 10 patients with Nelson's syndrome treated with sodium valproate (Epilin), although pigmentation lightened in six patients and a reduction in the size of the tumor was demonstrated in one of 10 patients treated with valproate (90).

Opioid agonist and antagonist have been used in patients with Cushing's and Nelson's syndrome, but there is conflicting evidence at present regarding their mode of action and their effectiveness for the treatment of syndromes associated with ACTH hypersecretion (196).

Inhibitors of Steroid Biosynthesis. Several pharmacological agents that block the synthesis of cortisol have been employed for the long-term management of Cushing's disease. These include *o,p'*-DDD (mitotane), aminoglutethimide (cytadren), metyrapone (metopyrone), and trilostane (Win 24540). Agents of this type have been used for long-term management of Cushing's as well as for the purpose of reducing cortisol synthesis in preparation for surgery and while awaiting the effects of pituitary radiation. Drug combinations (e.g., aminoglutethimide and metopyrone) at lower dose levels decrease the toxicity of both compounds and may improve their clinical utility (66). Mitotane (*o,p'*-DDD) has been reported to cause remission of Cushing's disease in 38 of 46 patients undergoing treatment with *o,p'*-DDD alone and in all patients ($n = 16$) who received the drug in combination with radiation. However, 60% of these patients subsequently relapsed, although additional treatment with *o,p'*-DDD and/or radiation was effective in 63% of patients with an average follow-up period of at least three years (234). Adrenal insufficiency occurs in approximately one-third of the patients; therefore, this type of therapy requires regular monitoring of plasma cortisol. Mitotane increases the excretion of 6-β-hydroxycortisol, which interferes with the determination of the 17-hydroxycorticosteroids (17 OHCS). Permanent adrenal failure requiring lifelong replacement with corticosteroids has been reported in some cases (232). Treatment with this drug is associated with a high incidence of side effects including anorexia, nausea, vomiting, and mental depression; therefore, this drug is usually reserved for the treatment of adrenal carcinomas and for the ectopic ACTH syndrome.

Aminoglutethimide is a competitive inhibitor of the mitochondrial enzyme cholesterol side-chain cleaving enzyme and therefore its primary effect is to inhibit the conversion of cholesterol to pregnenolone. Aminoglutethimide causes a reversible medical adrenalectomy. Most of the common side effects of aminoglutethimide are related to central nervous system toxicity; these side effects include lethargy, dizziness, blurred vision, and depression.

Metyrapone inhibits 11-β-hydroxylase activity and causes a rapid reduction of plasma cortisol. By blocking cortisol biosynthesis this group of drugs may cause a compensatory increase in ACTH, which may enhance steroid biosynthesis sufficiently to overcome the "block," and therefore close surveillance of treatment and careful adjustment of the dose is required for effective therapy. Hirsutism, nausea, abdominal discomfort, sedation, dizziness, and headache are the most common side effects (167). Recently, trilostane (Win 24540), a 3-β-hydroxy dehydrogenase inhibitor, was reported to be effective in six patients with pituitary-dependent Cushing's syndrome, and in one patient with adrenal carcinoma. The drug was well tolerated except for minor gastrointestinal complaints (189). In general, this group of drugs is seldom used for the treatment of adrenal carcinoma and for the ectopic ACTH syndrome.

Treatment of Adrenal Cushing's Syndrome. Surgery is the treatment of choice for adrenal Cushing's (348). Precise localization of the tumor by CT scan or other available techniques is important prior to surgery. Cortisol-secreting adrenal tumors cause suppression of ACTH and, therefore, the adrenal tissue surrounding the adenoma as well as the contralateral adrenal are atrophic. Therefore, these patients develop adrenal insufficiency following removal of the tumor. Parenteral corticosteroid replacement should be started prior to the induction of anesthesia and tapered down to maintenance doses postoperatively until the function of the remaining adrenal tissue returns to normal. Recovery of adrenal function may take several weeks, one year, or even longer. Recovery of adrenal reserve may take even longer. A unilateral posterior extraperitoneal, or flank approach, is the most tolerated procedure and is indicated when precise tumor localization has been accomplished. On the other hand, a transabdominal approach enables the surgeon to explore the contralateral adrenal to rule out micro- or macronodular hyperplasia for which bilateral adrenalectomy is the treatment of choice. Furthermore, in a case of adrenal carcinoma the transabdominal approach permits a more complete resection of the tumor as well as detection of intraabdominal metastatic spread. Metastases occur early in adrenal carcinomas and often are present at the time of diagnosis. The lungs and liver are the most common sites of metastasis. Adrenal carcinoma is a highly malignant tumor that is usually resistant to radiation therapy. In unresectable tumors or for metastatic adrenocortical carcinomas, drug therapy may offer symptomatic relief from the metabolic effects of hypercortisolism. Mitotane, aminoglutethimide, metopyrone, and trilostane have been used for treatment of adrenocortical carcinoma. Drug combinations and sequential use of these agents may be employed in refractory cases (66). However, use of these drugs has not been shown to prolong survival of patients with adrenal carcinoma (133,157,181). Mitotane (*o,p'*-DDD) has been used for treatment of adrenal carcinoma in over 250 patients. Inhibition of cortisol production occurs in about 60% of patients and, due to the cytotoxic effect of the drugs, tumor regression occurs in some cases (145,157), although dosages of up to 20 g/day may be required to inhibit steroid synthesis, a dosage that is associated with high incidence of intolerable side effects (145). There are isolated reports, however, of prolonged survival, and a documented cure in a patient with metastatic adrenocortical carcinoma treated with mitotane and fluorouracil (286).

Ectopic Cushing's. The treatment of choice for ectopic ACTH syndrome is surgical resection of the tumor, radiotherapy, or chemotherapy. Unfortunately, the most common cause of the syndrome is small cell anaplastic carcinoma of the lung and, therefore, complete removal or permanent eradication of the tumor is seldom possible. In less aggressive tumors, such as bronchial adenomas or thymomas, complete removal may result in total cure of the syndrome (221). In rare cases successful chemotherapy of lung carcinoma has been accompanied by normalization of plasma ACTH, correction of the metabolic abnormalities caused by hypercortisolism, and prolongation of life expectancy (308). In inoperable cases, correction of the water, electrolyte, and acid-base balance abnormalities, as well as the use of adrenal enzyme inhibitors, such as *o,p'*-DDD, aminoglutethimide, and metyrapone may provide temporary symptomatic relief from hypercortisolism (102).

Course and Prognosis

The course of Cushing's syndrome is usually progressive, although spontaneous remissions have been described in few patients (141,288). It has been estimated that if the condition is untreated, the 5-year mortality is approximately 50% (297). However, the course more accurately reflects the underlying cause of the syndrome. Patients with Cushing's disease may have a fluctuating clinical course with exacerbations and remissions, whereas patients with adrenal carcinomas and those with ectopic ACTH syndrome usually have a rapid downhill course. The most common causes of death in patients with Cushing's syndrome are infection and congestive heart failure secondary to hypertensive cardiovascular disease (297).

Complications of Therapy

With the availability of steroid replacement and broad spectrum antibiotics, complications of transsphenoidal surgery, such as adrenal insufficiency and meningitis are rare. Of 807 transsphenoidal surgical procedures in 786 patients reported by Laws et al. (213) there were seven fatal postoperative complications, four of which occurred in patients with pituitary adenomas and included hypothalamic and carotid injuries, and intracranial hematomas. Major postoperative complications occurred in 11 patients, including vascular lacerations and permanent visual loss due to optic nerve infarct or surgical trauma. Permanent diabetes insipidus occurred in 16 patients, eight of which were operated for pituitary adenomas. Cerebrospinal fluid rhinorrhea developed in five patients. Among the patients with ACTH-producing tumors there were no fatalities. However, one patient developed permanent diabetes insipidus postoperatively (213). Symptomatic empty sella is another complication seen less frequently. Complications of radiation therapy include transient localized loss of hair, radiation-induced neoplasia, brain necrosis, damage to the optic nerve or chiasma, and hypopituitarism. These complications may appear several months to years after completion of irradiation. In a review of the literature, Sheline (352) found 12 fibrosarcomas and two osteosarcomas developing in irradiated tissues following radiotherapy for pituitary adenomas. The average dose for these patients was 5,000 rads, but seven of the 14 patients had multiple courses of therapy and, therefore, the total radiation dose was higher. Brain necrosis is also rare and, according to Sheline (352), only two incidences of necrosis have been reported with the conventional use of 5,000 rads or less. Optic and chiasmatic injury and hypopituitarism are rare after conventional doses of radiation (352). Of 22 patients with various types of pituitary adenomas, only one developed evidence of hypoadrenalism and hypothyroidism after conventional doses of radiotherapy (168). However, this patient had evidence of pituitary dysfunction prior to radiation.

The most common complications of bilateral adrenalectomy include thrombophlebitis and thromboembolic phenomena. There is approximately 10% mortality associated with the operation (35,96). In addition, approximately 10%–16% of patients developed hyperpigmentation and enlargement of the sella turcica by an ACTH-producing tumor (241,252, 260,261). The syndrome has been called Nelson's syndrome and appeared to be more frequent in children than in adults (149). The cause of Nelson's syndrome has been attributed to the continued growth of a previously undetected microadenoma or to an increased hypothalamic stimulation of the pituitary corticotrophs following removal of the hyperfunctioning adrenal tissue. These tumors have been reported to develop 6 months to 16 years after adrenalectomy, and it appears that pituitary radiation before adrenalectomy does not prevent their development (252). On occasion these tumors undergo rapid growth, become locally invasive, and undergo malignant transformation (149). Pituitary apoplexy following massive hemorrhage is a life-threatening complication of pituitary tumors which causes damage to the hypothalamus, sudden loss of vision, and bilateral cavernous sinus compression. However, these catastrophic complications appear to be much less common in ACTH/β-LPH tumors than in other secretory or nonsecretory types of pituitary tumors (251).

VIRILIZING TUMORS OF THE ADRENAL

Virilizing adrenal tumors in the female are characterized by hirsutism, clitoral enlargement, deepening of the voice, acne, and breast atrophy. In a review of 34 virilizing adrenal adenomas and eight adrenal carcinomas occurring in adult women, Gabrilove et al. (112) found that hirsutism was present in 100% of the patients. Clitoral enlargement was found in 79% of patients with adenoma and 62% of patients with carcinoma. Amenorrhea and deepening of the voice occurred in approximately 50% of the patients with adenoma and carcinoma. Decreased breast size and increased libido may also be present, and hypertension occurs in approximately 20% of cases.

In children, virilizing adenomas are rare and most of the virilizing lesions are adrenal carcinomas. Accelerated bone age and sexual development are the most common initial manifestations of virilizing adrenal tumors in children. Hypertension occurs in approximately one-third of these children. In general, the clinical features of patients with virilizing adrenal adenomas do not differ from those of patients with virilizing adrenocortical carcinomas. Virilizing adrenal tumors may occur from early infancy to late in life. Marks et al. (240), reported a 3-cm (diam.) virilizing adenoma in a 10-month-old girl. Virilizing adenomas are slightly more frequent in the right side and range in size from a few centimeters diameter to large tumor masses (16−17 cm) palpable in the abdomen. Virilizing adrenal tumors produce excessive secretion of dehydroepiandrosterone which results in high plasma levels of this hormone and excessive excretion of 17-ketosteroids. High to very high 17-ketosteroids were found in 24 of 31 adult patients with virilizing adenomas for whom values were given, with levels ranging from 20−450 mg/24 hours. Similarly, urinary excretion of 17-ketosteroids was elevated in all eight female children with virilizing adenomas and in five of the patients with adrenal carcinoma in whom values were reported. The levels of 17-ketosteroids in patients with adrenal carcinoma ranged from 51−1227 mg/24 hours (112). The elevation of 17-ketosteroids is helpful in the differential diagnosis of adrenal tumors, since virilization produced by gonadal tumors does not result in such marked elevation of the 17-ketosteroids. On the other hand, in contrast to the widely accepted concept that testosterone elevations are more likely to be found in gonadal tumors, Gabrilove et al. (112) found that of the 16 adult patients with virilizing adrenal tumors in whom plasma testosterone was measured, it was found strikingly elevated in 14 and slightly elevated in two. Elevation of other adrenal androgens, such as androstenedione, dehydroepiandrosterone, dehydroepiandrosterone sulfate, as well as 17α-hydroxyprogesterone and progesterone has been present in some patients (112). It is of interest to notice that in one hypertensive patient with a virilizing adrenal adenoma reported by Gabrilove et al., the plasma level of aldosterone and corticosterone were normal but deoxycorticosterone was markedly elevated. Whether the elevation of deoxycorticosterone is responsible for the hypertension frequently found in this syndrome requires further investigation.

Suppression and Stimulation Test

In a review of the dexamethasone suppression test employing either 2 or 8 mg of dexamethasone/day and measuring the levels of plasma testosterone and the urinary excretion of 17-ketosteroids, Gabrilove et al. found slight suppression in five subjects, no effect in five, and some increase in one subject (112). Estrogen suppression had no effect in three subjects and lower plasma testosterone in two. ACTH stimulation caused mild to moderate stimulation of 17-ketosteroids and plasma testosterone in three subjects and had no effect on seven. On the other hand, human chorionic gonadotropin, (hCG) administration caused stimulation of 17-ketosteroids and plasma testosterone in six of seven patients. Therefore, an increase in the 17-ketosteroids and plasma testosterone after hCG cannot be interpreted as evidence for a gonadal lesion. In conclusion, it appears that neither the stimulation or suppression test help in the differential diagnosis of benign from malignant lesions or in the differentiation of gonadal versus adrenal origins of these tumors. In some difficult cases in which the lesion is not detectable by the usual techniques, venous catheterization and measurement of steroid content in the adrenal and ovarian venous afferens may establish the site of the lesion.

Localization of the tumor can now be accomplished by means of noninvasive as well as invasive procedures. Ultrasonography and CT scan of the adrenals are very sensitive methods for localization of these lesions. Isotopic scanning is another noninvasive approach, although the radiation dose delivered to the patient is usually larger than that delivered by CT scanning, in view of which some centers have abandoned their use in favor of CT scanning (128). Arteriography is another technique that is useful for diagnosis of small tumors.

Therapy of virilizing adrenal tumors consists of surgical removal. Differentiation of benign from malignant may be extremely difficult by clinical or laboratory evaluation. For benign tumors the prognosis is good; menses return in the majority of patients and hirsutism decreases although it may take several months, or even years, after surgery, and often there is not complete remission. Clitoromegaly may also improve in some cases and the levels of urinary 17-ketosteroids and plasma testosterone may return to normal. For malignant tumors that cannot be completely resected, or for metastatic lesions, chemotherapy with adrenal enzyme inhibitors can be used.

FEMINIZING TUMORS OF THE ADRENAL

Feminizing adrenal tumors are extremely rare. In a review of 52 cases by Gabrilove et al. (110), adrenal carcinoma accounted for 78% of the cases and adrenal adenoma for 22% of the cases. Carcinoma occurs more commonly between ages 25 and 45 years, whereas the few reported adenomas have occurred between ages 5 and 60 years. The most common clinical manifestations are gynecomastia, which has been found in 98% of the cases. A palpable tumor is the second most common sign and occurs in approximately 60% of the cases. Testicular atrophy and decreased libido occurs in about one-half of the patients. Pain at the site of the tumor, tenderness of breasts, pigmentation of the areola, and obesity are less frequently seen. Plasma estradiol is usually elevated. The urinary excretion of 17-ketosteroids may be normal or elevated but the urinary excretion of estrogens or estrogen precursors is always elevated. Adrenal feminizing tumors secrete an increased amount of androstenedione, which is peripherally converted to estrogens. The increased urinary estrogen excretion is predominantly due to increased estriol, although estradiol and estrone are also found in high quantities. These tumors usually do not respond to exogenous ACTH and do not suppress with dexamethasone (57). Plasma estradiol is usually elevated. The levels of FSH and LH are usually low and do not respond to LH-RH stimulation (30). These tumors are rare in children. In a recent review there were only eight reported cases of feminizing adrenocortical tumors in children and six of the eight cases were benign adenomas. Feminizing adrenal tumors can also occur in females, and in female children they may cause isosexual female precocity (57). The tumors are usually unilateral and the contralateral adrenal is normal. Feminizing adrenocortical carcinomas are usually very large and often can be palpated on physical examination. Most of the feminizing adrenal carcinomas can be detected by tomography of the suprarenal region, ultrasound, or CT scan of the adrenals. The presence of gynecomastia, a flank mass, and an increased urinary estrogen excretion is diagnostic of a feminizing adrenal tumor. Feminizing adrenal tumors are radioresistant, and the treatment of choice is surgical resection. Despite surgery, most patients with feminizing adrenocortical carcinomas died within 3 years of diagnosis. After successful resection the urinary level of estrogens fall to normal. Gynecomastia and increased estrogen excretion can also be seen with testicular neoplasms. Occasionally, the adrenal tumors may produce β-hCG which may increase estrogen secretion by the testicles. Periodic measurements of β-hCG and plasma and urinary estrogens is important in the follow-up of patients who have been successfully treated by surgery (110).

HYPOFUNCTION OF THE ADRENAL CORTEX

Definition and Historical Perspective

In 1849 Thomas Addison described the disease that bears his name as a condition characterized by "anemia, general languor, debility, remarkable feebleness of the heart action, irritability of the stomach, and a peculiar change of color in the skin." In his original description Addison did not clearly differentiate patients with Addison's disease from patients with pernicious anemia, a condition previously described by him (5). However, in a classic monograph published in 1855 he reported the clinical features and autopsy findings of 11 patients with Addison's disease, including five patients with tuberculous destruction of the adrenals, one case of adrenal atrophy, and one of metastatic destruction of the glands. The remaining four patients presented cases of unilateral destruction of the adrenals, which probably did not represent adrenal insufficiency (6). One year later Brown-Sequard demonstrated that death followed the removal of the adrenal glands of experimental animals (47). However, it was not until 1927 when Rogoff and Stewart (315), Hartman et al. (135), and subsequently Swindler and Pffeier (378), independently demonstrated the efficacy of crude adrenal extracts in extending the life of adrenalectomized animals. In 1931 the Hartman extract was reported to be effective in treating acute adrenal insufficiency in man as well as improving the health of patients with Addison's disease (136). Between 1930 and 1940, small quantities of steroids were isolated and identified from adrenal extracts by Reichstein (106) in Zurich and Kendall et al. (182) at the Mayo Clinic. In 1937 Steiger and Reichsten (369) first synthetized deoxycorticosterone (DOCA) which started a new era in the therapy of Addison's disease. This was followed by the partial synthesis of cortisone by Sarett in 1946 (330), which within three years was commercially available. Addition of cortisone to the therapy of Addison's disease caused a remarkable improvement in the energy, well-being, and appetite of patients with Addison's disease. Also during the early 1940s Brown (44) demonstrated activation of the adrenal cortex of hypopituitary patients given ACTH for several days. The subsequent commercial availability of ACTH and glucocorticoids permitted the extensive studies that elucidated the physiologic and pharmacologic effects of these substances. The most recent advances in the understanding of the function of the adrenal cortex was the isolation , characterization, and synthesis of aldosterone (357,358) and the discovery of the renin–angiotensin–aldosterone axis as one of the major factors involved in the regulation of aldosterone production (84,113,209).

Classification

Adrenal insufficiency can be classified into 1) primary adrenocortical insufficiency, or 2) Addison's disease and secondary adrenal insufficiency, which results from reduction of ACTH secretion due to lesions of the pituitary or the hypothalamus. Moreover, acute adrenocortical insufficiency or adrenal crisis may occur in patients with primary or secondary adrenal insufficiency, subject to episodes of acute illness, trauma, or other major stress.

Primary Adrenocortical Insufficiency, or Addison's Disease

Incidence. Primary adrenocortical insufficiency is a relatively rare disease. In the 1960s the prevalence of Addison's disease in London was about 39 cases/million (374) and in Denmark it was estimated to be 60 cases/million (265). Addison's disease may occur at any age. Idiopathic autoimmune Addison's disease is slightly more common in adult females and in children, whereas Addison's secondary to tuberculous destruction of the adrenal glands is more common in adults and affects both sexes equally.

Pathogenesis. Primary adrenal insufficiency results from progressive destruction of the adrenal glands, which must involve over 90% of the glands before clinical signs of adrenal insufficiency appears. Tuberculosis used to be the most common cause of Addison's disease, but because of the effective control of the disease the proportion of cases due to tuberculosis has declined from 79% of the cases in the decade 1928–1938 to only approximately 21% of the cases in the decade of 1962–1972 (163). At present, the most common cause of Addison's disease is autoimmune or idiopathic atrophy of the adrenal glands, which accounts for approximately 75% of the cases; other etiologies account for approximately 5%–7% of the cases (163).

Autoimmune, or Idiopathic, Addison's Disease. Idiopathic Addison's disease is the most common cause of adrenal insufficiency and is usually caused by autoimmune destruction and atrophy of the adrenal glands. The atrophy is usually confined to the adrenal cortex with little or no involvement of the medullary portion of the adrenal. Histology of the adrenal glands shows lymphocytic infiltration and fibrosis. In 1957 Anderson et al. (11) first detected antibodies against the adrenals in two of 10 patients with Addison's disease. Adrenal antibodies can be detected by complement fixation or by immunofluorescent techniques. In a review of 511 patients from eight large studies, Irvine and Barnes (164) found that 58% of 297 patients with idiopathic Addison's disease had specific adrenal autoantibodies, whereas only 12 of 154 patients (8%) with tuberculous Addison's had positive adrenal antibodies (Table 5). In Irvine's surveys a higher incidence of adrenal antibodies was found in females (72%) than in males (52%). The titers of antibodies tend to be lower than those found in patients with autoimmune thyroiditis and pernicious anemia, but similar to these conditions, the antibody titers persist for many years. In addition to adrenal-specific antibodies, some patients may show antibodies against steroid-producing cells that react with more than one steroid-producing tissue. Adrenal antibodies are rare in first-degree relatives of patients with idiopathic Addison's disease, provided that these relatives do not have idiopathic hypoparathyroidism. Besides Addison's disease,

TABLE 5. Incidence of Adrenal Antibodies in Addison's Disease

Author	Idiopathic Addison's		Tuberculous Addison's	
	No. of patients	Patients with positive antibodies (%)	No. of patients	Patients with positive antibodies (%)
Goudie et al. (1966)	35	51	27	18
Blizzard et al. (1967)	118	68	—	—
Andrada et al. (1968)	45	38	5	60
Wuepper et al. (1969)	22	64	9	11
Maisey et al. (1969)	32	70	8	0
Pousset et al. (1970)	15	53	41	7
Irvine et al. (1972)	174	63	46	0
Nerup et al. (1974)	70	74	18	0
Total	511	58	154	8

Source: Modified from Irvine, W.J., and Barnes, E.W. (1975) Clin. Endocrinol. Metab. 4:379. Author references are from this article.

idiopathic hypoparathyroidism is the only condition in which adrenal antibodies occur with high prevalence (163,364). Characterization of the adrenal antigens responsible for the autoimmune process has been difficult. It appears that these antigens are primarily located in the cells of the zona fasciculata and are particulate components of the cytoplasm which are predominately found in the microsomal and to a lesser extent in the mitochondrial fractions of adrenal extracts (36,122,162,265). The biochemical nature of the antigen appears to be a lipoprotein (122). Abnormalities of cell-mediated immunity are also found in patients with Addison's disease. Antiadrenal cellular hypersensitivity as assessed by leukocyte migration test was present in 40% of patients with idiopathic Addison's disease reported by Nerup and Bendixen (263,264) and in 80% of cases studied by Moulias and Goust (254). Peripheral lymphocytes from patients with idiopathic Addison's disease may show an impaired response to phytohemagglutinin suggesting that T-lymphocyte function may be abnormal but the proportion of T- and B-lymphocytes as well as the total lymphocyte count is normal. There is increasing evidence that the manifestations of autoimmunity in idiopathic Addison's disease reflect a defect in immune surveillance mechanisms, specifically, a genetically determined deficiency of suppressor cells that allows the persistence and proliferation of a forbidden clone of immunocytes directed against antigenic determinants in the adrenocortical cells. This type of abnormality is similar to that found in other autoimmune disorders, such as Hashimoto's thyroiditis, etc.

In a study of the histocompatibility antigens of 15 unrelated patients with idiopathic Addison's disease, Platz et al. (295) found that 12 (80%) were HLA-B8 positive, which is a highly significant increase incidence compared with the frequency of these antigens in the Danish population. These authors estimated that the relative risk of developing Addison's disease is approximately 12 times higher for HLA-B8 positive individuals than for HLA-B8 negative. This finding suggests the possibility that the HLA-B8 or some other genes controlling immune responses are closely linked or associated with the HLA-B8 and may be the common denominator for the development of organ specific autoimmune disease. Patients with idiopathic Addison's disease have a significant increased incidence of autoimmune disorders affecting other tissues. The term "Schmidt syndrome" has been used to describe the association of adrenal insufficiency and Hashimoto's thyroiditis, since Schmidt was the first to describe such an association (338). Table 6 shows the relative incidence of associated disorders from two large series of patients with idiopathic Addison's disease reported in the literature (163,265). Autoimmune thyroid disease in the form of Grave's disease, autoimmune Hashimoto's thyroiditis, or nontoxic goiter are the most commonly associated conditions. Amenorrhea due to premature ovarian failure and testicular failure are also commonly associated. These patients frequently have antibodies against steroid-producing cells and the ovaries show positive immunofluorescent stain reactions with the graphian follicles and the corpus luteum (164). Lymphocytic infiltration of the ovaries is a characteristic feature. Loss of libido, impotence, and gynecomastia are symptoms of testicular failure in male patients. Antibodies that react against the Leydig's cells have been found in some patients (164).

The association of diabetes mellitus and Addison's disease was first reported by Ogle in 1886 (274). The incidence of diabetes mellitus in Addison's disease is estimated to be about 18%. The type of diabetes is

TABLE 6. Clinical Disorders Associated with Addison's Disease in 332 Cases

Disorders	Idiopathic	TB	Other
Thyrotoxicosis	16	—	—
Hypothyroidism and Hashimoto's	19	—	1
Simple goiter	17	—	2
Pernicious anemia	12	—	—
Diabetes mellitus	31	1	—
Hypoparathyroidism	12	—	—
Gonadal failure	39	1	—
Vitiligo	17	2	—
Total number of patients	245	65	22

Source: Modified from Irvine, W.J., and Barnes, E.W. (1975) Clin. Endocrinol. Metab. 4:379.

predominantly insulin-dependent, or type I, diabetes. Pernicious anemia and hypoparathyroidism are also commonly associated. Idiopathic Addison's disease is sometimes familial. Also, the association of idiopathic Addison's with hypothyroidism and with hypoparathyroidism has been described in families and in both cases appears to be an autosomal recessive character. In a recent review of 295 patients with autoimmune Addison's from the world literature, Neufeld et al. (266) proposed that autoimmune Addison's disease associated with other diseases occurred in at least two distinct types. In type I polyglandular autoimmune disease (PGA), Addison's disease is associated with acquired hypoparathyroidism and/or mucocutaneous candidiasis. Whereas in type II polyglandular syndrome, Addison's disease is associated with insulin-dependent diabetes and/or autoimmune thyroid disease. Table 7 shows the incidence of other disorders associated with each type of polyendocrine syndrome. Type I PGA occurs in sporadic and familiar forms and is not associated with any specific HLA antigens. Patients with type I PGA appear to have an underlying defect in cell-mediated thymus-derived immunity (175). Suppressor T lymphocyte functions are defective in such patients (14) and abnormalities of delayed hypersensitivity and IgA deficiency have been reported in some patients implicating an abnormality of the thymus as the primary pathogenetic abnormality in this syndrome. In contrast, type II PGA appears to be linked to the HLA system, especially to the HLA-B8, A-1, and (DW3) haplotypes suggesting that the immunologic dysfunction seen in this type of polyglandular failure results from a gene (S) on chromosome 6 in linkage disequilibrium with the HLA-B8 allele (93).

TABLE 7. Addison's Disease in Type I and Type II Polyglandular Autoimmune Syndrome

Entity	Type I 71 Patients (%)	Type II 224 Patients (%)
Addison's disease	100	100
Hypoparathyroidism	76	—
Mucocutaneous Candidiasis	73	—
Autoimmune thyroid disease	11	69
Insulin-dependent diabetes	4	52
Chronic active hepatitis	13	—
Malabsorption	22	—
Alopecia	32	0.5
Pernicious anemia	13	0.5
Gonadal failure	17	3.6
Vitiligo	8	4.5
HLA Association	None	A-1, B-8, DW3

Source: Modified from Neufeld, M., et al. (1981) Medicine 60:355.

Tuberculosis and Other Infections. Tuberculous destruction of the adrenal gland is now the second most common cause and accounts for approximately 20% of cases. In contrast to the case in idiopathic Addison's, the adrenal medulla is destroyed by the tuberculous process. The disease may or may not be associated with active tuberculosis of other organs. The most common primary focus of tuberculosis is the lungs (329). Adrenal calcification is often seen in Addison's disease caused by tuberculosis, but it also occurs in other granulomatous infections and following adrenal hemorrhage. Other infectious causes of chronic adrenal insufficiency that are less common include histoplasmosis (75), blastomycosis (3), coccidiodomycosis (238), and cryptococcosis. Several other bacterial, viral, spirochetal, and parasitic diseases have occasionally been reported to cause Addison's disease (104).

Adrenal Hemorrhage. Adrenal hemorrhage from a variety of causes can lead to adrenal insufficiency. Shock, septicemia, fulminating purpura, and bilateral adrenal hemorrhages associated with meningococcal infections constitute the Waterhouse–Friderichsen syndrome (80). This syndrome is frequently fatal. Septicemia and endotoxin released from other pathogens can also cause bilateral adrenal hemorrhage. In fact, in a survey of 51 children dying from bilateral adrenal hemorrhage, meningococcemia was found in 18% of the cases, and *Pseudomonas aeruginosa* was the most prevalent pathogen isolated from 27% of the cases (239). Adrenal hemorrhage can occur during the newborn period, especially in large infants after traumatic deliveries.

In a review of 144 cases of adrenal hemorrhage in the adult, Xarli et al. (402) found a history of anticoagulant drug administration in 30% of the cases. Adrenal hemorrhage was highly prevalent in patients with several cardiovascular and respiratory diseases, including acute myocardial infarction, congestive heart failure, arteriosclerotic and hypertensive heart disease, pulmonary embolism, etc. Also, it has been reported postoperatively and especially after complicated pregnancies. Patients with acute myocardial infarction and pulmonary embolus who are on anticoagulants are particularly susceptible to adrenal hemorrhage. Experimental evidence indicates that prolonged ACTH administration may produce focal adrenal necrosis and an increase in adrenal blood flow that may predispose for a significant hemorrhage to occur (396). Therefore, it appears that the stressed adrenal under endogenous or exogenous ACTH stimulation is highly susceptible to hemorrhage. Calcification of the adrenal glands often develops within weeks of the adrenal hemorrhage and may be apparent in plane films of the abdomen.

Iatrogenic Adrenal Insufficiency. Because of the widespread use of corticosteroids for nonendocrine uses, iatrogenic adrenal insufficiency is a relatively common and important cause of adrenal insufficiency. Patients receiving large doses of corticosteroids for nonendocrine disorders are at high risk for developing chronic suppression of the hypothalamic–pituitary–adrenal axis and adrenal atrophy. Abrupt withdrawal of steroid therapy in these patients may cause an acute adrenal crisis. Dosages over 25–30 mg of cortisol/day may cause significant suppression of the hypothalamic–pituitary–adrenal axis.

The length of time necessary to produce atrophy of the adrenals is not known. In experimental animals atrophy and hypofunction of the adrenals can be demonstrated 12 hours after hypophysectomy or suppression of ACTH release by corticosteroids (39,389). However, the adrenals quickly regain their function and return to normal size after discontinuation of corticosteroid therapy. In humans, treatment with large doses of prednisone for 5 days causes significant decrease in the cortisol response to insulin-induced hypoglycemia and ACTH administration which lasts 5 days or longer after discontinuation of therapy (372). However, in patients receiving corticosteroid therapy for periods of months or years, adrenal atrophy may persist for several months after steroids are discontinued and these patients may potentially develop acute adrenal insufficiency when exposed to stressful situations. These patients may be able to secrete sufficient amounts of cortisol under normal circumstances but have a markedly diminished adrenal reserve (244). After withdrawal of exogenous corticosteroids, there is an initial recovery of ACTH secretion followed some time later by normal adrenocortical steroid production (123). The period of time necessary to achieve normal function of the hypothalamic–pituitary–adrenal axis (HPA) varies greatly among patients; however, in adults, full recovery is usually observed within one year of stopping medication. In children, recovery usually occurs 2–3 months after therapy has been discontinued. Several screening tests have been proposed to assess the integrity of the hypothalamic–pituitary axis. A morning plasma cortisol below 7 μg/dL is suggestive of adrenal atrophy. A rapid ACTH stimulation, the intravenous methopyrone test, and, in particular, the cortisol response to insulin-induced hypoglycemia are helpful in establishing the recovery of the HPA. However, when in doubt it is safer to administer supplementary corticosteroid therapy to patients who are under stress within 1 year of discontinuing long-term steroid therapy. Administration of ACTH with the corticosteroids in attempts to maintain adrenal responsiveness is undesirable since the recovery of the hypothalamic–pituitary function may be further delayed (89). Adrenal atrophy and suppression of the hypothalamic–pituitary–adrenal axis may be minimized by using an intermediately acting steroid given as a single morning dose on alternate days.

Metastatic Destruction of the Adrenals. Breast cancer is perhaps the most common tumor leading to metastatic destruction of the adrenal glands and adrenal insufficiency. Bronchogenic carcinoma often metastasizes to the adrenal glands but rarely causes adrenal insufficiency. Addison's disease secondary to metastatic disease may develop as a result of complete replacement of the adrenal cortex by tumor or as a result of adrenal infarction owing to obstruction of the vascular supply to the adrenals. The incidence of Addison's disease in metastatic cancer is low. In a review of 566 patients with Addison's disease only three cases (0.5%) were secondary to metastatic cancer (130). On the other hand, metastatic involvement of the adrenal glands is relatively frequent, ranging from 5%−40% in two large autopsy series of patients with cancer (325,398).

Other Familial Types of Addison's Disease. Several familial types of adrenal insufficiency have been described. These syndromes are usually transmitted as either autosomal recessive, or X-link recessive traits.

Familial Unresponsiveness to ACTH. The syndrome was first delineated as a distinct clinical entity by Migeon et al. in 1968 (250), although there were few earlier reports of patients with this condition (353,397). This syndrome is characterized by an impaired production of cortisol in the presence of high circulating levels of ACTH. There is normal production of aldosterone and normal sodium balance. Clinically, these children present with feeding problems, hypoglycemia, hyperpigmentation, lethargy, and convulsions. In contrast to patients with congenital adrenal hyperplasia, there is no accumulation of cortisol precursors and no enzymatic abnormalities of cortisol biosynthesis have been demonstrated. Patients with this condition do not increase the plasma cortisol or the urinary excretion of cortisol metabolites after the injection of ACTH. Until 1972 approximately 20 patients from 16 families had been described in the literature (180,184). Although an X-link recessive mode of inheritance has been suggested, Verhoeven and Wilson (388) found no evidence of male preponderance and suggested that the more likely pattern of inheritance is autosomal recessive. Little is known about the pathophysiology of this syndrome. The lack of response to exogenous ACTH makes it improbable that a structural abnormality of ACTH is responsible for the disease. On pathological examination the adrenal glands are atrophic with dominance of the glomerulosa cells and occasional fasciculata reticularis cells (180,250).

Adrenoleukodystrophy. Adrenoleukodystrophy (ALD) is an X-link recessive disorder characterized by a progressive neurological disorder associated with adrenal insufficiency. The disease is thought to be caused by an abnormality of fatty acid metabolism leading to accumulation of very long chain, unbranched, saturated, or monounsaturated fatty acids. Fatty acids of carbon lengths 20−30 accumulate in cholesterol esters and gangliosides of the cerebral white matter and the adrenal cortex (253). Adrenoleukodystrophy is manifested by adrenal insufficiency and central and peripheral demyelinization. Characteristically, trilaminar cytoplasmic inclusions (lamellar lipid profile) are found in adrenocortical cells and macrophages in brain white matter. In the majority of cases of ALD, clinical and laboratory evidence of adrenal insufficiency can be demonstrated sometime during the illness and may precede the onset of neurological manifestations by several years. Many ALD phenotypes have been described. Typically, ALD occurs in childhood, affecting males 4–8 years of age; the disease is characterized by cortical blindness, deafness, and progressive dementia associated with mild to moderate adrenal insufficiency. A second variant, called adrenomyeloneuropathy, affects adult males and is characterized by spastic paraparesis, peripheral neuropathy, moderate adrenal insufficiency, and testicular failure. A "mix" and a neonatal form have also been described (279). In addition, X-linked Addison's disease without neurological involvement has been reported. These patients have elevated C-26 fatty acids in skin fibroblasts (279). Also, spastic paraparesis in female carriers without adrenal disease has been reported. The accumulation of C-26 fatty acids (hexacosanoate), a saturated unbranched fatty acid, is unique to ALD. Cultured skin fibroblasts accumulate C-26 fatty acids and the ratio of the C-26/C-22 have been used for diagnosing as well as for detecting carriers. Also, a significant increase in the plasma concentration of C-25 and C-26 fatty acids occurs in patients and carriers and can be detected by gas liquid chromatography (279).

Familial Cytomegalic Adrenocortical Hypoplasia. Familial cytomegalic adrenocortical hypoplasia is a rare X-linked syndrome associated with pubertal failure due to hypogonadotropic hypogonadism, probably secondary to deficiency of gonadotropin-releasing hormone (140).

In homozygous hypobetalipoproteinemia, basal cortisol production is normal but the cortisol response to ACTH is impaired, presumably due to decreased plasma low-density lipoprotein which, in turn, serves as an important source of cholesterol for adrenal steroidogenesis (158). Also, patients with homozygous familial hypercholesterolemia, especially the receptor negative type, have normal basal adrenocortical function but show a subnormal cortisol response to ACTH (158a).

Clinical Manifestations and Pathophysiology

Chronic adrenocortical insufficiency is characterized by an insidious onset of symptoms and signs. The most common symptoms of Addison's disease are weakness and easy fatigability (Table 8). Characteristically, the patients wake up feeling relatively well but develop increasing weakness and fatigue as the day goes on. This cycle is in contrast to depressed patients in whom weakness and fatigability start from the time they wake up. Early in the disease the weakness, asthenia, and fatigability may occur only after periods of stress or after exertion; also, symptoms are exacerbated by hot weather. With advancing disease, symptoms may be permanent. The pathophysiological mechanism for the weakness and asthenia is not understood. Alleviation of the symptoms requires correction of both mineralocorticoid and glucocorticoid deficiencies. Muscle weakness and achiness may be present. Hyperkalemic periodic paralysis has been reported in a few cases (126). Anorexia and weight loss occur in a great majority of patients. Other common gastrointestinal complaints are

TABLE 8. Incidence of Symptoms in 255 Patients with Addison's Disease

Weakness	100%
Weight loss	98%
Hyperpigmentation	91%
Hypotension	83%
Gastrointestinal symptoms	81%

nausea, vomiting, diarrhea, and abdominal pain. In patients with adrenal crisis the gastrointestinal complaints may be the most prominent feature. Erroneous diagnosis of "gastroenteritis" or "acute abdomen" can lead to a fatal outcome. The mechanism of the gastrointestinal symptoms of Addison's disease is not known, but the symptoms respond promptly to the administration of cortisol. Salt craving, probably resulting from sodium depletion, is reported by some patients. Hyperpigmentation is one of the classic signs of Addison's disease. It occurs particularly in exposed areas of the skin, in the creases of the hands, in scars, and in the mucosal surfaces, especially in the oral cavity. A generalized tanning of the skin which is exacerbated by sunlight is commonly seen. The hyperpigmentation results from the markedly elevated levels of ACTH and other POMC-derived peptides with high melanotropic activity, such as β-LPH and γ-LPH (26,119,195). Vitiligo occurs in 10%–20% of patients with Addison's disease and has been attributed to autoimmune destruction of the melanocytes. Decreased axillary and pubic hair owing to decreased production of adrenal androgens is common in female patients since the adrenal gland is the main source of androgens in women. This usually does not occur in males because of continued production of testosterone by the testicles.

Hypotension is extremely frequent, especially in moderate to advanced stages. Postural hypotension and syncope may be early signs of adrenal insufficiency. The mechanism whereby hypotension occurs is multifactorial. Volume depletion resulting from sodium wasting by the kidney owing to deficiency of aldosterone is an important factor. Decreased cardiac output and dysfunction of the peripheral vascular system are also important factors in the pathogenesis of hypotension. The renin–angiotensin system plays an important role in blood pressure regulation during adrenal insufficiency. Plasma renin concentration is markedly elevated in adrenalectomized animals and patients with adrenal insufficiency (310,371). There is also a marked increase in plasma renin activity (PRA) despite the accompanying decrease in plasma renin substrate which results from deficiency of glucocorticoids (310,371). The increased renin concentration results from volume depletion secondary to aldosterone deficiency. Angiotensin II levels are two- to threefold higher than normal in dogs with adrenal insufficiency (346) and the infusion of the angiotensin II antagonist, saralasin, causes a decrease in blood pressure in glucocorticoid and mineralocorticoid deficient dogs (22). Moreover, it has recently been shown that plasma vasopressin increases by approximately fourfold after withdrawal of steroid treatment in conscious adrenalectomized dogs and that the infusion of an antagonist of the pressor effects of antidiuretic hormone causes a rapid and significant decrease in mean arterial pressure (346). These results indicate that angiotensin II and vasopressin play an important role in blood pressure regulation during adrenal insufficiency and may partly explain the increased peripheral vascular resistance found in adrenal insufficiency (311,392). Decreased cardiac output and decrease in the inotropic action of the heart is common in Addison's disease and is corrected by replacing the deficiency of glucocorticoids and mineralocorticoids. Patients with Addison's disease characteristically have a small heart (165).

Calcification of the ear cartilage may be seen in some patients with Addison's disease. Similarly, there appears to be an increased incidence of calcification of the costal cartilages in addisonian patients. Patients with adrenal insufficiency are particularly prone to develop hypoglycemia during prolonged fasting or after the ingestion of alcohol. Hypoglycemia in patients with Addison's is due to impairment in gluconeogenesis resulting from deficiency of cortisol. Personality changes in the form of irritability, restlessness, and mental sluggishness are frequent.

Laboratory Findings

Patients with advanced Addison's disease typically have hyponatremia, hyperkalemia, and mild hyperchloremic acidosis. Also, they may have a disproportionate elevation of the BUN relative to the plasma creatinine as a result of prerenal azotemia due to volume depletion and decreased cardiac output. The serum sodium is usually low, but may be normal in mild cases. In severe, long-standing, untreated Addison's, the serum sodium rarely may be as low as 100 mEq/L. Hyponatremia in Addison's disease is partly the result of sodium wasting by the kidney due to deficiency of aldosterone but another important factor is the markedly elevated levels of antidiuretic hormone which develop as a compensatory mechanism for the decreased circulating blood volume. The increased ADH levels cause a decreased free-water clearance resulting in water retention and dilution of the serum sodium. Another mechanism involved in the pathogenesis of hyponatremia is a decreased delivery of filtrate to the diluting segments of the nephron as a result of decreased glomerular filtration rate (GFR) and/or increased proximal reabsorption (187). When glucocorticoid deficiency predominates, as in the case of hypopituitarism, there is usually no evidence of absolute decrease in circulating blood volume. However, hemodynamic alterations caused by decreased cardiac output and peripheral vascular dysfunction lead to a decrease in the "effective" circulating blood volume which, in turn, is a stimulus to antidiuretic hormone release (365). The increased ADH levels in adrenal insufficiency lead to an impaired capacity to maximally dilute the urine. As a result, patients with adrenocortical insufficiency are unable to excrete a water load. Glucocorticoid administration usually corrects the impaired water excretion in these patients. However, the defect in urinary diluting capacity requires the addition of mineralocorticoids (124). The ability to generate a maximally concentrated urine is also impaired in adrenal insufficiency. This concentration defect is partly the result of the absence of adrenal steroids which play a permissive effect on the ADH-induced reabsorption of water across the collecting duct (345). Hyperkalemia in adrenal insufficiency is due to decreased cation exchange by the distal convoluted tubule resulting from the lack of aldosterone. Other factors responsible for the hyperkalemia are the decreased GFR and the mild acidosis which allows potassium to shift from the intracellular to extracellular space. Elevation of serum potassium varies from patient to patient but may be severe and cause cardiac arrhythmias. Hyperkalemia does not occur in secondary adrenal insufficiency since aldosterone secretion is primarily controlled by the renin-angiotensin system which is usually intact in patients with secondary adrenal insufficiency. However, under situations of volume depletion a decreased aldosterone secretion is seen in these patients as compared with normal individuals. Mild acidosis is common in advanced cases. Acidosis usually results from impairment of ammonia and, in particular, hydrogen ion secretion by the renal tubules. The acidosis is corrected by adequate mineralocorticoid replacement. The increased levels of BUN and creatinine are largely the result of decreased GFR and renal blood flow owing to hypotension and decreased cardiac output. Hypoglycemia may be seen during fasting. Hypercalcemia may occur in some patients and is thought to be secondary to the loss of the antagonist effect of glucocorticoids on calcium absorption in the gut. Pharmacological doses of glucocorticoids antagonize the effect of vitamin D on calcium absorption from the gut and calcium reabsorption from bone (98). Adrenalectomized rats have been found to have an increase in free ionized calcium, protein-bound calcium, and calcium complex in the plasma (302).

Mild to moderate eosinophilia and relative lymphocytosis are common in Addison's disease. Anemia is frequently seen in these patients and may become more prominent after correction of the dehydration. Pernicious anemia may also be seen in patients with autoimmune Addison's and polyglandular autoimmune syndrome.

Diagnosis of Addison's Disease

The diagnosis of adrenal insufficiency is based on the demonstration of decreased cortisol production under basal (complete adrenal insufficiency) or stimulated conditions (partial adrenal insufficiency). In cases of severe adrenal insufficiency, the plasma cortisol levels and the urinary excretion of free cortisol, 17-OHCS and 17-KS, are low. A single plasma cortisol level over 25 μg/dL may be useful to rule out adrenal insufficiency (262). However, levels in the 5–20 μg/dL range may be seen in patients with partial adrenal insufficiency whose adrenals are functioning at maximal capacity, but these patients have no adrenal reserve to increase cortisol levels during periods of stress. By the same reason, the urinary free cortisol and the excretion of 17-OHCS and 17-KS may be normal under basal conditions. Therefore, basal plasma or urinary corticosteroid levels are not sensitive enough to rule out the diagnosis of adrenal insufficiency. The measurement of ACTH in plasma has been useful for the differential diagnosis of adrenal insufficiency. Patients with Addison's disease have a marked elevation of plasma ACTH as well as high levels of β-LPH, γ-LPH, and β-endorphins, which derive from the common ACTH precursor, POMC (26,119,195). An elevation of the plasma ACTH level ($>$ 200 pg/dL) associated with a low plasma cortisol level is diagnostic of primary adrenal insufficiency or Addison's disease. However, similar findings can be seen in patients with congenital adrenal hyperplasia. In secondary adrenal insufficiency the plasma ACTH and plasma cortisol are usually low. However, proof of the diagnosis of adrenal insufficiency will rest upon the demonstration of a failure to increase cortisol secretion following stimulation by ACTH.

Rapid ACTH Stimulation Test. The rapid ACTH stimulation test is a simple outpatient screening test. The test consists of the administration of 0.250 mg of synthetic α^{1-24}ACTH intravenously or intramuscularly with determination of the plasma cortisol before the injection and 30 and 60 minutes later. In normal subjects the plasma cortisol usually doubles and the absolute increment is greater than 7–10 μg/dL above control levels (397). Also, it has been postulated that this simple screening test may be helpful in establishing the integrity of the hypothalamic pituitary axis since an abnormal cortisol response to ACTH can be demonstrated in hypopituitary patients 8–12 days after ACTH deprivation (144). An abnormal response of the plasma cortisol to ACTH cannot be interpreted as proof of the diagnosis of adrenal insufficiency and in these patients prolonged ACTH stimulation test is necessary to establish the diagnosis.

Prolonged ACTH Stimulation. This test is the most sensitive and definitive test for the diagnosis of adrenal insufficiency. At least two baseline 24-hour urine collections for determinations of urinary free cortisol, 17-OHCS, and creatinine should be obtained and then 40–50 units of aqueous ACTH or 0.250 mg of synthetic α_{1-24} ACTH are dissolved in 500 mL of 5% dextrose in 0.9% sodium chloride and infused intravenously over an 8-hour period. The ACTH infusion should be repeated for 3–4 consecutive days and daily 24-hour urines should be collected for measurements of urinary free cortisol, 17-OHCS, and creatinine. In patients with primary adrenal insufficiency urinary 17-OHCS excretion does not increase by more than 1–2 mg/24 hours above the baseline levels. An increase of 10 mg/24 hours or more over the baseline level is an indication of adequate adrenal reserve (262). In patients with secondary adrenal insufficiency a "staircase" response with successive daily increments in steroid excretion leading to a 10 mg/24 hour increase or more over the baseline levels by the third or fourth day of ACTH infusion. Increases of less than 10 mg/24 hours may be seen in chronically ill or debilitated patients without adrenal insufficiency, requiring repeated testing or additional laboratory parameters for a definitive diagnosis.

The Rapid Metyrapone Test. The oral administration of 30 mg/kg of metyrapone at 11 P.M. followed by the measurement of 11-deoxycortisol (compound S) at 8:00 A.M. on the following morning has been used by some investigators for the diagnosis of Addison's disease. An increase of at least 7 μg/dL in the plasma level of 11-deoxycortisol is an indication of adequate stimulation and responsiveness of the adrenal gland by endogenous ACTH (394). In a study of 10 patients with Addison's disease and 134 normal subjects, there was no overlap in the levels of 11-deoxycortisol between normals and addisonian patients. However, a number of drugs interfere with the metabolism of metyrapone (dilantin, phenobarbital, estrogens) leading to false/negative results. In addition, this test is of no use if corticosteroids are simultaneously being administered to the patient. Moreover, metyrapone blocks cortisol production and, therefore, may aggravate adrenal insufficiency or precipitate an adrenal crisis. Also, this test requires the measurement of plasma 11-deoxycortisol which is not as readily available as the plasma cortisol assay. In view of the above reasons the rapid ACTH stimulation test is the screening test of choice for the diagnosis of Addison's disease.

A number of protocols have been devised for the simultaneous diagnosis and treatment of suspected adrenal insufficiency (222,354); however, treatment should never be delayed in severe cases and it is usually safer to start the conventional treatment of acute adrenal insufficiency and postpone the diagnostic test until the patient is stable. Nonetheless, a blood sample for later measurement of plasma cortisol and ACTH can usually be obtained when the diagnosis of adrenal insufficiency is suspected, but should not interfere with or delay the administration of proper treatment.

Test Used for the Differential Diagnosis of Adrenal Insufficiency

The Metyrapone Test. The metyrapone test was originally used for the measurement of pituitary ACTH reserve and has been useful for the differential diagnosis of primary from secondary adrenal insufficiency. After collection of two baseline 24-hour urines for measurements of 17-OHCS, 750 mg of metyrapone are given orally every 4 hours for six doses and daily 24-hour urines are collected for measurement of 17-OHCS. In normal individuals, a two- to fourfold increase in 17-OHCS occurs on the day of administration of metyrapone or the day after. A less than twofold increase may indicate a limited ACTH reserve. Plasma ACTH levels can also be measured and in normal individuals show a significant increase. However, as stated before, metyrapone inhibits 11-β-hydroxylase and thereby blocks the synthesis of cortisol, and in patients with adrenal insufficiency may precipitate an acute adrenal crisis. Therefore, this test has to be used with extreme caution in patients with suspected adrenal insufficiency.

Insulin Hypoglycemia. The ACTH and cortisol response to insulin-induced hypoglycemia has become the most commonly used test for the evaluation of ACTH reserve. Insulin is usually administered in conjunction with TRH and LHRH, permitting a complete evaluation of anterior pituitary function in a short time. Crystalline insulin, 0.05–0.1 units/kg of body weight are given intravenously and blood is obtained for plasma glucose, ACTH, cortisol, growth hormone, prolactin, TSH, LH, and FSH levels at zero time and at 15, 30, 45, 60, and 90 minutes after the injection of insulin and the other releasing factors. A drop in the plasma glucose to below 40 mg/dL is usually considered an adequate hypoglycemic stimulus. Preliminary results with the use of synthetic CRF and growth hormone releasing factor (GHRF) suggest that in the future injection of these two releasing factors may obviate the use of insulin hypoglycemia as the stimulus for ACTH and growth hormone release.

Vasopressin Stimulation Test. The intramuscular injection of 10 units of lysine vasopressin has also been used as a stimulus for ACTH release. In this test blood for ACTH and cortisol levels is obtained before and 30, 60, 90, and 120 minutes after the injection of vasopressin.

Differential Diagnosis. In view of the fact that weakness, fatigue, and gastrointestinal complaints are common complaints in the general population, the diagnosis of early adrenocortical insufficiency is frequently difficult. The presence of weight loss associated with weakness and anorexia may be useful in some cases to differentiate adrenal insufficiency from mental depression since in depressed patients weight gain is often seen in association with these symptoms. Hyperpigmentation may be difficult to evaluate in blacks and in members of other dark-skinned races. However, a recent and progressive increase in pigmentation is usually reported by the addisonian patients. Differentiation from other diseases presenting with increased pigmentation may be difficult, although the appearance and distribution of pigmentation of Addison's disease is characteristic. However, when in doubt, the ACTH stimulation test provides clear differentiation between these conditions and adrenal insufficiency.

Therapy

Patients with adrenal insufficiency have to be thoroughly educated regarding their disease and should understand the need for lifelong therapy. Also, they should be instructed about the need to increase their steroid dose during periods of stress. It is also advisable to educate them in the parenteral self-administration of steroids and they should be instructed to carry an identification card or medical alert bracelet or necklace stating their diagnosis, physician's name and telephone number. All patients with adrenal insufficiency should receive replacement steroid therapy. Cortisone or hydrocortisone is the drug of choice. Cortisone doses vary from 12.5–50 mg/day but the majority of patients require between 25 and 37.5 mg/24 hours. In order to simulate the normal diurnal variation of plasma cortisol it is advisable to take two-thirds of the daily dosage in the morning and one-third in the late afternoon. Patients should be told not to take the evening dosage of cortisone close to their bedtime since it may cause insomnia in some patients. To minimize gastric irritation it is best to take the cortisone with meals. In children, the initial maintenance dosage of hydrocortisone is 20 mg/m^2 of body surface, but careful adjustment of the dosage is necessary to prevent growth retardation, which is a very sensitive index of glucocorticoid excess and which may occur in the absence of other signs of excess cortisol, such as weight gain or cushingoid features. Doses of cortisone below 75 mg/day do not have sufficient sodium-retaining activity; hence, for proper replacement, it is usually necessary to add small quantities of mineralocorticoids. This is best accomplished by the administration of 9α-fluorohydrocortisone in dosages of 0.05–0.2 mg/day. Adjustments of the dosage of cortisol in the individual patient is done largely on empirical basis. Patients who are undertreated may continue to experience anorexia, weakness, and fatigue. On the other hand, patients receiving too much cortisone may show an increased appetite, progressive weight gain, euphoria, and sometimes frank manic symptoms. A normal level of plasma ACTH is used by some as an indication of adequate replacement therapy. Patients with Addison's disease have been shown to have a decreased number of glucocorticoid receptors in lymphocytes and a twofold increase in binding affinity. The change in affinity is corrected after six months of conventional therapy but normalization of the number of glucocorticoid receptors requires longer time (336). The physiologic implications of these changes are not known. Patients receiving lower than required dosages of 9α-fluorohydrocortisone may continue to experience an increased salt appetite and may exhibit significant postural hypotension. Normalization of PRA has been used by some investigators as an indicator of adequate mineralocorticoid replacement (230). On the other hand, overtreatment with mineralocorticoids may lead to hypertension, edema, headaches, muscle cramps, and weakness secondary to hypokalemia. Patients with Addison's disease should take a normal diet, containing at least 150 mEq of sodium/day and should be advised to increase salt intake or increase mineralocorticoid replacement during periods of hot weather, heavy perspiration, or in the event of diarrhea. Similarly, they should be instructed to double their cortisol dosage in the event of any minor infection and to seek prompt medical attention in the case of a major illness or trauma. Addisonian patients undergoing surgery or during delivery should receive supplemental steroids. For minor surgical procedures, such as dilatation and curettage, excision biopsies, etc., 100 mg of cortisol acetate should be given intramuscularly 1 hour before the procedure and a repeat dosage should be given every 8 hours thereafter. The day after the procedure if the patient is afebrile and there are no complications the oral maintenance regime may be resumed. For patients undergoing major surgery under general anesthesia, the following protocol is useful:

- *Evening before procedure*—100 mg of cortisone acetate intramuscularly;
- *Day of the operation*—100 mg of cortisone acetate intramuscularly 1 hour before the procedure and 50 mg every eight hours thereafter.

Intravenous infusion with 1,000 mL of 5% dextrose in normal saline containing 100 mg of hydrocortisone succinate should be started before operation and infused over the ensuing 8–12 hours;

- *First postoperative day*—cortisone acetate, 50 mg q.6h. intramuscularly;
- *Second postoperative day*—cortisone acetate, 50 mg q.8h. intramuscularly;
- *Third postoperative day*—cortisone acetate, 30 mg q.6h. intramuscularly;
- *Fourth postoperative day*—cortisone acetate, 25 mg q.8h., either orally or intramuscularly;
- *Fifth postoperative day*—cortisone acetate, 25 mg b.i.d.; florinef, 0.1 mg/day;
- *Sixth postoperative day*—cortisone acetate, 25 mg in the A.M. and 12.5 mg in the P.M.; florinef, 0.1 mg/day.

If the patient is able to take pills by mouth and has no nausea, the replacement with cortisone acetate can be given by mouth starting on the third day postoperatively. In the event of complications of surgery, fever, or infection, the patient should be maintained on a dosage of approximately 150–200 mg of cortisone acetate until the febrile process or infection is controlled. After that, steroids should be tapered as indicated.

Course and Prognosis

Untreated Addison's disease is a chronic and progressive disease. However, with adequate treatment the prognosis is good and the patient should expect to have a fully active life. Patients with autoimmune Addison's may develop other autoimmune-associated disorders and the physician should be alerted to these possibilities. The main danger to addisonian patients is the development of adrenal crisis during periods of stress. However, proper education and treatment helps to prevent this complication.

Secondary Adrenocortical Insufficiency

Deficiency of pituitary ACTH secretion causes secondary adrenal insufficiency. This deficiency may be selective, as in the case of isolated ACTH deficiency, or after chronic treatment with glucocorticoids, or generalized as seen in panhypopituitarism. The most common causes of secondary adrenocortical insufficiency are listed in Table 9.

Chromophobe adenomas and craniopharyngiomas are frequent causes of secondary adrenal insufficiency. Hyperfunctioning pituitary tumors can sometimes cause secondary adrenal insufficiency, but it is rare. On the other hand, successful removal of basophilic microadenomas causing Cushing's syndrome is followed by the rapid onset of secondary adrenal insufficiency. Postpartum necrosis of the pituitary (Sheehan's syndrome) is a common cause of pituitary failure. Isolated ACTH deficiency is a rare cause of secondary adrenocortical insufficiency. There are only 43 cases of isolated ACTH deficiency reported in the literature and it appears that

TABLE 9. Causes of Secondary Adrenocortical Insufficiency

1. Pituitary tumors: chromophobe adenomas
   craniopharyngioma
   hyperfunctioning tumors
2. Pituitary infarction
3. Hypophysectomy
4. Irradiation of the pituitary
5. Metastatic destruction of pituitary
6. Infection
7. Granulomatous destruction of the pituitary gland
8. Isolated ACTH deficiency
9. Chronic treatment with glucocorticoids for nonendocrine uses

this entity represents a heterogeneous group of disorders of ACTH secretion (368). One of the most common causes of secondary adrenocortical insufficiency is the chronic administration of glucocorticoids for nonendocrine diseases.

Clinical Manifestations. The clinical manifestations of secondary adrenocortical insufficiency are similar to those found in primary adrenocortical insufficiency or Addison's disease with the exception that hyperpigmentation does not occur in secondary adrenal insufficiency since the levels of ACTH/β-LPH, γ-LPH are characteristically low. Another distinguishing feature in secondary adrenal insufficiency is the finding of normal to low-normal levels of aldosterone under basal conditions, since the renin-angiotensin system is usually normal in these patients. Similarly, and by the same reason, hyperkalemia does not occur in secondary adrenal insufficiency. On the other hand, dilutional hyponatremia resulting from excess antidiuretic hormone (ADH) and decreased GFR is a common finding. Increased ADH levels and decreased GFR results from a decrease in the "effective" circulating blood volume owing to decreased cardiac output. This abnormality is rapidly corrected after cortisol administration. Adrenal insufficiency secondary to panhypopituitarism may be associated with symptoms and signs caused by the lack of other trophic pituitary hormones, such as hypothyroidism and hypogonadism. However, some patients with polyglandular autoimmune syndrome may also present with adrenal insufficiency, hypothyroidism, and hypogonadism. However, in this latter group of patients, hyperpigmentation is not present.

Diagnosis. The plasma cortisol and the urinary excretion of free cortisol, 17-OHCS, and 17-ketosteroids are low in secondary adrenal insufficiency. Plasma ACTH is also low and prolonged ACTH testing of these patients shows the typical "staircase" increase in urinary steroids. Metyrapone testing may be dangerous and usually shows no increase in 17-

OHCS. Patients with panhypopituitarism may be more sensitive to insulin-induced hypoglycemia and usually fail to increase ACTH and cortisol levels after adequate hypoglycemic stimulus.

Therapy. Substitution therapy with glucocorticoids is similar to that used for primary adrenal insufficiency. On the other hand, mineralocorticoid replacement is not necessary since in these patients aldosterone secretion is usually unimpaired. Patients with secondary adrenal insufficiency should follow the same guidelines outlined for addisonian patients while under periods of stress, surgery, or infection.

Acute Adrenocortical Insufficiency

Acute adrenal insufficiency or adrenal crisis may develop in addisonian patients who are subject to stress, trauma, surgery, or in patients with adrenal atrophy from rapid withdrawal of steroids secondary to chronic steroid treatment who have suffered rapid withdrawal of steroids. It can also develop acutely in patients without a previous history of adrenal insufficiency as a result of adrenal hemorrhage associated with anticoagulant therapy, particularly in patients with myocardial infarction or pulmonary embolus. Adrenal hemorrhage may also develop in patients with overwhelming septicemia (Waterhouse–Friderichsen syndrome). In patients with a previous history of adrenal insufficiency, adrenal crisis presents as a rapid exacerbation of the symptoms of chronic adrenal insufficiency. Severe nausea, vomiting, and abdominal pain are usually present. High fever is usually seen but the absence of fever does not rule out the diagnosis. Severe dehydration secondary to intractable vomiting, diarrhea, and sodium wasting by the kidney is usually present. The pulse is rapid and feeble. Severe hypotension and shock rapidly develop. Extreme prostration, somnolence, and lethargy are common. Patients in adrenal crisis secondary to rapid withdrawal of steroids may not initially show dehydration or hypotension since aldosterone secretion is usually preserved. In patients with adrenal hemorrhage, pain in the flank and epigastrium is a frequent complaint and if the hemorrhagic process extends into the abdomen signs of peritoneal irritation may be present. Unexplained hypotension in a patient on anticoagulant therapy may be a presenting symptom of adrenal hemorrhage.

Therapy. Acute adrenal insufficiency is a life-threatening condition that requires immediate therapy. Extremely ill patients should be given an intravenous bolus of 100 mg of soluble hydrocortisone succinate followed by the rapid infusion of 1,000 mL of 5% dextrose in normal saline containing 100 mg of hydrocortisone succinate. The initial 250–500 mL should be infused over 30 to 60 minutes according to the levels of blood pressure and the degree of dehydration of the patient. After the blood pressure is restored the rate of infusion can be slowed down so that the remainder of the first liter of fluid is administered over the ensuing 2–4 hours. The majority of patients in addisonian crisis require 2–4 L of intravenous fluids and 300–400 mg of hydrocortisone in the initial 24 hours of treatment. After the blood pressure is restored, and in patients with poor veins, it is advisable to administer 100 mg of cortisone acetate intramuscularly to avoid possible interruptions of therapy due to infiltration of the infusion. Hypertonic saline replacement should be avoided and 5% dextrose in normal physiological saline is the treatment of choice. In patients with severe long-standing hyponatremia, rapid correction of the serum sodium should be avoided since it may precipitate severe, and sometimes irreversible, neurologic damage. It has been shown that in long-standing severe hyponatremic states, rapid correction of the serum sodium may lead to central pontine myelolysis, a condition that may cause permanent neurological damage (211). There is usually no need for mineralocorticoid replacement during the treatment of adrenal crisis as the large doses of cortisol will contain sufficient mineralocorticoid activity. Usually, the serum potassium decreases gradually after the onset of therapy. A search for a precipitating cause, such as infection, etc., and proper cultures and antibiotic coverage, should be administered. In uncomplicated cases and if there is no evidence of infection, steroids can gradually be tapered down, as indicated previously, and in approximately 4–6 days the patient can be placed back on maintenance dosages of steroids.

REFERENCES

1. Abe, K., Island, D. P., Liddle, G. W., Fleischer, N., and Nicholson, W. E. (1967) Radioimmunologic evidence for an α-MSH (melanocyte stimulating hormone) in human pituitary and tumor tissues. J. Clin. Endocrinol. Metab. 27, 46–52.
2. Abe, K., Nicholson, W. E., Liddle, G. W., Orth, D. N., and Island, D. P. (1969) Normal and abnormal regulation of β-MSH in man. J. Clin. Invest. 48, 1580–1585.
3. Abernathy, R. S., and Melby, J. C. (1961) Addison's disease in North American blastomycosis. N. Engl. J. Med. 54, 189.
4. Aco, Z., and Stark, E. (1978) Possible role of GABA synthesis in the mechanism of dexamethasone-feedback action. J. Endocrinol. 77, 137.
5. Addison, T. (1849) Anemia–disease of the suprarenal capsules. London Med. Gaz. N.S. 43, 517.
6. Addison, T. (1855) On the Constitutional and Local Effects of Disease of the Supra-renal Capsules. Highley, London.
7. Albright, F. (1942-1943) Cushing's syndrome. Harvey Lect. 38, 123–186.
8. Allolio, B., Winkelmann, W., Kaulen, D., Hipp, F. X., and Miles, R. (1982) Valproate in Cushing's syndrome. Lancet i, 171.
9. Ambrosi, B., Gaggini, M., Secchi F., and Faglia, G. (1979) Lack of effect of antiserotoninergic and/or dopaminergic treatment in patients with pituitary-dependent Cushing's syndrome. Horm. Metab. Res. 11, 318.
10. Anderson, E., Haymaker, W., and Joseph, M. (1938) Hormone and electrolyte studies of patients with hyperadrenocortical syndrome (Cushing's syndrome). Endocrinology 23, 398.
11. Anderson, J. R., Goudie, R. B., Gray, K. G., and Timbury, G. C. (1957) Autoantibodies in Addison's disease. Lancet i, 1123.
12. Aron, D. C., Findling, J. W., Fitzgerald, P. J., Brooks, R. M., Fisher, F. E., Forsham,

P. H., and Tyrrel, J. B. (1981) Pituitary ACTH dependency of nodular adrenal hyperplasia in Cushing's syndrome. Am. J. Med. 71, 302–306.

13. Aron, D. C. Findling, J. W., Fitzgerald, P. A., Forsham, P. H., Wilson, C. B., and Tyrrel, J. B. (1982) Cushing's syndrome: Problems in management. Endocr. Rev. 3, 229–249.

14. Arulanatham, K., Dwyer, J. M., and Genel, M. (1979) Evidence for defective immunoregulation in the syndrome of familial candidiasis endocrinopathy. N. Engl. J. Med. 300, 164–168.

14a. Asa, S. L., Kovacs, K., Tindall, G. T., Barrow, D. L., Horvath, E., and Vecsei, P. (1984) Cushing's disease associated with an intrasellar gangliocytoma producing corticotrophin-releasing factor. Ann. Int. Med. 101, 789–793.

15. Asfeldt, V. H. (1969) Simplified dexamethasone suppression test. Acta Endocrinol. 61, 219–231.

16. Ashcraft, M. W., Van Herle, A. J., Vener, S. L., and Geffner, D. L. (1982) Serum cortisol levels in Cushing's syndrome after low- and high-dose dexamethasone suppression. Ann. Intern. Med. 97, 21–26.

17. Azzopardi, J. G., and Williams, G. D. (1968) Pathology of non-endocrine tumors associated with Cushing's syndrome. Cancer 22, 274–286.

18. Bailey, R. E. (1971) Periodic hormonogenesis—a new phenomenon. Periodicity in function of a hormone-producing tumor in man. J. Clin. Endocrinol. Metab. 32, 317–327.

19. Baylin, S. B., and Mendelsohn, G. (1980) Ectopic (inappropriate) hormone production by tumors, mechanisms involved, and the biological and clinical implications. Endocr. Rev. 1, 45.

20. Beck-Nielsen, H., De Pirro, R., and Pedersen, O. (1980) Prednisone increases in the number of insulin receptors on monocytes from normal subjects. J. Clin. Endocrinol. Metab. 50, 1.

21. Beierwaltes, W. H., Lieberman, L. M., Ansari, A. N., and Nishiyama, H. (1971) Visualization of human adrenal glands in vivo by scintillation scanning. JAMA 216, 275.

22. Berns, A. S., Pluss, R. G., Erickson, A. L., Anderson, R. J., McDonald, K. M., and Schrier, R. W. (1977) Renin-angiotensin system and cardiovascular homeostasis in adrenal insufficiency. Am. J. Physiol. 233, F509.

23. Berson, S. A., and Yalow, R. S. (1968) Radioimmunoassay of ACTH in plasma. J. Clin. Invest. 47, 2725–2751.

24. Bertagna, C., and Orth, D. N. (1981) Clinical and laboratory findings and results of therapy in 58 patients with adrenocortical tumors admitted to a single medical center (1951-1978). Am. J. Med. 71, 855–875.

25. Bertagna, X. Y., Nicholson, W. E., Sorenson, G. D., Pettengill, O. S., and Orth, D. N. (1978) Endorphin, corticotropin and lipotropin production by a human nonpituitary tumor in tissue culture: Evidence for a common precursor (Abst.). Clin. Res. 26, 489A.

26. Bertagna, X. Y., Stone, W. J., Nicholson, W. E., and Mount, C. D. (1981) Simultaneous assay of immunoreactive β-lipotropin, γ-lipotropin, and β-endorphin in plasma of normal human subjects, patients with ACTH/lipotropin hypersecretory syndromes and patients undergoing chronic hemodialysis. J. Clin. Invest. 67, 124.

27. Besser, G. M., Edwards, C. R. W. (1972) Cushing's syndrome. Clin. Endocrinol. Metab. 1, 451–490.

28. Bethge, H., Nahmer, D., and Zimmerman, H. (1967) The insulin tolerance test in assessment of the hypothalamic–pituitary–adrenal axis. I. Normal persons. Acta Endocrinol. 54, 668–680.

29. Bethge, H., Bayer, J. M., and Winkelmann, W. (1969) Diagnosis of Cushing's syndrome. The differentiation between adrenocortical hyperplasia and adrenocortical adenoma by means of lysine–vasopressin. Acta Endocrinol. 60, 47–59.

30. Bhettay, E., and Bonnici, F. (1977) Pure estrogen-secreting feminizing adrenocortical adenoma. Arch. Dis. Child. 52, 241-243.

31. Biglieri, E. G., and Lopez, J. M. (1976) Clinical and laboratory diagnosis of adrenocortical hypertension. Cardiovasc. Med. 1, 335–341.
32. Bigos, S. T., Somma, M., Rasio, E., Eastman, R. C., Lanthier, A., Johnston, J. J., and Hardy, J. (1980) Cushing's disease; management by transsphenoidal pituitary microsurgery. J. Clin. Endocrinol. Metab. 50, 384.
33. Birkenhäger, J. C., Timmermans, H. A. T., and Lamberts, S. W. J. (1976) Depressed plasma FFA turnover rate in Cushing's syndrome. J. Clin. Endocrinol. Metab. 42, 28–32.
34. Blan, N., Miller, W. E., Miller, E. R., Jr., and Cerri-Skinner, S. J. (1975) Spontaneous remission of Cushing's syndrome in a patient with an adrenal adenoma. J. Clin. Endocrinol. Metab. 40, 659–663.
35. Blichert-Tott, M., Bagerskov, A., and Lockwood, K., et al. (1972) Operative treatment, surgical approach, and related complications in 195 operations upon the adrenal glands. Surg. Gynecol. Obstet. 135, 261–266.
36. Blizzard, R. M., and Kyle, M. (1963) Studies of the adrenal antigens and antibodies in Addison's disease. J. Clin. Invest. 42, 1653.
37. Bloomfield, G. A., and Scott, A. P. (1974) β-Melanocyte stimulating hormone. Proc. R. Soc. Med. 67, 748–749.
38. Bocuzzi, G. Angeli, A., Bisbocci, D., Fonzo, D., Gaidano, G. P., and Ceresa, F. (1975) Effect of synthetic luteinizing releasing hormone (LH-RH) on the release of gonadotropins in Cushing's disease. J. Clin. Endocrinol. Metab. 40, 892–895.
39. Bohus, B., Endroczi, E., and Lissak, K. (1965) Adrenal system: Stress and humoral feed-back control. Acad. Sci. Hung. 27, 279.
40. Bondy, P. K. (1980) Endocrine and metabolic effects of cancer. In: P. K. Bondy and L. E. Rosenberg (eds.) , Metabolic Control and Disease, W. B. Saunders, Philadelphia, pp. 1815–1841.
41. Boyar, R. M., Witkin, M., Carruth, A., and Ramsey, J. (1979) Circadian cortisol secretory rhythms in Cushing's disease. J. Clin. Endocrinol. Metab. 48, 760.
42. Brannstein, G. D., and Loriaux, D. L. (1971) Proton beam therapy. N. Engl. J. Med. 284, 332–336.
43. Bressot, C., Meunier, P. J., Chapuy, M. C., Lejeune, E., Edouard, C., and Darby, A. J. (1979) Histomorphometric profile, pathophysiology and reversibility of corticosteroid-induced osteoporosis. Metab. Bone Dis. Relat. Res. 1, 303–311.
44. Brown, J. S. L. (1943) The effect of adrenocorticotrophic hormone on the excretion of cortin-like substances and 17-ketosteroids and on carbohydrates tolerance and nitrogen balance. Conference on Metabolic Aspects of Convalescence, Josiah Macy, Jr. Foundation Report, 4th Meeting, New York, June 11–12, p. 88.
45. Brown, R. D., and Strott, C. A. (1971) Plasma deoxycorticosterone in man. J. Clin. Endocrinol. Metab. 32, 744-750.
46. Brown, R. D., Van Loon, G. R., Orth, D. N., and Liddle, G. W. (1973) Cushing's disease with periodic hormonogenesis: One explanation for paradoxical response to dexamethasone. J. Clin. Endocrinol. Metab. 36, 445–451.
47. Brown-Sequard, E. (1856) Les capsules surrenales. Arch. Gen. Med. 8, 385.
48. Brown, W. H. (1928) A case of pluriglandular syndrome: Diabetes of bearded women. Lancet ii, 1022–1023.
49. Bullock, G. R., Carter, E. E., Eliot, P., Peters, R. F., Simpson, P., and White, A. M. (1972) Relative changes in the function of muscle ribosomes and mitochondria during the early phase of steroid-induced catabolism. Biochem. J. 127, 881.
50. Burke, C. W. and Beardwell, C.G. (1973) Cushing's syndrome. Q. J. Med. 42, 175–204.
51. Burke, C. W., Doyle, F. H., Joplin, G. F., Arnot, R. N., Macerlean, D. P. and Fraser, T. R. (1973) Cushing's disease: Treatment by pituitary implantation of radioactive gold or yttrium seeds. Q. J. Med. 42, 693–714.
52. Butler, P. W. P., and Besser, G. M. (1968) Pituitary-adrenal function in severe depressive illness. Lancet i, 1234–1236.

53. Cahill, G. (1971) Action of adrenal cortical steroids on carbohydrate metabolism. In: N. P. Christy (ed.), The Human Adrenal Cortex, Harper and Row, New York, p. 205.

54. Canalis, E. (1983) Effect of glucocorticoids on type I collagen synthesis, alkaline phosphatase activity, and deoxyribonucleic acid content in cultured rat calvariae. Endocrinology 112, 931–939.

55. Carmalt, M. H. B., Dalton, G. A., Fletcher, R. F., and Smith, T. (1977) The treatment of Cushing's disease by transsphenoidal hypophysectomy. Q. J. Med. 66 (181), 119– 134.

56. Caro, J. F., Meikle, A. W., Check, J. H., et al. (1978) Normal suppression to dexamethasone in Cushing's disease: An expression of decreased metabolic clearance for dexamethasone. J. Clin. Endocrinol. Metab. 47, 667–670.

57. Case Record of the Massachusetts General Hospital (Case 23-1979) (1979) N. Engl. J. Med. 1322–1328.

58. Cassar, J., Doyle, F. H., Lewis, P. D., Mashiter, K., Van Noorden, S., and Joplin, G. F. (1976) Treatment of Nelson's syndrome by pituitary implantation of yttrium-90 or gold-198. Br. Med. J. 2, 269-272.

59. Cassidy, C. E., Rosenfeld, P. S., and Bokat, M. A. (1966) Suppression of activity of the adrenal cortex by dexamethasone in Cushing's syndrome. J. Clin. Endocrinol. Metab. 26, 1181–1184.

60. Cavagnini, F., Raggi, U., Micossi, P., Di Landro, A., and Invitti, C. (1976) Effect of an antiserotoninergic drug, metergoline, on the ACTH and cortisol response to insulin hypoglycemia and lysine-vasopressin in man. J. Clin. Endocrinol. Metab. 43, 306.

61. Cerny, J. C., Nesbit, R. M., Conn, J. W., Bookstein, J. D., Rouner, D. R., Cohen, E. L., Lucas, C. D., Warshawsky, A., and Southwell, T. (1970) Preoperative tumor localization by adrenal venography in patients with primary aldosteronism: A comparison with operative findings. J. Urol. 103, 521–528.

62. Chajek, T., and Romanoff, H. (1976) Cushing syndrome with cyclical edema and periodic secretion of corticosteroids. Arch. Intern. Med. 136, 441–443.

63. Chan, J. S. D., Seidah, N. G., and Chretien, M. (1981) Human N-terminal fragment of pro-opiomelanocortin in plasmas of normal subjects, patients with Cushing's disease, Nelson's syndrome, and ectopic tumor measured by radioimmunoassay. Proc. 63rd Annual Meeting of the Endocrine Society, Cincinnati, OH, p. 183.

64. Chayen, J., Loveridge, N., and Daly, J. R. (1972) A sensitive bioassay for ACTH in human plasma. Clin. Endocrinol. 1, 219-233.

65. Chihara, K., Kato, Y., Maeda, K., Matsukura, S., and Imura, H. (1976) Suppression by cyproheptadine of human growth hormone and cortisol secretion during sleep. J. Clin. Invest. 57, 1393.

66. Child, D. F., Burke, C. W., Burley, D. M., Rees, L. H., and Fraser, T. R. (1976) Drug control of Cushing's syndrome. Combined aminoglutethamide and metyrapone therapy. Acta Endocrinol. (Copenh.) 82, 330.

67. Choi, Y., Werk, E. E., and Sholiton, L. J. (1970) Cushing's syndrome with dual pituitary–adrenal control. Arch. Intern. Med. 125, 1045–1049.

68. Christy, N. P. (1971) Iatrogenic Cushing's syndrome. In: N P. Christy (ed.), The Human Adrenal Cortex, Harper and Row, New York, pp. 395–425.

68a. Chrousos, G. P., Schulte, H. M., Oldfield, E. D., Gold, P. W., Cutler, G. B., Jr., and Loriaux, L. (1984) The corticotropin releasing factor stimulation test. An aid in the evaluation of patients with Cushing's syndrome. N. Engl. J. Med. 310, 622–626.

69. Cochet, M., Chang, C. Y., and Cohen, S. N. (1982) Characterization of the structural gene and putative 5′-regulatory sequences for human proopiomelanocortin. Nature 297, 335.

70. Cope, C. L., and Black, E. G. (1958) The behavior of ^{14}C cortisol and estimation of cortisol production rate in man. Clin. Sci. 17, 147–163.

71. Copeland, P. M. (1983) The incidentally discovered adrenal mass. Ann. Int. Med. 98, 940–945.

72. Corrigan, D. F., Schaaf, M., Whaley, R. A., et al. (1977) Selective venous sampling to differentiate ectopic ACTH secretion from pituitary Cushing's syndrome. N. Engl. J. Med. 296, 861–862.
73. Crane, M. G., and Harris, J. J. (1966) Desoxycorticosterone secretion rates in hyperadrenocorticism. J. Clin. Endocrinol. Metab. 26, 1135–1143.
74. Crapo, L. (1979) Cushing's syndrome: A review of diagnostic tests. Metabolism 28, 955–977.
75. Crispell, E. R., Parson, W., Hamlin, J., et al. (1956) Addison's disease associated with histoplasmosis: Report of four cases and review of the literature. Am. J. Med. 20, 23.
76. Currie, R. A., and Cidlowski, J. A. (1982) Identification of modified forms of human glucocorticoid receptors during the cell cycle. Endocrinology 110, 2192.
77. Cushing, H. (1912) The Pituitary Body and its Disorders. Lippincott, Philadelphia, London.
78. Cushing, H. (1932) The basophilic adenomas of the pituitary body and their clinical manifestations (pituitary basophilism). Bull. of the Johns Hopkins Hosp. 50 (3), 137–195.
79. Cushing, H. (1934) Hyperactivation of the neurohypophysial as the pathological basis of eclampsia and other hypertensive states. Am. J. Pathol. 10, 145–176.
80. D'Agati, V. C., and Marangoni, B. A. (1945) The Waterhouse–Fridericksen syndrome. N. Engl. J. Med. 232, 1.
81. Dalakos, T. G., Elias, A. N., Anderson, G. H., Streeten, D. H. P., and Schroeder, E. T. (1978) Evidence for an angiotensinogenic mechanism of the hypertension in Cushing's syndrome. J. Clin. Endocrinol. Metab. 46, 114–118.
82. Daly, J. R., Fleisher, M. R., Chambers, D. J., et al. (1974) Application of the cytochemical bioassay for ACTH to clinical and physiological studies in man. Clin. Endocrinol. 3, 335–345.
83. Daughaday, W. H., Jaffe, H. and Williams, R. H. (1948) Adrenocortical hormone excretion in endocrine and non-endocrine disease as measured by chemical assay. J. Clin. Endocrinol. Metab. 8, 244–256.
84. Davis, J. O., Carpenter, C. C. J., Ayers, C. R., et al. (1961) Evidence for secretion of an aldosterone-stimulating hormone by the kidney. J. Clin. Invest. 40, 684–696.
85. DeMoor, P., Steeno, O., Raskin, M., et al. (1960) Fluorimetric determination of free plasma 11-hydroxycorticosteroids in man. Acta Endocrinol. 33, 297–307.
86. DePirro, R., Green, A., Yung-Chin Kao, M., and Olefsky, J. (1981) Effects of prednisolone and dexamethasone in vivo and in vitro: Studies of insulin binding, deoxyglucose uptake, and glucose oxidation in rat adipocytes. Diabetologia 21, 149.
87. Dluhy, R. G., and Williams, G. H. (1982) Cushing's syndrome and the changing times. Ann. Intern. Med. 97, 131–133.
88. Dohan, F. C., Raventos, A., Boucot, N., and Rose, E. (1957) Roentgen therapy in Cushing's syndrome without adrenocortical tumor. J. Clin. Endocrinol. Metab. 17, 8.
89. Donald, R. A., and Espiner, E. A. (1975) The plasma cortisol and corticotrophin response to hypoglycemia following adrenal steroid and ACTH administration. J. Clin. Endocrinol. Metab. 41, 1.
90. Dornhorst, A., Jenkins, J. S., Lamberts, S. W., Abraham, R. R., Wynn, V., Beckford, V., Gillham, B., and Johns, M. T. (1983) The evaluation of sodium valproate in the treatment of Nelson's syndrome. J. Clin. Endocrinol. Metab. 56, 985.
91. Dunnick, N. R., Schaner, E. G., Doppman, J. L., et al. (1979) Computed tomography in adrenal tumors. Am. J. Roentgenol. 132, 43–46.
92. Eddy, R. L., Jones, A. L., Gilliland, P. F., et al. (1973) Cushing's syndrome: A prospective study of diagnostic methods. Am. J. Med. 55, 621–630.
93. Eisenbarth, G. S., Wilson, P. W., Ward, F., Buckley, C., and Lebovitz, H. (1979) The polyglandular failure syndrome: Disease inheritance, HLA type and immune function. Ann. Int. Med. 91, 528–533.

94. Eisenhardt, L., and Thompson, K. W. (1939) A brief consideration of the present status of the so-called pituitary basophilism. Yale J. Biol. Med. 11, 507–522.

95. Elijovich, F., and Krakoff, L. R. (1980) Effect of converting enzyme inhibition on glucocorticoid hypertension in the rat. Am. J. Physiol. 238, H844–H848.

96. Ernest, I., and Ekman, H. (1972) Adrenalectomy in Cushing's disease: A long-term follow-up. Acta Endocrinol. 69 (suppl. 160), 5–41.

97. Fantus, I., Ryan, J., Hiraka, N., and Gorden, P. (1981) The effect of glucocorticoids on the insulin receptor: An in vivo and in vitro study. J. Clin. Endocrinol. Metab. 52, 953.

98. Farrell, P. M., Rikkers, H., and Moel, D. (1976) Cortisol-dihydrotachysterol antagonism in a patient with hypoparathyroidism and adrenal insufficiency: Apparent inhibition of bone resorption. J. Clin. Endocrinol. Metab. 42, 953–957.

99. Fehm, H. L., Voigt, K. H., Kummer, G., and Pfeiffer, E. F. (1979) Positive rate-sensitive corticosteroid feedback mechanism of ACTH secretion in Cushing's disease. J. Clin. Invest. 64, 102.

100. Fitzgerald, P. A., Aron, D. C., Findling, J. W., Brooks, R. M., Wilson, C. B., Forsham, P. H., and Tyrrell, J. B. (1982) Cushing's disease: Transient secondary adrenal insufficiency after selective removal of pituitary microadenomas; evidence for a pituitary origin. J. Clin. Endocrinol. Metab. 54, 413.

101. Frajria, R., and Angeli, A. (1977) Alcohol-induced pseudo-Cushing's syndrome. Lancet i, 1050.

102. Franco-Saenz, R. (1982) Endocrine syndromes. In: R. T. Skeel (ed.), Manual of Cancer Chemotherapy, Little, Brown and Co., Boston, pp. 231–248.

103. Fraser, R., James, V. H. T., Landon, J., Peart, W. S., Rawson, A., Giles, C. A., and McKay, A. M. (1968) Clinical and biochemical studies of a patient with a corticosterone-secreting adrenocortical tumor. Lancet ii, 1116–1120.

104. Frawley, T. F. (1967) Adrenal cortical insufficiency. In: A. B. Eisenstein (ed.), The Adrenal Cortex, pp. 439.

105. Freeman, R. H., and Rostorfer, H. H. (1972) Hepatic changes in renin substrate biosynthesis and alkaline phosphatase activity. Am. J. Physiol. 233, 364-370.

106. Fremery, P., Laqueur, Reichstein, T., Spanhoff, R. W., and Uyldert, I. E. (1937) Corticosterone, a crystallized compound with the biological activity of the adrenal cortical hormone. Nature 139, 26.

107. Frost, H. M., and Villaneuva, A. R. (1961) Human osteoblastic activity. III. The effect of cortisone on lamellar osteoblastic activity. Henry Ford Hosp. Bull. 9, 97.

108. Fukushima, D. K., Bradlow, H. L., Hellman, L., et al. (1960) Metabolic transformation of hydrocortisone-4-C^{14} in normal men. J. Biol. Chem. 235, 2246–2252.

109. Gabcke, C. E. (1931) Uber einen Fall vom primarem-Spindelzellen-sarkom des Thymus. Inaugural dissertation. Kiel, P. Peters. Quoted by D. Leyton, H. M. Turnbull, A. B. Bratton. J. Pathol. Bacteriol. 34, 635.

110. Gabrilove, J. L., Sharma, D. C., Wotiz, H. H., and Dorman, R. I. (1965) Feminizing adrenocortical tumors in the male: A review of 52 cases including a case report. Medicine 44, 37.

111. Gabrilove, J. L., Nicolis, G. L., and Sohval, A. R. (1974) The testis in Cushing's syndrome. J. Urol. 112, 95–99.

112. Gabrilove, J. L., Seman, A. T., Sabet, R., Mitty, H. A., and Nicolis, G. L. (1981) Virilizing adrenal adenoma with studies of steroid content of the adrenal venous effluent and a review of the literature. Endocr. Rev. 2, 462–470.

113. Ganong, W. F., and Mulrow, P. J. (1961) Evidence of secretion of an aldosterone-stimulating substance by the kidney. Nature 190, 1115–1116.

114. Garcia, J. H., Kalimo, H., and Givens, J. R. (1976) Human adenohypophysis in Nelson's syndrome. Arch. Pathol. Lab. Med. 100, 253.

115. George, W. F., Jasain, M., Lock, J. P., and Katz, F. H. (1982) Failure of cyproheptadine to inhibit vasopressin-stimulated cortisol release in a patient with Cushing's disease. Horm. Res. 7, 308.

116. Gershengorn, M. C., Arevalo, C. O., Geras, E., and Rebecchi, M. J. (1980) Thyrotropin-releasing hormone stimulation of adrenocorticotropin production by mouse pituitary tumor cells in culture. J. Clin. Invest. 65, 1294.

117. Gewirtz, G., and Yalow, R. S. (1974) Ectopic ACTH production in carcinoma of the lung. J. Clin. Invest. 53, 1022–1032.

118. Gifford, S., and Gunderson, J. B. (1970) Cushing's disease as a psychosomatic disorder: a selective review of the clinical and experimental literature and a report of ten cases. Perspect. Biol. Med. 13, 169–221.

119. Gilkes, J. J. H., Rees, L. H., and Besser, G. M. (1977) Plasma immunoreactive corticotrophin and lipotrophin in Cushing's syndrome and Addison's disease. Br. Med. J. 1, 996–998.

120. Gold, E. M. (1979) Cushing's syndrome: Changing views of diagnosis and treatment. Ann. Int. Med. 90, 829–844.

121. Goldberg, M. B., Sheline, G. E., and Malamurd, N. (1963) Malignant intracranial neoplasms following radiation therapy for acromegaly. Radiology 80, 465–470.

122. Goudie, R. B., McDonald, E., Anderson, J. R., and Gray, K. (1968) Immunological features of idiopathic Addison's disease: Characterization of the adrenocortical antigens. Clin. Exper. Immunol. 3, 119.

123. Graber, A. L., Ney, R. L., Nicholson, W. E., et al. (1965) Natural history of pituitary-adrenal recovery following long-term suppression with corticosteroids. J. Clin. Endocrinol. Metab. 25, 11–16.

124. Green, H. H., Harrington, A. R., and Valtin, H. (1970) On the role of antidiuretic hormone in the inhibition of acute water diuresis in adrenal insufficiency and the effects of gluco- and mineralocorticoids in reversing the inhibition. J. Clin. Invest. 49, 1724–1736.

125. Green, J. R. B., and Van'T Hoff, W. (1975) Cushing's syndrome with fluctuation due to adrenal adenoma. J. Clin. Endocrinol. Metab. 41, 235–240.

126. Greipp, P. R. (1978) Hyperpigmentation syndromes (diffuse hypermelanosis). Arch. Intern. Med. 138, 356–357.

127. Gross, M. D., Valk, T. W., Freitas, J. A., Swanson, D. P., Schteingart, D. E., and Beierwalters, W. H. (1981) The relationship of adrenal cholesterol uptake to indices of adrenal cortical function in Cushing's syndrome. J. Clin. Endocrinol. Metab. 52, 1062.

128. Guerin, C. K., Wahner, H. W., Gorman, C. A., Carpenter, P. C., and Sheedy, P. F. (1983) Computed tomographic scanning versus radioisotope imaging in adrenocortical diagnosis. Am. J. Med. 75, 653.

129. Guillemin, R., Vargo, T., Rossier, J., Minick, S., Ling, N., Rivier, C., Vale, W., and Bloom, F. (1977) β-endorphin and adrenocorticotropin are secreted concomitantly by the pituitary gland. Science 197, 1367–1369.

130. Guttman, P. H. (1930) Addison's disease: A statistical analysis of 566 cases and a study of the pathology. Arch. Pathol. (Chicago) 10, 742, 895.

131. Gwinup, G. (1965) Studies on the mechanism of vasopressin-induced steroid secretion in man. Metabolism 14, 1282–1286.

132. Hahn, T. J. (1978) Corticosteroid-induced osteopenia. Arch. Intern. Med. 138, 882–885.

133. Haijar, R. A., Hickey, R. C., and Samaan, N. A. (1975) Adrenal cortical carcinoma: Study of 32 patients. Cancer 35, 549–554.

134. Hardy, J. (1982) Cushing's disease: 50 years later. Can. J. Neurol. Sci. 9, 375–380.

135. Hartman, F. A., MacArthur, C. G., and Hartman, W. E. (1927) A substance which prolongs the life of adrenalectomized cats. Proc. Soc. Exp. Biol. Med. 25, 69.

136. Hartman, F. A., Bown, B. D., Thorn, G. W., and Greene, C. (1931) Vital hormone of adrenal cortex. Ann. Intern. Med. 5, 539.

137. Hassoun, J., Charpin, C., Jaquet, P., Lissitzky, J. C., Grisoli, F., and Toga, M. (1982) Corticolipotropin immunoreactivity in silent chromophobe adenomas. Arch. Pathol. Lab. Med. 106, 25.

138. Hassoun, J., Charpin, C., Jaquet, P., Oliver, C., Lissitzky, J. C., Lucas, C., and Toga, M. (1978) Histological immunocytochemical and ultrastructural aspects of basophilic adenomas. A study of four cases. International Symposium on Pituitary Microadenomas, Serono, Milan, Italy.
139. Hausberger, F. X., and Hausberger, B. C. (1958) Effect of insulin and cortisone on weight gain, protein and fat content of rats. Am. J. Physiol. 193, 455.
140. Hay, I. D., Smail, P. J., and Forsyth, C. C. (1981) Familial cytomegalic adrenocortical hypoplasia: X-linked syndrome of pubertal failure. Arch. Dis. Child. 56, 715–721.
141. Hayslett, J. P., and Cohn, G.L. (1967) Spontaneous remission of Cushing's disease. Report of a case. N. Engl. J. Med. 276, 968.
142. Herrera, M. G., Cahill, G. F., Jr., and Thorn, G. W. (1964) Cushing's syndrome: diagnosis and treatment. Am. J. Surg. 107, 144–152.
143. Heuschle, R., and Lampe, I. (1967) Pituitary irradiation for Cushing's syndrome. Radiol. Clin. Biol. 36, 27.
144. Hjortrup, A., Kehlet, H., Lindholm, J., and Stentoft, P. (1983) Value of the 30 minute adrenocorticotropin (ACTH) test in demonstrating hypothalamic–pituitary–adrenocortical insufficiency after acute ACTH deprivation. J. Clin. Endocrinol. Metab. 57, 668.
145. Hoffman, D. L., and Mattox, V. R. (1972) Treatment of adrenocortical carcinoma with o,p¸-DDD. Med. Clin. North Am. 56, 999–1012.
146. Holdaway, I. M., Rees, L. H., and Landon, J. (1973) Circulating ACTH levels in severe hypopituitarism and in the neonate. Lancet ii, 1170–1172.
147. Hollt, V., Muller, O. A., and Fahlbusch, R. (1979) β-endorphin in human plasma: basal and pathologically elevated levels. Life Sci. 25, 37.
148. Hope, J., Ratter, S. J., Estivariz, F. E., McLoughlin, L., and Lowry, P. J. (1981) Development of a radioimmunoassay for an amino-terminal peptide of pro-opiocortin containing the γ-MSH region: Measurement and characterization in human plasma. Clin. Endocrinol. 15, 221.
149. Hopwood, N. J., and Kenny, F. M. (1977) Incidence of Nelson's syndrome after adrenalectomy for Cushing's disease in children. Am. J. Dis. Child. 131, 1353–1356.
150. Horvath, E., Kovacs, K., Killinger, D. W., Smith, H. S., Platts, M. E., and Singer, W. (1980) Silent corticotropic adenomas of the human pituitary gland. Am. J. Pathol. 98, 617.
151. Hough, A. J., Hollifield, J. W., Page, D. L., Scott, H. W., and Hartmann, W. H. (1979) Prognostic factors in adrenocortical tumors: A mathematical analysis of clinical and morphologic data. Am. J. Clin. Pathol. 72, 390–399.
152. Hough, S., Tettelbaum, S. L., Bergfeld, M. A., and Avioli, L. Y. (1981) Isolated skeletal involvement in Cushing's syndrome. Response to therapy. J. Clin. Endocrinol. Metab. 52, 1033.
153. Houser, O. W., Baker, H. L., Jr., Reese, D. F., and Homan, C. B. (1982) Radiographic evaluation of the sella turcica and the pituitary gland. In: E. R. Laws, Jr., R. V. Randall, E. B. Kern, and C. F. Abboud (eds.), Management of Pituitary Adenomas and Related Lesions with Emphasis on Transsphenoidal Microsurgery, Appleton Century-Crofts, New York, pp. 85–109.
154. Hsu, T. H., Gann, D. S., Tsan, K. W., and Russell, R. P. (1981) Cyproheptadine in the control of Cushing's disease. Johns Hopkins Med. J. 149, 77.
155. Huff, T. A. (1977) Clinical syndromes related to disorders of adrenocorticotropic hormone. In: M. B. Allen, Jr., and V. B. Mahesh (eds.), The Pituitary: A Current Review, Academic Press, New York, pp. 153–168.
156. Hutter, A. M., and Kayhoe, D. E. (1966) Adrenal cortical carcinoma: Clinical features of 138 patients. Am. J. Med. 41, 572–580.
157. Hutter, A. M., Jr., and Kayhoe, D. E. (1966) Adrenal cortical carcinoma: Results of treatment with *o,p'*-DDD in 138 patients. Am. J. Med. 41, 581-592.

158. Illingworth, D. R., Kenny, T. A., and Orwoll, E. S. (1982) Adrenal function in heterozygous and homozygous hypobetalipoproteinemia. J. Clin. Endocrinol. Metab. 54, 27.

158a. Illingworth, D. R., Lees, A. M., and Lees, R. S. (1983) Adrenal cortical function in homozygous familial hypercholesterolemia. Metabolism 30, 1045–1052.

159. Imura, H. (1980) Ectopic hormone syndrome. J. Clin. Endocrinol. Metab. 9, 235–260.

160. Imura, H., Matsukura, S., Yamamoto, H., Hirata, Y., Nakai, Y., Endo, J., Tanaka, A., and Nakamura, M. (1975) Studies on ectopic ACTH-producing tumors. II. Clinical and biochemical features of 30 cases. Cancer 35, 1430–1437.

161. Imura, H., Nakai, Y., Nakao, K., Oki, S., Matsukura, S., Hirata, Y., Fukase, M., Hattori, M., Yoshimi, H., and Sueoka, S. (1978) Functioning tumors with special reference to ectopic hormone producing tumors. Protein, Nucleic Acid and Enzyme 23, 641–656.

162. Irvine, W. J., Chan, M. M. W., and Scarth, L. (1969) The further characterization of auto-antibodies reactive with extra-renal steroid-producing cells in patients with adrenal disorders. Clin. Exper. Immunol. 4, 489.

163. Irvine, W. J., and Barnes, E. W. (1972) Adrenocortical insufficiency. Clin. Endocrinol. Metab. 1, 549–594.

164. Irvine, W. J., and Barnes, E. W. (1975) Addison's disease, ovarian failure and hypoparathyroidism. Clin. Endocrinol. Metab. 4, 379.

165. Jarvis, J. L., Jenkins, D., Sosman, M. C., et al. (1954) Roentgenologic observations in Addison's disease. A review of 120 cases. Radiology 62, 16.

166. Jee, W. S. S., Park, H. Z., Roberts, W. E., and Kenner, G. H. (1970) Corticosteroid and bone. Am. J. Anat. 129, 477–479.

167. Jeffcoate, W. J., Rees, L. H., Tomlin, S., Jones, A. E., Edwards, C. R. W., and Besser, G. M. (1977) Metyrapone in long-term management of Cushing's disease. Br. Med. J. 2, 215–217.

168. Jenkins, J. S., Ash, S., and Bloom, H. J. G. (1972) Endocrine function after external pituitary irradiation in patients with secreting and nonsecreting pituitary tumors. Q. J. Med. 41, 57–69.

169. Jennings, A. S., Liddle, G. W., and Orth, D. N. (1977) Results of treating childhood Cushing's disease with pituitary irradiation. N. Engl. J. Med. 297, 957.

170. Jones, M. T., Hillhouse, E. W., and Burden, J. L. (1976) The effect of various putative neurotransmitters on the release of CRF from the rat hypothalamus in vitro. J. Endocrinol. 69, 1.

171. Jordan, R. M., Jacobson, J. M, and Young, R. L. (1979) Alcohol induced Cushing's syndrome. South. Med. J. 72, 1347–1348.

172. Jowsey, J., and Riggs, B. L. (1970) Bone formation in hypercortisolism. Acta Endocrinol. (Copenh.) 63, 21.

173. Jubiz, W., Meikle, A. W., Levinson, R. A., et al. (1970) Effect of diphenylhydantoin on the metabolism of dexamethasone. N. Engl. J. Med. 283, 11–14.

174. Julesz, J., Laczi, F., Janaky, T., and Laszlo, F. (1980) Effects of somatostatin and bromocryptine on the plasma ACTH level in bilaterally adrenalectomized patients with Cushing's disease. Endokrinologie 76, 68.

175. Kaffe, S., Pettigrow, C. S., Cahill, L. T., Perlman, D., Moloshok, R. E., Hirschhorn, K., and Papageorgiou, P. S. (1975) Variable cell-mediated immune defects in a family with "Candida endocrinopathy syndrome." Clin. Exp. Immunol. 20, 397–408.

176. Kahn, P. C. (1967) The radiologic identification of functioning adrenal tumors. Radiol. Clin. North. Am. 5, 221–234.

177. Kahn, R., Goldfine, I., Neville, D., and De Meyts, P. (1978) Alteration in insulin binding induced by changes in vivo in the levels of glucocorticoids and growth hormones. Endocrinology 103, 1054.

178. Kapcala, L. P., and Jackson, I. M. D. (1982) Long term bromocriptine therapy in Cushing's disease. J. Endocrinol. Invest. 91, 117.
179. Kaplan, N. M., and Shires, G. T. (1972) Apparent cure of Cushing's disease by bilateral adrenalectomy and autotransplantation. Am. J. Med. 53, 377.
180. Kelch, R. P., Kaplan, S. L., Biglieri, E. G., et al. (1972) Hereditary adrenocortical unresponsiveness to adrenocorticotropic hormone. J. Pediatr. 81, 726–736.
181. Kelly, W. F., Barnes, A. J., Cassar, J., White, M., Mashiter, K., Loizou, S., Welbourn, R. B., and Joplin, G. F. (1979) Cushing's syndrome due to adrenocortical carcinoma. A comprehensive clinical and biochemical study of patients treated by surgery and chemotherapy. Acta Endocrinol. 91, 303–318.
182. Kendall, E. C., Mason, H. L., Hoehn, W. M., and McKenzie, B. F. (1937) Studies in chemistry of suprarenal cortex: Structure and physiologic activity of compound B: its relation to compound A and Reichstein's corticosterone. Proc. Mayo Clin. 12, 136.
183. Kennedy, A. L., Sheridan, B., and Montgomery, D. A. D. (1978) ACTH and cortisol response to bromocriptine and results of long-term therapy in Cushing's disease. Acta Endrocrinol. 89, 461.
184. Kershnar, A. K., Roe, T. F., and Kogut, M. D. (1972) Adrenocorticotropic hormone unresponsiveness: Report of a girl with excessive growth and review of 16 reported cases. J. Pediatr. 80, 610–619.
185. Kimberg, D. V., Baerg, R. D., Gershon, E., and Gracidusius, R. T. (1971) Effect of cortisone treatment on the active transport of calcium by the small intestine. J. Clin. Invest. 50, 1309.
186. Kjellberg, R. N., and Kliman, B. (1973) A system for therapy of pituitary tumors. In: P. O. Kohler and G. T. Ross (eds.), Diagnosis and Treatment of Pituitary Tumors, Elsevier, New York, p. 234.
187. Kleeman, C. R., Maxwell, M. H., and Rockney, R. E. (1958) Mechanisms of impaired water excretion in adrenal and pituitary insufficiency. I. The role of altered glomerular filtration rate and solute excretion. J. Clin. Invest. 37, 1799–1808.
188. Kliman, B., and Peterson, R. E. (1960) Double isotope derivative assay of aldosterone in biological extracts. J. Biol. Chem. 235, 1639–1648.
189. Komanicky, P., Spark, R. F., and Melby, J. C. (1978) Treatment of Cushing's syndrome with trilostane (WIN 24,540), an inhibitor of adrenal steroid biosynthesis. J. Clin. Endocrinol. Metab. 47, 1042–1051.
190. Krakoff, L. (1973) Measurement of plasma renin substrate by radioimmunoassay of angiotensin I: Concentration in syndromes associated with steroid excess. J. Clin. Endocrinol. Metab. 37, 110–117.
191. Krakoff, L. R., and Elijovich, F. (1981) Cushing's syndrome and exogenous glucocorticoid hypertension. J. Clin. Endocrinol. Metab. 10, 479.
192. Kricheff, I. I., and Schotland, D. L. (1964) Tumor stain in a pituitary adenoma. Radiology 82, 11.
193. Krieger, D. T., Allen, W., Rizzo, F., et al. (1971) Characterization of the normal temporal pattern of plasma corticosteroid levels. J. Clin. Endocrinol. Metab. 32, 266–284.
194. Krieger, D. T. (1978) The central nervous system and Cushing's disease. Med. Clin. North Am. 62, 261–268.
195. Krieger, D. T., Liotta, A. S., Suda, T., Goodgold, A., and Condon, E. (1979) Human plasma immunoreactive lipotropin and adrenocorticotropin in normal subjects and in patients with pituitary adrenal disease. J. Clin. Endocrinol. Metab. 48, 566.
196. Krieger, D. T. (1983) Physiopathology of Cushing's disease. Endocr. Rev. 4, 22–43.
197. Krieger, D. T., and Glick, S. (1972) Growth hormone and cortisol responsiveness in Cushing's syndrome: Relation to a possible central nervous system etiology. Am. J. Med. 52, 25.
198. Krieger, D. T., Liotta, A., and Li, C. H. (1977) Human plasma immunoreactive β-

lipotropin: Correlation with basal and stimulated plasma ACTH concentrations. Life Sci. 21, 1771.

199. Krieger, D. T., and Luria, M. (1977) Plasma ACTH and cortisol responses to TRF, vasopressin or hypoglycemia in Cushing's disease and Nelson's syndrome. J. Clin. Endocrinol. Metab. 44, 361.
200. Kwun Tang, C., and Gray, G. F. (1975) Adrenocortical neoplasms, prognosis and morphology. Urology 5, 691.
201. Lagerquist, L. G., Meikle, A. W., West, D. C., and Tyler, R. S. (1974) Cushing's disease with cure by resection of a pituitary adenoma: Evidence against a primary hypothalamic defect. Am. J. Med. 57, 826.
202. Lamberts, S. W. J., and Birkenhäger, J. C. (1976) Body composition in Cushing's disease. J. Clin. Endocrinol. Metab. 42, 864–866.
203. Lamberts, S. W. J., and Birkenhäger, J. C. (1976) Effect of bromocriptine in pituitary-dependent Cushing's syndrome. J. Endocrinol. 70, 315.
204. Lamberts, S. W. J., Klijn, J. G. M., De Jong, F. H., and Birkenhäger, J. C. (1979) Hormone secretion in alcohol-induced pseudo-Cushing's syndrome: Differential diagnosis with Cushing's disease. JAMA 242, 1640–1643.
205. Lamberts, S. W. J., Stefanko, S. Z., Fermin, Salh, Van Der Vijyer, J. M., Weber, R. F. A. and De Jong, F. H. (1980) Failure of clinical remission after transsphenoidal removal of a microadenoma in a patient with Cushing's disease: Multiple hyperplastic and adenomatous cell nests in surrounding pituitary tissue. J. Clin. Endrocrinol. Metab. 50, 793.
206. Lamberts, S. W. J., De Lange, S. A., and Stefanko, S. K. (1982) Adrenocorticotropin-secreting-pituitary adenomas originate from the anterior or the intermediate lobe in Cushing's disease: Differences in the regulation of hormone secretion. J. Clin. Endocrinol. Metab. 54, 286.
207. Landon, J., James, V. H. T., and Stoker, D. J. (1965) Plasma cortisol response to lysine-vasopressin: Comparison with other tests of human pituitary–adrenocortical function. Lancet ii, 1156–1159.
208. Lankford, H. V., Tucker, H. S. G., and Blackard, W. G. (1981) A cyproheptadine-reversible defect in ACTH control persisting after removal of the pituitary tumor in Cushing's disease. N. Engl. J. Med. 305, 1244–1248.
209. Laragh, J. H., Angers, M., Kelly, W. G. (1960) The effect of epinephrine, norepinephrine, angiotensin II, and others on the secretory rate of aldosterone in man. JAMA 174, 234–240.
210. Launois, P. E., Pinard, M., and Gallais, A. (1911) Syndrome adiposo-génital avec hypertrichose. Troubles Nerveux et Mentaux Gaz. d. Hop. 84, 649–654.
211. Lauren, O. R. (1983) Central pontine myelinolysis following rapid correction of the hyponatremia. Ann. Neurol. 13, 232–242.
212. Lawrence, J. H., Tobias, C. A., Linfoot, J. A., Born, J. L., and Chong, C. Y. (1976) Heavy-particle therapy in acromegaly and Cushing's disease. JAMA 235, 2307–2310.
213. Laws, E. R., and Kern, E. B. (1982) Complications of transsphenoidal surgery. In: E. R. Laws, Jr., R. Y. Randall, E. B. Kern, and C. F. Abboud (eds.), Management of Pituitary Adenomas and Related Lesions with Emphasis on Transsphenoidal Microsurgery, Appleton-Century-Crofts, New York, pp. 329–346.
214. Laws, Jr., E. R., Ebersold, M. J., Piepgras, D. G., Randall, R. V., and Salassa, R. M. (1982) The result of transsphenoidal surgery in specific clinical entities. In: E. R. Laws, Jr., R. V. Randall, E. B. Kern, and C. F. Abboud (eds.), Management of Pituitary Adenomas and Related Lesions with Emphasis on Transsphenoidal Microsurgery, Appleton-Century-Crofts, New York, pp. 277–305.
215. Lefkowitz, R. J., Roth, J., and Pastan, I. (1970) Radioreceptor assay of adrenocorticotropic hormone: New approach to assay of polypeptide hormones in plasma. Science 170, 633–635.
216. Liberman, B., Wajchenberg, B. L., Tambascia, M. A., et al. (1976) Periodic remission

in Cushing's disease with paradoxical dexamethasone response: An expression of periodic hormonogenesis. J. Clin. Endocrinol. Metab. 43, 913–918.

217. Liddle, G. W., Island, D., Lance, E. M., et al. (1958) Alterations of adrenal steroid patterns in man resulting from treatment with a chemical inhibitor of 11 β-hydroxylation. J. Clin. Endocrinol. Metab. 18, 906–912.

218. Liddle, G. W., Estep, H. L., Kendall, J. W., et al. (1959) Clinical application of a new test of pituitary reserve. J. Clin. Endocrinol. Metab. 19, 875–894.

219. Liddle, G. W. (1960) Tests of pituitary-adrenal suppressibility in the diagnosis of Cushing's syndrome. J. Clin. Endocrinol. Metab. 20, 1539–1560.

220. Liddle, G. W. (1967) Cushing's syndrome. In: A. B. Eisenstein (ed.), The Adrenal Cortex, Little, Brown and Co., Boston, pp. 523–552.

221. Liddle, G. W., Nicholson, W. E., Island, D. P., Orth, D. N., Abe, K., and Lowder, S. C. (1969) Clinical and laboratory studies of ectopic humoral syndromes. Rec. Prog. Horm. Res. 25, 283–314.

222. Liddle, G. W., (1981) The adrenals. In: R. H. Williams (ed.), Williams' Textbook of Endocrinology (6th ed.), W. B. Saunders, Philadelphia, p. 249.

223. Lieberman, L. M., Beierwaltes, W. H., Conn, J. W., Ansari, A., and Nishiyama, H. (1971) Diagnosis of adrenal disease by visualization of human adrenal glands with ^{131}I-19-iodocholesterol. N. Engl. J. Med. 285, 1387.

224. Linfoot, J. A. (1975) Heavy-ion therapy: α-particle therapy of pituitary tumors. In: J. A. Linfoot (ed.), Recent Advances in the Diagnosis and Treatment of Pituitary Tumors, Raven Press, New York, p. 254.

225. Linfoot, J. A. (1979) Heavy ion therapy. In: J. A. Linfoot (ed.), Recent Advances in the Diagnosis and Treatment of Pituitary Tumors, Raven Press, New York.

226. Lipscomb, H., and Nelson, D. H. (1959) Measurement of corticosterone in rat adrenal venous plasma as a bioassay for ACTH. Fed. Proc. 18, 95.

227. Lipscomb, H. S., and Nelson, D. H. (1962) A sensitive biologic assay for ACTH. Endocrinology 71, 13–23.

228. Lipsett, M. B., Hertz, R., and Ross, G. T. (1963) Clinical and pathophysiologic aspects of adrenocortical carcinoma. Am. J. Med. 35, 374–383.

229. Lipsett, M. B., and Wilson, H. (1962) Adrenocortical cancer: Steroid biosynthesis and metabolism evaluated by urinary metabolites. J. Clin. Endocrinol. Metab. 22, 906–915.

230. Lipton, H. L., Tan, S. Y., Noth, R., Mulrow, P. J., and Genel, M. (1977) Usefulness of plasma renin activity to monitor mineralocorticoid replacement in salt-losing congenital adrenal hyperplasia. In: P. A. Lee, L. P. Plotnick, A. A. Kowarski, and C. J. Migeon (eds.), Congenital Adrenal Hyperplasia, University Park Press, Baltimore, p. 127.

231. Lukert, B. P. and Adams, J. S. (1976) Calcium and phosphorus homeostasis in man: effect of corticosteroids. Arch. Int. Med. 136, 1249.

232. Luton, J. P., Remy, J. M., Valcke, J. C., Landat, P. H., and Bricaire, H. (1973) Cure or remission of Cushing's disease by prolonged therapy with *o,p'*-DDD: 17 cases. Ann. Endocrinol. 34, 351–376.

233. Luton, J. P., Thieblot, P., Valcke, J. C., Mahoudeau, J. A., and Bricaire, H. (1977) Reversible gonadotropin deficiency in male Cushing's disease. J. Clin. Endocrinol. Metab. 45, 488–495.

234. Luton, J. P., Mahoudeau, J. A., Bouchard, P. H., et al. (1979) Treatment of Cushing's disease by *o,p'*-DDD. Survey of 62 cases. N. Engl. J. Med. 300, 459–464.

234a. Lytras, N., Grossman, A., Tomlin, P. S., Wass, J. A. H., Coy, D. H., Schally, A. V., Rees, L. H., and Besser, G. M. (1984). Corticotrophin-releasing factor responses in normal subjects and patients with disorders of hypothalamus and pituitary. Clin. Endocrinol. (Oxe.) 20, 71–84.

235. MacErlean, D. P., and Doyle, F. H. (1976) The pituitary fossa in Cushing's syndrome: A retrospective analysis of 93 patients. Br. J. Radiol. 49, 820–826.

236. Mains, R. E., and Eippér, B. A. (1979) Synthesis and secretion of corticotropins, melanotropins and endorphins by rat intermediate pituitary cells. J. Biol. Chem. 254, 7885.

237. Mains, R. E., Eippér, B. A., and Ling, N. (1977) Common precursor to corticotropins and endorphins. Proc. Nat. Acad. Sci. (U.S.A.) 74, 3014–3018.

238. Maloney, P. J. (1952) Addison's disease due to chronic disseminated coccidiodomycosis. Arch. Intern. Med. 90, 869.

239. Margaretten, W., Hisayo, N., and Landing, B. H. (1963) Septicemic adrenal hemorrhage. Am. J. Dis. Child. 105, 346.

240. Marks, T. M., Thomas, J. M., and Warkany, J. (1940) Adrenocortical obesity in children. Am. J. Dis. Child. 60, 923.

241. Marks, V. (1959) Cushing's syndrome occurring with pituitary chromophobe tumors. Acta Endocrinol. 32, 527–535.

242. Mattingly, D. (1962) A simple fluorimetric method for the estimation of free 11-hydroxycorticoids in human plasma. J. Clin. Pathol. 15, 374–379.

243. Meador, C. K., Liddle, G. D., Island, D. P., Nicholson, W. E., Lucas, C. P., Nuckton, J. G., and Luetscher, J. A. (1962) Cause of Cushing's syndrome in patients with tumors arising from "nonendocrine" tissue. J. Clin. Endocrinol. Metab. 22, 693–703.

244. Meakin, J. W., Tantongco, M. S., Crabbe, J., et al. (1960) Pituitary-adrenal function following long-term steroid therapy. Am. J. Med. 29, 459–464.

245. Meikle, J. W., Jubiz, W., Matsukura, S., et al. (1969) Effect of diphenylhydantoin on the metabolism of metyrapone and release of ACTH in man. J. Clin. Endocrinol. Metab. 29, 1553–1558.

246. Meikle, A. W., Jubiz, W., Matsukura, S., et al. (1970) Effect of estrogen on the metabolism of metyrapone and release of ACTH. J. Clin. Endocrinol. Metab. 30, 259–263.

247. Meikle, A. W., Lagerquist, L. G., and Tyler, F. H. (1975) Apparently normal pituitary-adrenal suppressibility in Cushing's syndrome: dexamethasone metabolism and plasma levels. J. Lab. Clin. Med. 86, 472–478.

248. Melby, J. C. (1971) Therapeutic possibilities in Cushing's syndrome (Editorial). N. Engl. J. Med. 285, 288–289.

249. Mendlowitz, M., Naftchi, N., Weinreb, H. L., and Gitlow, S. E. (1961) Effect of prednisone on digital vascular reactivity in normotensive and hypertensive subjects. J. Appl. Physiol. 16, 89–94.

250. Migeon, C. J., Kenny, F. M., Kowarski, A., et al. (1968) The syndrome of congenital adrenocortical unresponsiveness to ACTH. Report of six cases. Pediatr. Res. 2, 501–513.

251. Mohr, G., and Hardy, J. (1982) Hemorrhage, necrosis and apoplexy in pituitary adenomas. Surg. Neurol. 18, 181–189.

252. Moore, T. J., Dluhy, R. G., Williams, G. H. et al. (1976) Nelson's syndrome: Frequency, prognosis, and effect of prior pituitary irradiation. Ann. Intern. Med. 8, 731–734.

253. Moser, H. W., Moser, A. B., Kawamura, N., Murphy, J., Suzuki, K., Schaumburg, H., and Kisimoto, Y. (1980) Adrenoleukodystrophy: Elevated C_{26} fatty acid in cultured skin fibroblasts. Ann. Neurol. 7, 542, 429.

254. Moulias, R., and Goust, M. J. (1971) Contribution a l'étude d'un neouveau test d'hypersensibilitet retardée in vitro chez l'homme: Le test de migration des leucocytes (TML). Thése, Université de Paris, faculté de Médicine, Petite-Salpetriére.

255. Murphy, B. P., Engelberg, W., and Pattee, C. J. (1963) Simple method for the determination of plasma corticoids. J. Clin. Endocrinol. Metab. 23, 293–300.

256. Murphy, B. E. P. (1968) Clinical evaluation of urinary cortisol determinations by competitive protein-binding radioassay. J. Clin. Endocrinol. Metab. 28, 343–348.

257. Nakahara, M., Shibasaki, T., Shizume, K., Kiyosawa, Y., Odagiri, E., Suda, T.,

Yamaguchi, H., Tsushima, T., Demura, H., Marda, T., Wakabashi, I., and Ling, N. (1983) Corticotropin-releasing factor test in normal subjects and patients with hypothalamic–pituitary–adrenal disorders. J. Clin. Endocrinol. Metab. 57, 963–968.

258. Nelson, D. H., Samuels, L. T., Willardson, D. G., and Tyler, F. H. (1951) The levels of 17-hydroxycorticosteroids in peripheral blood of human subjects. J. Clin. Endocrinol. Metab. 11, 1021.

259. Nelson, D. H., Meakin, J. W., Dealy, Jr., J. B., et al. (1958) ACTH producing tumors of the pituitary gland. N. Engl. J. Med. 259, 161–164.

260. Nelson, D. H., and Meakin, J. W. (1959) A new clinical entity in patients adrenalectomized for Cushing's syndrome. J. Clin. Invest. 38, 1028–1029.

261. Nelson, D. H., Meakin, J. W., and Thorn, G. W. (1960) ACTH-producing pituitary tumors following adrenalectomy for Cushing's syndrome. Ann. Intern. Med. 52, 560–569.

262. Nelson, D. H. (1980) Addison's disease (primary adrenal insufficiency). In: D. H. Nelson (ed.), The Adrenal Cortex: Physiological Function and Disease, Major Problems in Internal Medicine, Vol. 18, W. B. Saunders, Philadelphia, p. 113.

263. Nerup, J., and Bendixen, G. (1969A) Antiadrenal cellular hypersensitivity in Addison's disease. III. Species-specificity and subcellular localization of the antigen. Clin. Exper. Immunol. 5, 355.

264. Nerup, J., and Bendixen, G. (1969B) Anti-adrenal cellular hypersensitivity in Addison's disease. II. Correlation with clinical and serological findings. Clin. Exper. Immunol. 5, 341–353.

265. Nerup, J. (1974) Addison's disease. Clinical studies. A report of 108 cases. Acta Endocrinol. 76, 127–141.

266. Neufeld, M., MacLaren, N. K., and Blizzard, R. M. (1981) Two types of autoimmune Addison's disease associated with different polyglandular autoimmune (PGA) syndrome. Medicine 60, 355.

267. Neville, A. M., and Symington, T. S. (1972) Bilateral adrenocortical hyperplasia in children with Cushing's syndrome. J. Pathol. 107, 95–106, 268.

268. Neville, A. M. and Symington, T. (1967) The pathology of the adrenal gland in Cushing's syndrome. J. Pathol. Bacteriol. 93, 19–35.

269. Nichols, T., Nugent, C. A., and Tyler, F. H. (1968) Steroid laboratory test in the diagnosis of Cushing's syndrome. Am. J. Med. 45, 116–128.

270. Nicolis, G. L., Mitty, H. A., Modlinger, R. S., and Gabrilove, J. L. (1972) Percutaneous adrenal venography. A clinical study of 50 patients. Ann. Intern Med. 76, 899–909.

271. Norymberski, J. K., Stubbs, R. D., and West, H. F. (1953) Assessment of adrenocortical activity by assay of 17-ketogenic steroids in urine. Lancet i, 1276–1281.

272. Nosadini, R., Del Prato, S., Tiengo, A., Valerio, A., Mugged, M., Opocher, G., Mantero, F., Duner, E., Marescotti, C., Mollo, F., and Belloni, F. (1983) Insulin resistance in Cushing's syndrome. J. Clin. Endocrinol. Metab. 57, 529–536.

273. Nugent, C. A., Nichols, T., and Tyler, F. H. (1965) Diagnosis of Cushing's syndrome—single dose dexamethasone suppression test. Arch. Intern. Med. 116, 172–176.

274. Ogle, J. W. (1866) On disease of the brain as a result of diabetes mellitus. St. George's Hosp. Rep. 1, 157.

275. Oki, S., Nakai, Y., Nakao, K., and Imura, H. (1980) Plasma β-endorphin reponses to somatostatin, thyrotropin-releasing hormone, or vasopressin in Nelson's syndrome. J. Clin. Endocrinol. Metab. 50, 194.

276. Olefsky, J. (1975) Effect of dexamethasone on insulin binding, glucose transport and glucose oxidation of isolated rat adipocytes. J. Clin. Invest. 56, 1499.

277. O'Mullane, N., Walker, B., Jefferson, J., Hipkin, L., Diver, M., and Davis, C. (1978) Lack of effect of bromocriptine on ACTH levels in patients with bilateral adrenalectomy for pituitary-dependent Cushing's syndrome. J. Endocrinol. Invest. 1, 355.

278. O'Neal, L. W. (1968) Correlations between clinical pattern and pathological findings in Cushing's syndrome. Med. Clin. North Am. 52, 313.
279. O'Neill, B. P., and Moser, H. W. (1982) Adrenoleukodystrophy. Can. J. Neurol. Sci. 9, 449–452.
280. Orth, D. N., and Liddle, G. W. (1971) Results of treatment in 108 patients with Cushing's syndrome. N. Engl. J. Med. 285, 243–247.
281. Orth, D. N. (1974) Adrenocorticotropic hormone and melanocyte stimulating hormone (ACTH and MSH). In: B. M. Jaffe and H. R. Behrman (eds.), Methods of Hormone Radioimmunoassay, Academic Press, New York, London, p. 125.
282. Orth, D. N., DeBold, C. R., DeCherney, S., Jackson, R. V., Alexander, A. N., Rivier, J., Rivier, C., Spiess, J., and Vale, W. (1982) Pituitary microadenomas causing Cushing's disease respond to corticotropin-releasing factor. J. Clin. Endocrinol. Metab. 55, 1017–1019.
283. Orth, D. W., Holscher, M. A., Wilson, M. G., Nicholson, W. E., Plue, R. E., and Mount, C. D. (1982) Equine Cushing's disease: Plasma immunoreactive proopiolipomelanocortin peptide and cortisol levels basally and in response to diagnostic test. Endocrinology 110, 1430–1441.
284. Orth, D. N., Guillemin, R., Ling, N., and Nicholson, W. E. (1978) Immunoreactive endorphins, lipotropins and corticotropins in a human non-pituitary tumor: Evidence for a common precursor. J. Clin. Endocrinol. Metab. 46, 849–852.
285. Orth, D. W., and Nicholson, W. E. (1982) Bioactive and immunoreactive adrenocorticotropin in normal equine pituitary and pituitary tumors of horses with Cushing's disease. Endocrinology 111, 559–563.
285a. Orth, D. N.(1984) The old and the new in Cushing's syndrome. N. Engl. J. Med. 310, 649–651.
286. Ostuni, J. A., and Roginsky, M. S. (1975) Metastatic adrenal cortical carcinoma. Documented cure with combined chemotherapy. Arch. Intern. Med. 135, 1257–1258.
287. Papapetroy, P. D., and Jackson, I. (1975) Cortisol secretion in Nelson's syndrome. Persistence after "total" adrenalectomy for Cushing's syndrome. JAMA 234, 847–849.
288. Pasqualini, R. Q., and Gurevich, N. (1956) Spontaneous remission in a case of Cushing's syndrome. J. Clin. Endocrinol. Metab. 16, 406.
289. Pavlatos, F. C., Smilo, R. P., and Forsham, P. H. (1965) A rapid screening test for Cushing's syndrome. JAMA 193, 720–723.
290. Pearse, A. G. E. (1975) Neurocristopathy, neuroendocrine pathology and the APUD concept. Z. Krebforsch 84, 1–18.
291. Peterson, R. E., and Wyngaarden, J. B. (1956) The miscible pool and turnover rate of cortisol in man. J. Clin. Invest. 35, 552–561.
292. Pieters, G. F. F. M., Smals, A. G. H., Benraad, T. J, and Kloppenborg, P. W. C. (1979) Plasma cortisol response to thyrotropin-releasing hormone and luteinizin hormone-releasing hormone in Cushing's disease. J. Clin. Endocrinol. Metab. 48, 874.
293. Pieters, G. F. F. M., Smals, A. G. H., Goerde, H. J. M., Pesman, G. J., Meyer, E., and Kloppenborg, P. W. C. (1982) adrenocorticotropin and cortisol responsiveness to thyrotropin-releasing hormone discloses two subsets of patients with Cushing's disease. J. Clin. Endocrinol. Metab. 55, 1188.
294. Pieters, G. F. F., Hermus, A. R. M. M., Smals, A. G. H., Bartelink, A. K. M., Benraad, T. H. J., and Kloppenborg, P. W. C. (1983) Responsiveness of the hypophyseal-adrenocortical axis to corticotropin-releasing factor in pituitary dependent Cushing's disease. J. Clin. Endocrinol. Metab. 57, 513.
295. Platz, P., Ryder, L., Nielsen, L. S., Svejgaard, A., Thomsen, M., Nerup, J., and Christy, M. (1974) HL-A and idiopathic Addison's disease. Lancet ii, 289.
296. Plonk, J., and Feldman, J. M. (1976) Modification of adrenal function by the antiserotonin agent cyproheptadine. J. Clin. Endocrinol. Metab. 42, 291.
297. Plotz, C. M., Knowlton, A. I. and Ragan, C. (1952) The natural history of Cushing's syndrome. Am. J. Med. 13, 597–614.

298. Porter, C. C., and Silber, R. H. (1950) A quantitative color reaction for cortisone and related 17, 21-dihydroxy-20-ketosteroids. J. Biol. Chem. 185, 201–207.

299. Powell, D. F., Baker, H. L., Jr., and Laws, E. R., Jr. (1974) The primary angiographic findings in pituitary adenomas. Radiology 110, 589.

300. Prunty, F. T. G., Brooks, R. V., Dupré, J., Gimlette, T. M. D., Hutchinson, J. S. M., McSwiney, R. R., and Mills, I. H. (1963) Adrenocortical hyperfunction and potassium metabolism in patients with "non-endocrine" tumors and Cushing's syndrome. J. Clin. Endocrinol. Metab. 23, 737–746.

301. Przewlocki, R., Höllt, V., Voigt, K. H., and Herz, A. (1979) Modulation of in vitro release of β-endorphin from the separate lobes of the rat pituitary. Life Sci. 24, 1601.

302. Raman, A. (1970) Effect of adrenalectomy on ionic and total plasma calcium in rats. Horm. Metab. Res. 2, 181–183.

303. Ratcliffe, J. G., Knight, R. A., Besser, G. M., Landon, J., and Stansfield, A. G. (1972) Tumor and plasma ACTH concentrations in patients with and without the ectopic ACTH syndrome. Clin. Endocrinol. 1, 27–44.

304. Ratcliffe, J. G., Scott, A. P., Bennett, H. P. J., Lowry, P. J., McMartin, C., Strong, J. A., and Walbaum, P. R. (1973) Production of a corticotrophin-like intermediate lobe peptide and of corticotrophin by a bronchial carcinoid tumour. Clin. Endocrinol. 2, 51–55.

305. Raux, M. C., Binoux, M., Luton, J.-P., Gourmelen, M., and Girard, F. (1975) Studies of ACTH secretion control in 116 cases of Cushing's syndrome. J. Clin. Endocrinol. Metab. 40, 186–197.

306. Rees, L. H., Ratcliffe, J. G., Besser, G. M., et al. (1973) Comparison of the redox assay for ACTH with previous assays. Nature New Biol. 241, 84–85.

307. Rees, L. H., and Landon, J. (1976) Adrenocorticotrophic hormone. In: J. A. Loraine and E. Trenor Bell (eds.), Hormone Assays and Their Clinical Applications, Churchill Livingston, Edinburgh, London, New York, pp. 193–220.

308. Rees, L. H. (1977) ACTH, lipotrophin and MSH in health and disease. J. Clin. Endocrinol. Metab. 6, 137–153.

309. Rees, L. H., Besser, G. M., Jeffcoate, W. J., Goldie, D. J., and Marks, V. (1977) Alcohol-induced pseudo-Cushing's syndrome. Lancet i, 726–728.

310. Reid, I. A., Tu, W. H., Otsuka, K., Assaykeen, T. A., and Ganong, W. F. (1973) Studies concerning the regulation and importance of plasma angiotensinogen concentration in the dog. Endocrinology 93, 107.

311. Reidenberg, M. M., Ohler, E. A., Sevy, R. W., and Harakal, C. (1963) Hemodynamic changes in adrenalectomized dogs. Endocrinology 72, 918.

312. Reuter, R. S., Blau, J. A., Schteingart, D. E., and Bookstein, J. J. (1967) Adrenal venography. Radiology 89, 805–814.

313. Rizza, R., Mandarino, L., and Gerich, J. (1982) Cortisol-induced insulin resistance in man: impaired suppression of glucose production and stimulation of glucose utilization due to a postreceptor defect of insulin action. J. Clin. Endocrinol. Metab. 54, 131.

314. Robert, F., Pelletier, G., and Hardy, J. (1978) Pituitary adenomas in Cushing's disease: A histologic, ultrastructural and immunocytochemical study. Arch. Pathol. Lab. Med. 102, 448.

315. Rogoff, J. M., and Steward, G. N. (1927) Suprarenal cortical extracts in suprarenal insufficiency (Addison's disease). JAMA 92, 1569–1571.

316. Romanoff, E. B., Hudson, P., and Pincus, G. (1953) Isolation of hydrocortisone and corticosterone from adrenal vein blood. J. Clin. Endocrinol. Metab. 13, 1546.

317. Rose, L. I., Williams, G. H., Jagger, P. I., Lauler, D. P., and Thorn, G. W. (1969) The paradoxical dexamethasone response phenomenon. Metabolism 18, 369–375.

318. Rosner, J. M., Cos, J. J., and Biglieri, E. G. (1963) Determination of urinary unconjugated cortisol by glass fiber chromatography in the diagnosis of Cushing's syndrome. J. Clin. Endocrinol. Metab. 23, 820–827.

319. Ross, E. J., Marshal-Jones, P., and Friedman, M. (1966) Cushing's syndrome: Diagnostic criteria. Q. J. Med. 35, 149–192.
320. Rossier, J., French, E., Gros, C., Miniek, S., Guillemin, R., and Bloom, F. E. (1979) Adrenalectomy, dexamethasone or stress alters opiod peptide levels in rat anterior pituitary but not in intermediate lobe or brain. Life Sci. 25, 2105.
321. Rovit, R. L., and Berry, R. (1965) Cushing's syndrome and the hypophysis. A reevaluation of pituitary tumors and hyperadrenalism. J. Neurosurg. 23, 270–295.
322. Ruder, H. J., Loriaux, D. L., and Lipsett, M. B. (1974) Severe osteopenia in young adults associated with Cushing's syndrome due to micronodular adrenal disease. J. Clin. Endocrinol. Metab. 39, 1138–1147.
323. Saeger, W. (1974) Zur Ultrastruktur der hyperplastischen und adenomatosen ACTH-Zellen beim Cushing-Syndrom hypothalamich–hypophysarer Genese. Virchows Arch. (Pathol. Anat.) 362, 73.
324. Saez, J. M., Dazord, A., and Gallet, D. (1975) ACTH and prostaglandin receptors in human adrenocortical tumors. Apparent modification of a specific component of the ACTH-binding site. J. Clin. Invest. 56, 536–547.
325. Sahagian-Edwards, A., and Holland, J. F. (1954) Metastatic carcinoma to the adrenal glands with cortical hypofunction. Cancer 7, 1242.
326. Salassa, R. M., Kearns, T. P., Kernohan, J. W., Sprague, R. G., and MacCarty, C. S. (1959) Pituitary tumors in patients with Cushing's syndrome. J. Clin. Endocrinol. Metab. 19, 1523–1539.
327. Salassa, R. M., Laws, E. R., Jr., Carpenter, P. C., and Northcutt, R. C. (1978) Transsphenoidal removal of pituitary microadenoma in Cushing's disease. Mayo Clinic Proc. 53, 24–28.
328. Sample, W. F. (1978) Adrenal ultrasonography. Radiology 127, 461–466.
329. Sanford, J. P., and Favour, C. B. (1956) The interrelationships between Addison's disease and active tuberculosis: A review of 125 cases of Addison's disease. Ann. Intern. Med. 45, 56.
330. Sarett, L. H. (1946) Partial synthesis of pregnen-4-triol-17 (B), 20 (B), 21-dione-3, 11 and pregnen-4-diol-17 (B), 21-trione, 3,11,20-monoacetate. J. Biol. Chem. 162, 601.
331. Sarkar, S. D., Cohen, E. L., Beierwaltes, W. H., Ice, R. D., Cooper, R., and Gold, E. N. (1977) A new and superior adrenal imaging agent ^{131}I-6β-iodomethyl-19-norcholesterol (NP-59). Evaluation in humans. J. Clin. Endocrinol. Metab. 45, 353.
332. Sawin, C. T., Bray, G. A., and Idelson, B. A. (1968) Overnight suppression test with dexamethasone in Cushing's syndrome. J. Clin. Endocrinol. Metab. 28, 422-424.
333. Sawyer, G., and Beall, R. J. (1973) Isolated adrenal cortex cells: hypersensitivity to ACTH after hypophysectomy. Science 179, 1330–1331.
334. Schambelan, M., Slaton, P. E. and Biglieri, E. G. (1971) Mineralocorticoid production in hyperadrenocorticism: Role in pathogenesis of hypokalemic alkalosis. Am. J. Med. 51, 299–303.
335. Scheithauer, B. W. (1982) Surgical pathology of the pituitary and sella region. In: E. R. Laws, Jr., R. V. Randall, E. B. Kern, and C. F. Abboud (eds.), Management of Pituitary Adenomas and Related Lesions with Emphasis in Transsphenoidal Microsurgery, Appleton-Century-Crofts, New York, pp. 129–218.
336. Schlechte, J. A., and Sherman, B. M. (1982) Decreased glucocorticoid receptor binding in adrenal insufficiency. J. Clin. Endocrinol. Metab. 54, 145.
337. Schletter, F. E., Clift, G. V., Meyer, R., et al. (1967) Cushing's syndrome in childhood: Report of two cases with bilateral adrenocortical hyperplasia, showing distinctive clinical features. J. Clin. Endocrinol. Metab. 27, 22–28.
338. Schmidt, M. B. (1926) Eine biflanduläre Erkrankung (Nebennieren und Schilddrüse) bei morbus Addisonii. Verhandlungen der Deutsche Gesellschaft für Pathologie 21, 212.
339. Schnall, A. M., Brodkey, J. S., Kaufman, B., and Pearson, O. H. (1978) Pituitary

function after removal of pituitary microadenomas in Cushing's disease. J. Clin. Endocrinol. Metab. 47, 410.

340. Schnall, A. M., Kovacs, K., Brodkey, J. S., and Pearson, O. H. (1980) Pituitary Cushing's disease without adenomata. Acta Endocrinol. 94, 297.

341. Schorr, I. S. and Ney, R. L. (1971) Abnormal hormone responses of an adrenocortical cancer to adenylate cyclase. J. Clin. Invest. 50, 1295–1300.

342. Schteingart, D. E., Oberman, H. A., Friedman, B. A., and Conn, J. W. (1968) Adrenocortical neoplasms causing Cushing's syndrome: A clinicopathologic study. Cancer 22, 1005.

343. Schteingart, D. E., Conn, J. W., Lieberman, L. M., and Beierwaltes, W. H. (1972) Persistent or recurrent Cushing's syndrome after total adrenalectomy: Adrenal photoscanning for residual tissue. Arch. Intern. Med. 130, 384.

344. Schteingart, D. E., Conn, J. W., Orth, D. N., et al. (1972) Secretion of ACTH and β-MSH by an adrenal medullary paraganglioma. J. Clin. Endocrinol. Metab. 34, 676–683.

345. Schwartz, M. J., and Kokko, J. P. (1980) Urinary concentrating defect of adrenal insufficiency, permissive role of adrenal steroids on the hydroosmotic response across the rabbit cortical collecting tubule. J. Clin. Invest. 66, 234–242.

346. Schwartz, J., Keil, L. C., Marselli, J., and Reid, I. A. (1983) Role of vasopressin in blood pressure regulation during adrenal insufficiency. Endocrinology 112, 234.

347. Scott, W. H., Jr., Liddle, G. W., Harris, A. P., and Foster, J. H. (1962) Diagnosis and treatment of Cushing's syndrome. Ann. Surg. 155, 696–710.

348. Scott, W. H., Jr., Foster, J. H., and Rhamy, R. K. (1971) Surgical management of adrenocortical tumors with Cushing's syndrome. Ann. Surg. 173, 892–905.

349. Scott, A. P., and Lowry, P. J. (1974) Adrenocorticotropic and melanocyte-stimulating peptides in the human pituitary. Biochem. J. 139, 593–602.

350. Seabold, J. E., Haynie, T. P., DeAsis, D. N., Samaan, N. A., Glenn, H. J., and Jahns, M. F. (1977) Detection of metastatic adrenal carcinoma using ^{131}I-β-iodo-methyl-19-norcholesterol total body scans. J. Clin. Endocrinol. Metab. 45, 788.

351. Shapiro, B., Britton, K. E., Hawkins, L. A., and Edwards, C. R. W. (1981) Clinical experience with ^{75}Se selenomethyl–cholesterol adrenal imaging. Clin. Endocrinol. 15, 19–27.

352. Sheline, G. E. (1979) Conventional radiotherapy in the treatment of pituitary tumors. In: G. T. Tindall and W. F. Collins (eds.), Clinical Management of Pituitary Disorders, Raven Press, New York, pp. 287–314.

353. Sheppard, R. H., and Meema, H. E. (1967) Skin thickness in endocrine disease. Ann. Int. Med. 66, 531–539.

354. Sheridan, P., and Mattingly, D. (1975) Simultaneous investigation and treatment of suspected acute adrenal insufficiency. Lancet ii, 676.

355. Shibasaki, T., Nakahara, M., Shizume, K., Kiyosawa, Y., Suda, T., Demura, H., Kuwayama, A., Kageyama, N., Benoit, R., and Ling, N. (1983) Pituitary adenomas that caused Cushing's disease or Nelson's syndrome are not responsive to ovine corticotropin-releasing factor in vitro. J. Clin. Endocrinol. Metab. 56, 414–416.

356. Silber, R. H., and Porter, C. C. (1954) The determination of 17, 21-dihydroxy-20-ketosteroids in urine and plasma. J. Biol. Chem. 923–932.

357. Simpson, S. A., Tait, J. F., and Bush, I. E. (1952) Secretion of salt-retaining hormone by mammalian adrenal cortex. Lancet ii, 226.

358. Simpson, S. A., Tait, J. F., Wettstein, A., Neher, R., von Euw, J., and Richstein, T. (1953) Isolierung eines neuen kristallisierten Hormons aus Nebennieren mit besonders hoher Wieksamkeit aus den Mineralstoffswechsel. Experientia 9, 33.

359. Sindler, B. H., Griffin, G. T., and Melby, J. C. (1983) The superiority of the metyrapone test versus the high-dose dexamethasone test in the differential diagnosis of Cushing's syndrome. Am. J. Med. 74, 657.

360. Smals, A., and Kloppenborg, P. (1977) Alcohol-induced pseudo-Cushing's syndrome (Letter). Lancet i, 1369.
361. Smals, A. G. H., Kloppenborg, P. W. C., and Benraad, T. J. (1977) Plasma testosterone profiles in Cushing's syndrome. J. Clin. Endocrinol. Metab. 45, 240–245.
362. Soffer, L. J., Iannacone, A., and Gabrilove, J. L. (1961) Cushing's syndrome: A study of fifty patients. Am. J. Med. 30, 129.
363. Sparagana, M., Fells, R. W., Stefani, S., and Jablokow, V. (1972) Osteogenic sarcoma of the skull: A rare sequela of pituitary irradiation. Cancer 29, 1376–1380.
364. Spinner, M. W., Blizzard, R. M., Gibbs, J., Abbey, H., and Childs, B. (1969) Familial distributions of organ-specific antibodies in the blood of patients with Addison's disease and hypoparathyroidism and their relatives. Clin. Exper. Immunol. 5, 461.
365. Spital, A. (1982) Hyponatremia in adrenal insufficiency: Review of pathogenetic mechanisms. South. Med. J. 75, 581.
366. Sprague, R. G., Randall, R. V., Salassa, R. M., et al. (1956) Cushing's syndrome, a progressive and often fatal disease: A review of 100 cases seen between July 1945 and July 1954. Arch. Intern. Med. 98, 389.
367. Sprague, R. G., Priestley, J. T., Weeks, R. E., and Salassa, R. M. (1961) Treatment of Cushing's syndrome by adrenalectomy. In: H. Gardiner-Hill (ed.), Modern Trends in Endocrinology: 2nd Series, Harper, New York, pp. 84–99.
368. Stacpoole, P. W., Interlandi, J. W., Nicholson, W. E., and Rabin, D. (1982) Isolated ACTH deficiency: A heterogeneous disorder. Critical review and report of four new cases. Medicine 61, 13.
369. Steiger, M., and Reichsten, T. (1937) Desoxycorticosterone (21-oxyprogesterone aus 5-3 oxyatio cholensaure). Helv. Chim. Acta 20, 1164.
370. Stitch, R. D., and Person, R. J. (1982) Effect of central catecholamine depletion on ^{3}H-dexamethasone binding in the dog. Neuroendocrinology 34, 410.
371. Stockigt, J. R., Hewett, M. J., Topliss, D. J., Higgs, E. J., and Taft, P. (1979) Renin and renin substrate in primary adrenal insufficiency. Contrasting effects of glucocorticoid and mineralocorticoid deficiency. Am. J. Med. 66, 915.
372. Streck, W. F., and Lockwood, D. H. (1979) Pituitary adrenal recovery following short-term suppression with corticosteroids. Am. J. Med. 66, 910.
373. Streeten, D. H. P., Stevenson, C. T., Dalakos, T. G., et al. (1969) The diagnosis of hypercortisolism. Biochemical criteria differentiating patients from lean and obese normal subjects and from females on oral contraceptives. J. Clin. Endocrinol. Metab. 29, 1191–1211.
374. Stuart-Mason, A., Meade, T. W., Lee, J. A. H., and Morris, J. N. (1968) Epidemiological and clinical picture of Addison's disease. Lancet ii, 744–747.
375. Studzinski, G. P., Hay, D. C. F., and Symington, T. (1963) Observations on the weight of the human adrenal gland and the effect of preparation of corticotrophin of different purity on the weight and morphology of the human adrenal gland. J. Clin. Endocrinol. Metab. 23, 248–254.
376. Suda, T., Demura, H., Demura, R., Jibiki, K., Tozawa, F., and Shizume, K. (1980) Anterior pituitary hormones in plasma and pituitaries from patients with Cushing's disease. J. Clin. Endocrinol. Metab. 51, 1048.
377. Suzuki, Y., Ichikawa, Y., Saito, E., and Homma, M. (1983) Importance of increased urinary calcium excretion in the development of secondary hyperparathyroidism of patients under glucocorticoid therapy. Metabolism 32, 151–156.
378. Swingle, W. W., and Pfiffner, J. J. (1930) An aqueous extract of the suprarenal cortex which maintains the life of bilaterally adrenalectomized cats. Science 71, 321–322.
379. Symington, T. S. (1969) Functional Pathology of the Human Adrenal Gland. E. and S. Livingston, Ltd., Edinburgh, London, pp. 120–121.
380. Tanaka, K., Nicholson, W. E., and Orth, D. N. (1978) Diurnal rhythm and disappearance half-time of endogenous plasma immunoreactive β-MSH (LPH) and ACTH in man. J. Clin. Endocrinol. Metab. 46, 883–890.

381. Thrall, J. H., Freitas, J. E., and Beierwaltes, W. H. (1978) Adrenal scintigraphy. Semin. Nucl. Med. 8, 23.

382. Tomori, N., Suda, T., Tozawa, F., Demura, H., Shizume, K., and Mouri, T. (1983) Immunoreactive corticotropin-releasing factor concentrations in cerebrospinal fluid from patients with hypothalamic pituitary adrenal disorders. J. Clin. Endocrinol. Metab. 57, 1305.

383. Tyler, F. H., and West, C. D. (1972) Laboratory evaluation of disorders of the adrenal cortex. Am. J. Med. 53, 664–672.

384. Tyrrell, J. B., Brooks, R. M., Fitzgerald, P. A., Cofoid, P. B., Forshman, P. H., and Wilson, C. B. (1978) Cushing's disease. Selective transsphenoidal resection of pituitary microadenomas. N. Engl. J. Med. 298, 753–758.

385. Tyrrell, J. B., Lorenzi, M., Gerich, J. E., and Forsham, P. H. (1975) Inhibition by somatostatin of ACTH secretion in Nelson's syndrome. J. Clin. Endocrinol. Metab. 40, 1125.

386. Upton, G. V., and Amatruda, T. T., Jr. (1971) Evidence for the presence of tumor peptides with corticotropin-releasing factor-like activity in the ectopic ACTH syndrome. N. Engl. J. Med. 285, 419–424.

387. Urbanic, R. C., and George, J. M. (1981) Cushing's disease—18 years experience. Medicine 660, 14–24.

388. Verhoeven, G. F. M., and Wilson, J. D. (1979) The syndrome of primary hormone resistance. Metabolism 28, 253.

389. Vernikos-Danellis, J. (1969) Sensitivity of the adrenal corticosterone response to ACTH as a function of time after hypophysectomy. Endocrinology 84, 1507.

390. Voccia, E., Saenger, P., Peterson, R. E., Rauh, W., Gottesdiener, K., Levine, L. S., and New, M. I. (1979) 6β-hydroxycortical excretion in hypercortisolemic states. J. Clin. Endocrinol. Metab. 48, 467.

391. Waltz, T. A., and Brownell, B. (1966) Sarcoma: A possible late result of effective radiation therapy for pituitary adenomas. J. Neurosurg. 24, 901–905.

392. Webb, W. R., Degerli, I. U., Hardy, J. D., and Unal, M. (1965) Cardiovascular responses in adrenal insufficiency. Surgery 58, 273.

393. Welbourn, R. B., Montgomery, D. A. D., and Kennedy, T. L. (1971) The natural history of treated Cushing's syndrome. Br. J. Surg. 58, 1–16.

394. West, C. D., and Dolman, L. I. (1977) Plasma ACTH radioimmunoassays in the diagnosis of pituitary-adrenal dysfunction. Ann. N.Y. Acad. Sci. 297, 205–219.

395. West, C. D., and Meikle, A. W. (1979) Laboratory test for the diagnosis of Cushing's syndrome and adrenal insufficiency and factors affecting this test. In: L. J. Groot et al. (eds.) Endocrinology, Vol. 2, Grune and Stratton, New York, pp. 1157–1178.

396. Wilbur, O. M., and Rich, A. R. (1953) A study of the role of adrenocorticotropic hormone (ACTH) in the pathogenesis of tubular degeneration of the adrenals. Bull. Johns. Hopkins Hosp. 93, 321.

397. Williams, G. H., Dluhy, R. G., and Thorn, G. W. (1977) Diseases of the adrenal cortex. In: G. W. Thorn, R. D. Adams, E. Braunwald, K. Isselbacher, and R. G. Petersdorf (eds.), Harrison's Principles of Internal Medicine (8th Ed.), McGraw Hill Co., New York, p. 520.

398. Willis, R. A. (1952) The Spread of Tumors in the Human Body, 2nd ed. C.V. Mosby, St. Louis.

399. Wilson, C. B., Tyrrell, J. B., Fitzgerald, P. A., and Pitts, L. (1979) Neurosurgical aspects of Cushing's disease on Nelson's syndrome. In: G. T. Turdall and W. F. Collins (eds.), Clinical Management of Pituitary Disorders, Raven Press, New York, pp. 229–238.

400. Wolfsen, A. R., McIntyre, H. B., and Odell, W. D. (1972) Adrenocorticotropin measurement by competitive binding receptor assay. J. Clin. Endocrinol. Metab. 34, 684–689.

401. Wool, I. G., and Weinshelbaum, E. I. (1959) Incorporation of C-14 amino acids into protein of isolated diaphragms: Role of the adrenal steroids. Am. J. Physiol. 197, 1089.
402. Xarli, V. P., Steele, A., Davis, P. J., Nuescher, E. S., Rios, C. N., and Garcia-Bunuel, R. (1978) Adrenal hemorrhage in the adult. Medicine 57, 211.
403. Yeh, H.-C., Mitty, H. A., Rose, J., et al. (1978) Ultrasonography of adrenal masses: Usual features. Radiology 127, 467–474.
404. Yeh, H.-C., Mitty, H. A., Rose, J., et al. (1978) Ultrasonography of adrenal masses: Unusual manifestations. Radiology 127, 475–483.

S.Y. TAN, M.D.

DISEASES OF HYPER- AND HYPOMINERALOCORTICOID PRODUCTION

HYPERMINERALOCORTICOIDISM

Primary Aldosteronism: Incidence and Clinical Manifestations

The discovery of primary aldosteronism due to a secreting adrenal adenoma by Conn (46,51) stimulated intense interest in the role of aldosterone in hypertension. It is now clear that increased aldosterone secretion may be present in a variety of hypertensive patients. In some, the excess production causes the hypertension; in others, it is secondary to hyperreninemia, e.g. in malignant hypertension. It is recognized also that primary aldosteronism can result from bilateral nodular hyperplasia of the adrenals as well as from a single aldosterone-producing adenoma (6,61).

The incidence of primary aldosteronism is a subject for vigorous debate. Certainly, the classic form of hypokalemic primary aldosteronism is a rare disease present in perhaps less than 1% of all hypertensives. Conn et al. contend that an earlier, more subtle form of the disease, normokalemic primary aldosteronism, is a common cause of hypertension (49a). Conn noted while reviewing his cases of classic hypokalemic primary

From the University of Hawaii, John A. Burns School of Medicine, Honolulu, Hawaii. Formerly of the Department of Medicine, Medical College of Ohio, Toledo, Ohio.

aldosteronism that many of the patients had normal serum potassiums for years before the diagnosis was made, yet they were hypertensive. Because of the incidence of adrenal adenoma in autopsy studies of hypertensive patients, he has speculated that the incidence of primary aldosteronism may be as high as 20% in the hypertensive population. From his own series of hypertensive patients, he has found an incidence of 7% of normokalemic primary aldosteronism (52).

Another report did not find an increased incidence of adrenal adenoma in hypertensive patients at autopsy (116), and several studies report the infrequent occurrence of excess aldosterone secretion in patients with benign hypertension (74,114,131). Nevertheless, it is clear that mild cases of primary aldosteronism with normal serum potassium concentrations do exist. Some investigators feel that normokalemia may be encountered in up to 25% of all cases of primary aldosteronism (227). Aldosterone excretion may be increased only slightly or may be in the normal range because of the inhibitory effect of hypokalemia, although it may not respond to the procedures which usually raise or lower it.

The clinical symptoms of primary aldosteronism are due to hypertension and hypokalemia. Aldosterone excess leads to renal sodium and water retention and kaliuresis. The chief symptoms are polyuria, polydipsia, nocturia, weakness, intermittent paresthesia and tetany, and occasionally paralysis. The physical examination reveals only benign hypertension; malignant hypertension is rarely associated with primary aldosteronism (113). There is no edema, unless the patient develops heart failure from the hypertension. Occasionally, arrhythmias and sensitivity to digitalis are present. Some patients with primary aldosteronism have a sharp fall in blood pressure in assuming the upright position. The response to the Valsalva maneuver may be abnormal (14). If potassium depletion is profound, the deep tendon reflexes may be diminished or absent. In the less advanced case only mild general asthenia is present, which may be worsened by diuretic therapy.

In the classic case the laboratory findings are quite characteristic. The blood electrolyte studies reveal a low serum potassium and elevated serum bicarbonate, pH, and sodium concentration. Magnesium concentration may occasionally be low; the blood urea nitrogen is usually normal. The urine is dilute and neutral, and the concentrating ability of the kidney is reduced because of hypokalemia. Although urinary pH is near 7.0 with a low titratable acidity, ammonium excretion is increased. Occasionally, proteinuria may be present.

Carbohydrate tolerance is impaired in 50% of the patients (49). The potassium deficiency interferes with the peripheral action of insulin as well as the release of insulin from the pancreas. Potassium repletion corrects the abnormalities.

Aldosterone secretion and excretion are elevated and are not suppressed with salt loading. In rare cases, the values are within the normal range while the patient is potassium depleted; they become elevated only when the potassium deficit is corrected. Plasma renin concentrations are depressed because of volume expansion, and are poorly responsive to posture and salt restriction.

Although aldosterone enhances renal sodium reabsorption, patients with primary aldosteronism do not have edema. It has been clearly demonstrated that the continuous administration of aldosterone to normal subjects does not produce progressive edema (5). After a few days of sodium retention, the patient escapes from the sodium-retaining effect of aldosterone but continues to lose potassium.

Diagnosis (Table 1)

Normal subjects on diets containing over 100 mEq sodium secrete between 50 to 200 μg of aldosterone per day. The secretion rate of aldosterone may be calculated by injecting a tracer dose of radioactive aldosterone and measuring the specific activity of one of its metabolites. The plasma concentration of aldosterone can also be measured by a radioimmunoassay technique (11,220). The concentration of aldosterone/100 ml plasma in normal subjects on unrestricted diets is between 5 and 15 ngs.

Plasma aldosterone fluctuates considerably during the day in response to a variety of stimuli (231). An elevated aldosterone secretion rate with a low plasma renin level is diagnostic of primary aldosteronism (47,136). The plasma renin concentration is reduced because the excess aldosterone results in plasma volume expansion and inhibition of renin production. The juxtaglomerular cells fail to respond to acute sodium depletion and the upright posture. A patient with primary aldosteronism who has been on diuretic therapy for an extended period may, however, have a normal or elevated plasma renin concentration. It should also be noted that a number of hypertensive patients have suppressed renin production on some basis other than primary aldosteronism. In these patients, the aldosterone secretion is not elevated.

The usual plan of study is to discontinue all diuretic therapy, prescribe a normal to high sodium diet (150–200 mEq/day) for 4–7 days, measure serum potassium at frequent intervals, as well as rates of aldosterone excretion and secretion toward the end of the period. Under ideal circumstances, careful balance studies can be performed. The patient with

TABLE 1. Evaluation for Suspected Primary Aldosteronism

1. Hypokalemia in hypertensive patients. If hypokalemia is unprovoked (e.g., by diuretics), 1° aldosteronism is likely.
2. Demonstrate hyperaldosteronism with plasma or urinary aldosterone measurements.
3. Document lack of suppressibility of aldosterone during saline loading, high-salt diet, or DOCA administration.
4. Is plasma renin activity low and nonstimulatable?
5. Differentiate between adenoma and bilateral hyperplasia with iodocholesterol scan, adrenal vein aldosterone levels, Luetscher test, or 18-hydroxycorticosterone measurements, or CAT scan.
6. Therapeutic trial with spironolactone. Surgery if adenoma present.

primary aldosteronism will have a negative potassium balance, a fall in serum potassium, and an elevated aldosterone production. In some patients these abnormalities may be mild and barely outside the normal range. The patient is then placed on a low sodium diet (10 mEq/day) and the plasma renin concentration measured after 3–5 days on the diet. Plasma samples are usually collected in the morning while the patient is still supine in bed and again 4 hours after rising. In contrast to the normal subject, patients with primary aldosteronism have low to undetectable levels of renin in the plasma. Aldosterone secretion also fails to increase in response to sodium depletion and upright posture.

There are simpler modifications of the diagnostic procedure, but the principles are the same. Failure of plasma aldosterone concentration to suppress below 10 ng after 2 L of normal saline infused over 4 hours indicates abnormal aldosterone production (98). Plasma renin activity can be assayed after the acute administration of a potent diuretic, such as furosemide plus upright activity (99,111). If the plasma aldosterone fails to suppress and the plasma renin activity fails to stimulate normally, the diagnosis of primary aldosteronism is established. Failure to reduce aldosterone levels into the normal range with deoxycorticosterone acetate (DOCA) and a high-salt diet also constitutes strong evidence for the disease.

Adrenal steroids other than aldosterone may also be produced in excess in primary aldosteronism. These include 11-deoxycorticosterone (DOC), corticosterone, 18-hydroxycorticosterone, and 18-hydroxydeoxycorticosterone (16).

Obviously, these studies cannot be carried out on every hypertensive patient. A less rigorous exclusion of primary aldosteronism may be obtained by several screening procedures. The patient is placed on a diet containing liberal quantities of sodium for 2 weeks and his serum potassium, blood pressure, and cardiac status are monitored carefully. If the serum potassium remains above 3.8 mEq/L, primary aldosteronism is unlikely. Care should be taken in withdrawing the blood. A tourniquet and muscle contraction should be avoided, because these maneuvers may increase the serum potassium concentration.

Failure of the plasma renin level to increase significantly after the administration of a potent diuretic such as furosemide should raise the possibility of primary aldosteronism. If the urinary potassium concentration is above 30 mEq/L in a patient with a low serum potassium who is not receiving diuretics or potassium supplements, or if the salivary sodium: potassium ratio is 0.25 or less (135), excess aldosterone secretion is probably present. All screening tests, however, should be viewed with caution.

Forms of Primary Aldosteronism

Primary aldosteronism is usually caused by an aldosterone-producing adrenal adenoma, or bilateral nodular hyperplasia.

Adrenal carcinoma has very rarely been associated with hyperaldosteronism (73); the usual picture is a hypermineralocorticoid state characterized by increased tumor deoxycorticosterone (DOC) production, hypertension, hypokalemia, and suppression of aldosterone. Aldosteronism has also been described in a case of ovarian carcinoma (218).

Preoperative distinction between an aldosterone-producing adenoma and bilateral nodular hyperplasia is critical, since the former condition is surgically curable, whereas the latter is not (6,70). The relative incidence of adenoma versus bilateral adrenal hyperplasia is a controversial topic. An incidence of hyperplasia as high as 30%–50% has been reported (6). Preoperatively, it is important to decide which adrenal gland has the tumor or whether bilateral adrenal hyperplasia is present. The surgical results in patients with a single adenoma reveal approximately an 80% correction of the hypertension, but results are much less satisfactory in patients with bilateral adrenal hyperplasia. In general, the chemical abnormalities in patients with hyperplasia are less pronounced than in patients with adenomas, but the values overlap considerably. By taking into account several different measurements and using quadric analysis, Atchison et al. (4) are able to predict which patient has adrenal hyperplasia. Other techniques are also used. Bilateral adrenal vein cannulation is a popular technique; it can locate the tumor by retrograde dye injection and collection of blood for aldosterone and cortisol (107,154,164,191). The aldosterone concentration is high on the side of tumor and low on the opposite side, whereas it is elevated in both adrenal veins when bilateral zona glomerulosa hyperplasia is present. Because it may cause adrenal hemorrhage, retrograde dye injection is not routinely done.

Visualization of the adrenal glands by external photoscanning after the administration of ^{131}I-19-iodocholesterol has been reported (106). The radioactive cholesterol accumulates in the adenoma and the accumulation is not suppressed by dexamethasone. CAT scanning of the adrenal gland may localize the adenoma if its diameter is greater than 1 cm. Unfortunately many of the adenomas are smaller than 1 cm. Investigators (18,147) suggest that the measurement of plasma aldosterone in the supine position and after 4 hours of ambulation may be helpful in distinguishing tumor from hyperplasia (Luetscher Test). In the tumor case, upright aldosterone levels are lower than supine levels, whereas in patients with bilateral hyperplasia, the upright levels are unchanged or slightly higher. The precise explanation for these findings is obscure. One possibility is that in the case of an adenoma, the renin–angiotensin control system is completely unresponsive; aldosterone regulation is now ACTH-dependent, and the decline in ACTH at noon leads to the fall in aldosterone levels.

Biglieri and Schambelan (20) have suggested that 18-hydroxycorticosterone (18 OH-B), a glomerulosa steroid, may be an effective discriminator of an adenoma. Plasma 18 OH-B was found to be markedly elevated at 8 A.M. in patients with adenoma, being some six times higher than in patients with hyperplasia. A value of 100 ng/dL or greater distinguishes an adenoma from hyperplasia without overlap.

In addition to these two most common forms of primary aldosteronism, at least two other types have been described. One of these has been termed indeterminate hyperaldosteronism and the other glucocorticoid-remediable hyperaldosteronism. The distinguishing features of indeterminate hyperaldosteronism is the ability of DOCA administration to suppress aldosterone into the normal range, a finding not observed in the other types of primary aldosteronism (19). Glucocorticoid-remediable hyperaldosteronism is a rare variant seen in children; its pathogenesis is unknown. Replacement dosage of glucorticoid hormones restores blood pressure to normal levels and corrects the hypokalemia and hyperaldosteronism (163,206). In the usual form of primary aldosteronism, dexamethasone decreases plasma aldosterone by 50% or more in 24 hours, but this effect is only transient and levels rise subsequently despite continued use of dexamethasone (77).

Differential Diagnosis (Table 2)

Hypokalemia in a hypertensive patient should always raise the suspicion of primary aldosteronism. Diuretic drugs are the most common cause of hypokalemia, and their effects may persist 1 week or more after cessation of therapy. Gastrointestinal losses of potassium must also be considered; the chronic use of laxatives is often overlooked.

Accelerated or malignant hypertension is frequently associated with secondary aldosteronism and hypokalemia (133). In this condition, the aldosteronism is due to the increased renin caused by severe vascular damage in the kidney. Primary aldosteronism can usually be excluded by the severity of the hypertension, especially the hemorrhage, exudates, and papilledema in the retina, a low serum sodium, and an elevated plasma renin concentration (33,48). Patients treated for malignant hypertension may go through a phase lasting several months in which aldosterone secretion remains high while plasma renin activity is suppressed (151). This suggests a condition of tertiary aldosteronism but is often confused with primary aldosteronism. A similar biochemical phenomenon might develop if large supplements of potassium are administered, because potassium loading can directly decrease renin release and increase aldosterone secretion.

Occasionally the clinical picture in patients with unilateral renovascular disease simulates primary aldosteronism. These patients have hypokalemia and increased aldosterone secretion, but an elevated plasma renin. The serum sodium is often low; the hypertension is usually severe and accelerated. Correction of the renal lesion relieves the hypertension and the secondary aldosteronism (126,234). Most patients, however, with unilateral renal vascular disease and benign hypertension do not have significantly elevated peripheral venous renin concentrations and secondary aldosteronism, or evidence of potassium depletion (31,34,117,159). The renal vein renin concentration from the affected kidney may be increased (158,168,232) and become useful in predicting a favorable blood pressure response to surgery, but the total production from both kidneys may not be elevated.

TABLE 2. Differential Diagnosis of Primary Aldosteronism

Diagnosis	Plasma renin activity	Aldosterone	Other
Diuretic drugs	High	High	K often low; most common cause of hypokalemia in the hypertensive patient
Malignant hypertension	High	High	BP severe; K ↓
Renal artery stenosis	High	High	BP severe; K sometimes ↓
Salt-losing nephritis	High	High	BUN high; acidosis
Cushing's syndrome	Variable	Variable	Cortisol high; DOC occasionally ↑; K sometimes ↓
Oral contraceptives	High	High	Normal K; BP ↑ occasionally
Juxtaglomerular hyperplasia (Bartter's syndrome)	High	High	BP normal and resistant to angiotensin; K ↓
Renin-secreting tumor	High	High	Renal arteriogram abnormal; renal vein renin high on tumor side; BP ↑; K ↓
Congenital adrenal hyperplasia			
11-β-hydroxylase deficiency	N or low	Low	High 17 KS; DOC; and "S," BP ↑; K ↓
17-α-hydroxylase deficiency	Low	Low	High DOC, B; Low 17 KS; low 17 OHCS; BP ↑; K ↓
DOC and 18-OH-DOC excess	Low	Low	Seen rarely in adrenal tumors; BP ↑; K ↓
Liddle's syndrome	Low	Low	Hypokalemia, hypertension, familial; responds to triamterene
Low renin essential hypertension	Low	N	Normal K; mineralocorticoid excess on rare occasion
Licorice	Low	Low	Active agent: glycyrrhizic acid, BP ↑, K ↓
Nasal spray (Biorinal)	Low	Low	Active agent 9α-fluoroprednisolone

N = normal
DOC = deoxycorticosterone
B = corticosterone
18-OH-DOC = 18-hydroxydeoxycorticosterone
"S" = 11-deoxycortisol
17KS = 17 ketosteroids
17OHCS = 17 hydroxycorticoids
BP = blood pressure

Chronic pyelonephritis, medullary cystic disease, or other forms of renal disease with sodium wasting may lead to secondary aldosteronism and hypokalemia. The blood urea nitrogen is elevated, the serum bicarbonate reduced, and the renin levels elevated. Sodium repletion corrects the aldosteronism.

Cushing's syndrome occasionally presents with hypertension and hypokalemia and only mild signs of classic Cushing's syndrome. This is especially true of nonendocrine tumors producing ACTH. The hypokalemia is due to the high cortisol and DOC production (56); aldosterone secretion is low (23,173).

Hypertension and hypokalemia can result from a congenital deficiency in 17α-hydroxylase enzyme affecting both gonadal and adrenal tissue. Deoxycorticosterone and corticosterone production rates are increased. This leads to sodium retention and hypervolemia, which inhibits renin production and subsequently aldosterone secretion by the zona glomerulosa (15,91). A congenital deficiency in 11β-hydroxylase activity is also associated with hypertension and hypokalemia (66). The latter may not always be present, however. Excess DOC production is believed to be the cause of the hypertension, suppressed renin, and aldosterone. Compound "S," another 11-deoxysteroid, is also elevated in this condition. A mild form of the 11β-hydroxylase deficiency syndrome has been described in adults (76,213a).

Hypersecretion of 18-hydroxydeoxycorticosterone (18-OH DOC) has been reported as causing hypertension and hypokalemia. Because 18-OH DOC secretion is regulated by ACTH, dexamethasone suppression corrected the hypertension and hypokalemia (153). Adenoma secreting the mineralocorticoid DOC or corticosterone may also simulate primary aldosteronism. Excess licorice ingestion can induce hypokalemic alkalosis and hypertension with suppressed plasma renin and aldosterone. The active mineralocorticoid-like substance in the licorice is ammonium glycyrrhizate (53). A new syndrome of factitious mineralocorticoid excess has been described. A nasal spray preparation (Biorinal) containing a potent mineralocorticoid 9α-fluoroprednisolone was found to be responsible for hypertension, hypokalemia, and a suppressed renin-aldosterone system in 20 patients (149).

Juxtaglomerular cell hyperplasia (Bartter's syndrome) may produce hypokalemic alkalosis and hyperaldosteronism, but hypertension is not present even though plasma renin concentrations are markedly increased (7,40). Liddle's syndrome is a rare familial condition characterized by increased Na−K exchange, hypokalemia, Na^+ retention, and hypertension. It responds to triamterene but not to spironolactone.

Oral contraceptive medications (104,132,228) can increase plasma renin levels and aldosterone secretion. In a hypertensive patient, the elevated aldosterone secretion raises the suspicion of primary aldosteronism, but the elevated plasma renin activity is the important factor ruling out the diagnosis. Hypokalemia is usually absent.

A renin-secreting tumor may cause hypokalemia and hypertension (179,189). These juxtaglomerular cell tumors may be small and only visualized by renal angiography. The peripheral plasma renin levels are elevated as well as the renal venous renin on the side of the tumor. Nephrectomy corrects the hyperreninemia, hypertension and hypokalemia.

Treatment of Primary Aldosteronism

The treatment of choice for primary aldosteronism is surgery (84,162, 172,193). The adrenal tumors are quite small and are rarely identified by retroperitoneal gas studies or angiograms. An intravenous pyelogram with nephrotomogram suffices to rule out the rare case of adrenal carcinoma. The surgeon must be experienced in adrenal gland surgery. A pathologist familiar with adrenal pathology should also be present. Both adrenal glands must be exposed and the gland carefully dissected and examined for small nodules. Serial sectioning of the adrenal gland may be necessary to locate the small tumor. The tumors are usually single; occasionally multiple and bilateral tumors occur, or adrenal hyperplasia may be all that is found (6,61,70). Unfortunately, bilateral adrenalectomy is sometimes necessary; grossly, the tumors are encapsulated and orange in color on crosssection. The histology is not specific; in fact, many of the tumors are composed of fasciculata-like cells (25,172).

In preparation for surgery, the potassium depletion should be corrected by prescribing a low-sodium diet, potassium supplements, and aldactone (spironolactone). The serum potassium and blood urea nitrogen should be followed closely. Aldactone should be stopped a few days before surgery because of the body's tendency to retain potassium after removal of the adenoma. Postoperatively, the tendency to waste sodium and retain potassium because of resulting hypoaldosteronism can be managed easily by saline infusions for the first few days. The hypoaldosteronism may persist for several weeks, or even months (24) but a liberal sodium intake is all that is necessary to prevent sodium depletion. The blood pressure may remain elevated for several weeks, and occasionally months, before returning to normal.

If surgery is inadvisable, aldactone and a low-sodium diet will control the potassium wasting and the symptoms caused by hypokalemia. Frequently, the degree of hypertension is also reduced (29,101). If the blood pressure does not fall, standard antihypertensive therapy should be added and the medical therapy continued indefinitely.

Aldactone treatment may be used to predict the outcome of surgery (32,199). If the blood pressure is not lowered by the administration of large dosages of aldactone (300–400 mg daily for 3–5 weeks), it will not be lowered by surgical removal of adenoma. Not all patients need such large dosages for maintenance; not infrequently, dosages as low as 50 mg/day are sufficient. Those patients with primary aldosteronism caused by bilateral adrenal hyperplasia are best treated with aldactone plus other antihypertensive therapy if needed. Aldactone therapy may be associated with gynecomastia in males and irregular menses in females.

In addition to its well-known aldosterone-antagonizing action, aldactone is believed also to directly inhibit aldosterone biosynthesis by the adrenal cortex. In addition to in vitro animal data, observations in patients with primary aldosteronism treated with this drug support such a hypothesis. Early in the course of aldactone therapy, plasma and urinary aldosterone decrease sharply despite a rise in plasma renin activity and serum potassium. Spironolactone bodies, which are laminated intracytoplasmic bodies seen within a white halo, can be demonstrated in the tumor cells but not in the inactive glomerulosa cells or in the zona fasciculata. They are believed to be the morphological expression of a block in aldosterone biosynthesis, probably the conversion of corticosterone to aldosterone. With prolonged therapy (i.e., more than 1 month), aldosterone production may increase above baseline levels, and spironolactone bodies begin to diminish in number, disappearing by 70 days (54).

LOW RENIN HYPERTENSION: A MINERALOCORTICOID EXCESS SYNDROME?

With the ability to quantitate many of the pathophysiologic changes involved in the development and maintenance of hypertension has come the realization that not all patients with "essential" hypertension are alike. When renin measurements became available, investigators reported that 10–50 per cent of essential hypertensive patients had low renin (41,112,118,148). Although various etiologies have been proposed to explain the occurrence of low renin levels, a minority of these patients with low-renin hypertension (LRH) appear to have an inappropriately increased secretion of mineralocorticoids, either singly or in combination. Since aldosterone secretion is low in normal subjects with low renin, the normal or rarely high normal values seen in LRH may be inappropriate to the level of renin and angiotensin II in these patients. Recent data suggest an increased sensitivity of the adrenals of patients with LRH to angiotensin II (216). Certain patients with LRH fail to suppress aldosterone secretion normally in response to sodium loading (45a). The metabolic clearance of aldosterone usually has been found to be normal in essential hypertension (142); this is true also in LRH (36). Total body sodium has been reported to be elevated in patients with low renin, but only when compared with hypertensive patients with normal renin. This finding, however, has not been reproduced (138). The unusually rapid excretion of an acute sodium load by patients with LRH has suggested to many investigators that plasma volume is at least functionally expanded (120,187). Actual increases in plasma volume have been reported by some, but not all investigators (112,187). Aminoglutethimide, an inhibitor of adrenal steroid biosynthesis, causes a modest reduction in blood pressure in patients with LRH, but essentially no reduction in those with normal renin hypertension (233). This effect of aminoglutethimide has been confirmed in a recent study (140) that showed, in addition, that metyrapone was ineffective in LRH, whereas it lowered the blood pressure in patients with primary aldosteronism. This latter finding was interpreted as evidence against aldosterone being of etiologic importance in LRH. Dexamethasone has no hypotensive effect in both LRH and 1° aldosteronism; this implies that the steroid involved is not ACTH-dependent. However, adrenalectomy has been reported to cure LRH (100). Over two-thirds of patients with LRH respond to aldosterone antagonists (58,200), a somewhat higher response rate than in normal or high renin patients. Their equally good response to spironolactone and hydrochlorthiazide suggests that volume contraction rather than specific aldosterone antagonism is the more important factor (1).

Actual identification of mineralocorticoids in LRH has been more difficult. Cortisol and corticosterone are not involved. 11-Deoxycorticosterone and 18-OH-DOC are normally present in plasma, but in extremely minute quantities, making measurement difficult. Using a gas chromatographic technique, Brown et al. (35) reported elevated plasma DOC levels in six of 21 patients with LRH (35). The mean serum potassium in six patients was normal, but intermittent hypokalemia was observed. Spironolactone was effective in controlling their hypertension. Two of the six patients were believed to have adenomas secreting only DOC in excess. In other small series, secretion of DOC has usually been normal. Plasma DOC and urinary-free DOC levels were found to be normal in patients with essential hypertension irrespective of renin profile when assayed by a specific radioimmunoassay method incorporating prior Sephadex LH-20 chromatography (209). The disparity in results among the various reports may be attributed to factors such as the population studied, the steroid assay, and possible drug interference in the assay procedure (210). It should be noted that in patients with aldosteronomas, secretion of DOC is elevated (16,211) and early 1° aldosteronism may present as LRH (97). Even when it is possible to demonstrate elevation of DOC in plasma, the question remains whether DOC itself is the cause of hypertension. Deoxycorticosterone has certainly been implicated in several animal models of hypertension (44a,45) and pharmacologic dosages can cause a hypertensive response in human subjects with labile hypertension (17). The potency of DOC and 18-OH-DOC in stimulating sodium transport is only about 2%−10% that of aldosterone. The assumption is that prolonged exposure of a susceptible individual to DOC or another mineralocorticoid, even at only slightly higher levels, may cause gradual elevation of the blood pressure. Other factors, such as salt intake and sympathetic nervous system activity, also play at least a permissive role (62).

In a group of 12 patients with LRH, an increased excretion of 18 hydroxy-tetrahydro-deoxycorticosterone (18-OH-TH-DOC) was noted (155). Secretion of DOC was normal in these patients. Although levels of 18-OH-TH-DOC were elevated five- to tenfold in one patient, five of the 12 patients with LRH had only a twofold increase. Additionally, patients with adrenal adenomas and hyperplasia have been shown to have increased levels of 18-OH-DOC in adrenal vein blood.

A genetic model of low LRH has been developed in rats selectively bred for salt sensitivity (109). At least one of the factors involved in their low renin and hypertension appears to be an increased adrenal secretion of 18-OH-DOC (175).

Several adrenal steroids have been identified in various hypertensive states, thus serving as potential candidates for the "unknown mineralocorticoid" in LRH. These steroids include 16β-hydroxydehydroepiandrosterone, 16α,18 dihydroxy-DOC, 19 nor-DOC, 17α,20α-dihydroxyprogesterone, and 5α-dihydrocortisol. Questions regarding some of these compounds are: 1) Are they produced in excess in LRH? 2) How much in excess? 3)How potent are they as mineralocorticoids? Using a radioreceptor assay to measure "total plasma mineralocorticoid activity," Baxter et al. (10) failed to detect increased activity in patients with essential hypertension, including those with LRH. Increased activity, however, was demonstrable in patients with 1° aldosteronism.

Many other mechanisms have been proposed to explain the low renin state and these may be operative in some patients. In general, an increase in blood pressure would be expected to lower renin by its direct effect on the juxtaglomerular apparatus. However, this does not explain evidence of increased mineralocorticoid function in some of these patients, nor does it explain why blood pressure tends to be lower in the low renin group than in the normal and high renin group. Diminished autonomic function has been reported in a few patients with low renin but in most patients it is normal (118). Hypertensive diabetics with neuropathy or nephropathy tend to have low renin (44,180), and in alloxan-diabetic rats, low-renin hypertension is present (43). The mechanism for suppressed renin in the hypertensive diabetic remains to be elucidated.

SECONDARY ALDOSTERONISM

Excessive secretion of aldosterone resulting from a primary abnormality of the adrenal cortex, usually an adenoma, was termed "primary aldosteronism" by Conn, whereas "secondary aldosteronism" denotes excessive aldosterone production due to an extraadrenal stimulus, most commonly angiotensin. Thus, the factor distinguishing primary from secondary aldosteronism is renin production; in the former, it is suppressed, whereas in the latter it is increased. Various examples of secondary aldosteronism are shown in Table 3. Some of these conditions are accompanied by edema, indicating a failure of the escape mechanism; in other conditions, edema is not a factor, thus more closely mimicking primary aldosteronism.

Very rarely, the stimulus to aldosterone production may lead to the development of an adenoma in the adrenal gland, which may ultimately become autonomous. This situation has been termed "autonomous secondary" or "tertiary" aldosteronism (184).

Aldosterone During the Menstrual Cycle and in Pregnancy

Menstrual Cycle. During the luteal phase of the normal menstrual cycle, a ten- to twenty-fold increase in plasma progesterone may occur (205).

TABLE 3. Secondary Aldosteronism

Physiological Increases In Renin:	Diseases without Edema:
Upright posture	Bartter's and Pseudo-Bartter's syndrome
Low Na+ diet	Oral contraceptive use
Dehydration	Renovascular hypertension
Hemorrhage	Malignant hypertension
Pregnancy	Renin-secreting tumor
Diseases with Edema:	
Liver cirrhosis	
Nephrotic Syndrome	
Congestive heart failure	
Idiopathic edema	

Plasma renin activity, angiotensin II formation, and aldosterone secretion rate all increase about twofold (28,95,197). Administration of progesterone to males in dosages that attain plasma progesterone levels similar to the levels seen during the normal luteal phase will increase plasma renin activity and aldosterone secretion (204). This increase in aldosterone can be inhibited by sodium loading the subjects. The data, therefore, support the concept that the natriuresis produced by progesterone (128) stimulates renin release and angiotensin II formation with subsequent increase in aldosterone secretion to compensate for the natriuresis.

During the luteal phase of the normal menstrual cycle there is also an increase in plasma estrogens. Although estrogen administration can increase renin substrate and lead to increased plasma renin activity and aldosterone secretion (57,103), it does not appear that the substrate concentration is significantly increased during the luteal phase.

The increase in aldosterone production during the luteal phase may play a role in the premenstrual edema that occurs in some patients. But other factors must also be important, there being no correlation between the extent of edema and the levels of renin and aldosterone (95).

Normal Pregnancy. Aldosterone secretion is markedly elevated in pregnancy (110,194). The secretion rate is increased as early as the 15th week of gestation and reaches very high levels during the last trimester (greater than 1000 μg/day). This increased secretion rate has its origin in the maternal adrenal, because the levels of aldosterone excretion are low or undetectable in the urine of adrenalectomized pregnant women (9,125). Furthermore, aldosterone secretion responds appropriately to sodium loading and depletion in the pregnant woman.

The physiological significance of the high aldosterone secretion in pregnancy is not clear. There is a significantly positive sodium balance for the development of the fetus, the uterus, and the expansion of maternal blood volume. Total exchangeable sodium increases by about 400 mEq, and the blood volume may be increased by as much as 50%. Heparinoid-induced inhibition of aldosterone biosynthesis in pregnancy results in natriuresis even though the aldosterone excretion remains at nongravid levels. This natriuresis suggests that sodium conservation during pregnancy is dependent upon augmented secretion of aldosterone (67). Yet pregnancy may be continued successfully in adrenalectomized women maintained on cortisone (55).

The exact mechanism of the increased secretion is not known. There is the increased need for a positive sodium balance. Moreover, the marked increase in progesterone production during pregnancy may inhibit the renal tubular effects of aldosterone, and hence a compensatory increase is necessary to overcome this inhibition. Aldosterone secretion does appear to have the same time course as progesterone production; it increases early in pregnancy and continues to increase through the pregnancy. Administration of progesterone to normal males results in increased plasma renin activity and aldosterone excretion which can be prevented by sodium-loading the subjects (194). Another explanation is that the placenta and fetus behave like an arteriovenous fistula and, although the blood volume is increased, the arterial tree remains poorly filled and undistended, thus resulting in a compensatory activation of the renin system.

Regardless of the cause, the renin–angiotensin system appears to be the major mechanism regulating the secretion of aldosterone. High concentrations of renin in the plasma of pregnant women have been reported (26). Plasma renin substrate and angiotensin II concentrations also are increased in pregnancy (178,229). It is perplexing that the renin concentrations are highest during the first trimester, whereas aldosterone secretion is highest in the third trimester. It may be that hypertrophy of the zona glomerulosa occurs and, for a given concentration of renin, more aldosterone is produced. Supporting this concept is the fact that dogs that are sodium depleted for approximately 2 weeks become more sensitive to the aldosterone-stimulating effects of ACTH and angiotensin (78).

The source of the plasma renin during pregnancy has been a subject of investigation. The uterus of both humans and animals contains a renin-like enzyme (160,201) that is actually synthesized in the uterus. During the normal pregnancy, however, the circulating renin probably originates in the kidney, because the plasma renin responds in the same fashion to stimuli that increase plasma renin in nonpregnant women: sodium depletion and the upright posture (22). The high plasma renin levels observed during molar pregnancies and in the pregnant rabbit postnephrectomy imply that the uterus may contribute to plasma renin activity under certain conditions.

Two puzzling questions arise concerning aldosterone in pregnancy. Why do pregnant women not develop potassium depletion from such high rates of aldosterone secretion? In this respect, pregnant women are similar to patients with nephrosis, cirrhosis, and those on a low-sodium diet, all of whom have high aldosterone secretion rates but who do not waste potassium. These patients have one thing in common: increased reabsorption of sodium in the proximal tubule of the kidney. Hence, little sodium is delivered to the distal ion exchange site for exchange with potassium. Indeed, a low-sodium diet will prevent potassium wasting even when large doses of a mineralocorticoid are administered (177). This cannot be the explanation in pregnancy, because plenty of sodium is excreted. Perhaps the best explanation is that an antagonist to aldosterone, progesterone, is produced in large quantities during pregnancy. The inhibition of aldosterone action probably occurs in the distal ion exchange site where aldosterone stimulates secretion of potassium for sodium ions. In a recent report (68), a marked dissociation between the antinatriuretic and kaliuretic effects of mineralocorticoids in pregnancy was noted. A similar response was observed in nonpregnant volunteers given progesterone.

Another question that arises is why all pregnant women do not become hypertensive from the high concentrations of circulating renin and aldosterone. The answer is unknown.

Toxemia of Pregnancy. This complication of late pregnancy is usually seen in primigravidas and is characterized by hypertension, edema, proteinuria, and, on occasion, convulsions. The etiology of toxemia is unknown. The renin–angiotensin–aldosterone system has been implicated owing to the fact that pregnancy is associated with marked increases in plasma renin concentration, renin substrate, angiotensin II, and aldosterone levels. Numerous studies, however, have confirmed that the renin–angiotensin–aldosterone axis is not more active in toxemic than in normotensive pregnancies. Indeed, most studies indicate that all components of this system are depressed rather than elevated (30, 194,229).

Most authors believe that uteroplacental insufficiency secondary to reduced uterine blood flow constitutes the initiating insult in toxemia. Uterine ischemia has been shown to result in the release of uterine renin (71), although the latter's role is undefined. It is known, however, that the infusion of angiotensin II into the uterine circulation leads to vasodilatation and increased blood flow, an effect opposite to that seen in other vascular beds (3,71). Prostaglandin E, a potent vasodilator produced in substantial amounts by the uterus, may be the mediator of angiotensin II–induced vasodilation. Angiotensin II stimulates the release of uterine prostaglandins (75,217); furthermore, uterine blood flow can be significantly reduced with the inhibition of prostaglandin biosynthesis (222). Impaired prostaglandin production by the uteroplacental unit in toxemia, however, remains to be proven.

It can be deduced from studies on the clearance of dehydroepiandrosterone sulphate (DHEA-S) by the uteroplacental unit, a measurement correlating well with uterine blood flow (79), that the underlying abnormality of toxemia precedes its clinical manifestations. Toxemic pregnancies are characterized by a reduced DHEA-S clearance. More importantly, this reduction is apparent in early pregnancy in those women who subsequently develop toxemia (81). A second abnormality in toxemia is the augmented pressor response, or increased sensitivity, to angiotensin II (80). This abnormality also is apparent before the onset of clinical toxemia, representing a loss of the usual vascular refractoriness to angiotensin II seen in normal pregnancy (82).

Secondary Aldosteronism with Edema

Edema develops when the balance between capillary filtration and resorption of fluid and electrolytes is disturbed. Many factors are involved: capillary filtration pressure, the oncotic pressure of plasma proteins, venous and lymphatic pressure, muscular activity, cardiac output, aldosterone secretion, renal function, and the failure of the escape mechanism. After its initial discovery, aldosterone was thought to play the central role in edema formation. It is now clear that aldosterone is only one such factor. Other important mechanisms that signal the kidney to rid the body of excess sodium are vitally involved in the development of edema. Some of these are still poorly understood (e.g., natriuretic or third factor). The failure of the escape mechanism in the face of aldosterone excess in some cases of secondary aldosteronism is a mystery. The daily administration of large doses of mineralocorticoids, like DOC, 9-alpha-fluorohydrocortisone, and aldosterone, to normal dogs or humans results in several days of sodium retention and then an escape from the sodium-retaining effect (5,59). The body content of sodium remains elevated, but the subjects no longer continue to retain sodium (escape mechanism). Three explanations of this phenomenon have been proposed: an intrinsic mechanism of the kidney responding to expansion of the extracellular fluid volume; stimulation of secretion of a salt-losing hormone by volume expansion; and inhibition of a salt-retaining hormone that normally enhances sodium reabsorption by the kidney.

In contrast to healthy subjects, patients with edema from heart failure, liver cirrhosis, or nephrosis do not escape, and this is true as well of dogs with thoracic inferior vena caval constriction, arteriovenous fistulas, or heart failure (59,60). Obviously, the underlying illness is the reason for the failure of the escape mechanism in edematous states. How this happens is still obscure. Possibly, it is the underdistention of the arterial tree at certain critical sites that signals the body into believing there is insufficient salt and water.

Liver Cirrhosis. The metabolism of aldosterone occurs mostly in the liver. Extrahepatic metabolism accounts for about 15% of the total clearance (146). The half-life of aldosterone in the plasma is prolonged from an average of 30 minutes in normal subjects up to 90 minutes in patients with hepatic cirrhosis (54a). The proportion of the secreted aldosterone that is excreted as the 18-glucuronide is increased while that of the tetrahydroaldosterone fraction is decreased (54a). Since the tetrahydroaldosterone metabolite is made chiefly in the liver, liver disease reduces its formation, and more of the circulating aldosterone is then available to be metabolized to the 18-glucuronide by the kidney (146).

In addition to the decreased metabolic clearance of aldosterone, there is a fairly consistent increase in the aldosterone secretion rate in patients with cirrhosis and ascites (2,54a); the plasma concentration of aldosterone is markedly elevated (170). Where both metabolic clearance and blood secre-tion rates have been measured, the reduction in the former was modest compared to the marked elevation in the latter (182). It thus appears that marked aldosterone hypersecretion is the predominant factor in producing very elevated blood aldosterone levels in the cirrhotic patients with ascites.

The plasma renin concentrations may be very high in patients with cirrhosis and ascites but are usually normal in those with cirrhosis without ascites (27,223). That the pressor and aldosterone-stimulating actions of infused angiotensin are reduced in cirrhotic patients with ascites also suggests that these patients have high endogenous angiotensin blood levels (130).

The abnormal transudation of fluid out of the vascular compartment during the formation of edema and ascites is associated with a reduction in effective arterial volume. The decreased volume stimulates renin release, which in turn increases aldosterone secretion. Plasma renin activity can be shown to be inversely correlated with outer renal cortical blood flow (181). The raised aldosterone secretion rate and decreased metabolism result in an elevated aldosterone blood level that enhances sodium retention. Unlike normal subjects, the cirrhotic patient fails to escape from the sodium-retaining effect. Aldosterone antagonists (e.g., spironolactone) are frequently useful in the treatment of the edema of cirrhosis.

The elevated plasma renin activity and plasma aldosterone are only minimally affected by posture, dietary sodium restriction, and diuretic administration (182). Although aldosterone excess may explain the ascites and edema of the cirrhosis, it is not the whole explanation. Portal hypertension and hypoalbuminemia certainly play important roles. During spontaneous diuresis, some cirrhotic patients continue to show markedly elevated aldosterone levels, and in three patients treated with aminoglutethimide and dexamethasone, steroidogenesis including aldosterone biosynthesis was markedly inhibited, yet significant diuresis did not occur (182). Immersion studies in cirrhotic patients also demonstrate an absent or markedly blunted natriuretic response despite aldosterone suppression.

A report suggested that renal prostaglandins are produced in excess in the cirrhotic patient (235). This may mediate the hyperreninemia and hyperaldosteronism since indomethacin or ibuprofen, known prostaglandin inhibitors, were effective in lowering plasma renin activity and aldosterone levels (235).

Cardiac Failure. In congestive heart failure there is an abnormal tendency to retain dietary sodium, which results in edema. Increased proximal tubular reabsorption of sodium appears to be the primary and principal abnormality of renal handling of sodium in congestive heart failure; aldosteronism adds a secondary difficulty in promoting sodium excretion. Initial studies reported increased urinary aldosterone secretion. However, estimates of aldosterone secretion as well as excretion rates have shown wide variation in untreated subjects on normal electrolyte intake, with most cases within the normal range (38,55,105,185,208). The rates rise with diuresis. Nevertheless, the peripheral blood concentration of aldosterone may be elevated. The metabolic clearance rate of aldosterone by the liver is diminished (38,105,208); hepatic extraction of aldosterone is only about 70% in patients with severe congestive heart failure compared with 95%–100% in normal subjects. Therefore, even though the secretion rate of aldosterone may be within the normal range, plasma concentrations may be higher than normal in subjects with severe congestive heart failure (38).

There are only a few reports of renin or angiotensin blood levels in congestive heart failure (27,150,223). Like the aldosterone secretion data, the renin concentrations were inconsistently elevated. Sodium intake and diuretic therapy were not always controlled in these studies.

Nephrotic Syndrome. Hypersecretion of aldosterone has been reported in the edematous phase of nephrosis and decreased secretion in the diuretic phase (129,144). Reports of plasma renin or angiotensin levels in nephrosis are few (150,223). Raised plasma renin activity and plasma angiotensin concentration have been reported by some but not by others. Renin substrate is known to be decreased in the nephrotic syndrome. The importance of blood volume and renal perfusion can be demonstrated in the nephrotic patient with edema and a markedly reduced serum albumin. The infusion of concentrated human albumin expands plasma volume, increases renal blood flow and glomerular filtration rate, and decreases renin production and hence aldosterone secretion, and perhaps activates the escape mechanism. A diuresis ensues, but owing to the continued urinary loss of albumin the edematous state returns.

Idiopathic Edema. Idiopathic edema is a common form of dependent edema that may occur in women with no obvious history or physical signs of diseases of the heart, liver, kidneys, veins, or thyroid (145). Mild to moderate obesity may be present. The edema may worsen premenstrually, but in most instances swelling is continuous, but with cyclical fluctuations. Many of these patients are emotionally disturbed and have a long "allergic" history that is not always substantiated by allergy tests. The edema frequently disappears on bed rest and is worsened by the upright position. Some patients show cycles of edema and diuresis not related to the menstrual cycle. The serum potassium is normal.

The pathogenesis of idiopathic edema is unknown. Aldosterone excretion has been reported to be elevated in some of these patients during the sodium-retaining phase (96,145,183,202). On the other hand, Sims et al. (195) reported normal aldosterone excretion, although this may be inappropriate in view of the expanded ECF volume and edema. Idiopathic edema has even been observed in an Addisonian patient whose aldosterone levels were negligible, and who was not on mineralocorticoid therapy. Aldosterone may be important in at least a permissive way, but certainly other factors are important too. Increased capillary permeability and thickened capillary basement membranes have been described in some cases (195). An increased incidence of abnormal carbohydrate tolerance has raised the possibility that latent diabetes mellitus is the cause of the abnormal capillary permeability. Gill et al. reported abnormal albumin metabolism in patients with idiopathic edema (86,87). The changes are subtle and not easily recognized, and the cause is unknown. Serum albumin concentration, total circulatory albumin and plasma volume are diminished. In most cases, the diminished total circulating albumin could be attributed to either accelerated degradation or decreased synthesis. The hypovolemia leads to an increase in sympathetic nerve activity, slightly increased renin and aldosterone production, and decreased excretion of sodium by the kidney.

Abnormalities in the sympathetic nervous system have been described in patients with idiopathic edema. Increased urinary norepinephrine excretion may be present, although this has been refuted by others (86,121,122). Plasma but not urinary cAMP may be elevated, perhaps reflecting an excessive β-adrenergic tone (122). Decreased dopamine production has been suggested as a pathogenetic factor (123), since this catecholamine has recently been recognized to have natriuretic activity.

Treatment with bed rest, elastic stockings, low-caloric diet, limitation of sodium intake, intermittent diuretics, and aldosterone antagonists is usually satisfactory. Diuretics commonly lead to further activation of the renin–aldosterone system and can result in rebound edema when discontinued. With time, however, some of the edema will recede as aldosterone levels decline. Potassium supplements are sometimes necessary to prevent the weakness and fatigue as well as other complications of the potassium depletion that may follow diuretic therapy. In some cases, vasopressor agents such as ephedrine or neosynephrine are useful. In rare instances of prolonged and intractable edema, nodular hyperplasia or adenomas (183,202) are found in the adrenal cortex. Excision of the abnormal tissue may be helpful. In most cases, however, the adrenal gland is normal histologically, and in some cases the edema disappears spontaneously.

It should be emphasized that idiopathic edema is a diagnosis of exclusion. In many of the patients in whom this diagnosis has been made, an underlying cause of the edema has been found after careful study. Subtle forms of heart disease (85), hypothyroidism, lymphedema, and venous insufficiency may be uncovered. Treatment of the primary condition may alleviate the symptoms.

Premenstrual edema is a frequent cause of mild edema and differs from idiopathic edema in that it is specifically related to the menstrual cycle. Many factors are involved in the pathogenesis of the edema. Aldosterone may play a contributing role, because its secretion rate and plasma renin levels are increased in the luteal phase of the cycle. However, the secretion rates are as high in the luteal phase of women without premenstrual edema (94,176).

Secondary Aldosteronism without Edema

Bartter's Syndrome. In 1962, Bartter and his associates described an unusual form of secondary hyperaldosteronism in which hypertrophy and hyperplasia of the juxtaglomerular cells were associated with a normal blood pressure and hypokalemic alkalosis in the absence of edema (7). Surgical exploration documented the absence of an adrenal tumor to account for the hyperaldosteronism. Many patients with this unusual disorder have dwarfism and mental retardation, and although the diagnosis has been established at the ages 2.5–25 years, most patients appear to have become ill during late infancy or early childhood.

A variety of complaints have brought these patients to medical attention. The most frequent complaint is weakness, small stature, or vomiting. The latter is occasionally accompanied by significant dehydration. Metabolic alkalosis with hypokalemia coupled with hyponatremia and hypochloremia is the typical pattern of the plasma electrolyte disturbances. Hyperactivity of the renin–angiotensin system appears to be primarily responsible for aldosteronism in patients with this syndrome. Reduced concentrations of renin substrate have been reported (40); this may reflect an increased generation of angiotensin II by the large amounts of circulating renin.

One of the hallmarks of Bartter's syndrome is a resistance or subnormal vasopressor response to the pressor effect of angiotensin II but not of noradrenaline (7). Whether this is unique to the syndrome is debatable, since many states of secondary aldosteronism manifest resistance to the pressor effect of angiotensin II (40).

There are studies showing that the oversecretion of renin and aldosterone in Bartter's syndrome could not be completely prevented by expansion of plasma volume by albumin or by high-sodium intake (7,40). These observations suggest that with juxtaglomerular cell hyperplasia, the release of renin by the kidney is relatively, but not completely, independent of hemodynamic stimuli (40). The state of potassium balance is another significant factor influencing the rate of aldosterone secretion in Bartter's syndrome. In most of the patients reported (40,93) rises or falls in the rate of aldosterone secretion occurred when potassium supplements were administered or withdrawn. This probably indicates a direct effect of potassium in augmenting adrenal secretion of aldosterone since the infusion of potassium is known to stimulate secretion of this hormone. Potassium can produce greater alterations in aldosterone secretion when the adrenal glands are already hyperactive. In patients with Bartter's syndrome the adrenal glands may respond excessively to altered potassium balance because they have an abnormally high secretory capacity to start with (39).

The nature of the defective control of renin release is poorly understood. In some patients, balance studies reveal defective sodium conservation and high rates of urinary excretion of potassium and hydrogen ion (39). Study of the renal histology has suggested the possibility of renal injury in the perinatal period. This lesion, by producing renal salt wasting may lead to reduced arterial volume and diminished stretch on the afferent arteriole with subsequently increased renin secretion. Altered sodium transport in Bartter's syndrome has also been demonstrated in the erythrocytes of patients and siblings (83). Another possibility is decreased arterial receptors, including the juxtaglomerular cells, for angiotensin II. This concept implies that angiotensin II has an important physiological role in maintaining arteriolar tone and feedback inhibition of renin secretion.

Most recently, overproduction of renal prostaglandins has been shown to be present in Bartter's syndrome, and this is believed to mediate the hyperreninemia (72,88). During short-term treatment with prostaglandin inhibitors (e.g., indomethacin or aspirin), many of the biochemical abnormalities, including hypokalemia, can be corrected. Pressor responses to angiotension II are restored. Hypokalemia, however, apparently returns with continued therapy. A renal tubular chloride-leak hypothesis has also been advanced as being the primary defect in Bartter's syndrome (89).

Spironolactone and propranolol may be useful in correcting the potassium wasting of Bartter's syndrome. More recently, indomethacin and other nonsteroidal antiinflammatory drugs have been shown to be effective as well.

Occasionally, patients with surreptitious vomiting or diuretic ingestion can present with the biochemical findings of Bartter's syndrome (115, 226). This condition is called pseudo-Bartter's syndrome and is more commonly encountered than true Bartter's syndrome. The diagnosis may be difficult to establish since these patients may be extremely clever in hiding their malfeasance.

Oral Contraceptives. Oral contraceptive therapy is well known to increase plasma renin levels and aldosterone secretion via a marked increase in renin substrate. The estrogen component of oral contraceptives is believed to be the active principle responsible for the increase in renin substrate, and similar changes have also been observed in estrogen treated rats (12,57,103,104,132,134,197,228). Plasma renin concentration is consistently decreased, and is inversely correlated with the level of plasma renin substrate (156,157). Plasma angiotensin II levels rise within 5 days, remain elevated throughout the course of treatment, and return to normal levels within 1 month after discontinuing use (37). Presumably the increased angiotensin II inhibits renin secretion (short-loop inhibition), thus minimizing the changes in the renin activity from the alterations in renin substrate. The renin–angiotensin–aldosterone system remains responsive to sodium loading and depletion although operating from a higher baseline (161). Renin and angiotensin II levels, however, fail to return all the way to normal. This failure may be one of the mechanisms contributing to the development of hypertension during therapy with oral contraceptive agents. A prospective study of women taking oral contraceptives revealed that those who became hypertensive had somewhat higher levels of renin substrate, renin activity, and renin concentration than those who remained normotensive (186).

The mechanism of the hypertension is still not entirely clear (134). Although most subjects treated with oral contraceptive agents have increased plasma angiotensin II concentrations, only a few develop hypertension (37). It is possible that genetic and other factors play a role. In those subjects developing hypertension, there is a higher prevalence of hypertension in their families and frequently a history of toxemia of pregnancy.

Renovascular Hypertension, Malignant Hypertension, and Renin Secreting Tumor. These are also examples of secondary aldosteronism without accompanying edema. Both renin activity and aldosterone production are elevated. These conditions have been briefly described in the section on primary aldosteronism.

HYPOMINERALOCORTICOIDISM

Adrenal Insufficiency

In Addison's disease and following bilateral adrenalectomy, aldosterone secretion is deficient or absent. The deficiency of cortisol, however, leads to the acute problems. The Addisonian patient may be maintained adequately, although not optimally, on cortisol and a liberal salt diet. Usually a mineralocorticoid is added to the regimen. Aldosterone is not effective by mouth so that another mineralocorticoid such as 9-alpha-fluorhydrocortisone (florinef) may be used. The usual dosage is 0.1 mg/day; in some patients, even this small dosage may cause edema or hypertension. In adrenal insufficiency secondary to pituitary failure, aldosterone secretion is relatively well preserved, and mineralocorticoid replacement is usually unnecessary.

Selective Hypoaldosteronism

This disorder was once thought to be rare (108,127,169,196,221), but its true incidence may have been underestimated. In a review of 100 cases of hyperkalemia, selective hypoaldosteronism was present in 10% (see Table 4 for causes of hypoaldosteronism). As many as 50% of all patients with "unexplained" hyperkalemia may have this syndrome (212). The biochemical hallmark of the disease is low aldosterone production. Cortisol production is generally within normal limits and an ACTH test should be done to rule out a more general adrenal insufficiency. Most patients have asymptomatic hyperkalemia but some may come to medical attention because of hyperkalemia-induced cardiac abnormalities (e.g., heart block with Stokes-Adams attacks). Frequently, mild renal disease, especially diabetic nephropathy, is present. Mild acidosis with impaired ammonium excretion has been documented (207). Salt loss is not a prominent feature despite hypoaldosteronism. Orthostatic hypotension has been emphasized in the past, but occurs only occasionally. Indeed, many patients are hypertensive, possibly because of renal disease (102,190).

TABLE 4. Causes of Hypoaldosteronism

Low Plasma Renin Activity
Primary hyporeninemia
Autonomic neuropathy
Prostaglandin deficiency
Normal or High Plasma Renin Activity
Addison's disease
Bilateral total adrenalectomy
Potassium deficiency
Heparin administration
Congenital adrenal hyperplasia
Postresection of aldosteronoma
Chronic hypopituitarism
18-hydroxylase deficiency
Pseudohypoaldosteronism

Hyporeninemia appears to be the primary defect in most cases of hypoaldosteronism, hence the commonly used term "hyporeninemic hypoaldosteronism" (188). The low plasma renin activity is poorly repsonsive to the usual stimuli (e.g., upright posture, low salt diet, etc.).

Hyporeninemic hypoaldosteronism has recently been observed in patients with impaired renal prostaglandin biosynthesis (e.g., during indomethacin therapy) (124,165,214,215). Prostaglandins appear to be essential for the full expression of the renin response, and hyporeninemia can result from the inhibition of prostaglandin biosynthesis (213). In the correct clinical setting (e.g., mild renal insufficiency), the full-blown picture of hyporeninemic hypoaldosteronism with frank hyperkalemia may result. Impaired prostaglandin E_2 production has also been documented in a few cases of hyporeninemic hypoaldosteronism not caused by nonsteroidal antiinflammatory drugs (165,214). Infusion of prostaglandin into a patient with this disease resulted in the reversal of many of the metabolic abnormalities including hyperkalemia (165). Since it now appears that prostaglandins may mediate the renin response to many if not all stimuli (e.g., posture, furosemide, low-salt diet, or hemorrhage), the hypothesis that impaired renal prostaglandin production may be etiologic in hyporeninemic hypoaldosteronism has been advanced (165, 215). Not all such patients, however, have low prostaglandin E_2 production; whether other prostaglandins (e.g., PGI_2) are involved remains to be established (214). Hahn et al. (102) have recently measured urinary kallikrein in patients with hyporeninemic hypoaldosteronism; they found its excretion to be markedly suppressed. In Bartter's syndrome (hyperreninemic hyperaldosteronism with hypokalemia), which is in many respects the mirror-image of hyporeninemic hypoaldosteronism, kallikrein and prostaglandin excretion are known to be elevated (224). Since kallikrein mediates the generation of kinins which in turn can stimulate the biosynthesis of prostaglandins, there is good reason to feel that abnormalities in these linked systems may well play important pathogenetic roles in these syndromes.

It is now recognized that renin exists in at least two forms, namely active and inactive renin. The latter may be a proenzyme and can be converted to active renin by acid, cold, or protease exposure (198,214). Recently, Tan et al. (214) have shown that whereas plasma renin activity and active renin are clearly low in hyporeninemic hypoaldosteronism, total renin production (i.e., inactive plus active renin) was normal and the ratio of inactive to active renin was significantly elevated). These results contrast with the situation in primary aldosteronism where both active and inactive renin are low. These findings suggest that the primary lesion in hyporeninemic hypoaldosteronism may be a defect of renin conversion or activation rather than of total renin production (188).

Many patients with hyporeninemic hypoaldosteronism are insulin-dependent diabetics, often with diabetic nephropathy (188). It is unclear why the diabetic should be particularly predisposed to this complication. According to one hypothesis (63), insulinopenia leads to failure of glucose and K^+ to enter the intracellular compartment. Hyperkalemia then results in renin suppression and hypoaldosteronism. This hypothesis, however, does not explain why other hyperkalemic states may not be associated with a suppressed renin–angiotensin system (e.g., in the Addisonian patient where renin is markedly elevated). Additionally, renin responses do not return to normal when patients are rendered normokalemic (188).

A subtle abnormality in renal sodium excretion has also been suggested as the primary lesion leading to hyporeninemia and hypoaldosteronism (167). In support of this hypothesis is the finding of increased extracellular volume in this disease. Subtle defects in aldosterone biosynthesis have also been reported to be present in hyporeninemic hypoaldosteronism (139) (Table 5).

Most cases of hyporeninemic hypoaldosteronism have been described in elderly patients with mild nonoliguric renal disease and asymptomatic hyperkalemia. It should be recognized that impaired potassium excretion leading to hyperkalemia occurs only in the face of severely compromised renal function [e.g. GFR 10 mL/minute (92,137)]. Hyperkalemia in the

TABLE 5. Proposed Mechanisms for Hyporeninemic Hypoaldosteronism

1. Diminished renin production is the primary lesion
   Hypoaldosteronism is secondary to hyporeninemia (ref. 188)
2. Insulinopenia leads to hyperkalemia which in turn suppresses renin (ref. 63)
3. Sodium and volume retention initiates the syndrome (ref. 167)
4. Renal prostaglandin deficiency causes renin inhibition (ref. 215)
5. A disease of impaired conversion of prorenin to active renin rather than of total renin production (ref. 214)
6. Defects in the adrenal aldosterone biosynthetic pathway play contributory role (ref. 139)

absence of overt renal failure should therefore alert the clinician to the diagnosis of hypoaldosteronism.

One form of selective hypoaldosteronism occurs after the removal of an aldosteronoma (24). The residual adrenal tissue has an atrophied zona glomerulosa that responds poorly to angiotensin or ACTH. This form of hypoaldosteronism may persist for several weeks and even months after surgery despite a rise in plasma renin activity and serum potassium (24). Hypoaldosteronism has also been described in patients with postural hypotension secondary to autonomic insufficiency, presumably because of inadequate renin stimulation (192).

Long-term heparin administration results in depressed aldosterone production by a mechanism that is not completely understood. The evidence suggests that heparin has a direct effect on the biosynthesis of aldosterone in the adrenal gland (50). Chronic hypopituitarism may result in diminished aldosterone biosynthesis, especially in response to sodium depletion (141,230). Prolonged potassium deficiency inhibits aldosterone secretion by interfering with biosynthesis and zona glomerulosa cell growth. Hyperkalemia may develop during repletion with potassium.

Hypoaldosteronism is treated with replacement doses of mineralocorticoid (e.g., 0.1 mg daily of florinef). Some patients cannot tolerate this dosage and may develop sodium retention and congestive heart failure. Therapy with loop diuretics such as furosemide has also been effective and may be preferable in patients with significant renal or cardiac compromise (190).

Congenital Adrenal Hyperplasia

The most common type of congenital adrenal hyperplasia results from 21-hydroxylase deficiency. This type may be divided into the salt losers and the nonsalt losers. In the untreated stage of the nonsalt losers, aldosterone and plasma renin levels are elevated (8,90,119). This hyperaldosterone state is probably secondary to the overproduction of cortisol precursors such as 17α-hydroxyprogesterone, which can block aldosterone action on the kidney. A similar, secondary hyperreninemia and hyperaldosteronism occur following treatment with the aldosterone antagonist, spironolactone. The salt-losing form has low aldosterone secretion, probably the result of a more severe 21-hydroxylase deficiency, because these cases have the lowest cortisol secretion rates (119,143). Salt loss with low aldosterone also occur in the rare 3β-ol-dehydrogenase-isomerase and desmolase enzyme deficiencies (21). In 11β- and 17α-hydroxylase deficiency, aldosterone is low; DOC is elevated, leading to salt retention and decrease in renin production. Hypokalemia with hypertension may be present (15,66).

A defect in aldosterone biosynthesis has been observed in infants with dehydration, hyponatremia, and hyperkalemia; the defect cannot be attributed to general adrenal insufficiency or the usual forms of congenital adrenal hyperplasia. One group demonstrated a block in biosynthesis between 18-hydroxycorticosterone and aldosterone, while another found a block between corticosterone and aldosterone (219,225). In contrast to the far more common form of hypoaldosteronism (i.e., hyporeninemic hypoaldosterone), patients with the biosynthetic block are usually markedly salt-depleted and have elevated plasma renin activity.

Pseudohypoaldosteronism

In 1958, a syndrome of congenital renal salt loss associated with insensitivity to mineralocorticoids was described (42). This disorder is now known as pseudohypoaldosteronism, with the clinical hallmarks of hyponatremia, hyperkalemia, renal salt loss, and failure to thrive (174). Salt loss is characteristically transient and it spontaneously resolves within several months. Saline but not deoxycorticosterone administration leads to dramatic clinical improvement.

A partial defect in the aldosterone receptor of the renal tubule has been proposed as the underlying mechanism, since renin activity and aldosterone levels are elevated, and adrenal function and usual parameters of renal function are all within normal limits. A deficiency in Na, K-ATPase in microdissected renal tubules has been reported (13). Aldosterone action on the sweat and salivary glands and the colon may also be impaired (166). However, in one study, no abnormality in nuclear binding of radioactive aldosterone in a colon biopsy was demonstrable (171).

An impaired response to mineralocorticoids has also been described in cases of hyperkalemia following renal transplantation (64).

REFERENCES

1. Adlin, V. E., Marks, A. D., and Channick, B. J. (1972) Spironolactone and hydrochlorothiazide in essential hypertension; blood pressure response and plasma renin activity. Arch. Intern. Med. 130, 855–858.
2. Ames, R. P., Barkowski, A. J., Sicinski, A. M., and Laragh, J. H. (1965) Prolonged infusions of angiotensin II and norepinephrine on blood pressure, electrolyte balance, and aldosterone and cortisol secretion in normal man and in cirrhosis with ascites. J. Clin. Invest. 44, 1171–1186.
3. Assali, N. S., Holm, L. W., and Segal, N. (1962) Regional blood flow and vascular resistance of the fetus in uterine action of vasoactive drugs. Am. J. Obstet. Gynecol. 83, 809–817.
4. Atchison, J., Brown, J. J., Ferriss, J. B., Fraser, R., Kay, A. W., Lever, A. F., Neville, A. M., Symington, T., and Robertson, J. I. S. (1971) Quadric analysis in the preoperative distinction between patients with and without adrenocortical tumors in hypertension with aldosterone excess and low plasma renin. Am. Heart J. 82, 660–671.
5. August, J. T., Nelson, D. H., and Thorn, G. W. (1958) Response of normal subjects to large amounts of aldosterone. J. Clin. Invest. 37, 1549–1555.
6. Baer, L., Sommers, S. C., Krakoff, L. R., Newton, M. A., and Laragh, J. H. (1970) Pseudo-primary aldosteronism: An entity distinct from true primary aldosteronism. Circ. Res. 24, 203–220.
7. Bartter, F. C., Ponove, P., Gill, J. R., and MacCardle, R. C. (1962) Hyperplasia of the juxtaglomerular complex with hyperaldosteronism and hypokalemic alkalosis. Am. J. Med. 33, 811–828.

8. Bartter, F. C., Henkin, I., and Bryan, G. (1968) Aldosterone hypersecretion in the "non-salt-losing" congenital adrenal hyperplasia. J. Clin. Invest. 47, 1742–1752.
9. Baulieu, E. E., de Vigan, M., Bricaire, H., and Hayle, M. D. (1957) Lack of plasma cortisol and urinary aldosterone in a pregnant woman with Addison's disease. J. Clin. Endocrinol. 17, 1478–1482.
10. Baxter, J. D., Schambelan, M., Matulich, D. T., Spindler, B. J., Taylor, A. A., and Bartter, F. C. (1976) Aldosterone receptors and the evaluation of plasma mineralocorticoid activity in normal and hypertensive states. J. Clin. Invest. 58, 579–589.
11. Bayard, F., Beitins, I. Z., Kowarski, A., and Migeon, C. J. (1970) Measurement of plasma aldosterone by radioimmunoassay. J. Clin. Endocrinol. Metab. 31, 1–6.
12. Becker Hoff, R., Vetter, W., Armbruster, H., Luetscher, J. A., and Siegenthaler, W. (1973) Plasma aldosterone during oral-contraceptive therapy. Lancet i, 1218–1219.
13. Bierich, J. R., and Schmidt, U. (1976) Tubular, Na, K-ATPase deficiency, the cause of the congenital renal salt-losing syndrome. Eur. J. Pediatr. 121, 81–87.
14. Biglieri, E. G., and Slaton, P. E., Jr. (1964) Aldosterone in clinical medicine. Calif. Med. 101, 191–195.
15. Biglieri, E. G., Herron, M. A., and Burst, N. (1966) 17α-Hydroxylation deficiency in man. J. Clin. Invest. 45, 1946–1954.
16. Biglieri, E. G., Slaton, P. E., Schambelan, M., and Kronfield, S. J. (1968) Hypermineralocorticoidism. Am. J. Med. 45, 170–175.
17. Biglieri, E. G., Schambelan, M., Slaton, P. E., and Stockigt, J. R. (1970) The intercurrent hypertension of primary aldosteronism. Circ. Res. 27 (Supp. I), 195–202.
18. Biglieri, E. G., Schambelan, M., Brust, N., Chang, B., and Hogan, M. (1974) Plasma aldosterone concentration: Further characterization of aldosterone-producing adenomas. Circ. Res. 34,35 (Supp. I), 183–191.
19. Biglieri, E. G., Stockigt, J. R., and Schambelan, M. (1974) Adrenal mineralocorticoid hormones causing hypertension. In: J. H. Laragh, (ed.), Hypertension Manual. Dun-Donnelley, New York, pp. 461–483.
20. Biglieri, E. G., and Schambelan, M. (1979) The significance of elevated levels of plasma 18-hydroxycorticosterone in patients with primary aldosteronism. J. Clin. Endocrinol. Metab. 49, 87–91.
21. Bongiovanni, A. M. (1972) Disorders of adrenocortical steroid biosynthesis. In: J. B. Stanbury, J. B. Wyngaarden, and D. S. Frederickson, (eds.), The Metabolic Basis of Inherited Disease. McGraw-Hill, New York, pp. 857–885.
22. Boonshaft, B., O'Connell, J. M. B., Hayes, J. M., and Schriener, G. E. (1968) Serum renin activity during normal pregnancy. Effect of alterations of posture and sodium intake. J. Clin. Endocrinol. Metab. 28, 1641–1644.
23. Bornstein, P., Nolan, V., and Bernanke, D. (1961) Adrenocortical hyperfunction in association with anaplastic carcinoma of the respiratory tract. N. Engl. J. Med. 264, 363–370.
24. Bravo, E. L., Dustan, H. P., and Tarzai, R. C. (1975) Selective hypoaldosteronism despite prolonged pre- and postoperative hyperreninemia in primary aldosteronism. J. Clin. Endocrinol. Metab. 41, 611–617.
25. Brode, E., Grant, J. K., and Symington, T. (1962) A biochemical and pathological investigation of adrenal tissues from patients with Conn's syndrome. Acta Endocrinol. (Copenh) 41, 411–431.
26. Brown, J. J., Davies, D. L., Doak, P. B., Lever, A. F., and Robertson, J. I. S. (1963) Plasma renin in normal pregnancy. Lancet ii, 900–901.
27. Brown, J. J., Davies, D. L., Lever, A. F., and Robertson, J. I. S. (1964) Variations in plasma renin concentration in several physiological and pathological states. Can. Med. Assoc. J. 90, 201–206.
28. Brown, J. J., Davies, D. L., Lever, A. F., and Robertson, J. I. (1964) Variations in plasma renin during the menstrual cycle. Brit. Med. J. 2, 1114–1115.

29. Brown, J. J., Davies, D. L., Lever, A. F., Peart, W. S., and Robertson, J. I. S. (1965) Plasma concentration of renin in a patient with Conn's syndrome with fibrinoid lesions of the renal arterioles: The effect of treatment with spironolactone. J. Endocrinol. 33, 279–293.
30. Brown, J. J., Davies, D. L., Doak, P. B., Lever, A. F., and Robertson, J. I. S. (1966) Plasma renin concentration in the hypertensive diseases of pregnancy. J. Obstet. Gynaecol. 73, 410–417.
31. Brown, J. J., Lever, A. F., and Robertson, J. I. S. (1967) Plasma renin concentration in human hypertension. Am. Heart J. 74, 413–418.
32. Brown, J. J., Chinn, R. H., Ferriss, J. B., Fraser, R., Robertson, J. I. S., and Lever, A. F. (1970) Hypertension with hyperaldosteronism and low plasma renin concentration: The effect of prolonged treatment with spironolactone. J. Med. 39, 631–633.
33. Brown, J. J., Fraser, R., Lever, A. F., and Robertson, J. I. S. (1971) Hypertension: A review of selected topics. Abst. World Med. 45, 549–559.
34. Brown, J. J., Fraser, R., Lever, A. F., and Robertson, J. I. S. (1972) Hypertension with aldosterone excess. Br. Med. J. 2, 391–396.
35. Brown, J. J., Fraser, R., Love, D. R., Ferris, J. B., Lever, A. F., Robertson, J. I. S., and Wilson, A. (1972) Apparently isolated excess deoxycorticosterone in hypertension. Lancet ii, 243–247.
36. Brown, R. D. (1976) Aldosterone metabolic clearances is normal in low-renin essential hypertension. J. Clin. Endocrinol. Metab. 42, 661–666.
37. Cain, M. D., Walters, W. A., and Catt, K. J. (1971) Effects of oral contraceptive therapy on the renin–angiotensin system. J. Clin. Endocrinol. 33, 671–676.
38. Camargo, C. A., Dowdy, A. J., Hancock, E. W., and Luetscher, J. A. (1965) Decreased plasma clearance and hepatic extraction of aldosterone in patients with heart failure. J. Clin. Invest. 44, 356–365.
39. Cannon, P. J., Ames, R. P., and Laragh, J. H. (1966) Relation between potassium balance and aldosterone secretion in normal subjects and in patients with hypertensive or renal tubular disease. J. Clin. Invest. 45, 865–879.
40. Cannon, P. J., Lemming, J. M., Sommers, S. C., Winters, R. W., and Laragh, J. H. (1968) Juxtaglomerular cell hyperplasia and secondary hyperaldosteronism (Bartter's syndrome): A reevaluation of the pathophysiology. Medicine 47, 107–131.
41. Channick, B. J., Adlin, E. V., and Marks, A. D. (1969) Suppressed plasma renin activity in hypertension. Arch. Intern. Med. 123, 131–140.
42. Cheek, D. B., and Perry, J. W. (1958) A salt-wasting syndrome in infancy. Arch. Dis. Child. 33, 252–256.
43. Christlieb, A. R. (1974) Renin, angiotensin, and norepinephrine in alloxan diabetes. Diabetes 23, 962–970.
44. Christlieb, A. R., Kaldany, A., and D'Elia, J. A. (1976) Plasma renin activity and hypertension in diabetes mellitus. Diabetes 25, 969–974.
44a. Colby, H. D., Skelton, F. R., and Brownie, A. C. (1970) Testosterone-induced hypertension in the rat. Endocrinology 86, 1093–1101.
45. Colby, H. D., Skelton, F. R., and Brownie, A. C. (1973) Metyrapone-induced hypertension in the rat. Endocrinology 86, 620–628.
45a. Collins, R. D., Weinberger, M. H., Dowdy, A. J., Nokes, G. W. et al. (1970) Abnormally sustained aldosterone secretion during salt loading in patients with various forms of benign hypertension: Relation to plasma renin activity. J. Clin. Invest. 49, 1415–1426.
46. Conn, J. W. (1955) Primary aldosteronism, a new clinical syndrome. J. Lab. Clin. Med. 45, 3–17.
47. Conn, J. W., Cohen, E. L., and Rovner, D. R. (1964) Suppression of plasma renin activity in primary aldosteronism. Importance in distinguishing primary from secondary aldosteronism in hypertensive disease. J.A.M.A. 190, 213–221.

48. Conn, J. W., Knopf, R. F., and Nesbit, R. M. (1964) Primary aldosteronism: Present evaluation of its clinical characteristics and of the results of surgery. In: E. E. Balieu, and P. Robel (eds.), Aldosterone—A Symposium. Oxford, Blackwell Scientific Publication, pp. 327–352.

49. Conn, J. W., (1965) Hypertension, potassium ion and impaired carbohydrate tolerance. N. Engl. J. Med. 273, 1135–1143.

49a. Conn, J. W., Cohen, E. L., and Rovner, D. R. (1965) Normokalemic primary aldosteronism. A detectable cause of essential hypertension. J.A.M.A. 193, 300–306.

50. Conn, J. W., Rovner, D. R., Cohen, E. L., and Anderson, J. R., Jr. (1966) Inhibition by heparinoid of aldosterone biosynthesis in man. J. Clin. Endocrinol. 26, 527–532.

51. Conn, J. W. (1967) The evolution of primary aldosteronism: 1954–1967. Harvey Lecture, pp. 257–291.

52. Conn, J. W. (1967) Diagnosis of normokalemic primary aldosteronism, a new form of primary aldosteronism. Science 158, 525–526.

53. Conn, J. W., Rovner, D. R., and Cohen, E. L. (1968) Licorice-induced pseudoaldosteronism. JAMA 205, 492–496.

54. Conn., J. W., and Hinerman, D. L. (1977) Spironolactone-induced inhibition of aldosterone biosynthesis in primary aldosteronism: Morphological and functional studies. Metabolism 26, 1293–1307.

54a. Coppage, W. S., Island, D. P., Cooner, A. E., and Liddle, G. W. (1962) The metabolism of aldosterone in normal subjects and in patients with hepatic cirrhosis. J. Clin. Invest. 41, 1672–1680.

55. Cox, J. R., Davies-Jones, A. B., and Leonard, P. J. (1964) Sodium content and urinary aldosterone excretion in patients with congestive heart failure before and after treatment and comparison with normal subjects undergoing salt restriction. Clin. Sci. 26, 177–184.

56. Crane, M., and Harris, J. J. (1966) Deoxycorticosterone secretion rates in hyperadrenocorticism. J. Clin. Endocrinol. Metab. 26, 1135–1143.

57. Crane, M. G., and Harris, J. J. (1969) Plasma renin activity and aldosterone excretion rate in normal subjects. I. Effect of ethinyl estradiol and medroxyprogesterone acetate. J. Clin. Endocrinol. 29, 550–557.

58. Crane, M. G., and Harris, J. J. (1970) Effect of spironolactone in hypertensive patients. Am. J. Med. Sci. 260, 311–330.

59. Davis, J. O. (1963) The role of the adrenal cortex and the kidney in the pathogenesis of cardiac edema. Yale J. Biol. Med. 35, 402–428.

60. Davis, J. O. (1964) Two important frontiers in renal physiology. Circulation 30, 1–6.

61. Davis, W. W., Newsome, H. H., Wright, L. D., Hammond, W. G., Easton, J., and Bartter, F. C. (1967) Bilateral adrenal hyperplasia as a cause of primary aldosteronism with hypertension, hypokalemia and suppressed renal activity. Am. J. Med. 42, 642–647.

62. DeChamplain, J., and Van Ameringen, M. R. (1972) Regulation of blood pressure by sympathetic nerve fibers and adrenal medulla in normotensive and hypertensive rats. Circ. Res. 31, 617–628.

63. DeFronzo, R. A. (1977) Non-uremic diabetic hyperkalemia. Arch. Intern. Med. 137, 842–843.

64. DeFronzo, R. A., Goldberg, M., Cooke, C. R., Barker, C., Grossman, R. A., and Augus, Z. S. (1977) Investigations into the mechanisms of hyperkalemia following renal transplantation. Kidney Int. 11, 357–365.

65. Drucker, W. D., Hendrikx, A., Laragh, J. H., Christy, N. P., and Vander Wiele, R. L. (1963) Effect of administered aldosterone upon electrolyte excretion during and after pregnancy in two women with adrenal cortical insufficiency. J. Clin. Endocrinol. 23, 1247–1255.

66. Eberlein, W. R., and Bongiovanni, A. M. (1955) Congenital adrenal hyperplasia with

hypertension: Unusual steroid pattern in blood and urine. J. Clin. Endocrinol. Metab. 15, 1531–1534.

67. Ehrlich, E. N. (1971) Heparinoid-induced inhibition of aldosterone secretion in pregnant women. Am. J. Obstet. Gynecol. 109, 963–970.
68. Ehrlich, E. N., and Lindheimer, M. D. (1972) Effect of administered mineralocorticoids or ACTH in pregnant women. J. Clin. Invest. 51, 1301–1309.
69. Epstein, M., Levinson, R., Sancho, J., Haber, E., and Re, R. (1977) Characterization of the renin–aldosterone system in decompensated cirrhosis. Circ. Res. 41, 818–829.
70. Ferriss, J. B., Brown, J. J., Fraser, R., Haywood, E., Davies, D. L., Kay, A. W., Lever, A. F., Robertson, J. I. S., Owen, K., and Peart, W. S. (1975) Results of adrenal surgery in patients with hypertension, aldosterone excess, and low plasma renin concentration. Brit. Med. J. 1, 135–138.
71. Ferriss, T. F., Stein, J. H., and Kauffman, J. (1972) Uterine blood flow and uterine renin secretion. J. Clin. Invest. 51, 2827–2833.
72. Fichman, M. P., Telfer, N., Zia, P., Speckart, P., Golub, M., and Rude, R. (1976) Role of prostaglandins in the pathogenesis of Bartter's Syndrome. Am. J. Med. 60, 785–797.
73. Filipecki, S., Feltynowski, T., Poplawska, W., Lapinska, K., Krus, S., Wocial, B., and Januszewicz, W. (1972) Carcinoma of the adrenal cortex with hyperaldosteronism. J. Clin. Endocrinol. Metab. 35, 225–229.
74. Fishman, L. M., Kuchel, O., Liddle, G. W., Michelakis, A. M., Gordon, R. D., and Chick, W. T. (1968) Incidence of primary aldosteronism in uncomplicated "essential" hypertension. J.A.M.A. 295, 497–502.
75. Franklin, G. O., Dowd, A. J., Caldwell, B. V., and Speroff, L. (1974) The effect of angiotensin II on plasma renin activity and prostaglandins A, E and F levels in the uterine vein of the pregnant monkey. Prostaglandins 6, 271–280.
76. Gabrilove, J. L., Sharma, D. C., and Dorfman, R. I. (1965) Adrenocortical 11β-hydroxylase deficiency and virilism first manifest in adult women. N. Engl. J. Med. 272, 1189–1194.
77. Ganguly, A., Chavarri, M., Luetscher, J. A., and Dowdy, A. J. (1977) Transient fall and subsequent return of high aldosterone secretion by adrenal adenoma during continued dexamethasone administration. J. Clin. Endocrinol. Metab. 44, 775–779.
78. Ganong, W. F., Biglieri, E. G., and Mulrow, P. J. (1966) Mechanisms regulating adrenoocortical secretion of aldosterone and glucocorticoids. Rec. Prog. Horm. Res. 22, 381–430.
79. Gant, N. F., Hutchinson, H. T., Siiteri, P. K., and MacDonald, P. C. (1971) Study of the metabolic clearance rate of dehydroisoandrosterone sulfate in pregnancy. Am. J. Obstet. Gynecol. 111, 555–563.
80. Gant, N. F., Daley, G. L., Chand, S., Whalley, P. J., and MacDonald, P. C. (1973) A study of angiotensin II presor response throughout primigravid pregnancy. J. Clin. Invest. 52, 2682–2689.
81. Gant, N. F., Chand, S., Worley, R. J., Whalley, P. T., Crosby, V. D., and MacDonald, P. C. (1974) A clinical test useful for predicting the development of acute hypertension in pregnancy. Am. J. Obstet. Gynecol. 120, 1-7.
82. Gant, N., Chand, S., Cunningham, S. G., and MacDonald, P. C. (1976) Control of vascular reactivity to angiotensin II in human pregnancy. In: M. D. Lindheimer, A. I. Katz, and F. P. Zuspan, (eds.), Hypertension in Pregnancy. Wiley Medical, New York, pp. 377–389.
83. Gardner, J. D., Simopoulos, A. P., Lapey, A., and Shibolet, S. (1972) Altered membrane sodium transport in Bartter's Syndrome. J. Clin. Invest. 51, 1565–1571.
84. George, J. M., Wright, L., Bell, N. H., Bartter, F. C., and Brown, R. (1970) The syndrome of primary aldosteronism. Am. J. Med. 48, 343–356.
85. Gill, J. R., Mason, D. T., and Bartter, F. C. (1964) "Idiopathic" edema resulting from occult cardiomyopathy. Am. J. Med. 38, 475–480.

86. Gill, J. R., Jr., Cox, J., Delea, C. S., and Bartter, F. C. (1972) Idiopathic edema. II. Am. J. Med. 52, 452–456.

87. Gill, J. R., Jr., Waldmann, T. A., and Bartter, F. C. (1972) Idiopathic edema. I. Am. J. Med. 52, 444–451.

88. Gill, J. R., Frolich, J. C., Bowden, R. E., Taylor, A. A., Keiser, H. R., Seyberth, H. W., Oates, J. A., and Bartter, F. C. (1976) Bartter's syndrome: A disorder characterized by high urinary prostaglandins and a dependence of hyperreninemia on prostaglandin synthesis. Am. J. Med. 61, 43–61.

89. Gill, J. R., Bartter, F. C., Taylor, A. A., and Radfar, N. (1977) Impaired tubular chloride reabsorption as a proximal cause of Bartter's syndrome. Clin. Res. 25, 526A.

90. Godard, C., Riondel, A. M., Veyrat, R., Megevand, A., and Muller, A. F. (1968) Plasma renin activity and aldosterone secretion in congenital adrenal hyperplasia. Pediatrics 41, 883–986.

91. Goldsmith, O., Solomon, D. H., and Horton, R. (1967) Hypogonadism and mineralocorticoid excess. N. Engl. J. Med. 277, 673–677.

92. Gonick, H. C., Kleeman, C. R., Rubine, M. E., and Maxwell, M. M. (1971) Functional impairment in chronic renal disease. III. Studies of potassium excretion. Am. J. Med. Sci. 261, 281–290.

93. Goodman, A. D., Vagnucci, A. H., and Hartroft, P. M. (1969) Pathogenesis of Bartter's Syndrome. N. Engl. J. Med. 281, 1435–1439.

94. Gray, M. J. (1967) Aldosterone secretion in women. Bull. Sloane Hosp. Women XIII, 100–105.

95. Gray, M. J., Strausfeld, K. S., Watanabe, M., Sims, E. A. H., and Solomon, S. (1968) Aldosterone secretory rates in the normal menstrual cycle. J. Clin. Endocrinol. 28, 1269–1275.

96. Greenough, W. B., Sonnenblick, E. H., Januszewicz, V., and Laragh, J. H. (1962) Correction of hyperaldosteronism and of massive fluid retention of unknown cause by sympathomimetic agents. Am. J. Med. 33, 603–614.

97. Grim, C. E. (1975) Low renin "essential" hypertension. A variant of classic primary aldosteronism? Arch. Intern. Med. 135, 347–350.

98. Grim, C. E., Weinberger, M. H., and Higgins, J. T. (1976) A rapid way to diagnose primary aldosteronism. Endocrine Soc., 58th Ann. Meeting (abst.) 565, 339.

99. Grim, C. E., Weinberger, M. H., Higgins, J. T., and Kramer, N. J. (1977) Diagnosis of secondary forms of hypertension. J.A.M.A. 237, 1311–1335.

100. Gunnells, J. C., McGuffin, W. L., Robinson, R. R., Grim, C. E., Wells, S., Silver, D., and Glenn, J. F. (1970) Hypertension, adrenal abnormalities and alterations in plasma renin activity. Ann. Intern. Med. 73, 901–911.

101. Gwinup, G., and Steinberg, T. (1967) Differential response to thiazides and spironolactone in primary aldosteronism. Arch. Intern. Med. 120, 436–443.

102. Hahn, J. A., Zipser, R. D., Stone, R. A., Zia, P. K., Horton, R. (1979) Vasoactive systems in hyporeninemic hypoaldosteronism (HH): Deficiency of kallikrein. Clin. Res. 27, 313A.

103. Helmer, O. M., and Griffith, R. S. (1952) The effect of the administration of estrogens on the renin-substrate (hypertensinogen) content of rat plasma. Endocrinology 51, 421–426.

104. Helmer, O. M., and Judson, W. E. (1967) Influence of high renin substrate levels on renin-angiotensin system in pregnancy. Am. J. Obstet. Gynecol. 99, 9–17.

105. Hickie, J. B., and Lazarus, L. (1966) Aldosterone metabolism in cardiac failure. Aust. Ann. Med. 15, 289–300.

106. Hogan, M. J., McRae, J., Schambelan, M., and Biglieri, E. G. (1976) Location of aldosterone-producing adenomas with ^{131}I-19-Iodocholesterol. N. Engl. J. Med. 294, 410–414.

107. Horton, R., and Finck, E. (1972) Diagnosis and localization in primary aldosteronism. Ann. Intern. Med. 76, 885–890.

108. Hudson, J. B., Chobanian, A. V., and Relman, A. S. (1957) Hypoaldosteronism. A clinical study of a patient with an isolated adrenal mineralocorticoid deficiency, resulting in hyperkalemia and Stokes-Adams attacks. N. Engl. J. Med. 257, 529–536.

109. Iwai, J., Dahl, L. K., and Knudsen, K. D. (1973) Genetic influence on the renin–angiotensin system. Circ. Res. 32, 678–684.

110. Jones, K. M., Lloyd-Jones, R., Riondel, A., Tait, J. F., Tait, S. A. S., Bulrock, R. D., and Greenwood, F. C. (1959) Aldosterone secretion and metabolism in normal men and women in pregnancy. Acta Endocrinol. (Copenh) 30, 321–342.

111. Jose, A., and Kaplan, N. M. (1969a) Plasma renin activity in the diagnosis of primary aldosteronism. Arch. Intern. Med. 123, 141–146.

112. Jose, A., Crout, J. R., and Kaplan, N. M. (1970) Suppressed plasma renin activity in essential hypertension. Ann. Intern. Med. 72, 9–15.

113. Kaplan, N. M. (1963) Primary aldosteronism with malignant hypertension. N. Engl. J. Med. 269, 1282–1286.

114. Kaplan, N. M. (1967) The steroid content of adrenal adenomas and measurements of aldosterone production in patients with essential hypertension and primary aldosteronism. J. Clin. Invest. 46, 728–734.

115. Katz, F. H., Eckert, R. C., and Geboth, M. D. (1972) Hypokalemia caused by surreptitious self-administration of diuretics. Ann. Intern. Med. 76, 85–90.

116. Kokko, J. P., Brown, T. C., and Berman, M. M. (1976) Adrenal adenoma and hypertension. Lancet i, 468–470.

117. Kotchen, T. A., Lytton, B., Morrow, L. B., Mulrow, P. J., Shutkin, P. M., and Stansel, H. C. (1970) Angiotensin and aldosterone in renovascular hypertension. Arch. Intern. Med. 125, 265–272.

118. Kotchen, T. A., Mulrow, P. J., Morrow, L. B., Shutkin, P. M., and Marieb, N. (1971) Renin and aldosterone in essential hypertension. Clin. Sci. 41, 321–331.

119. Kowarski, A., Finklestein, J. W., Spaulding, J. S., Hozman, G. H., and Migeon, C. J. (1965) Aldosterone secretion rate in congenital adrenal hyperplasia. J. Clin. Invest. 44, 1505–1513.

120. Krakoff, L. R., Goodwin, F. J., Baer, L., Torres, M., and Laragh, J. N. (1970) The role of renin in the exaggerated natriuresis of hypertension. Circulation 42, 335–345.

121. Kuchel, O., Horky, K., Gregorova, I., Marek, J., Kopecka, J., and Kobilkova, J. (1970) Inappropriate response to upright posture. A precipitating factor in the pathogenesis of idiopathic edema. Ann. Intern. Med. 73, 245–252.

122. Kuchel, O., Hamet, P., Coche, J. L, Tolis, G., Fraysse, J., and Genest, J. (1975) Urinary and plasma cyclic AMP in patients with idiopathic edema. J. Clin. Endocrinol. Metab. 41, 282–289.

123. Kuchel, O., Cuche, J. L., Buu, N. T., Guthrie, Jr., G. P., Unger, T., Nowoczynski, W., Boucher, R., and Genest, J. (1977) Catecholamine excretion in "idiopathic" edema: Decreased dopamine excretion, a pathogenic factor? J. Clin. Endocrinol. Metab. 44, 639–646.

124. Kutyrina, I. M., Androsova, S. O., Tareyeva, I. E. (1979) Indomethacin-induced hyporeninaemic hypoaldosteronism. Lancet i, 785.

125. Laidlaw, J. C., Cohen, M., and Gornall, A. G. (1958) Studies on the origin of aldosterone during human pregnancy. J. Clin. Endocrinol. 18, 222–225.

126. Laidlaw, J. C., Yendt, E. R., and Gornall, A. G. (1960) Hypertension caused by renal artery occlusion simulating primary aldosteronism. Metabolism 9, 612–623.

127. Lambrew, C. T., Carver, S. T., Peterson, R. E., and Horwith, M. (1961) Hypoaldosteronism as a cause of hyperkalemia and syncopal attacks in a patient with complete heart block. Am. J. Med. 31, 81–86.

128. Landau, R. L., and Lugibihl, K. (1958) Inhibition of the sodium-retaining influence of aldosterone by progesterone. J. Clin. Endocrinol. 18, 1237–1245.

129. Laragh, J. H. (1962) Hormones and the pathogenesis of congestive heart failure: Vasopressin, aldosterone, and angiotensin II. Further evidence for renal-adrenal interaction from studies in hypertension and in cirrhosis. Circulation 25, 1015–1023.

130. Laragh, J. H., Cannon, P. J., and Ames, R. P. (1964) Interaction between aldosterone secretion, sodium and potassium balance, and angiotensin activity in man. Studies in hypertension and cirrhosis. Can. Med. Assoc. J. 90, 248–256.

131. Laragh, J. H., Sealey, J. E., and Sommers, S. C. (1966) Patterns of adrenal secretion and urinary excretion of aldosterone and plasma renin activity in normal and hypertensive subjects. Circ. Res. (Supp. I) 18, 158–174.

132. Laragh, J. H., Sealey, J. E., Ledingham, J. G. G., and Newton, M. A. (1967) Oral contraceptives. J.A.M.A. 201, 918–922.

133. Laragh, J. H., Ulick, S., Januszewicz, V., Deming, Q. B., and Kelly, W. G. (1969) Aldosterone secretion in primary and malignant hypertension. J. Clin. Invest. 39, 1091–1106.

134. Laragh, J. (1976) Oral contraceptive-induced hypertension–nine years later. Am. J. Obstet. Gynecol. 126, 141–157.

135. Lauler, D. P., Hickler, R. B., and Thorn, G. W. (1962) The salivary sodium-potassium ratio. N. Engl. J. Med. 267, 1136–1137.

136. Lauler, D. P. (1966) Preoperative diagnosis of primary aldosteronism. Am. J. Med. 41, 855–863.

137. Leaf, A. Z., and Camara, A. (1949) Renal tubular secretion of potassium in man. J. Clin. Invest. 28, 1526–1533.

138. LeBel, M., Schalekamp, M. A., Beevers, D. G., Brown, J. J., Davies, D. L., Fraser, R., Kremer, D., Lever, A. F., Morton, J. J., Robertson, J. I. S., Tree, M., and Wilson, A. (1974) Sodium and the renin-angiotensin system in essential hypertension and mineralocorticoid excess. Lancet ii, 308–310.

139. LeBel, M., and Grose, J. H. (1976) Selective hypoaldosteronism: A study of steroid biosynthetic pathways under adrenocorticotrophin and angiotensin II infusion. Clin. Sci. Mol. Med. 51, 335s–337s.

140. Liddle, G. W., Hollifield, J. W., Slaton, P. E., and Wilson, H. M. (1976) Effects of various adrenal inhibitors in low-renin essential hypertension. J. Ster. Biochem. 7, 937–940.

141. Lieberman, A. H., and Luetscher, J. A., Jr. (1960) Some effects of abnormalities of pituitary, adrenal or thyroid function on excretion of aldosterone and the response to corticotropin or sodium deprivation. J. Clin. Endocrinol. 20, 1004–1016.

142. Lommer, D., Distler, A., Phillipp, T., and Wolff, H. P. (1972) Secretion distribution and turnover of aldosterone in essential hypertension, primary aldosteronism, and hypertension associated with renal artery stenosis. In: J. Genest, E. Koiw, (eds.), Hypertension '72, Springer-Verlag, New York, pp. 255–262.

143. Loras, B., Haour, F., and Bertrand, J. (1970) Exchangeable sodium and aldosterone secretion in children with congenital adrenal hyperplasia due to 21-hydroxylase deficiency. Pediatr. Res. 4, 145–156.

144. Luetscher, J. A., and Johnson, B. B. (1954) Observations on the sodium-retaining corticoid (aldosterone) in the urine of children and adults in relation to sodium balance and edema. J. Clin. Invest. 33, 1441–1446.

145. Luetscher, J. A., Dowdy, A. J., Arnstein, A. R., Lucas, C. P., and Murray, C. L. (1965) Idiopathic edema and increased aldosterone secretion. In: E. E. Baulieu and P. Robel (eds.), Aldosterone—A symposium, Blackwell Scientific Publications, London, pp. 487–498.

146. Leutscher, J. A., Hancock, E. W., Camargo, C. A., Dowdy, A. J., and Nokes, G. W. (1965) Conjugation of 1,2-^{3}H-Aldosterone in human liver and kidney and renal extraction of aldosterone and labelled conjugates from blood plasma. J. Clin. Endocrinol. Metab. 25, 628–638.

147. Luetscher, J. A., Weinberger, M. H., Dowdy, A. J., Nokes, G. W., Balikian, H., Brodie, A., and Willoughby, S. (1969) Effects of sodium loading, sodium depletion and

posture on plasma aldosterone concentration and renin activity in hypertensive patients. J. Clin. Endocrinol. 29, 1310–1318.

148. Luetscher, J. A., Ganguly, A., Melada, G. A., and Dowdy, A. J. (1974) Pre-operative, differentiation of adrenal adenoma from idiopathic adrenal hyperplasia in primary aldosteronism. Circ. Res. 34,35 (Supp. I), 175–182.

149. Mantero, F., Faglia, G., Adam, W. R., Funder, J. W., and Ulick, S. (1979) A new syndrome of factitious mineralocorticoid excess (Abst.). Presented at Endocrine Society Meeting, Anaheim, Calif., June 13-15, 1979, p. 279.

150. Massami, Z. M., Finkielman, S., Worcel, M., Agrest, A., and Paladini, A. C. (1966) Angiotensin blood levels in hypertensive and non-hypertensive diseases. Clin. Sci. 30, 473–483.

151. McAllister, R. G., Jr., Van Way, C. W., Dayani, K., Anderson, W. J., Temple, E., Michelakis, A., Coppage, W. S., and Oates, J. A. (1971) Malignant hypertension: Effect of therapy on renin and aldosterone. Circ. Res. (Supp. II) 28, 160–173.

152. Melby, J. C., Spark, R. F., Dale, S. L., Egdahl, R. H., and Kahn, P. C. (1967) Diagnosis and localization of aldosterone-producing adenomas by adrenal vein catheterization. N. Engl. J. Med. 277, 1050–1056.

153. Melby, J. C., Dale, S. L., and Wilson, T. E. (1971) 18-hydroxydeoxycorticosterone in human hypertension. Circ. Res. (Supp. II) 28, 143–152.

154. Melby, J. C. (1972) Identifying the adrenal lesion in primary aldosteronism. Ann. Intern. Med. 76, 1039–1041.

155. Melby, J. C., Dale, S. L., Grekin, R. J., Gaunt, R., and Wilson, T. E. (1972) 18-hydroxy-11-deoxycorticosterone (18-OH-DOC) secretion in experimental and human hypertension. Rec. Prog. Horm. Res. 38, 287–351.

156. Menard, J., Malmejac, A., and Milliez, P. (1970) Influence of diethylstilbesterol on the renin-angiotensin system of male rats. Endocrinology 86, 774–780.

157. Menard, J., Cain, M. D., and Catt, K. J. (1971) Rapid effects of estrogen on the renin-angiotensin system. Clin. Res. 19, 377.

158. Michelakis, A. M., Foster, J. H., Liddle, G. W., Rhamy, R. K., Kuchel, O., and Gordon, R. D. (1967) Measurement of renin in both renal veins. Arch. Intern. Med. 120, 444–448.

159. Mulrow, P. J., Lytton, B., and Stansel, H. C. (1966) The role of renin–angiotensin system in the hypertension associated with renal vascular disease. International Club on Arterial Hypertension, Vol. I, Expansion Scientifique Francaise, Paris, pp. 296–304.

160. Mulrow, P. J., Ferris, T. F., Gorden, P., Anderson, R. C., and Herbert, P. N. (1969) Properties and origin of uterine renin. In: H. Salhanick, D. Kipnis, and R. Vander Wiele (eds.), Metabolic Effects of Gonadal Hormones and Contraceptive Steroids. Plenum Press, New York, pp. 464–470.

161. Mulrow, P. J. (1971) Renin-angiotensin-aldosterone and toxemia of pregnancy. In: F. Fuchs and A. Klopper (eds.), Endocrinology of Pregnancy. Harper and Row, New York, pp. 167–183.

162. Nesbit, R. M. (1967) Primary aldosteronism: Its diagnosis and surgical management. J. Urol. 97, 404–408.

163. New, M. I., and Peterson, R. E. (1967) A new form of congenital adrenal hyperplasia. J. Clin. Endocrinol. Metab. 27, 300–305.

164. Nicolis, G. L., Mitty, H. A., Modlinger, R. S., and Gabrilove, J. L. (1972) Percutaneous adrenal venography. Ann. Int. Med. 76, 899–909.

165. Norby, L. H., Weidig, J., Ramwell, P., Slotkoff, L., Flamenbaum, W. (1978) Possible role for impaired renal prostaglandin production in pathogenesis of hyporeninaemic hypoaldosteronism. Lancet ii, 1118–1121.

166. Oberfield, S. E., Levine, S. L., Carey, R. M., Bejar, R., New, M. I. (1979) Pseudohypoaldosteronism: Multiple target organ unresponsiveness to mineralocorticoid hormones. J. Clin. Endocrinol. Metab. 48, 228–234.

167. Oh, M. S., Carroll, H. J., Clemmons, J. E., Vagnucci, A. H., Levison, S. P., and Whang, S. M. (1974) A mechanism for hyporeninemic hypoaldosteronism in chronic renal disease. Metabolism 23, 1157–1166.

168. Oparil, S., and Haber, E. (1971) Renin in differential diagnosis of hypertension. Am. Heart J. 82, 568–570.

169. Perez, G., Siegel, L., and Schreiner, G. E. (1972) Selective hypoaldosteronism with hyperkalemia. Ann. Intern. Med. 76, 757–763.

170. Peterson, R. E. (1964) Determination of peripheral plasma aldosterone. In: E. E. Baulieu and P. Robel (eds.), Aldosterone—A Symposium, Blackwell Scientific Publications, Oxford, pp. 145–161.

171. Postel-Vinay, M. C., Alberti, G. M., Ricour, C. et al. (1974) Pseudohypoaldosteronism: Persistence of hyperaldosteronism and evidence for renal tubular and intestinal responsiveness to endogenous aldosterone. J. Clin. Endocrinol. Metab. 39, 1038–1044.

172. Priestly, J. T., Ferris, D. W., ReMine, W. H., and Woolner, L. B. (1968) Primary aldosteronism: Surgical management and pathological findings. Mayo Clin. Proc. 43, 761–775.

173. Prunty, F. T. G., Brooks, R. V., Dupre, J., Gimlette, T. M. D., Hutchison, J. S. M., McSwiney, R. R., and Mills, I. H. (1963) Adrenocortical hyperfunction and potassium metabolism in patients with "non-endocrine" tumors and Cushing's syndrome. J. Clin. Endocrinol. 23, 737–746.

174. Rampini, S., Furrer, J., Keller, H. P. et al. (1978) Congenital pseudohypoaldosteronism: Case report and review. Effect of indomethacin during sodium chloride depletion. Helv. Padiatr. Acta 33, 153–168.

175. Rapp, J. P. (1971) Adrenal steroidogenesis in rats bred for susceptibility and resistance to the hypertensive effect of salt. Endocrinology 88, 52-65.

176. Reich, M. (1962) The variations in urinary aldosterone levels of normal females during their menstrual cycle. Aust. Ann. Med. 11, 41-49.

177. Relman, A. S., and Schwartz, W. B. (1952) Effect of DOCA on electrolyte balance in normal man and its relation to sodium chloride intake. Yale J. Biol. Med. 24, 540–558.

178. Robertson, J. I. S., Weir, R. J., Dusterdieck, G. O., Fraser, R., and Tree, M. (1971) Renin, angiotensin and aldosterone in human pregnancy and the menstrual cycle. Scott. Med. J. 16, 183–196.

179. Robertson, P. W., Klidjian, A., Harding, L. K. et al. (1967) Hypertension due to renin secreting tumor. Am. J. Med. 43, 963–976.

180. Roginsky, M., Abesamis, C., and Asad, S. (1973) The renin–angiotensin–aldosterone system in the hypertensive diabetic. Clin. Res. 21, 501.

181. Rosoff, Jr., L., Williams, J., Moult, P., Williams, H., and Sherlock, S. (1979) Renal hemodynamics and the renin–angiotensin system in cirrhosis. Am. J. Dig. Dis. 24, 25–32.

182. Rosoff, Jr., L., Zia, P., Reynolds, T., and Horton, R. (1975) Studies of renin and aldosterone in cirrhotic patients with ascites. Gastroenterology 69, 698–705.

183. Ross, E. J., Crabbe, J., Renold, A. E., Emerson, K., and Thorn, G. W. (1958) A case of massive edema in association with an aldosterone secreting adrenocortical adenoma. Am. J. Med. 25, 278–292.

184. Ross, E. J. (1975) "Autonomous" secondary or "tertiary" aldosteronism. In: Aldosterone and Aldosteronism, Lloyd-Luke (Medical Books) Ltd., London, pp. 296–297.

185. Sanders, L. L., and Melby, J. C. (1964) Aldosterone and the edema of congestive heart failure. Arch. Intern. Med. 113, 331–341.

186. Saruta, M., Saade, C. A., and Kaplan, N. M. (1970) A possible mechanism for hypertension induced by oral contraceptives. Arch. Intern. Med. 126, 621–630.

187. Schalekamp, M. A. D. H., Krauss, X. H., Schalekamp-Kuykan, M. P. A., Kolsters, G., and Birkenhager, W. H. (1971) Studies on the mechanism of hypernatriuresis in

essential hypertension in relation to measurements of plasma renin concentration, body fluid compartments and renal function. Clin. Sci. 41, 219–231.

188. Schambelan, M., Stockigt, J. R., and Biglieri, E. G. (1972) Isolated hypoaldosteronism in adults: A renin deficiency syndrome. N. Engl. J. Med. 287, 573–578.

189. Schambelan, M., Howes, E. L., Stockigt, J. R., Noakes, C. A., and Biglieri, E. G. (1974) Role of renin and aldosterone in hypertension due to a renin-secreting tumor. Am. J. Med. 55, 86–92.

190. Schambelan, M., and Sebastian, A. (1979) Hyporeninemic hypoaldosteronism. Adv. Intern. Med. 24, 385–405.

191. Scoggins, B. A., Oddie, C. J., Hare, W. S. C., and Coghlan, J. P. (1972) Preoperative lateralization of aldosterone-producing tumours in primary aldosteronism. Ann. Intern. Med. 76, 891–897.

192. Seaton, P. E., and Biglieri, E. (1967) Reduction in aldosterone excretion in patients with autonomic insufficiency. J. Clin. Endocrinol. Metab. 27, 37–45.

193. Silen, W., Biglieri, E. G., Slaton, P., and Galante, M. (1966) Management of primary aldosteronism: evaluation of potassium and sodium balance, technic of adrenalectomy and operative results in 24 cases. Ann. Surg. 164, 600–610.

194. Sims, E. A. H., Meeker, C. I., Gray, M. M., Watanabe, M., and Solomon, S. (1964) The secretion of aldosterone in normal pregnancy and in preeclampsia. In: E. E. Baulieu and P. Robel (eds.), Aldosterone—A Symposium. Blackwell, Scientific Publications, Oxford, pp. 499–508.

195. Sims, E. A. H., MacKay, B. R., and Shirai, T. (1965) The relation of capillary angiopathy and diabetes mellitus to idiopathic edema. Ann. Int. Med. 63, 972–987.

196. Skanse, B., and Hokfelt, B. (1958) Hypoaldosteronism with otherwise intact adrenocortical function resulting in a characteristic clinical entity. Acta Endocrinol. (Copenh) 28, 29–36.

197. Skinner, S. L., Lumbers, E. R., and Symonds, E. M. (1969) Alteration by oral contraceptives of normal menstrual changes in plasma renin activity, concentration and substrate. Clin. Sci. 36, 67–76.

198. Slater, E. E., Haber, E. (1978) A large form of renin from normal human kidney. J. Clin. Endocrinol. Metab. 47, 105–109.

199. Spark, R. F., and Melby, J. C. (1968) Aldosteronism in hypertension. Ann. Intern. Med. 69, 685–691.

200. Spark, R. F., and Melby, J. C. (1971) Hypertension and low plasma renin activity: Presumptive evidence for mineralocorticoid excess. Ann. Intern. Med. 75, 831–836.

201. Speroff, L. (1970) Toxemia and the renin-angiotensin system: Progress in the sixties. Bull. Sloane Hosp. Women 16, 33–48.

202. Streeten, D. H. P., Luis, L. H., and Conn, J. W. (1960) Secondary aldosteronism in idiopathic edema. Trans. Assoc. Am. Physicians 73, 227–239.

203. Sundsfjord, J. A., and Aakvaag, A. (1970) Plasma angiotensin II and aldosterone excretion during the menstrual cycle. Acta Endocrinol. (Copenh) 64, 452–458.

204. Sundsfjord, J. A. (1971) Plasma renin activity and aldosterone excretion during prolonged progesterone administration. Acta Endocrinol. (Copenh) 67, 483–490.

205. Sundsfjord, J. A., and Aakvaag, A. (1972) Plasma renin activity, plasma renin substrate and urinary aldosterone excretion in the menstrual cycle in relation to the concentration of progesterone and estrogens in the plasma. Acta Endocrinol. (Copenh) 71, 519–529.

206. Sutherland, D. J. A., Ruse, J. L., and Laidlaw, J. C. (1966) Hypertension, increased aldosterone secretion and low plasma renin activity relieved by dexamethasone. Can. Med. Assoc. J. 95, 1109–1119.

207. Szylman, P., Better, O. S., Chaimowitz, C., and Rosler, A. (1976) Role of hyperkalemia in the metabolic acidosis of isolated hypoaldosteronism. N. Engl. J. Med. 294, 361–365.

208. Tait, J. F., Bougas, J., Little, B., Tait, S. A. S., and Flood, C. (1965) Splanchnic extraction and clearance of aldosterone in subjects with minimal and marked cardiac dysfunction. J. Clin. Endocrinol. 25, 219–228.

209. Tan, S. Y., and Mulrow, P. J. (1979) Low renin hypertension: Failure to demonstrate excess II-deoxycorticosterone production. J. Clin. Endocrinol. Metab.

210. Tan, S. Y., and Mulrow, P. J. (1975) Interference of spironolactone in 11-deoxycorticosterone radioassays. J. Clin. Endocrinol. Metab. 41, 791–792.

211. Tan, S. Y., Noth, R. H., and Mulrow, P. J. (1976) The role of DOC in human hypertension. Clin. Sci. Mol. Med. 51, 311S–314S.

212. Tan, S. Y., and Burton, M. (1977) Hyporeninemic hypoaldosteronism: An overlooked cause of hyperkalemia. Clin. Res. 25, 567A.

213. Tan, S. Y., and Mulrow, P. J. (1977) Inhibition of the renin-aldosterone response to furosemide by indomethacin. J. Clin. Endocrinol. Metab. 45, 174–176.

213a. Tan, S. Y., Noth, R. H., and Mulrow, P. J. (1978) Deoxycorticosterone and 17 ketosteroids. Elevated levels in adult hypertensives. J.A.M.A. 240, 123–126.

214. Tan, S. Y., Antonipillai, I., and Mulrow, P. J. (1979) Inactive renin and impaired prostaglandin production in hyporeninemic hypoaldosteronism. Clin. Res. 27, 452A.

215. Tan, S. Y., Shapiro, R., Franco, R., Stockard, H., and Mulrow, P. J. (1979) Indomethacin-induced prostaglandin inhibition with hyperkalemia. Ann. Intern. Med. 90, 783–785.

216. Taylor, A., Pool, J., Rosen, R., Snodgrass, W., Rollins, D., McWlurty, R., Bartter, F., and Mitchell, J. (1977) Major abnormality in low renin hypertension: Exaggerated aldosterone reponse to angiotensin. Clin. Res. 25, 446A.

217. Terragno, N. A., Terragno, D. A, Pacholczyk, D., and McGiff, J. C. (1974) Prostaglandins and the regulation of uterine blood flow in pregnancy. Nature 279, 57–58.

218. Todesco, S., Terribile, V., Borsatti, A., and Mantero, F. (1975) Primary aldosteronism due to a malignant ovarian tumor. J. Clin. Endocrinol. Metab. 41, 809–819.

219. Ulick, S., Gautier, E., Vetter, K. K., Markello, J. R., Yaffe, S., and Low, C. U. (1965) An aldosterone biosynthetic defect in a salt-losing disorder. J. Clin. Endocrinol. 14, 669–672.

220. Underwood, R. H., and Williams, G. H. (1972) Simultaneous measurement of aldosterone, cortisol and corticosterone in peripheral plasma by displacement analysis technique. J. Lab. Clin. Med. 79, 848–862.

221. Vagnucci, A. H. (1969) Selective aldosterone deficiency. J. Clin. Endocrinol. Metab. 29, 279–289.

222. Venuto, R., O'Dorisio, T., Stein, J. H., and Ferris, T. F. (1975) Uterine prostaglandin E secretion and uterine blood flow in the pregnant rabbit. J. Clin. Invest. 55, 193–197.

223. Veyrat, R., deChamplain, J., Boucher, R., and Genest, J. (1964) Measurement of human arterial renin activity in some physiological and pathological states. Can. Med. Assoc. J. 90, 215–220.

224. Vinci, J. M., Gill, J. R., Jr., Bowden, R. E., Pisano, J. J., Izzo, J. L., Radfar, N., Taylor, A. A., Zusman, R. M., Bartter, F. C., and Keiser, H. R. (1978) The kallikrein-kinin system in Bartter's syndrome and its response to prostaglandin synthetase inhibition. J. Clin. Invest. 61, 1671–1682.

225. Visser, H. K. and Cost, W. S. (1964) A new hereditary defect in the biosynthesis of aldosterone-urinary C_{21} corticosteroid pattern in three related patients with a salt-losing syndrome suggesting an 18-oxidation defect. Acta Endocrinol. (Copenh) 47, 589–612.

226. Wallace, M., Richards, P., Chesser, E., and Wrong, O. (1968) Persistent alkalosis and hypokalaemia caused by surreptitious vomiting. Q. J. Med. 37, 577–588.

227. Weinberger, M. H., Grim, C. E., Hollifield, J. W., Kem, D. C., Ganguly, A., Kramer, N. J., Yune, H. Y., and Wellman, H. (1979) Primary aldosteronism. Diagnosis, localization and treatment. Ann. Intern. Med. 90, 386–395.

228. Weinberger, M. H., Collins, R., Dowdy, A. J., Nokes, G. W., and Leutscher, J. A. (1969) Hypertension induced by oral contraceptives containing estrogen and gestagen. Ann. Intern. Med. 71, 891–902.

229. Weir, R. J., Paintin, D. B., Brown, J. J., Fraser, R., Lever, A. F., Robertson, J. I. S., and Young, J. (1971) A serial study in pregnancy of the plasma concentrations of renin, corticosteroids, electrolytes and proteins and of hematocrit and plasma volume. J. Obstet. Gynaecol. Br. Commonwlth. 78, 590–602.

230. Williams, G. H., Rose, L. I., Dluhy, R. G., Dingman, J. F., and Lauler, D. P. (1971) Aldosterone response to sodium restriction and ACTH stimulation in panhypopituitarism. J. Clin. Endocrinol. Metab. 32, 27–35.

231. Williams, G. H., Cain, J. P., Dluhy, R. G., and Underwood, R. H. (1972) Studies of the control of plasma aldosterone concentration in normal man. J. Clin. Invest. 51, 1731–1742.

232. Winer, B. M., Lubbe, W. F., Simon, M., and William, J. A. (1967) Renin in the diagnosis of renovascular hypertension. J.A.M.A. 202, 121–128.

233. Woods, J. W., Liddle, G. W., Stant, E. G., Jr., Michelakis, A. M., and Brill, A. B. (1969) Effect of an adrenal inhibitor in hypertensive patients with suppressed renin. Arch. Intern. Med. 123, 366–370.

234. Wrong, O. (1964) Hyperaldosteronism secondary to renal ischemia. In: E. E. Baulieu and P. Robel (eds.), Aldosterone—A Symposium. Blackwell Scientific Publications, Oxford, pp. 377–392.

235. Zipser, R. D., Hoefs, J. C., Speckart, P. F., Zia, P. K., and Horton, R. (1979) Prostaglandins: Modulators of renal function and pressor resistance in chronic liver disease. J. Clin. Endocrinol. Metab. 48, 895–900.

PAUL V. DeLAMATER, M.D.

CONGENITAL ADRENAL HYPERPLASIA

HISTORY

Virilization of the external genitalia in association with congenitally hyperplastic adrenals, known previously as adrenogenital syndrome, was probably first reported by DeCrecchio (16) in 1865. This work, cited by New and Levine (61), describes a patient (post mortem) with a penis, first degree hypospadius, and normal female internal genitalia with hyperplastic adrenals.

The first clinical description of a living patient who was undoubtedly afflicted with congenital adrenal hyperplasia (CAH) was made by Wilkins et al. (95) in 1940. Since that time the syndrome has come to include seven distinct clinical forms. Studies of patients with these various forms have resulted in greater understanding of adrenal steroidogenesis and the roles of adrenal androgens, glucocorticoids, and mineralocorticoids. Investigations of these clinical forms identified enzyme deficiencies in the steroid pathways.

Studies of such deficiencies in steroidogenesis have contributed significantly to an understanding of many related issues. Discoveries by Wilkins et al. (96) and Bartter et al. (3) regarding the effectiveness of cortisone

From the Department of Pediatrics, Medical College of Ohio, Toledo, Ohio; Mercy Hospital, Toledo, Ohio.

administration in decreasing the urinary 17-ketosteroid excretion in patients with the syndrome were a foundation to the understanding of cortisol's feedback role on ACTH.

Further elucidation of the adrenal steroidogenesis pathways was provided by Prader (70) in his description of "lipoid" adrenal hyperplasia characterized by lack of virilization due to a very proximal steroidogenic block in the pathway. This lethal block was demonstrated at the desmolase step in conversion of cholesterol to Δ5 pregnenolone.

Bongiovanni and Eberline (9) made observations that defined another form of this syndrome. They described patients who were hypertensive with the adrenogenital syndrome. Later, the excess of deoxycorticosterone was shown by Bongiovanni and Root (10) to be the result of deficient 11-hydroxylation and to produce the hypertension seen in this subgroup of patients.

Other subgroups, described as new phenotypes, were studied biochemically. Bongiovanni (8), reported several cases of incompletely virilized males who, he theorized, had deficiency of 3β-hydroxysteroid dehydrogenase, resulting in a virtual absence of cortisol synthesis. Adrenal tissue enzyme analysis by Goldman et al. (29) confirmed this theory by direct measurement.

Biglieri et al. (6) described a group of sexually infantile females with hypertension, who appeared to have a block in steroid synthesis at 17-α-hydroxylation that involved adrenal and ovarian steroid synthesis. This block was later shown by New (60) to be a cause of incomplete virilization in the male.

The final two biosynthetic steps in aldosterone production have been the subject of recent study. Deficiency of 18-hydroxylase (89) was clinically described in children with isolated hypoaldosteronism, salt-loss, failure to grow, bouts of dehydration, and fever. A similar phenotype (88,31) has been shown to result from deficiency of 18-dehydrogenase resulting in deficient aldosterone production.

Many contributions to our knowledge of steroid synthesis have come as a result of observations made of patients with congenital adrenal hyperplasia. As Dr. Fredric Bartter has aptly said (2), we continue to learn from this "splendid teacher."

GENETICS

All of the subgroups of congenital adrenal hyperplasia (CAH) identified to date (with the possible exception of dexamethasone suppressible hyperaldosteronism) conform to the autosomal recessive mode of inheritance. The incidence varies widely in published reports of geographic population studies. The highest incidence is 1 in 490 live births reported by Hirschfeld and Fleshman (32) among Alaskan Eskimos. In Zurich, Switzerland, Prader (68) reported 1 in 5,000 affected, while Child et al. (13), reviewing experience in the state of Maryland, reported an incidence of 1 in 67,000 births.

Of current interest is the recent discovery by Dupont et al. (20) that there appears to be close genetic linkage between 21-hydroxylase deficiency and the major histocompatibility portion of chromosome 6. Levine et al. (48) has further characterized this linkage as very close to the HLA-B locus. Genetics studies are currently underway to determine if other rarer subgroups of CAH are linked with the HLA loci. These studies would contribute to further mapping chromosome 6. HLA genotyping, in conjunction with hormonal studies, have allowed detection of the asymptomatic heterozygote carrier of CAH (52). Similar genetic studies have allowed a method for prenatal diagnosis of CAH by HLA typing of cultured amniotic cells (67). This tool has allowed the clear identification of a mild form of 21-hydroxylase deficiency in several adults and children with only minimal clitoromegaly and slight posterior labial fusion, as typical CAH. This report (15) demonstrated the typical CAH heterozygote hormonal responses in parents and sibs and close HLA-B locus linkage.

New et al. (62) and others have employed HLA genotyping to demonstrate that an adolescent female with an "acquired" 21-hydroxylase deficiency and adrenal hyperplasia had a disorder different from classical CAH. Her HLA identical sister was unaffected and her father failed to respond hormonally like an obligate heterozygote.

CLINICAL PRESENTATION AND DIAGNOSIS

Each subgroup of CAH presents distinctive biochemical and clinical findings. These are summarized in Figure 1 and Table 1.

21-Hydroxylase Deficiency, Simple Virilized

This is by far the most common inborn error of adrenal steroidogenesis responsible for CAH. There are two "subgroups" that may actually be two extremes of a clinical spectrum. The first subgroup, accounting for some 60% of CAH patients, demonstrates impaired cortisol synthesis (36). Since cortisol is the major hormone feeding back to inhibit ACTH, circulating concentrations of the trophic hormone are clearly elevated (50,87). More recently it has been appreciated that levels of cortisol may be near normal (22,57) but only at the expense of greatly increased ACTH drive, subsequent increase in cortisol precursors proximal to the 21-hydroxylation step, and marked increase in adrenal androgen production (22,53,55,57,81,85) (which do not require 21 hydroxylation). It is this elevation of adrenal androgens that, in utero, results in varying degrees of masculinization of the external genitalia of the female fetus, and postnatally results in progressive virilization of the male or female child. This disorder may not be suspected in the affected male at birth. The affected female infant, on the other hand, must be clinically detected because of ambiguity of the external genitalia present. This can be quite variable, ranging from minimal clitoromegaly and slight posterior labial fusion to complete labioscrotal fusion and "penile" urethra (91). The reasons for this spectrum of masculization are not entirely clear. It could be explained

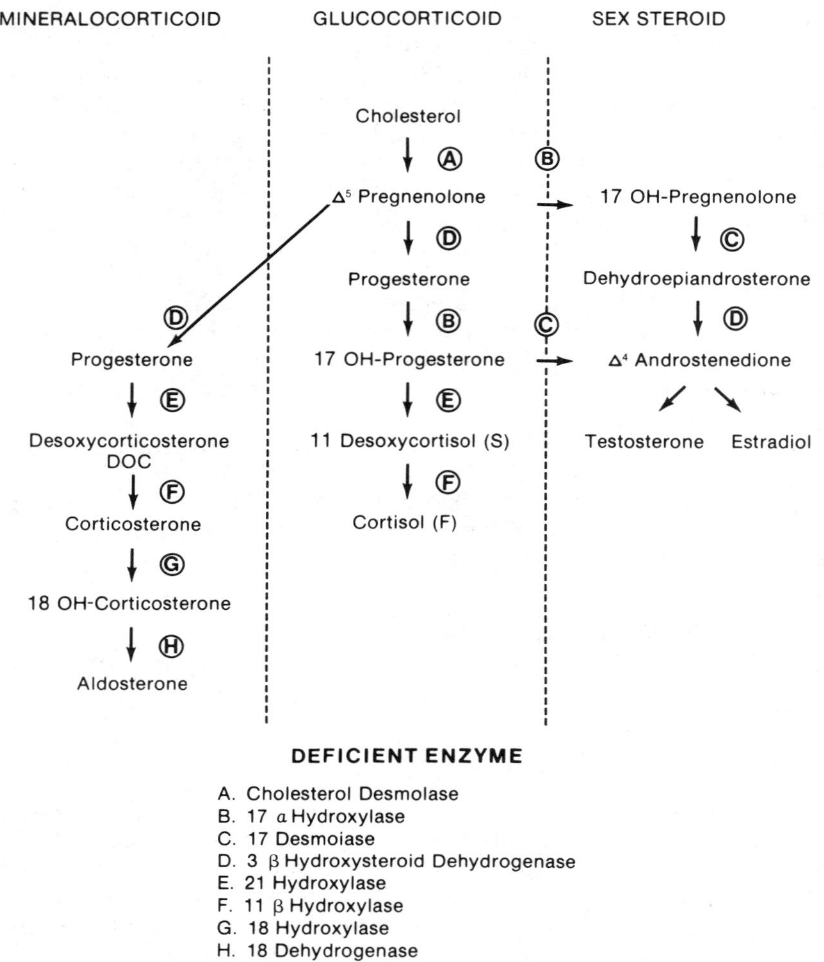

FIGURE 1. Adrenal steroidogenic pathways showing enzymatic steps involved.

by the severity of the 21-hydroxylase block and the greater increase in ACTH and adrenal androgens, and perhaps by an individual androgen-binding difference in the target organs. Other systemic effects of androgens include increasing linear growth, skeletal maturation, and hyperplasia of muscles. In untreated CAH of this type, the effects of increased adrenal androgens are appreciated clinically as: ambiguous genitalia of female infants at birth (see Figure 2); progressive virilization; rapid linear growth and increased muscle mass in childhood; and stunted ultimate height due to premature skeletal epiphyseal closure. The primary feature separating this subgroup from the one which will follow is the maintenance of salt and water homeostasis. These patients are termed "non-salt-

TABLE 1. Summary of Hormonal and Clinical Findings in CAH

Enzyme deficient	Hormone deficient	Hormone excess	Clinical manifestations
Desmolase	Glucocorticoids Mineralocorticoids Sex steroids	Cholesterol	Lipoid adrenal Hyperplasia Adrenal insufficiency
17-α-Hydroxylase	Sex steroids Cortisol Aldosterone	Corticosterone DOC	Hypokalemic alkalosis Sexual infantilism in female Ambiguous genitalia in male Hypertension
3-β Hydroxysteroid Dehydrogenase	Cortisol Aldosterone	Dehydroepi-androsterone	Salt loss Ambiguous genitalia in both males and females
21-Hydroxylase			
Partial	Cortisol	Androgens	Ambiguous genitalia in female Postnatal virilization in male
Complete	Cortisol Aldosterone	Androgens	Virilization Salt loss
11-β-Hydroxylase	Cortisol Aldosterone	11-desoxycortisol (compound S) DOC Androgens	Ambiguous genitalia in female Postnatal virilization in male Hypertension
18-hydroxylase	Aldosterone	Corticosterone	Salt loss
18-dehydrogenase	Aldosterone	18-hydroxy-corticosterone	Salt loss

losers," since under most conditions they can conserve salt and water and maintain normal sodium and potassium levels. Indeed, they are able to attain normal (45,77) and even elevated circulating levels of aldosterone on a low-salt diet (77). When, however, the most sensitive measurement of salt and water depletion was employed (i.e., plasma renin activity determinations) (18,26,84), Roslet (77) appreciated the fact that even the so-called "non-salt-losers" show excessively high renin response, which they concluded indicated a "sodium-losing tendency."

For this reason, a number of investigators (75,77,90) have believed that no definitive separation on the basis of sodium wasting can be made since there appears to be a clinical spectrum from mild sodium losing, appreciated only by excessive renin response, to the salt-wasting type, which will next be described.

21-Hydroxylase Deficiency, Salt-Wasting, and Virilizing

Since salt wasting can present an acute medical emergency, this subgroup of patients deserves additional discussion. Accounting for 30–40% of patients with CAH, these patients usually present early in life, from the

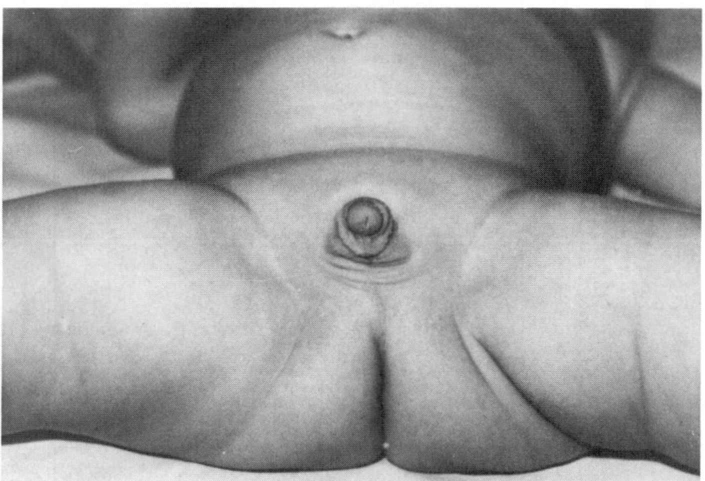

FIGURE 2. External genitalia of a two-week-old genotypic female demonstrating marked clitoral hypertrophy and hyperpigmentation. She presented in severe salt-losing crisis and proved to have 21-hydroxylase deficiency.

second to seventh week (98). Occasional cases are diagnosed earlier during the first week of life (44). Clinical features at the time of diagnosis may include weight loss, anorexia, vomiting, diarrhea, and circulatory collapse. Progressive hyponatremia, hyperkalemia, and metabolic acidosis are constant laboratory findings of this life-threatening crisis and require vigorous management. Females tend to be masculinized to a greater extent than in the non-salt-wasting form. Males may have an enlarged penis, but this is not often appreciated as abnormal (see Figure 3). Hyperpigmentation of the external genitalia can be seen i both sexes, but is not a constant finding.

The mechanism of salt-wasting is the subject of considerable debate. Initial observations by Crigler et al. (14) that treatment with ACTH resulted in sodium loss and that mineralocorticoid requirements were decreased when ACTH was suppressed with cortisone, led to the first theory of salt loss. The theory was that the salt-wasting patient produced an ACTH-dependent adrenal salt-losing hormone. Substantiating this theory was the previous finding by Barrett and McNamara (1): that these patients require higher dose mineralocorticoid therapy than do patients with Addison's disease.

The second theory to explain salt-wasting was advanced by Bongiovanni and Eberlein (9). They proposed that the non-salt-loser had a milder form of the disease (partial 21-hydroxylase deficiency) and was able to produce more aldosterone and cortisol and that these steroids had a synergistic effect: to maintain sodium homeostasis. In contrast, the salt-loser had a more complete block at 21-hydroxylation with resulting cortisol and aldosterone insufficiency.

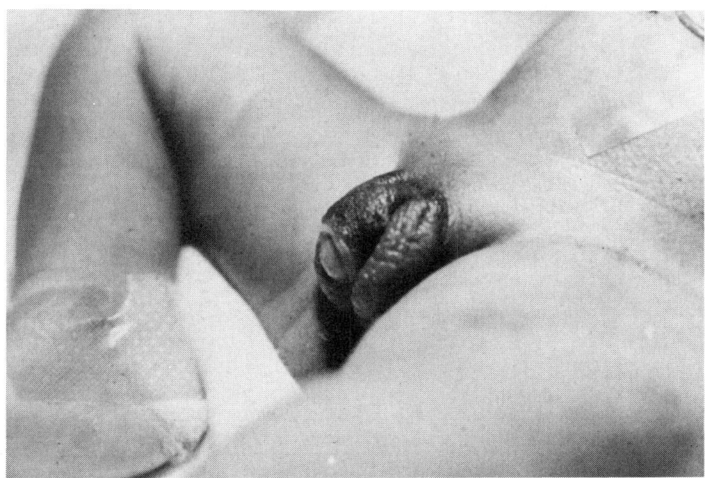

FIGURE 3. External genitalia of an untreated male with 21-hydroxylase deficiency presenting at age 7 years.

An alternative concept was first proposed by Bryan et al. (12) in 1965. They pointed to impaired aldosterone production in "salt-losing" CAH patients and the apparent aldosterone hypersecretion in the "non-salt-losing" variety as evidence that the two forms were genetically and biochemically distinct. Their theory required two 21-hydroxylase isoenzymes, each with different substrates: namely, 17-hydroxyprogesterone and progesterone. A deficiency of the former isoenzyme was seen in all CAH patients, and additionally of the latter isoenzyme in the salt-losing CAH patients. Other work tended to support the two isoenzyme theory (4,17).

A synthesis of the one-enzyme-deficiency theory and the aldosterone antagonist theory was advocated by Kowarski et al. (45) in 1965. In essence, this theory explains the salt loss by an "overproduction of aldosterone antagonists and a decreased ability to synthesize aldosterone." The non-salt-losers are in a compensated state, able to secrete enough aldosterone to overcome the antagonists by virtue of a much milder enzyme deficiency.

11-β-Hydroxylase Deficiency

The discovery of patients with a hypertensive form of CAH was made by Bongiovanni and Eberlein (9). They defined a new group, characterized by masculinization and continued virilization, as in 21-hydroxylase deficiency, but who produced large amounts of what was later shown to be 11-deoxycortisol (S) and 11-deoxycorticosterone (DOC) (10). Presumably, the excessive DOC secretion, itself a mineralocorticoid, produced the hypertension. The hypertension may not be apparent until early adulthood (23), or not at all (5,24). This inconsistency of hypertension has yet to be adequately explained. The apparent failure of excessive DOC production to result in hypertension in 18-hydroxylase deficiency (see below) and the report by Holcomb et al. (33) leads to further questions about the role of DOC in hypertension.

The affected female fetus has varying degrees of masculinization at birth and presents as a female pseudohermaphrodite. The internal genitalia are normal female.

These patients, like the 21-hydroxylase deficient patients, have rapid osseous maturation and premature fusion of epiphyses if not treated adequately.

3-β-Hydroxysteroid Dehydrogenase Deficiency

Ambiguityof the genitalia in *both* sexes is the prominent feature in this group of CAH patients. First described by Bongiovanni (7) in 1961, this syndrome results in impairment in the synthesis of mineralocorticoids, glucocorticoids and androgens. The defect occurs in the adrenal and in the male testis; hence the inability to produce testosterone. It is this lack of potent androgens in the male that leads to incomplete masculinization of the external genitalia. In the female, it is thought that DHEA, a mild androgen (28), produced in large quantities in this condition, accounts for the clitoromegaly.

Salt wasting in this group can be severe and life threatening. As in the complete form of 21-hydroxylase deficiency, early and aggressive treatment is necessary.

It is of great interest (and as yet without adequate explanation) that some males have appeared to have normal testicular production of testosterone at puberty (66,78). Clearly, they were deficient of potent androgens in utero, evidenced by ambiguous genitalia; but when studied during puberty they demonstrated normal testosterone response to HCG.

17-α-Hydroxylase Deficiency

This group of patients, first described by Biglieri et al. (6) shows evidence of hypertension, especially in young adult life, in association with hypokalemic alkalosis. Further, there is lack of production of sex hormones and, thus, these individuals remain infantile. The males affected with this disorder usually are poorly virilized and have ambiguity of the external genitalia. They are classified as male pseudohermaphrodites. New (60) reported gynecomastia in one such affected male with this disorder. Laboratory findings include hypokalemia, which is attributed to the excess of DOC production, a mild mineralocorticoid. It is not clear why these individuals have diminished aldosterone production. A reasonable hypothesis is that excessive DOC causes excessive sodium resorption, increasing plasma volume. This in turn suppresses renin, and the production of aldosterone. In support of this hypothesis is New's demonstration (60) of prolonged ACTH suppression with dexamethasone, resulting in decreased DOC followed by sodium loss and then an increase in aldosterone secretion to normal and even elevated levels.

The infantilism in the female and the ambiguity of the external genitalia in the male are due to deficient androgens and estrogens. Since 17-hydroxylation is diminished in both the gonadal and adrenal cortex, there is lack of production of precursor androgens and estrogens. The female patient, therefore, usually presents with normal female external genitalia, primary amenorrhea, and sexual infantilism. Pubic and axillary hair usually are scanty.

In patients with the suggestive clinical picture, the diagnosis can be confirmed, by showing decreased, or absence of, urinary 17-ketosteroids and 17-hydroxysteroids and elevated amounts of tetrahydrocorticosterone and tetrahydro DOC in the urine. Plasma levels of corticosterone and DOC are elevated while the concentration of cortisol is diminished.

The treatment is similar to the treatment of patients with 21-hydroxylase deficiency and 11-hydroxylase deficiency, but for feminization in females exogenous estrogens and progestagens in a cyclic fashion are necessary.

Cholesterol Desmolase Deficiency

Another extremely rare form of congenital adrenal hyperplasia was described by Prader and Gurtner (69). With few exceptions, all of these patients die in early infancy of early salt-losing adrenal crisis. At autopsy, the adrenals are enlarged and filled with a lipoid material. The biochemical defect appears to be in the conversion of cholesterol to pregnenolone, hence lack of all adrenocortical steroid production. The genotypic males have incomplete masculinization due to lack of androgens and lack of mineralocorticoid production results in severe salt-wasting and death.

Treatment involves early recognition and vigorous steroid replacement. Several such children have been reported to have survived. The report of Kirkland et al. (42) exemplifies one such case.

18-Hydroxylase Deficiency

Visser and Cost (89) described children with isolated hypoaldosteronism, salt loss, failure to grow, and bouts of dehydration and fever. Several other case reports demonstrated hyponatremia and hyperkalemia. The conversion of corticosterone to 18-hydroxycorticosterone was shown by Visser and Cost (89) to be deficient.

Other steroid pathways in the production of cortisol and sex hormones are unaffected. The growth and development of some of these individuals are normal; since no sex steroid abnormalities occur, the genital differentiation is also normal.

The salt loss that occurs in this condition in the face of DOC overproduction is still unexplained. In other conditions where DOC is overproduced, it exerts mineralocorticoid effect. It is possible that there may be some renal insensitivity to the DOC, especially early in life. The diagnosis can be confirmed by demonstrating elevated levels of corticosterone and tetrahydrocorticosterone in the urine while at the same time 18-hydroxycorticosterone and aldosterone and tetrahydro-18-hydroxycorticosterone are low in the urine. ACTH levels are not elevated in this condition but plasma renin levels have been reported to be elevated and are perhaps the mechanism by which DOC is stimulated.

18-Dehydrogenase Deficiency

First described by Ulick et al.(88) and later by Hamilton et al. (31), this condition was described in a child who demonstrated failure to thrive, short stature, and evidence of mineralocorticoid deficiency with dehydration, hyperkalemia, and hyponatremia. As in 18-hydroxylase deficiency, there is no impairment of sex hormone secretion, and thus the external genitalia differentiate along normal lines. In addition, and like 18-hydroxylase deficiency, the glucocorticoid pathway is not impaired. The final step in aldosterone biosynthesis is impaired and has been demonstrated to be deficient, leading to decreased vascular volume with stimulation of renin and stimulation of the aldosterone pathway.

Diagnosis is confirmed by laboratory studies showing an increase in urinary metabolites of tetrahydro-18-hydroxycorticosterone in the face of decreased levels of aldosterone. Again, levels of cortisol and sex hormones are normal as are ACTH levels.

Treatment is similar to the 18-hydroxylase deficiency syndrome with replacement of mineralocorticoid.

Dexamethasone-suppressible Hyperaldosteronism

In 1967, New and Peterson (63) described a 12-year-old male who was found to have hypertension associated with hyperaldosteronism. The hyperaldosteronism was dexamethasone-suppressible, raising the possibility of yet another congenital adrenal hyperplasia. The subsequent studies of this patient and several others reported in the literature (25,58,64,86) demonstrate that this rare disorder is inherited probably by an autosomal dominant genetic mechanism. With dexamethasone treatment at 1 mg/day, the blood pressure of the younger patients returns to normal as does aldosterone production.

It is not clear, however, as to which steroid is responsible for the hypertension. Studies (64) in a patient with this syndrome suggest that aldosterone and DOC may not be the steroids responsible for the hypertension, in view of the fact that when either of these steroids were infused in the patient during dexamethasone suppression, hypertension did not result. However, when either metyrapone or ACTH was infused, the hypertension promptly returned.

Grim and Weinberger (30) have suggested that patients with aldosteronism have an enhanced adrenal receptor on the aldosterone-producing adrenal cells for ACTH. The mechanism by which these patients develop hypertension is the subject of current controversy.

Acquired 21-Hydroxylase Deficiency, Partial 11- and 21-Hydroxylase Deficiency

Hirsutism associated with menstrual disturbances has been attributed to excessive adrenal androgen production. Some studies suggest adrenal enzyme deficiency (11,23).

Prolonged ACTH infusions in a group of 31 hirsute women studied by Newmark et al. (65) evoked a significantly greater tetrahydro compound S and/or pregnanetriol 24-hour urinary excretion in 13 of the patients. These data suggested partial deficiencies of 11- and 21-hydroxylase enzymes. In these hirsute women, long-term glucocorticoid suppression may result in a decrease in adrenal androgen precursors and hence a decrease in the stimulation of terminal hair growth.

Some of these patients may have a mild homozygous form of congenital virilizing adrenal hyperplasia, as suggested by Jones et al. (38) and Rosenwaks et al. (76). However, it is also clear by HLA typing in family studies (62) that some of these women with "acquired adrenal hyperplasia" have a disorder genetically different from congenital adrenal hyperplasia.

TREATMENT

The management may be outlined in three important general areas: hormonal, surgical, and psychologic.

Hormonal Treatment

First, hormonal treatment can be crucial in the first days of life and during stress conditions in those patients with the salt-losing types of CAH. Glucocorticoid and mineralocorticoid replacement are essential in patients affected with complete 21-hydroxylase, 3β-hydroxysteroid dehydrogenase, or desmolase deficiencies.

Glucocorticoid replacement alone is required for patients with partial 21-hydroxylase, 11-hydroxylase, and in the prepubertal child with 17-hydroxylase deficiencies. For pubertal development, the patients affected with 17-hydroxylase deficiency will need additional sex steroids.

Mineralocorticoid treatment alone is required for patients with both 18-hydroxylase and 18-dehydrogenase deficiencies, since only the aldosterone pathway is affected. The potent long-acting glucocorticoid dexamethasone may prove helpful in long-term management of the dexamethasone-suppressible hyperaldosteronism, as it has been in the acute situation. But this as yet remains to be demonstrated.

Glucocorticoids. Most authors favor the use of cortisol (cortisone acetate, hydrocortisone) over the longer acting and more potent synthetic glucocorticoids. The timing and dosage for chronic administration is the subject of considerable debate (43,47,72,73,82,83). In general, the oral administration of 25 mg/m^2/day in three divided doses has been effective. When doses in excess of 30–50 mg/m^2 of cortisol are used chronically, Cushingoid features and poor linear growth may result.

To determine adequacy of the dose, various biochemical parameters have been used. Urinary excretion of 17-ketosteroids and pregnanetriol have been useful in the past. More recently, the use of blood levels of 17-hydroxyprogesterone, dehydroepiandrosterone-sulfate, androstenedione, in males and females, and testosterone levels in females and prepubertal males have been advocated because of ease in obtaining these specimens compared with obtaining a 24-hour urine collection (19,27,35,55,97). To ensure adequate suppression of androgens and at the same time avoid excessive glucocorticoid effects, one should administer the smallest dose of cortisol that will suppress the 24-hour urinary 17-ketosteroids to normal and the 17-hydroxyprogesterone concentration in blood to 200 ng/dl. To attempt greater suppression than this frequently results in Cushingoid features and slowing of bone growth (19,27, 35,55,97). Height velocity and bone age should also be assessed periodically since overtreatment will result in slowing of height velocity and bone maturation and undertreatment will result in an increase in these parameters.

Inadequate glucocorticoid control may result in disorders of pubertal development in both males and females with CAH. Women with CAH often develop menstrual disorders, and girls frequently experience delayed menarche (39). Wentz et al. (92) have demonstrated in well-controlled patients an appropriate gonadotropin response to LRH, whereas girls with primary and secondary amenorrhea, who had histories of poor control, demonstrated prepubertal gonadotropin responses to LRH. It is currently felt that postnatal exposure of the female hypothalamus to increased androgens can disrupt the normal hypothalamic–pituitary–gonadal axis (40,74).

Males who are untreated or inadequately controlled with glucocorticoids may develop precocious puberty (93,94). Reiter et al. (74) have suggested that chronically increased adrenal androgens may induce early hypothalamic maturation and decreased negative feedback to sex steroids.

Another complication of inadequate control in the male is the development of bilateral testicular tumors (46,79). The origin of these tumor cells is somewhat obscure. Landing and Gold (46) suggest these tumors are of Leydig cell origin, while Shanklin et al. (80) suggest a multipotential cell derived from the adrenogenital ridge. It seems clear from work by Kirkland et al. (41) that these tumors are stimulated by ACTH to produce high levels of 17-hydroxyprogesterone and Δ^4- androstenedione, and thus act more like cells of adrenal origin, sharing the enzyme deficiency seen in adrenal tissue. However, these authors do not exclude a role for LH in stimulating the growth of these tumors since elevated levels of LH were noted in their patient. Adequate glucocorticoid suppression will cause the testicular tumors to regress.

During acute stress of infection with high fever, the glucocorticoid dose should be doubled. This in effect mimics the normal adrenal response to febrile illness. During major traumatic or surgical stress the dose should be tripled or quadrupled and the route of administration should be parenteral.

Mineralocorticoid. For the maintenance of salt and water homeostasis, exogenous mineralocorticoids are essential in the salt-losing forms of CAH. In the face of very high levels of 17-hydroxyprogesterone and 16-hydroxyprogesterone, both naturally occurring natriuretic steroids (56), patients are resistant to the usual doses of these hormones. This may be particularly true in the first few days following diagnosis in infants. They may require large doses transiently.

For infants, desoxycorticosterone acetate (DOCA) can be injected intramuscularly in a dosage of 1–2 mg/day or can be implanted in the subcutaneous tissue as 125 mg pellets, which allow slow absorption for up to 12 months. Two to three grams of additional salt should be given daily, but care should be taken to monitor the blood pressure since excessive mineralocorticoid and salt can result in profound hypertension. The orally effective synthetic mineralocorticoid 9-α-fluorohydrocortisone (Florinef^{R}) can be used in infants and certainly better accepted in the older child. This is given as a single, oral dose (0.05–0.1 mg/day).

The adequacy of mineralocorticoid replacement has been assessed (51) by plasma renin activity (PRA). Lipton et al. demonstrate that, if mineralocorticoid therapy is interrupted or inadequate, volume depletion results in stimulation of the PRA and normalization of PRA could be brought about by appropriate mineralocorticoid doses.

Horner et al. (34) have emphasized the importance of continued mineralocorticoid treatment for life in salt-losing 21-hydroxylase deficiency. They point out that better suppression of 17-hydroxyprogesterone is achieved in salt-losers who receive both mineralocorticoid and glucocorticoid as contrasted with salt-losers receiving only glucocorticoid. Presumably, a lower glucocorticoid dose could be utilized in treating salt-losers if mineralocorticoid is added, decreasing the likelihood of developing Cushingoid features and improving linear growth.

Surgical Treatment

The second aspect of treatment is surgical management. It is necessary in the cases of ambiguity of the external genitalia. In the virilized female infant the enlarged clitoris and varying degrees of labial fusion require surgical correction, usually during the first year of life. Currently, a procedure that reduces the size of the clitoris (71) and at the same time, or at a second procedure, exteriorization of the vaginal orifice is performed (37). The poorly virilized male usually will be reared as a female and appropriate surgical procedures done early on as well. The exception here is that, for the vaginoplasty required in these cases, better results are obtained when the patient is operated on during or after puberty. This delay allows for adequate pelvic size and the dilatation procedures often required.

Psychological Treatment

The third aspect of treatment is psychology. For both the parents and the patient, this issue needs to be addressed early and effectively.

What is said in the delivery room regarding the initial assignment of sex in cases of ambiguous genitalia has profound and long-reaching effects on the parents, family members, friends and, most importantly, the patient. It is critical that an error not be made at this point. Money and Lewis (59) and others have given us important insights into this crucial problem. He suggests that obstetricians and delivery room personnel not attempt assignment of sex in the case of ambiguous genitalia, explaining to the parents that ". . . they have waited nine months to learn the sex of the baby and in this case they will unfortunately have to wait two to three more days"(49). In the virilized female it is important to share with the parents that the internal genitalia are perfectly normal female and are reproductively functional. It is only the external genitalia, clitoris, vulva, and distal vagina that may require surgical correction. When these abnormalities of the genitalia can be explained as a birth defect of the external sex organs and said to be "unfinished" (49) the parents often can accept the problem as well as the therapeutic course ahead.

An all too frequent error made at delivery is to announce that a baby born with ambiguous genitalia is a male with hypospadius and cryptorchidism. In addition to delaying the diagnosis of a potentially life-threatening crisis, the parents assign a male name that is rapidly transmitted to relatives and friends making a later change difficult and indirectly damaging to the sexual identity of the patient.

FIGURE 4. External genitalia of a genotypic female with complete masculinization. No gonads were palpable at birth. The patient was diagnosed as having 21-hydroxylase deficiency after two salt-losing crises at age 2 months.

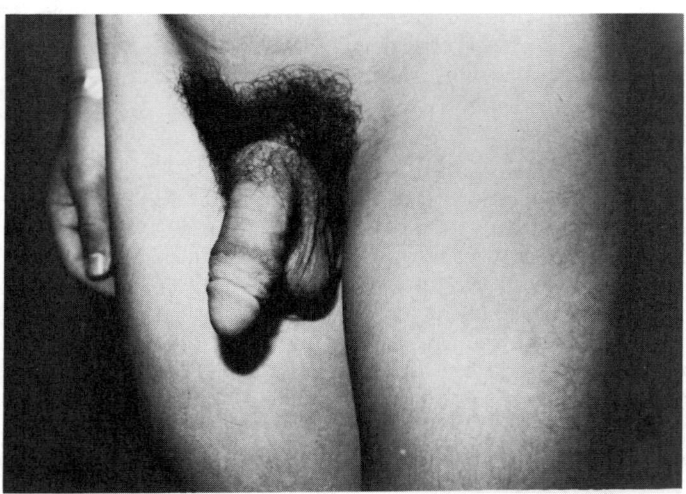

In the rare instance of a 46XX individual who has a completely virilized penile urethra (see Figure 4), some have been successfully reared as males. It is necessary, of course, to remove the internal female organs, implant testicle prostheses, and, at puberty, to treat adequately with testosterone for development of male secondary sexual characteristics. They should also be counselled as to their infertility.

Another interesting fact observed repeatedly in these children is the tendency to higher I.Q. performance (21,54,59). However, it appears that this increased I.Q. is not different from that of siblings or parents of patients.

In general, good management from the psychological standpoint, especially for the female, includes early recognition of the diagnosis, appropriate information for the family, and continued psychologic support for the family and patient.

REFERENCES

1. Barnett, H. L., and McNamara, H. (1949) Electrolyte balance in a male infant with adrenocortical insufficiency and virilism. The effect of desoxycorticosterone acetate and salt therapy with special reference to potassium. J. Clin. Invest. 28, 1498.
2. Bartter, F. C. (1977) Adrenogenital syndromes from physiology to chemistry (1950–1975). In: P. A. Lee, L. P. Plotnick, A. A. Kowarski, and C. J. Migeon (eds.), Congenital Adrenal Hyperplasia, Univ. Park Press, Baltimore, Maryland, pp. 9–18.
3. Bartter, F. C., Albright, F., Forbes, A. P., Leaf, A., Dempsey, E., and Carroll E. (1951) The effects of adrenocorticotropic hormone and cortisone in the adrenogenital syndrome associated with congenital adrenal hyperplasia: An attempt to explain and correct its disordered hormonal pattern. J. Clin. Invest. 30, 237–251.
4. Bartter, F. C., Henkin, R. I., and Bryan, G. T. (1968) Aldosterone hypersecretion in "non-salt-losing" congenital adrenal hyperplasia. J. Clin. Invest. 47, 1742–1752.
5. Bergstraud, C. G., Birke, G., and Plantin, L. O. (1959) Corticosteroid excretion pattern in infants and children with adrenogenital syndrome. Acta Endocrinol. 30, 500.
6. Biglieri, E. G., Herron, E. G., and Brust, N. (1966) 17-Hydroxylation deficiency in man. J. Clin. Invest. 45, 1946–1957.
7. Bongiovanni, A. M. (1961) Unusual steroid pattern in congenital adrenal hyperplasia: Deficiency of 3β hydroxydehydrogenase. J. Clin. Endocrinol. 21, 860.
8. Bongiovanni, A. M. (1962) Adrenogenital syndrome with deficiency of 3β-hydroxysteroid dehydrogenase. J. Clin. Invest. 41, 2086–2092.
9. Bongiovanni, A. M., and Eberlein, W. R. (1958) Defective steroidal biogenesis in congenital adrenal hyperplasia. Pediatrics 21, 661–672.
10. Bongiovanni, A. M., and Root, A. W. (1963) The adrenogenital syndrome. N. Engl. J. Med. 268, 1283–1289.
11. Brooks, R. V., Mattingly, D., Mills, I. H. et al. (1960) Postpubertal adrenal virilism with biochemical disturbance of congenital type of adrenal hyperplasia. Brit. Med. J. 1, 1294.
12. Bryan, G. T., Kliman, B., and Bartter, F. C. (1965) Impaired aldosterone production in "salt-losing" congenital adrenal hyperplasia. J. Clin. Invest. 44, 957–965.
13. Childs, B., Grambach, M. M., and VanWyk, J. J. (1956) Virilizing adrenal hyperplasia: A genetic and hormonal study. J. Clin. Invest. 35, 213.
14. Crigler, J. R. Jr., Silverman, S. H., and Wilkins, L. (1952) Further studies on the treatment of congenital adrenal hyperplasia with cortisone. IV. Effect of cortisone and compound B in infants with disturbed electrolyte metabolism. Pediatrics 10, 397.
15. Dean, H. J., and Winter, J. S. D. (1979) A mild form of congenital adrenal hyperplasia (21-OH deficiency) without prenatal virilization. Pediatr. Res. 13:4 Abs. 311.

16. DeCrecchio, L. (1865) Sopra un caso di apparenze virile in una donna. Morgagni 7, 1951.
17. Degenhart, H. J., Visser, H. K. A., Wilmink, R., and Croughs, W. (1965) Aldosterone and cortisol secretion rates in infants and children with congenital adrenal hyperplasia suggesting different 21-hydroxylation defects. Acta Endocrinol. 48, 587.
18. Dillon, M. J. (1975) Plasma renin activity and aldosterone concentration in children: Results in salt wasting states. Arch. Dis. Child. 50, 330.
19. Duck, S. C. (1980) Acceptable linear growth in congenital adrenal hyperplasia. J. Pediatr. 97, 93–96.
20. Dupont, B., Oberfield, S. E., Smithwick, E. M., Lee, T. D., and Levine, L. S. (1977) Close genetic linkage between HLA and congenital adrenal hyperplasia (21-hydroxylase deficiency). Lancet ii, 1309–1312.
21. Ehrhardt, A. A., and Baker, S. W. (1974) Fetal androgens, human central nervous system differentiation, and behavior sex differences. In: R. C. Friedman, R. M. Richart, and R. L. VandeWiele (eds.), Sex Differences in Behavior, John Wiley and Sons, Inc., New York, pp. 33–51.
22. Franks, R. C. (1974) Plasma 17-hydroxyprogesterone, 21-deoxycortisol, and cortisol in congenital adrenal hyperplasia. J. Clin. Endocrinol. Metab. 39, 1099.
23. Gabrilove, J. L., Sharma, P. C., and Dorfman, R. I. (1965) Adrenocortical 11β-hydroxylase deficiency and virilism first manifest in the adult woman. N. Engl. J. Med. 272, 1189–1194.
24. Gandy, H. M., Keutmann, E. H., and Izzo, A. J. (1960) Characterization of urinary steroids in adrenal hyperplasia: Isolation of metabolites of cortisol, compound-S, and deoxycorticosterone from normotensive patient with adrenogenital syndrome. J. Clin. Invest. 39, 364.
25. Giebink, G. S., Gotlin, R. W., Biglieri, E. G. et al. (1973) A kindred with familial glucocorticoid-suppressible aldosteronism. J. Clin. Endocrinol. Metab. 36, 715.
26. Godard, C., Riondel, A. M., Veyrat, R., Megevand, A., and Muller, A. F. (1968) Plasma renin activity and aldosterone in congenital adrenal hyperplasia. Pediatrics 41, 883.
27. Golden, M. P., Lippe, B. M., Kaplan, S. A., Lavin, N., and Slavin, J. (1978) Management of congenital adrenal hyperplasia using serum dehydroepiandrosterone sulfate and 17-hydroxyprogesterone concentrations. Pediatrics 61, 867–871.
28. Goldman, A. S. (1970) Virilization of the external genitalia of the female rat fetus by dehydroepiandrosterone. Endocrinology 87, 432.
29. Goldman, A. S., Bongiovanni, A. M., Yakovac, W. C., and Prader, A. (1964) Study of 3β-hydroxysteroid dehydrogenase in normal, hyperplastic, and neoplastic cortical tissue. J. Clin. Endocrinol. 24, 894–909.
30. Grim, C. E., and Weinberger, M. D. (1980) Familial dexamethasone-suppressible normokalemic hyperaldosteronism. Pediatrics 65, 597–604.
31. Hamilton, W., McCandless, A. E., Ireland, J. T., and Gray, C. E. (1976) Hypoaldosteronism in three sibs due to an 18-dehydrogenase deficiency. Arch. Dis. Child. 51, 576.
32. Hirschfeld, J. A., and Fleshman, J. K. (1969) An unusually high incidence of salt-losing congenital adrenal hyperplasia in the Alaskan Eskimo. J. Pediatr. 75, 492.
33. Holcombe, J. H., Keenan, B. S., Nichols, B. L., Kirkland, R. T., and Clayton, G. W. (1980) Neonatal salt loss in the hypertensive form of congenital adrenal hyperplasia. Pediatrics 65, 777.
34. Horner, J. M., Hintz, R. L., and Luetscher, J. A. (1979) The role of renin and angiotensin in salt-losing 21-hydroxylase-deficient congenital adrenal hyperplasia. J. Clin. Endocrinol. Metab. 48, 776–783.
35. Hughes, I. A., and Winter, J. S. D. (1978) The relationship between serum concentrations of 17-OH-progesterone and other serum and urinary steroids in patients with congenital adrenal hyperplasia. J. Clin. Endocrinol. Metab. 46, 98–104.
36. Jailer, J. W., Gold, J. J., van de Wiele, R., and Lieberman, S. (1955) 17-α-hydroxy-

progesterone and 21-desoxycorticosterone: Their metabolism and possible role in congenital adrenal hyperplasia. J. Clin. Invest. 34, 1639.

37. Jones, H. W. Jr., Garcia, S. C., and Klingensmith, G. J. (1977) Necessity for and the technique of secondary surgical treatment of the masculinized external genitalia of patients with virilizing adrenal hyperplasia. In: P. A. Lee, L. P. Plotnick, A. A. Kowarski, and C. J. Migeon (eds.), Congenital Adrenal Hyperplasia, Univ. Park Press, Baltimore, Maryland, pp. 347–352.
38. Jones, H. W. Jr., and Jones, G. E. S. (1954) The gynecological aspects of adrenal hyperplasia and allied disorders. Am. J. Obstet. Gynecol. 68, 1330.
39. Jones, H. W. Jr., and Verkauf, B. S. (1971) Congenital adrenal hyperplasia: Age at menarche and related pubertal events. Am. J. Obstet. Gynecol. 109, 292.
40. Kirkland, J., Kirkland, R., Librik, L., and Clayton, G. (1974) Serum gonadotropin levels in female adolescents with congenital adrenal hyperplasia. J. Pediatr. 84, 411–414.
41. Kirkland, R. T., Kirkland, J. L., Kennan, B. S., Bongiovanni, A. M., Rosenberg, H. S., and Clayton, G. W. (1977) J. Clin. Endocrinol. Metab. 44, 369–378.
42. Kirkland, R. T., Kirkland, T. T., Johnson, C. M., Hroning, M. G., Librik, L., and Clayton, G. W. (1973) Congenital lipoid adrenal hyperplasia in an eight-year-old phenotypic female. J. Clin. Endocrinol. 36, 488.
43. Klingensmith, G. J., Garcia, S. C., Jones, H. W., Migeon, C. J., and Blizzard, R. M. (1977) Glucocorticoid treatment of girls with congenital adrenal hyperplasia: Effects on height, sexual maturation and fertility. J. Pediatr. 90, 996–1004.
44. Kowarski, A. A. (1977) Mechanism of salt loss in congenital virilizing adrenal hyperplasia. In: P. H. Lee, L. P. Plotnick, A. A. Kowarski, and C. J. Migeon (eds.), Congenital Adrenal Hyperplasia, Univ. Park Press, Baltimore, Maryland, pp. 113–124.
45. Kowarski, A., Finkelstein, J. W., Spaulding, J. S. et al. (1955) Aldosterone secretion rate in congenital adrenal hyperplasia. A discussion of the theories on the pathogenesis of the salt-losing form of the syndrome. J. Clin. Invest. 44, 1505.
46. Landing, B. H., and Gold, E. (1951) The occurrence and significance of Leydig cell proliferation in familial adrenocortical hyperplasia. J. Clin. Endocrinol. Metab. 11, 1436.
47. Laron, Z., and Pertzelan, A. (1968) The comparative effect of 6-α-fluoroprednisolone, 6-α-methylprednisolone, and hydrocortisone on linear growth of children with congenital adrenal virilism and Addison's disease. J. Pediatr. 73, 774.
48. Levine, L. S., Zachmann, M., New, M. I., Prader, A., Pollack, M. S., O'Neill, G. J., Yang, S. Y., Oberfield, S. F., and Dupont, B. (1978) Genetic mapping of the 21-hydroxylase-deficiency gene within the HLA linkage group. N. Engl. J. Med. 299 (17), 911–915.
49. Lewis, V. G., and Money, J. (1977) Adrenogenital syndrome, the need for early surgical feminization in girls. In: P. H. Lee, L. P. Plotnick, A. A. Kowarski, and C. J. Migeon (eds.), Congenital Adrenal Hyperplasia, Univ. Park Press, Baltimore, Maryland, pp. 463–466.
50. Liddle, G. W., Islands, D. et al. (1962) Recent Progr. Hormone Res. 18, 125.
51. Lipton, H. L., Tan, S. Y., Noth, R., Mulrow, P. J., and Genel, M. (1977) Usefulness of plasma renin activity to monitor mineralocorticoid replacement in salt-losing congenital adrenal hyperplasia. In: P. H. Lee, L. P. Plotnick, A. A. Kowarski, and C. J. Migeon (eds.), Congenital Adrenal Hyperplasia, Univ. Park Press, Baltimore, Maryland, pp. 127–139.
52. Lorenzen, F., Pang, S., New, M. I., Dupont, B., Pollack, M., Chow, D. M., and Levine, L. S. (1979) Hormonal phenotype and HLA genotype in families of patients with congenital adrenal hyperplasia (21-hydroxylase deficiency). Pediatr. Res. 13, 1356–1360.
53. Loriaux, D. L., Ruder, H. H., and Lipsett, M. B. (1974) Plasma steroids in congenital adrenal hyperplasia. J. Clin. Endocrinol. Metab. 39, 627–630.
54. McGuire, L. S., and Omenn, G. S. (1975) Congenital adrenal hyperplasia. I. Family Studies of I.Q. Behav. Genet. 5, 165–173.

55. McKenna, T. J., Jennings, A. S., Liddle, G. W., and Burr, I. M. (1975) Pregnenolone, 17-OH-progesterone, and testosterone in plasma of patients with congenital adrenal hyperplasia. J. Clin. Endocrinol. Metab. 42, 918–925.
56. Meyer, W. J., III, Gutai, J. P., Keenan, B. S., Davis, G. R., Kowarski, A. A., and Migeon, C. J. (1977) A chronobiological approach to the treatment of congenital adrenal hyperplasia. In: P. H. Lee, L. P. Plotnick, A. A. Kowarski, and C. J. Migeon (eds.), Congenital Adrenal Hyperplasia, Univ. Park Press, Baltimore, Maryland, pp. 203–215.
57. Migeon, C. J. (1977) Diagnosis and management of congenital adrenal hyperplasia. Hosp. Pract. March 75–82.
58. Miura, K., Yoshinaga, K., Goto, K. et al. (1968) A case of glucocorticoid-responsive hyperaldosteronism. J. Clin. Endocrinol. Metab. 28, 1807.
59. Money, J., and Lewis, V. (1966) I.Q. genetics and accelerated growth: Adrenogenital syndrome. Bull. Johns Hopkins Hosp. 118, 365–373.
60. New, M. (1970) Male pseudohermaphroditism due to 17-α-hydroxylase deficiency. J. Clin. Invest. 49, 1930–1939.
61. New, M. I., and Levine, L. S. (1973) Congenital adrenal hyperplasia. Adv. Hum. Genet. 4, 251–326.
62. New, M. I., Lorenzen, F., Pang, S., Gunczler, P., Dupont, B., and Levine, L. S. (1979) "Acquired" adrenal hyperplasia with 21-hydroxylase deficiency is not the same genetic disorder as congenital adrenal hyperplasia. J. Clin. Endocrinol. Metab. 48, 356–359.
63. New, M. I., and Peterson, R. E. (1967) A new form of congenital adrenal hyperplasia. J. Clin. Endocrinol. Metab. 27, 300.
64. New, M. I., Peterson, R. E., Saenger, P., and Levine, L. S. (1976) Evidence for an unidentified ACTH-induced steroid hormone causing hypertension. J. Clin. Endocrinol. Metab. 43, 1283.
65. Newmark, S., Dluhy, R. G., Williams, G. H., Pochi, P., and Rose, L. I. (1977) Partial 11- and 21-hydroxylase deficiencies in hirsute women. Am. J. Obstet. Gynecol. 127, 594.
66. Parks, G. A., Bermudez, J. A., Anast, C. A., Bongiovanni, A. M., and New, M. I. (1971) A pubertal boy with 3β-hydroxysteroid dehydrogenase defect. J. Clin. Endocrinol. 33, 269.
67. Pollack, M., Levine, L. S., Duchon, M., Pang, S., Merkatz, I., Dupont, B., and New, M.I. (1979) Prenatal diagnosis of CAH due to 21-hydroxylase deficiency by HLA typing of cultured amniotic cells. Abst. 349, Pediat. Res. 13, 4.
68. Prader, A. (1958) Die haufigkeit des kongenitalen adrenogenitalen syndroms. Helv. Paediat. Acta 13, 426.
69. Prader, A., and Gurtner, H. P. (1955) Das Syndrom des Pseudohermaphroditismus masculinus bei kongenitales nebennie reninden-hyperplasie ohne. Androgen Überproduktion (adrenaler pseudohermaphroditismus masculinus). Helv. Paediat. Acta 10, 398.
70. Prader, A., Spahr, A., and Neher, R. (1955) Erhohte aldosteron-ausscheidung beim kongenitalen androgenitalen syndrom. Schweiz. Med. Wochenschr. 85, 1085–1088.
71. Randolph, J. G., and Hung, W. (1970) Reduction clitoroplasty in females with hypertrophied clitoris. J. Pediatr. Surg. 5, 224.
72. Rappaport, R., Bouthreuil, E., Marti-Henneberg, C., and Basmaciogullar, A. (1973) Linear growth rate, bone maturation and growth hormone secretion in prepubertal children with congenital adrenal hyperplasia. Acta Paediat. Scand. 62, 513–519.
73. Rappaport, R., Cornu, G., and Royer, P. (1968) Statural growth in congenital adrenal hyperplasia treated with oral hydrocortisone. J. Pediatr. 73, 760.
74. Reiter, E. O., Grumbach, M. M., Kaplan, S. L., and Conte, F. A. (1975) The response of pituitary gonadotropes to synthetic LRF in children with glucocorticoid-treated congenital adrenal hyperplasia: Lack of intrauterine and neonatal androgen excess. J. Clin. Endocrinol. Metab. 40, 318–325.
75. Rosenbloom, A. L., and Smith, D. W. (1966) Varying expression for salt losing in related patients with congenital adrenal hyperplasia. Pediatrics 38, 215.

76. Rosenwaks, Z., Lee, P. A., Jones, G. S., Migeon, C. J., and Wentz, A. C. (1979) An attenuated form of congenital virilizing adrenal hyperplasia. J. Clin. Endocrinol. Metab. 49, 335–339.
77. Rosler, A., Levine, L. S., Schneider, B., Novogradei, M., and New, M. I. (1977) The interrelationship of sodium balance, plasma renin activity, and ACTH in congenital adrenal hyperplasia. J. Clin. Endocrinol. Metab. 45, 500–512.
78. Saez, T. M., Frederich, A., and Bertraud, T. (1971) Endocrine and metabolic studies in children with male pseudohermphroditism. J. Clin. Endocrinol. Metab. 32, 611.
79. Schoen, E. J., DiRaimondo, V. C., and Domiguez, O. V. (1961) Bilateral testicular tumors complicating congenital adrenal hyperplasia. J. Clin. Endocrinol. Metab. 21, 518.
80. Shanklin, D. R., Richardson, A. P., and Rothstein, G. (1963) Testicular hilar nodules in adrenogenital syndrome. Am. J. Dis. Child. 106, 243.
81. Simopolous, A. P., Marshall, J. R., Delea, C. S., and Bartter, F. C. (1971) Studies on the deficiency of 21-hydroxylation in patients with congenital adrenal hyperplasia. J. Clin. Endocrinol. Metab. 32, 438.
82. Sperling, M. A., Kenny, F. M., Schutt-Aine, J. C., and Drash, A. L. (1971) Linear growth and growth hormonal responsiveness in treated congenital adrenal hyperplasia. Am. J. Dis. Child. 12, 408–413
83. Steryptel, R. S., Sheikholislam, B. M., Lebovitz, H. E., Allen, E., and Franks, R. C. (1968) Pituitary growth hormone suppression with low-dosage, long-acting corticoid administration. J. Pediatr. 73, 767.
84. Strickland, H. L., and Kotchen, T. A. (1972) A study of the renin–aldosterone system in congenital hyperplasia. J. Pediatr. 81, 962.
85. Strott, C. A., Yoshimi, T., and Lipsett, M. B. (1969) Blood levels and production rate of 17-hydroxypregnenolone in man. J. Clin. Invest. 48, 930.
86. Sutherland, D. J. A., Ruse, R. L., and Laidlow, J. C. (1966) Hypertension increased aldosterone secretion and low plasma renin activity relieved by dexamethasone. Can. Med. Assoc. J. 95, 1109.
87. Sydnor, K. L., Kelly, V. C., Raile, R. B., Ely, R. S., and Sayers, G. (1953) Blood adrenocorticotrophin in children with congenital adrenal hyperplasia. Proc. Soc. Exp. Biol Med. 82, 695.
88. Ulick, S. E., Gautier, K. K., Vette et al. (1964) An aldosterone biosynthetic defect in a salt-losing disorder. J. Clin. Endocrinol. Metab. 24, 669.
89. Visser, H. K. A., and Cost, W. S. (1964) A new hereditary defect in the biosynthesis of aldosterone. Acta Endocrinol. 47, 589.
90. Visser, H. K. A., and Degenhart, H. J. (1967) Salt losing in an infant with congenital adrenal hyperplasia and normal aldosterone production. Acta. Pediatr. Scand. 56, 216.
91. Weldon, V. V., Blizzard, R. M., and Migeon, C. J. (1966) Newborn girls misdiagnosed as bilaterally cryptorchid males. N. Engl. J. Med. 274, 829.
92. Wentz, A. C., Garcia, S. C., Klingensmith, G. J., Migeon, C. J., and Jones, G. S. (1976) Gonadotropin output and response to LRH administration in congenital virilizing adrenal hyperplasia. J. Clin. Endocrinol. Metab. 42, 239–246.
93. Wilkins, L., and Cara, J. (1954) Further studies on the treatment of congenital adrenal hyperplasia with cortisone. Pt. V. Effects of cortisone therapy on testicular development. J. Clin. Endocrinol. Metab. 14, 287–296.
94. Wilkins, L., Crigler, J. F., Silverman, S. H., Gardner, L. I., and Migeon, C. J. (1952) Further studies on the treatment of congenital adrenal hyperplasia with cortisone. Pt. II. The effects of cortisone on sexual and somatic development with a hypothesis concerning the mechanism of feminization. J. Clin. Endocrinol. Metab. 12, 277–295.
95. Wilkins, L., Fleischmann, W., and Howard, J. E. (1940) Macrogenitosomia precox associated with hyperplasia of the androgenic tissue of the adrenal and death from corticoadrenal insufficiency. Endocrinology 26, 385–395.
96. Wilkins, L., Lewis, R. A., Klein, R., and Rosenberg, E. (1950) The suppression of

androgen secretion by cortisone in a case of congenital adrenal hyperplasia. Bull. Johns Hopkins Hosp. 86, 249–255.

97. Winter, J. S. D. (1980) Marginal comment: Current approaches to the treatment of congenital adrenal hyperplasia. J. Pediatr. 87, 81-82.

98. Zurbrugg, R. P. (1975) Congenital adrenal hyperplasia. In: L. I. Gardner (eds.), Endocrine and Genetic Diseases of Childhood and Adolescence, W. B. Saunders, Philadelphia, p. 484.

DAVID JUAN, M.D.

PHEOCHROMOCYTOMA

INTRODUCTION

Pheochromocytoma is a catecholamine-producing tumor that arises from chromaffin cells in the adrenal medulla and the extraadrenal paraganglion system. It constitutes an uncommon but curable form of secondary hypertension. The disproportionate interest in pheochromocytoma on the part of many physicians is due to its dramatic presentation. Clinically, it is a maverick capable of mimicking a variety of diseases such as hyperthyroidism, essential hypertension, and emotional disorders. It can remain silent only to explode under stressful situations, such as surgery. Because of its evasive nature, pheochromocytoma can present itself to physicians of different specialties before a definitive diagnosis is achieved. With the present knowledge of catecholamine biochemistry and sophisticated radiological techniques in the localization of adrenal tumor, there is no excuse for missing the diagnosis. Once diagnosed, surgery can cure about 90% of the patients.

From Northwestern University Medical School, Clinical Pharmacology Center, Department of Medicine, Chicago, Illinois.

HISTORY

The year 1976 marked the 50th anniversary of the first successful removal of pheochromocytoma by Dr. Charles Mayo. Although L'abbé et al. (111) are frequently cited for the first clinical description of this tumor, the credit should go to Frankel, who first described pheochromocytoma in 1886 in an 18-year-old girl who died suddenly (58). He recorded that this young patient suffered from recurrent episodes of palpitations, headache, vomiting, and pallor accompanied by a hard, noncompressing pulse and retinitis. At autopsy, she had bilateral adrenal tumors, hypertensive vascular changes in her kidneys, and cardiac hypertrophy. In 1893, a second case was reported by Manasse, who later showed that these tumors have an affinity for bichromate salts (118). In 1902 Kohn described the "chromaffin system," which includes the adrenal medulla, the carotid body, the abdominal paraganglia, and the organ of Zuckerkandl (106). In 1912 Pick coined the term "pheochromocytoma," derived from the Greek phaios (dusky) phio chroma (color) (144). Since then, many investigators, basic scientists as well as physicians, contributed greatly to our present understanding of the chemistry, pathophysiology, diagnosis, and treatment of this fascinating tumor.

INCIDENCE

It is estimated that 35 million Americans have diastolic hypertension. Only 5% of this group are deemed potentially curable. Primary hyperaldosteronism, Cushing's syndrome, renovascular disease, coarctation of the aorta, pheochromocytoma, and hypertension associated with birth control pills are the more common remedial forms of hypertension. Manger and Gifford estimated that about 36,000 persons in the United States have this tumor (119). This figure is based on an incidence of 0.1% in 18 million persons with sustained diastolic hypertension and, on the probability that 50% of patients with pheochromocytoma have paroxysmal hypertension.

An accurate mortality rate from pheochromocytoma is unknown because of the significant number of patients who die with the disease unrecognized. In 1951, Graham estimated that each year 600–800 patients die annually of pheochromocytoma-associated hypertension in the United States. This figure is based on an incidence of 0.47% in the hypertensive population and a mortality rate from hypertension of 175,000 individuals per year.

The exact incidence of pheochromocytoma is also unknown. In the literature, the incidence is as low as 0.09% to as high as 2.2% of patients with diastolic hypertension (50,87,104). Sutton et al. (180) from the Mayo clinic reviewed 54 autopsy-proved cases of pheochromocytoma between 1928 to 1977 and found the autopsy incidence to be 0.13%.

Gitlow et al. felt that the incidence of 0.7% they detected in 1500 consecutive hypertensive subjects was too high since many of these patients were referred to their laboratory to confirm or exclude the diagnosis (66).

ETIOLOGY

The etiology of pheochromocytoma is unknown at the present time. From animal and human data, the following factors may be of some pathogenetic importance: 1) aging; 2) sex; 3) irradiation; 4) genetic predisposition; and 5) hormonal milieu.

Pheochromocytoma is usually a tumor of middle age to elderly. Figure 1 shows the age distribution in 138 patients from the Mayo Clinic (126, 153). There is a preponderance of male over female subjects with pheochromocytoma before puberty. Similarly, in the Wistar rats, male rats are more prone to this tumor than female rats. Irradiated rats developed pheochromocytomas (195). This interesting study showed that 1) parabiosis reduced the incidence of these tumors, especially in female rats, and 2) irradiation sharply increased the incidence of pheochromocytoma in male rats (> 50% in rats 700 days old).

In 1947 Calkins and Howard first described two familial pheochromocytomas (23). By 1968, Steiner and his colleagues collected 75 patients with familial pheochromocytomas from 28 families and added another 10 patients from a single large family (174). The incidence of familial pheochromocytoma is around 10%. This figure is based on the fact that 10% of reported cases have bilateral pheochromocytomas, one-half being familial, and 50% of familial tumors being bilateral. Other characteristics of familial pheochromocytoma include younger age group and no preferential involvement of the right adrenal gland. The mode of inheritance in familial pheochromocytoma is autosomal dominant with a high degree of penetrance. In addition, other diseases with familial preponderance associated with pheochromocytoma include von Recklinghausen's disease, tuberous sclerosis, Sturge–Weber syndrome, and von Hippel-Lindau's disease.

Comparing adult and childhood pheochromocytoma, Hume noted that childhood tumors are characterized by higher incidence of bilateral,

FIGURE 1. Age distribution of 138 patients with pheochromocytoma (1926–1970). (From ref. 153 with permission.)

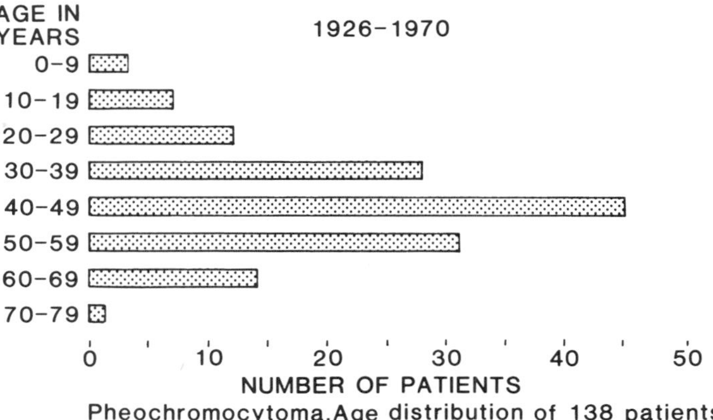

multiple, and ectopic pheochromocytoma with a more rapid and intense course (87). He speculated that endocrine factors associated with the onset of puberty may be of pathogenetic importance. The male predilection prior to puberty has been mentioned earlier. After puberty, most large series suggest a slight female preponderance.

PATHOLOGY

Pheochromocytoma is a tumor of neuroectodermal origin which arises from the chromaffin cells (pheochromocytes) of the sympathoadrenal system. In the past, various terms used to describe catecholamine-producing tumors have caused undue confusion. "Chromaffinoma" is used to describe a tumor that shows an affinity for chromium salts. "Paraganglioma" is used to describe a tumor arising from sympathetic ganglia or other extraadrenal chromaffin cells. To avoid this confusing terminology, many authors, such as Manger and Gifford, have suggested that the term pheochromocytoma be used for any tumor of the chromaffin cell regardless of site.

Embryology and Apudomas

An important concept that has made an impact on our present understanding of the ectopic hormone syndrome in general and the multiple endocrine adenomatosis in particular is the APUD concept which Pearse introduced in 1965 (141). The abbreviations have to do with the staining characteristics of the APUD cell series: flurogenic *A*mine content, amine *P*recursor *U*ptake and the presence of amino acid *D*ecarboxylase activity. The cells in this series all seem to be able to synthesize low molecular weight polypeptide hormones.

The tumors arise from the emigrated neuroectodermal cells comprising the so-called APUDomas (10). These neuroectodermal cells may reside in the adrenal medulla and paraganglia where they differentiate into sympathocytes and pheochromocytes and later transform into respective neoplasms. These neuroectodermal cells may also emigrate to the pituitary gland, pancreas, thyroid (parafollicular cells), stomach, intestine, carotid body, and lung as they accompany the endodermal cells destined to form the fore and midgut organs. These neural crest-derived cells (and their respective neoplasms) retain their original biochemical machinery for synthesis, storage, and release of the neurotransmitter biogenic amines. In support of the APUD concept, many polypeptides have been identified in pheochromocytoma, i.e. methionine-enkephalin, leucine-enkephalin, somatostatin-like immunoreactivity, calcitonin, ACTH, vasoactive intestinal polypeptide, corticotropin-releasing factor, dynorphin, neuropeptide Y, lipotrophin, β-endorphins (31,139,161,178,179). In Hassoun's series (7a), methionine-enkephalin was immunochemically identified in 11 out of 16 and somatostatin in 7 out of 16 patients with pheochromocytoma. Even though immunoreactive lipotrophin and β-endorphin were detected in all 10 patients with pheochromocytoma in

Bertagna's series (13), only three of these patients had clinical evidence of ectopic ACTH syndrome. Neuron specific enlase (NSE) is a potentially useful tumor marker since it is not normally present in adrenal cortex of adrenal cortical tumors (114). Yoshimasa and colleagues (198) reported that the methionine/leucine enkephalin ratio was lower in medullary than extramedullary pheochromocytoma. At the present time, the pathophysiologic significance of these polypeptides remains unclear, but they may assume clinical significance in the near future.

Location, Weight, and Size

It is well established that 85% –90% of all pheochromocytomas are located in the adrenal medulla. Melicow reviewed the experience of 100 patients at Columbia Medical Center; the distribution of these tumors in adults and children are depicted in Figures 2 and 3 (119). (It should be noted that childhood pheochromocyoma tends to be bilateral and multiple.) Manger and his associates claim that multiple pheochromocytoma is present in 8% of adults and 35% of children, a figure that agrees with the figure reported by Hermann and Mornex (80,119). Graham, in a collective review of 204 patients with pheochromocytoma, reported that unilateral (162) bilateral (19) lumbarparavertebral (12), in front of greater abdominal vessels (4), organ of Zuckerkandl (4), thoracic paravertebral (2) celiac ganglion (1) (72). In most of the large series, nonfamilial cases, pheochromocytomas occur more frequently in the right than in the left adrenal gland.

Intrathoracic pheochromocytoma occur in less than 2% of all cases; they usually occur in the posterior mediastinum and are paravertebral in location. An intrapericardial tumor has been reported (14). Other unusual locations include the neck (chemodectomas), intraspinal site, metastases to the skull, meninges and brain, and hilus of the liver.

The weight of pheochromocytoma varies from less than 5 g to 3600 g. In the Mayo Clinic series of 68 pheochromocytomas, the average weight was 100 g (63). Pheochromocytomas associated with paroxysmal hypertension on the average weighed less than those associated in the persistent hypertension. Zelch et al. (199) at the Cleveland Clinic reported that the average weight of pheochromocytoma in this series was around 90 g. Average size of pheochromocytomas in 46 patients was 4.5 cm, although it could reach the size of a football. There seems to be no correlation between size of the tumor and the severity of the pathophysiologic derangement. Although uncommon, it is recognized that even microscopic pheochromocytoma can cause hypertension, especially if it is palpated. Desai (41) reported such a case in a patient with paroxysmal hypertension who had sudden hypertensive episodes when the left adrenal gland was palpated.

Gross, Histological, and Ultrastructural Features

Usually, large tumors are well demarcated with a transparent, fibrous capsule. The cut surface appears yellowish brown or light gray with a

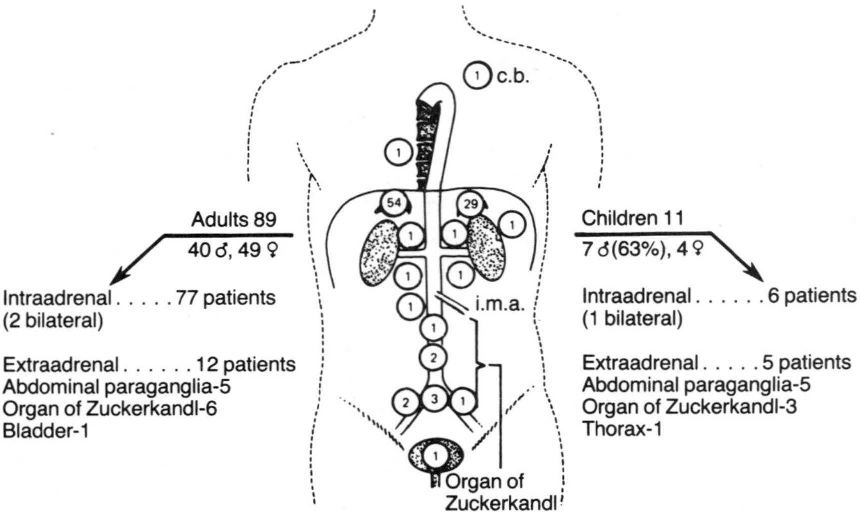

FIGURE 2. Distribution of 107 pheochromocytomas in 100 patients (47 male, 53 female) at Columbia Medical Center. Location: 98% in abdomen, and one tumor in thorax, one in bladder; 83 were intraadrenal and 17 were extraadrenal. Eighty-six percent were functioning, 14% possibly nonfunctioning, 7% malignant, 4% associated with neurofibromatosis. c.b. = carotid body; i.m.a. = inferior mesenteric artery. The numbers within the circles indicate the total number of tumors at that site. (Courtesy of Dr. M. M. Melicow, Columbia Medical Center, New York City, unpublished [123].)

compressible consistency, and it not uncommonly presents certain hemorrhagic, cystic, friable, necrotic areas. Calcium deposits are occasionally found. Larger tumors may have only gelatinous acellular tissue. Rarely, small tumors may be without a capsule but have a picture of adrenal medullary hyperplasia. Recent evidence supports the concept that familial pheochromocytoma and medullary thyroid carcinoma may originate on a background of adrenal medullary hyperplasia and C-cell hyperplasia of the thyroid, respectively. Thus, these small pheochromocytomas with predominant hyperplasic changes may represent an early asymptomatic stage of Sipple's syndrome or it may be a predecessor of the larger, fully encapsulated tumor. Some of the adrenal medulla frequently displaces the normal adrenal cortex to the periphery. The tumor is usually separated from the adrenal cortex by a fibrous capsule but tends to merge imperceptibly into normal medullary tissue.

Microscopically, there are several features that are characteristic of the pheochromocytoma. The cells tend to be larger and more pleomorphic; at times, multinucleated giant cells are found. In addition, colloid droplets are located in the cytoplasm; they vary in size from fine granules to large droplets. Alveolar pattern has been associated with tumor. Symington and Goodall (181) described three cellular patterns associated with pheochromocytomas.

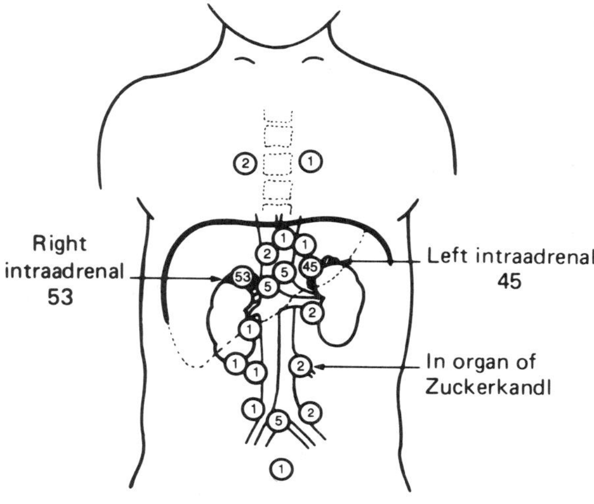

Tumor Incidence

Single tumors ....in 68 children
Multiple tumors ....in 32 children
Intraadrenal tumors only ....in 70 children
Extraadrenal tumors only ....in 22 children
Intra- and extraadrenal tumors ....in 8 children

FIGURE 3. Distribution of 140 pheochromocytomas in 100 children (69 boys, 31 girls). Note: The exact location of six extraadrenal tumors and the side of three intraadrenal tumors were not stated and not included in the diagram. (Courtesy of Dr. M. M. Melicow (with modification), Department of Pathology, Columbia Medical Center, New York, NY [123].)

In pheochromocytoma studies at the Mayo Clinic (153), three cellular patterns were described: epithelial (55%), pleomorphic (43%), and spindle cell (2%). For over a century pathologists have been trying to predict biologic behavior or prognosis on the basis of histologic pattern. Moreover, it is impossible to differentiate benign from malignant pheochromocytoma on the basis of cellular morphology.

It is agreed by most expert pathologists that the presence of metastases is the sole reliable criterion for malignancy. A predominant spindle element in pheochromocytoma has been cited by some authors as a characteristic of malignancy, although most pathologists would disagree with such a claim. Malignant pheochromocytoma metastasize mainly to lymph nodes, liver, and lung bone (123). Another criterion for malignancy is that chromaffin cells are found in sites where paraganglia are not usually found.

It has been known since the end of the 19th century that catecholamine-containing granules stain characteristically brown with chromium salt; thus the term chromaffin cell. Tumor cells in general tend to show a greater diffuse-chromium reaction than normal adrenal medullary cells, and Coupland (32) felt that it may be due to deficient adenosine triphosphate (ATP) binding capacity in the pheochromocytoma cells. More recently, it was found that serotonin and phenolic amines also give a positive reaction to chromium salts (166). Ljungberg et al. (113) found that medullary thyroid carcinoma tissue also gave a positive chromium response, a supporting piece of evidence for the common embryonic origin.

Tumor cells in familial pheochromocytomas are in general similar to the sporadic form in size, shape, nuclear pattern, cellular arrangement, and staining characteristics. They emphasized the point that unlike sporadic pheochromocytoma, moderately advanced pathology may exist in MEN-II (pheochromocytoma, medullary thyroid carcinoma, and hyperparathyroidism) without any detectable clinical or biochemical clue.

In 1970, Tannenbaum (182) reported the ultrastructural characteristics of pheochromocytomas and found a close correlation between the tissue concentration of catecholamines and the morphology of the granules containing these substances. Neither he nor other investigators could find any correlation between morphology and clinical symptomatology. In normal adrenals, these granules vary in length from 100 to 300 nm with a mean of 170 nm; in the pheochromocytoma cell, the mean length of granule is 270 nm. Other noticeable differences include: 1) greater number of mitochondria; 2) more prominent rough-surface endoplasmic reticulum; and 3) Golgi apparatus in juxtanuclear position. In general, tumors with a high epinephrine content tend to have less-dense granules or a greater proportion of granules with lesser density than tumors producing predominantly norepinephrine. Misugi et al. (129) made the observation that catecholamines granules are often associated with the Golgi apparatus and speculated that this intracellular organelle may be synthesizing catecholamines. This speculation was subsequently confirmed in normal chromaffin cells.

CLINICAL MANIFESTATIONS

Signs and Symptoms

It is increasingly clear that most patients with pheochromocytoma do not present in a classic manner with paroxysmal hypertension. Pheochromocytoma can manifest itself in such a kaleidoscopic fashion that it has earned itself the distinction of "The Great Mimic." The variable clinical manifestations in pheochromocytoma may be due to differences in the synthesis of catecholamines and/or differences in the storage and inactivation of catecholamines in the tumor itself.

The signs and symptoms of pheochromocytoma result from release of the catecholamines, epinephrine and norepinephrine. The symptoms and signs in adult patients with pheochromocytoma are shown in Table 1. In general, patients with paroxysmal hypertension have more severe symptomatology than those with sustained hypertension. This should be expected since those with paroxysmal hypertension have higher secretory surge of catecholamines. Recently, Bravo and colleagues from the Cleveland Clinic nicely demonstrated with both physical (head tilt) and

TABLE 1. Symptoms and Signs of Pheochromocytoma[a]

Common	Percent	Less Common	Percent
Hypertension	Over 98	Visual disturbance	3–21
Intermittent hypertens. only	2–50	Constipation	0–13
Sustained hypertens.	50–60	Paresthesias/pains in arms	0–11
Paroxysms superimposed	About 50	Flushing	About 18
Headache	72–92	Acrocyanosis	About 3
Fever	Up to 66	Dyspnea	11–19
Sweating	60–70	Dizziness	3–11
Palpitations ± tachycardia	51–73	Convulsions (grand mal)	3–5
Nervousness	35–40	Bradycardia (noted by patients)	3–8
Weight loss	40–70	Warmth ± heat intolerance	13–15
Funduscopic changes	50–70	Palpable mass in abdomen	10–14
Pallor	28–60	Tightness in throat	About 8
Chest/abdominal pains	22–48	Tinnitus/dysarthria/gagging	3
Nausea ± vomiting	26–43		
Weakness, fatigue	15–38		

[a]Data from Refs. 63,72,119,133,185.

pharmacologic (clonidine) means that the sympathetic nervous system in patients with pheochromocytoma is intact; but Bravo has shown that there are increased stores of norepinephrine at the nerve terminals (18). Any drugs or physical maneuvers which directly or reflexly increase sympathetic activity will cause a sudden release of catecholamines from the sympathetic nerve terminals with or without concomitant rise in the plasma catecholamines. Clinically, the most important and often difficult diagnosis to differentiate from pheochromocytoma is essential hypertension. There are several clinical clues that are characteristic of patients with pheochromocytoma. In untreated patients, up to 65% of patients with pheochromocytoma have orthostatic hypotension. Unlike patients with essential hypertension, the elevated blood pressure in pheochromocytoma patients remains unaltered during sleep (59). Besides, they often experience superimposed hyper/hypotension on top of existing hypertension. Their hypertension is often refractory to antihypertensive agents. Cubeddu et al. (36) recently pointed out another useful clue, namely, patients with pheochromocytoma are exquisitely sensitive to the hypotensive effect of the first dose of prazosin.

Ganguly et al. (60) described a 67-year-old male with catecholamine-secreting glomus jugular tumor who showed rapid cyclic fluctuation of blood pressure between 230/130 to 120/60 mmHg, and in whom fluid replacement plus α-adrenergic blocking agents were needed to stabilize his clinical status. These authors suggested that reflex neurogenic mechanism is involved in these cyclic changes of blood pressure in some patients with pheochromocytoma.

The majority of patients with pheochromocytoma do not secrete much dopamine even though the dopamine β-hydroxylase as well as the dopamine content in pheochromocytoma is higher than the normal adrenal medulla (54,61). Dopamine-secreting pheochromocytomas have been associated with normotension (115).

The most common symptom is headache, which occurs in 92% of patients with paroxysmal hypertension, and in 72% of patients with sustained hypertension in Manger and Gifford's series (119, pp. 88–94). The headache is characteristically throbbing in nature, bilateral, and quite severe during an attack, lasting hours to days. Most often it is occipital and frontal and may wake the patient from sleep. About 28% of patients with sustained hypertension may have a mild to moderate headache indistinguishable from the tension headache.

Sweating occurs in 60%–70% of patients. It is usually generalized, more so in the upper part of the body and occurs during the hypertensive episode. Those with paroxysmal hypertension have more profuse sweating. The exact cause of the sweating is not clear. It has been shown that cholinergic sweat glands can be stimulated by catecholamines, especially epinephrine and parasympathomimetic agents, and sweating can be blocked by parasympathetic blockade. Recent evidence suggests a beta-receptor component to the catecholamine-stimulated sweating (3). A central mechanism by which catecholamines directly affect the temperature-regulation center in the hypothalamus has also been suggested to explain the excess perspiration in pheochromocytoma.

Palpitations with or without tachycardia is the third-most common symptom, occurring in 73% and 51% of those patients with paroxysmal or sustained hypertension. Infusion of epinephrine, not norepinephrine, induces palpitations in normal subjects.

Some patients may have severe chest pain and electrocardiographic changes indistinguishable from a true myocardial infarction. In Graham's extensive review (72), chest pain occurred in 32.4% and 12.8% of patients with paroxysmal and sustained hypertension, respectively. It is well established that catecholamines, especially epinephrine, have a profound effect not only on myocardial blood flow but also on myocardial metabolism and may produce focal myocardial necrosis.

Gastrointestinal complaints such as nausea, vomiting, and epigastric pain are common; sometimes these abdominal complaints led to the misdiagnosis of peptic ulcer, cholecystitis, or acute abdomen. It is interesting that the incidence of cholelithiasis is markedly increased in pheochroocytoma. The mechanism of abdominal pain is unclear. Chronic elevation in catecholamines can impair intestinal motility leading to constipation in some patients.

In the Mayo Clinic series (63), patients with paroxysmal and persistant hypertension, 23% and 41%, respectively, were 10% below the standard body weight. Despite normal or even increased appetite, this weight loss is related to the hypermetabolic state caused by increased circulating catecholamines.

Epinephrine can induce tachycardia and myocardial instability; thus, patients with pheochromocytoma may often have higher pulse rates, especially during a paroxysmal attack. In the series reported by Thomas et al. (185), bradycardia was noted in 3% of patients. This is reflex bradycardia mediated by the vagus nerve during hypertensive episode.

Pallor of the face and upper part of the body was noted in 60% and 28% of patients with paroxysmal and sustained hypertension, respectively (64). In some patients, the flushing may be followed by pallor. In others, a flushed appearance was described even during normotensive periods. Raynaud's phenomena occurred in 3% of patients in Graham's series (72). These vasomotor phenomena could best be explained by the alpha- or beta-receptor stimulation, depending on which catecholamines, norepinephrine and/or epinephrine, predominate. It is possible that other vasoactive substances, serotonin or kallikrein, may be released from pheochromocytoma. Carcinoid tumors have been associated with malignant pheochromocytoma (131). In Manger and Gifford's series, of the patients with sustained hypertension, 53% had grade III, or IV, and 40% had grade I or II, and 5% had normal fundi (119). In those with paroxysmal hypertension, 50% had grade I–II retinopathy; the others were normal. In those with normal fundi, Hollenhorst (84) reported definite arteriolar spasm during paroxysmal attack. He has also pointed out that an important ophthalmologic clue to the diagnosis of pheochromocytoma is that hypertensive retinopathy exists without associated retinal arteriolar sclerosis, especially in a child with hypertension. Some authors reported lacrimation and dilated pupils during such an attack, and attributed these reactions to the effect of epinephrine (85). The retinal changes nearly always improve after the blood pressure is controlled and the pheochromocytoma is removed.

Smithwick et al.(171) found elevated temperature in two-thirds of the patients with pheochromocytoma. This temperature elevation may be present even when the patient is free from a paroxysmal attack. On rare occasions, the temperature may go as high as 105°F in association with marked leucocytosis, and be misdiagnosed as an acute infection (119). The elevation in temperature is due to the heat production of the hypermetabolic state and impaired heat loss due to peripheral vasoconstriction.

A palpable mass in the abdomen may be seen in 10%–14% of patients with pheochromocytoma (72,133). This mass could represent a displaced kidney or the pheochromocytoma itself. It is of diagnostic value but potentially hazardous to maneuver to see if mechanical squeezing of this mass would liberate enough catecholamines to elevate blood pressure and reproduce the patient's symptom. In fact, some physicians could precipitate an attack by mere palpation of the flank or having the patient roll over to one side (119).

A palpable neck mass in a pheochromocytoma patient may represent a chemodectoma, associated medullary thyroid carcinoma, or thyromegaly associated with pheochromocytoma.

There are a few patients with pheochromocytoma who demonstrate harsh systolic and low soft diastolic murmurs which probably result from an increased cardiac output stimulated by catecholamines. In fact, loud murmurs in the apical, pulmonic, and aortic areas have been reported which appeared during or shortly after a paroxysmal attack (119).

Moorhead et al. (133) have done a detailed study on the factors that might precipitate paroxysmal attack in patients with pheochromocytomas. It is especially important when taking a history from a patient with suspected pheochromocytoma to ask the question "Does bending over, stooping, or rolling over to one side in bed bring on these attacks?"

The key to any medical diagnosis is a heightened index of suspicion. Since pheochromocytoma is a curable disease in most cases, it is important to make the diagnosis.

Catecholamine Cardiomyopathy and Electrocardiographic Change

Catecholamines, especially norepinephrine, are known to cause focal myocardial necrosis. Myocarditis, cardiomyopathy, nonobstructive hypertrophic subaortic stenosis, and myocardial infarction have all been associated directly or indirectly with pheochromocytoma (30,76,93,105). Velasquez et al. (192) reported that only 17 out of 60 cases of catecholamine cardiomyopathy in their institution were diagnosed premortem. In their series, the first suggestion of cardiomyopathy in a patient with pheochromocytoma was during echocardiography when a mass was found in the inferior vena cava. Van Vliet et al. (190) at the Mayo Clinic reported that 58% of patients with pheochromocytoma who were autopsied had active myocarditis which they believed to be a direct result of catecholamines. Pathologic features of the myocarditis include focal areas of degeneration and necrosis of myocardial fibers with inflammatory cells, increased fibrosis in those foci, diffuse edema of myocardium, thickening of small- and medium-sized arteries due to edema of intima and media, and moderately severe degrees of coronary sclerosis. Similar pathologic lesions were observed in laboratory animals after repeated injections of catecholamines. Left ventricular failure is frequently associated with active myocarditis even in the absence of hypertension. In fact, hypotension refractory to treatment is seen in some of these patients (9). Surgical resection of pheochromocytoma led to improvement in the cardiomyopathy in some patients.

Myocardial infarction, even in the presence of normal coronary arteries, may occur in patients with pheochromocytoma (119). Radtke et al. (149) from the Mayo Clinic reported that two patients presented with transient cortical blindness and electrocardiographic evidence of transmural infarction and peripheral arterial spasm in whom the diagnosis of pheochromocytoma was later made. Reversal of clinical and biochemical abnormalities followed pharmacologic blockade and surgical resection of the tumor.

Sayer et al. (162) reviewed the electrocardiographic changes in patients with pheochromocytoma. They classified these changes as abnormalities of rhythm or of myocardial ischemia, damage, or strain. They found that arrhythmias most frequently occur during paroxysms of hypertension and may persist even after the blood pressure returned to normal. The changes due to myocardial dysfunction occur transiently during or between attacks and continued in some patients with sustained hypertension. Removal of pheochromocytoma led to complete reversal of the arrhythmias and partial or complete reversal of the electrocardiographic evidence of myocardial dysfunction. Interestingly, the electrocardiographic evidence of myocardial dysfunction may disappear spontaneously during an attack. Saint-Pierre et al. (159) found that ventricular extrasystoles occurred in 50% of pheochromocytoma patients. In general, they substantiated the findings of Sayer's series. These electrocardiographic changes are nonspecific. Recently, Huang (86) reported short PR interval (0.10 sec) narrow QRS and accelerated AV nodal conduction in a patient with pheochromocytoma. All these EKG abnormalities disappeared after tumor was resected. The physician confronting a patient with tachycardia, hypertension or hypotension, sweating, or headache, in addition to these electrocardiographic abnormalities, should think of pheochromocytoma in the differential diagnosis.

Pheochromocytoma in Pregnancy

The first case of pheochromocytoma in pregnancy was diagnosed at autopsy by Kawashima in 1911 (102). It was not until 1955 that the correct diagnosis was made preoperatively by Maloney (117). In Hume's review of the world literature (87), 37 of his 100 cases were associated with pregnancy. Pheochromocytoma could manifest itself in one of several ways: 1) severe preeclampsia; 2) paroxysmal hypertension with typical symptoms; 3) typical symptoms without hypertension; 4) sudden shock and death in the antipartum period; 5) hyperpyrexia after delivery; 6) shock after delivery occuring spontaneously, or induced by anesthesia or delivery itself. Hume pointed out that pheochromocytoma in pregnancy can be confused with toxemia preeclampsia and ruptured uterus; he admonished obstetricians to rule out pheochromocytoma whenever the above-mentioned diseases have been considered. Unlike toxemia, the hypertension of pheochromocytoma is seldom associated with edema or proteinuria, while glycosuria is often present. Congenital neuroblastoma from the fetus causing the typical symptoms of pheochromocytoma have also been reported (194). Peelen and DeGroat in 1955 (143) pointed out that pheochromocytoma if unrecognized in a pregnant woman can be associated with high maternal and fetal mortality, 45% and 32% respectively. The maternal mortality was 16% in Dean's series of 32 pregnancies (39). Symptoms of pheochromocytoma usually appear in the third trimester. Unlike nonpregnant subjects the evidence of paroxysmal hypertension is 80% in their series. In Gemmell's series, symptoms and signs developed in one-third of the patients between the onset of labor and 24 hours after delivery (62).

In Schenker and Chowers' series of 89 cases, two-thirds of the women were multiparas and the rest primigravidas (163). Remission of symptoms was seen in 17 cases. They have observed a higher incidence of visual complaints (17.7%) and convulsions (10%) in these patients when compared to nonpregnant subjects. Fetal movements and mechanical effect of the gravid uterus and uterine contractions (in the last trimester) are also precipitating factors in pregnant pheochromocytoma patients. In Schenker and Chowers' patients, 22% were correctly diagnosed during pregnancy, 35.5% diagnosed postpartum and 39% at postmortem examination. Compared with the maternal mortality of 48%, only 18% died in the group in which the correct diagnosis was made before term. Of this total of 112 pregnancies associated with pheochromocytoma, fetal death was 55%, 16 pregnancies terminated in spontaneous abortion, 23 died in utero, 23 died during birth and early postpartum period. Even among the 22 pregnancies in whom the diagnosis was made before term, fetal wastage was 50%. This high fetal mortality is felt by some authors to be due to the vasoconstrictive effect of maternal catecholamines on the fetal circulation.

Pheochromocytoma in Children

Pheochromocytoma is one of the most common endocrine tumors in children. The clinical manifestations, adrenal pathology, and malignant tendency are different from adult patients with pheochromocytoma. The age distribution described by Stackpole et al. is shown in Figure 4 (173). It occurs as soon as 1 week, with a peak age incidence of 10–12 years. There is male preponderance before puberty in children from Hume's series (71

FIGURE 4. Number of cases of pheochromocytoma in children, according to age. (Data from Stackpole et al. [176].)

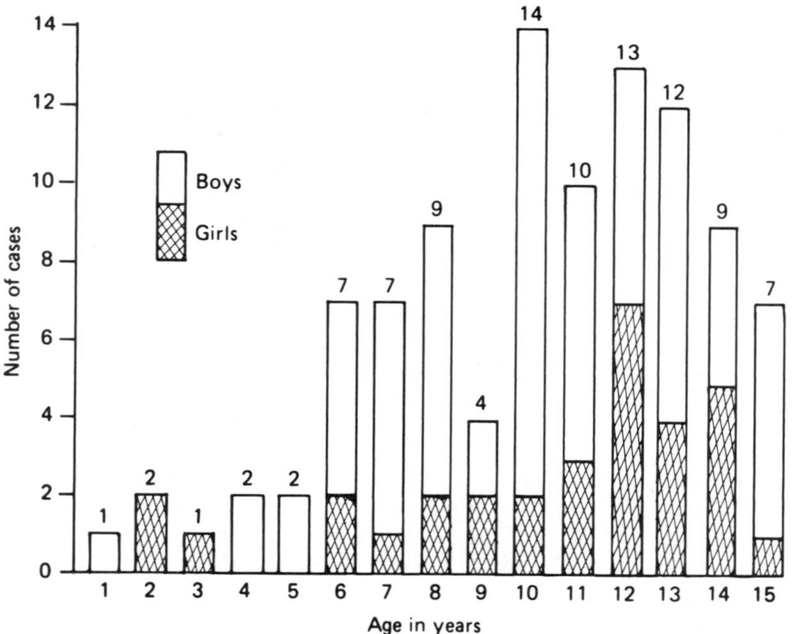

cases) and Stackpole's series (100 cases). The signs and symptoms are tabulated in Table 2.

In both series, sustained hypertension occurs in about 90% of cases in contrast to the 50% in adult pheochromocytoma.

In Hume's series, the average duration of symptoms was 1.5 years and varied between 2 weeks and 9 years. Symptoms which seem to occur more frequently in children than adults include nausea, vomiting, weight loss, sweating, visual changes. In Hume's series, 77% had retinal changes probably due to the high incidence of sustained hypertension. Polyuria and polydipsia are rarely observed in adult patients, whereas they occur in 25% of children with pheochromocytoma. Grand mal seizures and other types of convulsions occur in 23% of children but in less than 5% of adults. Puffy, red, cyanotic appearance of hands was seen in 11% of children but rarely if ever seen in adult patients.

In Stackpole's series, one-third of the 100 cases had multiple, often bilateral tumors and another one-third were extraadrenal in origin. Nine children had more than two tumors and one had as many as six. A 30-year survey (1954–1983) from the Mayo Clinic reemphasized the distinguishing features of childhood pheochromocytomas, namely fewer malignant tumors, more extraadrenal pheochromocytoma, greater bilaterality and multiplicity, increased incidence of familial and MEN syndrome (100). Familial dysautonomia (Riley–Day syndrome) and acrodynia may mimic childhood pheochromocytoma.

Pheochromocytoma of the Bladder

In the newborn child, Coupland (32) has been able to identify multiple chromaffin bodies associated with sympathetic nerve fibers in the perivesical and periprostatic tissues. The first case of true pheochromocytoma of the bladder was reported by Zimmerman et al. in 1953 (200). In a review

TABLE 2. Symptoms and Signs of Pheochromocytoma in Children

Symptoms/Signs	Hume [87](%)	Stackpole [173](%)
1. Hypertension	100	100
Sustained	90	88
Paroxysmal	10	12
2. Headache	81	75
3. Sweating	68	67
4. Nausea & Vomiting	56	48
5. Weight Loss	44	38
6. Visual disturbances	44	37
7. Abdominal pain	35	32
8. Polydipsia and polyuria	25	31
9. Convulsions	23	22
10. Acrocyanosis	11	22

Source: Data from Hume (87) and Stackpole (173).

of the world literature of pheochromocytoma of the bladder, Ochi et al. (138) found a female predominance with an age range between 7 to 78 years, peaking at the second decade. Common clinical manifestations included hypertension, hematuria, and micturitional attacks. The most common sites noted in this review were the trigone and dome. Cystoscopy demonstrated overlying mucosa either intact or with superficial ulcers and tumor in 77% and 84% of the cases, respectively. Typical symptoms of catecholamine release may be precipitated by manipulating the tumor through the cystoscope. Pugh et al. (148) reported a 36-year-old woman who died after cystoscopy, and at autopsy was found to have a bladder pheochromocytoma with metastases to the liver and regional lymph nodes. The most characteristic symptom is micturition-induced hypertension and it was present in 63%, although defecation or sexual intercourse induced hypertension occurred in about 6%. Only 28% had sustained hypertension.

Familial Pheochromocytoma and MEN Syndromes

Calkins and Howard in 1947 reported the first recognized occurrences of familial pheochromocytoma (23). In 1960, Carmen and Brasher (24) reported 10 kindreds with 25 cases of pheochromocytoma. These authors first alerted the medical community to the inherited nature of this disease. By 1968, Steiner et al. (174) collected 75 patients with familial pheochromocytoma from 28 families adding another 10 from a single large kindred. According to Page and Copeland (140), the mode of inheritance is autosomal dominant with a high degree of penetrance. Sporadic pheochromocytoma and familial pheochromocytoma have similar symptoms and signs. However, the two major differences include: 1) tumors in familial pheochromocytoma are usually bilateral; 2) familial pheochromocytoma is associated with other genetic diseases, i.e., neurocutaneous dysplasias and the multiple endocrine neoplasia (MEN) types IIa and III.

In 1932 Eisenberg and Wallerstein (49) first described the association of other endocrine tumors with pheochromocytoma. In 1961, Sipple (167) first described the association of pheochromocytoma with thyroid carcinoma and parathyroid adenomas or hyperplasia. By 1975, there were over 200 cases of Sipple's syndrome reported (119). Table 3 shows the MEN syndromes. As shown, pheochromocytoma is not part of MEN-I syndrome, whereas it definitely is part of types IIa and IIb and the neurocutaneous syndromes (von Recklinghausen's disease and von Hippel-Lindau disease.

Thyroid carcinoma is found in 23% of familial pheochromocytoma (174); it accounts for less than 10% of thyroid cancer. Recently, Minopoli and Bordi (128) pointed out the changing patterns of sex distribution in familial medullary thyroid carcinoma associated with pheochromocytoma. Prior to 1973, 49 kindreds with familial form of medullary thyroid carcinoma affecting 220 members showed a predominance of female subjects presenting with medullary thyroid carcinoma and male subjects presenting with pheochromocytoma. However, after 1973 this sex distri-

TABLE 3. Inherited Pheochromocytoma: MEN Syndromes

Tissue	MEN (Wermer's)	MEN-II or IIa (Sipple's)	MEN-III or IIb (mucosal neuroma syndrome)	Phakomatosis (von Recklinghausen's and von Hippel-Lindau's)
Adrenal	—	PHEO	PHEO	PHEO
Thyroid	—	Medullary carcinoma	Medullary carcinoma	—
Parathyroid	+	+	Rare	—
Nervous system	—		Neuromas, ganglioneuromas	Neurofibromas, retinal-cerebellar hemangioblastomas
Pancreas	Islet cell tumors (β and non-β cell)	—	—	—
Pituitary	Adenomas	—	—	—
Gut		—	—	—

bution pattern disappeared. These authors attributed this change to a different diagnostic approach, namely, the routine use of serum calcitonin to screen asymptomatic members of patients with medullary thyroid carcinoma. The same authors noted a decrease in the overall incidence of pheochromocytoma in kindreds reported from 1974 to 1979 as compared to earlier reports. It is possible that medullary thyroid carcinomas secrete vasoactive substances that counterbalance the hypertensive effect of circulating catecholamines. Hill et al. (81) at M. D. Anderson Hospital reported that pheochromocytoma in patients with medullary carcinoma of the thyroid is always located in the adrenal gland.

In Sipple's syndrome, pheochromocytomas develop upon a background of diffuse adrenal medullary hyperplasia analogous to the C-cell hyperplasia preceding medullary carcinoma of the thyroid. In Steiner's review in 1968 (174), parathyroid adenomas or chief cell hyperplasia occurred in 5 of 85 cases of pheochromocytoma whereas Catalona (28) reported an incidence of 50 percent in patients with Sipple's syndrome. Whether or not the parathyroid hyperplasia is secondary to hypocalcemia or part of the genetic aberration is still a controversial subject. Pearse (142) has presented evidence that the parathyroid gland is also derived from the neuroectoderm. Hypercalcemia due to excess parathyroid hormone has been associated with pheochromocytoma which is corrected upon surgical extirpation of the adrenal hormone (110). It has been suggested that catecholamines directly increase the secretion of parathyroid hormone. However, Miller et al. (126) felt that catecholamines do not have a stimulating effect on the parathyroid hormone secretion and that parathyroid disease seen in pheochromocytoma is a genetically determined part of MEN type II, syndrome.

Multiple mucosal neuromas of eyelids, conjunctiva, lips, or tongue have been described in some patients with Sipple's syndrome (103). Gorlin et al. (71) in 1968 reviewed the world's literature and found 17 patients with these neuromas, nine with medullary carcinoma of the thyroid and 10 others with pheochromocytoma. In addition, three patients had a marfanoid habitus, two had colonic diverticulosis, one presented with diffuse ganglioneuromatosis of the intestinal tract, and eight showed medullated corneal nerve. Occasionally, acromegalic facies has been described. Medullary carcinoma of the thyroid and alimentary tract ganglioneuromatosis are the major components of MEN type IIb as recently emphasized in a report by Carney et al. (26) from the Mayo Clinic. In this report, nine of 16 patients were found with diffuse ganglioneuromatosis extending from lips to rectum; six of these patients had diarrhea or constipation or both. Megacolon in five patients and diverticulosis in one was noted. In this report, 94% had bilateral adrenal medullary disease, 81% with skeletal anomalies (marfanoid habitus, pes cavus, slipped femoral capital epiphyses, pectus excavatum, and scoliosis). Carney et al. (27) emphasized the importance of recognizing these gastrointestinal manifestations of MEN syndrome because 14 of the 16 patients developed such symptoms prior to the discovery of the endocrine tumors. WDHA syndrome (watery diarrhea, hypokalemia, and achlorhydria), described by Verner and Morrison in 1958, is thought to be due to increased elaboration of vasoactive intestinal peptide (VIP) or prostaglandins by tumors or hyperplasia of the pancreatic islets (91). Since then, nonpancreatic tumors producing WDHA syndromes have been described in ganglioneuroma and pheochromocytoma (187). The watery diarrhea was associated with high serum and tumor levels of VIP. In these cases VIP levels and gut function returned to normal after surgical removal of the tumor. These findings further linked VIP with neural crest tissues and emphasize the importance of measuring catecholamines in patients with WDHA syndrome. In short, the recently recognized variant of MEN type II, namely the type IIb, consists of not only MCT, pheochromocytoma, hyperparathyroidism, but also neuromas, marfanoid habitus, characteristic facies, intestinal ganglioneuromatosis, skeletal abnormalities, and, rarely, myopathy. This association of mucosal and marfanoid habitus with pheochromocytoma and MCT is not seen in the usual MEN type II patients. Thus, this constellation of findings is now called MEN type III (or type IIB). The incidence of parathyroid abnormality is 2.4% in MEN type IIb, whereas it is as high as 54% in MEN type III. MEN type III can occur either sporadically or in an autosomal dominant pattern. Cerny et al. (29) and others pointed out that the histologic findings in MEN type II syndrome are consistent with Knudson's two mutational event theory for the initiation of neoplasia with adrenal medullary hyperplasia representing the first genetic mutational event. Recently, there are several reports of mixtures of MEN types I and II (2).

Malignant Pheochromocytoma

In 1924, Gravier (73) reported the first case of malignant pheochromocytoma. Graham's comprehensive review of the world literature (72) in 1951

(207 cases) reported the incidence of malignant pheochromocytoma to be around 9%. In 1955, Davis et al. (38) recommended that before the diagnosis of malignant pheochromocytoma was made, metastases should be demonstrated at a site where chromaffin tissue is not normally found, and hormonal function of the metastases proven. His criteria for malignancy have been widely accepted. In a review of 138 patients from the Mayo Clinic (153), the incidence of malignant pheochromocytoma was 13.1%. In Gittes and Mahoney's series of 38 patients with pheochromocytoma, they found an incidence of 19.1% (68). The incidence of malignant pheochromocytoma in children is lower than that in adults. Remine et al. reported a considerably higher incidence of malignancy in extra-adrenal pheochromocytoma as compared to adrenal pheochromocytoma, 28.6% and 11.3%, respectively (153). In addition, there seems to be a higher incidence of malignancy in familial pheochromocytoma than in sporadic cases. Carney et al. from the Mayo Clinic reported an incidence of 26.6% (25). One reason for this higher incidence may be due to the delay in diagnosis since in Carney's series six out of 15 patients were normotensive.

Remine et al. reported that 72.3% of their patients (18 cases) with malignant pheochromocytoma were female, the remainder were male (153). The role of estrogen in the possible pathogenesis of malignant pheochromocytoma remains unclear. Even though clinically it is almost impossible to differentiate malignant from benign pheochromocytoma, it is of some interest to note that tumors providing paroxysmal hypertension are rarely malignant. In addition, malignant pheochromocytoma may present as hypotensive crises (9). Melicow et al. presented a patient with malignant nonfunctional pheochromocytoma of the organ of Zuckerkandl masquerading as a primary carcinoma of the prostate with metastases (123).

Shapiro et al. (165) from the University of Michigan recently reviewed their experience with malignant pheochromocytoma. In their series, the mean time for diagnosis was 9.18 years and the mean duration of known metastasis was 3.71 years. Metastases to the skeletal system occurs most commonly in malignant pheochromocytoma. In Schonebeck's series of 41 patients with malignant pheochromocytoma, the distribution and frequency of metastases are: skeletal (44%), liver (37%), lymph node (37%), lungs (27%), central nervous system (10%), pleurae (10%), kidney (5%), pancreas (2%), and omentum (2%) (163a). Thus, in the preoperative evaluation of any patient with pheochromocytoma it is important to do appropriate radiologic studies looking for possible metastases. James et al. (92) reviewed the roentgenographic aspects of metastatic pheochromocytoma. The skeletal metastases are osteolytic-resembling metastases from thyroid, renal-cell carcinoma, and bronchogenic carcinoma. Pulmonary metastases appear as multiple, small, modular lesions with intermittent or recurrent pleural effusion.

Morphologically, all of the 30 patients in Shapiro's series had mitotic figures, pleomorphism, necrosis, capsular or vascular invasion. Unfortunately, there were no histological features which could predict the extent of the tumor spread. In this series, Zellballen pattern was found to be more prominent in the extraadrenal than intraadrenal pheochromocytoma.

Biochemically, malignant pheochromocytoma behaves the same as the benign tumor. Anton et al. (5) in 1967 reported that the presence of dopamine, or its precursor dopa, indicated malignancy but this has not been confirmed by subsequent studies. Recurrent pheochromocytoma symptoms and signs in a patient with surgical correction of the primary tumor is strongly suggestive of malignancy. In Remine's series (153), the mean time for recurrence was 5.6 years postoperatively. However, recurrences may appear as long as 20 years after excision of the primary tumor.

Neuroectodermal Dysplasias and Other Associated Diseases

Neuroectodermal dysplasias are disorders with central nervous system manifestations associated with skin lesions. Von Recklinghausen's disease, tuberous sclerosis, Sturge–Weber syndrome, and von Hippel-Landau's disease are associated with pheochromocytoma.

Von Recklinghausen's disease is characterized by multiple neurofibromas of peripheral nerves that are frequently associated with skin conditions such as cafe-au-lait spots, nevi, hairy nevi, and skin polyps. Neurofibromatosis occurs in about 5% of patients with pheochromocytoma although some authors claim it to be as high as 23% (119,158). Conversely, the incidence of pheochromocytoma in neurofibromatosis is low, between 1% and 2% at most. Neurofibromatosis is associated with many vascular anomalies, i.e., coarctation of the aorta, renal artery stenosis, or renal artery aneurysm which may cause hypertension in the absence of associated pheochromocytoma.

Retinal malformations, angiomatosis of retina associated with cystic cerebellar hemangioblastomas, is known as von Hippel-Landau's disease. Besides the association with pheochromocytoma, mucosal neuroma, and cafe-au-lait spots have also been described. Atuk et al. (7) reported a kindred with familial pheochromocytoma associated with von Hippel-Lindau disease in whom seven out of 13 of the affected members presented with pheochromocytoma. Recently, Ducatman et al. (46) presented 10 cases of renal cell carcinoma associated with pheochromocytoma and suggested that it may be a manifestation of von Hippel-Lindau disease. The Sturge–Weber syndrome is characterized by facial hemangioma or port wine stain over the distribution of trigeminal nerve associated with malformation of brain and meninges.

Many other endocrine diseases can be associated with pheochromocytoma. Acromegaly has been reported in a few patients with pheochromocytoma either concurrently or separately (4,125). The author is personally familiar with a patient presenting with diabetic ketoacidosis who was later discovered to have acromegaly and pheochromocytoma. As mentioned before, chronic administration of growth hormone in rats leads to the development of adrenal medullary tumors (132). In normal subjects, infusion of phenylsynephrine or methoxamine caused an increase in growth hormone levels (88). Elevated growth hormones have been noted by Nakano et al. in three patients with pheochromocytoma (135). It is speculative at this time to say that excessive catecholamines might induce an overproduction of growth hormone ultimately resulting in a pituitary tumor.

Cushing's syndrome, Addison's disease, and adrenal virilism have been reported in patients with pheochromocytoma (136,154,174). Adrenocorticotrophic hormone (ACTH) or ACTH-like material is known to originate from the pheochromocytoma itself, from MCT, or from pituitary tumors. In addition, pheochromocytoma can elaborate cortisol in vitro (134). A patient with both pheochromocytoma and adrenal cortical hyperplasia has been reported. It is well established that corticosteroids are required for norepinephrine to exert a vasoconstrictor effect. In theory, excess catecholamines can reduce the response of the adrenal cortex to ACTH. Mulrow et al. (134) reported two pheochromocytoma patients with diminished adrenocortical activity preoperatively who required both steroids and pressor agents postoperatively to maintain normal blood pressure. Ramsay and Langlands (150) pointed out the complexity of the corticomedullary relationship in patients with pheochromocytoma with much person-to-person variation. ACTH infusion precipitated hypertension in one pheochromocytoma patient.

Gallstones have been frequently associated with pheochromocytoma (104). Presence of gallstones in normal population is said to be about 6%, whereas the incidence triples in patients with pheochromocytoma. The explanation for this increased incidence is unclear.

DRUG-INDUCED HYPERTENSIVE CRISES

The drugs that can cause symptoms and signs indistinguishable from paroxysmal attacks of pheochromocytoma should be noted. Most notorious among them are the hypertensive crises in patients taking monoamine oxidase inhibitors, which are used to treat psychiatric illnesses, tuberculosis, and hypertension. Other drugs include clonidine withdrawal (usually within 12 hrs and after large doses), surreptitious administration of isoproterenol, ephedrine and theoephedrine, metaraminol, norepinephrine, antiemetics, and amphetamines. Tricyclic antidepressants produce pseudosymptoms of pheochromocytoma by their inhibition of the re-uptake and degradation of catecholamines by the adrenergic neurons (101). Chemotherapy for lymphoma, insulin hypoglycemia, and intravenously administered propanolol have been reported to precipitate hypertensive crises, pulmonary edema, and shock in patients with pheochromocytoma (170,184).

Adrenal glucocorticoids can precipitate a hypertensive paroxysm either by increasing the secretion of catecholamines directly or by potentiating the peripheral pressor effect to the catecholamines (37). Dunn et al. (47) recently reported that Saralasin, the angiotensin antagonist, precipitated a pheochromocytoma crisis. Therefore, it is very important for a clinician to elicit a drug history in anyone suspected of having symptoms and signs of pheochromocytoma. In an emotionally unstable patient who might have access to the above drugs, the index of suspicion should be high that the pheochromocytoma-like symptoms and signs are not due to a tumor, but instead self-induced. Ingestion of certain foods containing high concentrations of tyramine (sherry, beer, cheddar cheese, yeast extracts, pickled herring) or simultaneous use of sympathomimetic agents (amphetamines, ephedrine, imipramine, amitriptyline) plus MAO inhibitors, may precipitate these attacks (121).

DIAGNOSIS

The key to any medical diagnosis is a high index of suspicion on the part of the clinician. Howard's three Hs (hypermetabolism, hypertension, hyperglycemia) are well known to most physicians (85). As shown in the previous discussion, headache and palpitations should be added to the above clinical manifestations. In general, seven groups of patients need to be screened: 1) all symptomatic patients with sustained or paroxysmal hypertension; 2) asymptomatic patients, especially young patients or those with diseases associated with pheochromocytoma; 3) all patients with MEN types IIa and IIb and their first degree relatives even though they are asymptomatic and normotensive; 4) hypertensive patients refractory to the usual antihypertensive agents or who show paradoxical hypertensive responses; 5) patients who suddenly become hypertensive at delivery, during an invasive procedure surgery, or TRH testing; 6) patients who become hypertensive when treated with imipramine or desipramine; 7) hypertensive patients who develop symptomatic orthostatic hypotension after the single dose of prazosin.

The basis for laboratory diagnosis is to demonstrate abnormally high catecholamines and/or their metabolites in the urine or blood of a patient suspected of pheochromocytoma. Pioneer work by Engel and von Euler in 1950–1954 showed urinary catecholamines in patients with pheochromocytoma to be invariably high (50). Since then, extensive experience at the National Institutes of Health, Mayo Clinic, Cleveland Clinic, and at Mount Sinai Hospital in New York have substantiated the indisputable value of 24-hour urinary catecholamines or metabolites in confirming or excluding the diagnosis of pheochromocytoma (33,40,66,153). If these tests are done properly, the modern assays for catecholamines are not only specific but also sensitive. Even when normotensive, it is rare to have normal urinary free catecholamines, vanillylmandelic acid (VMA), and total metanephrines values in pheochromocytoma (Fig. 5). It is estimated that in only 1–2% of pheochromocytomas, the urinary catecholamines and metabolites are within normal limits. In these cases one needs to resort to provocative tests.

The methods for measuring catecholamines and their metabolites is beyond the scope of this chapter. Interested readers are referred to reviews on this topic (34,53,94,120,145,197). VMA is the oldest, cheapest, and most nonspecific test of all of the assays. The older colorimetric methods of measuring VMA often led to a high normal range of 10–15 mg/day. More specific and accurate methods using bidirectional paper chromatography and gas-liquid chromatography are used by most laboratories today. The normal adult excretion of VMA is less than 6.8 mg/day or

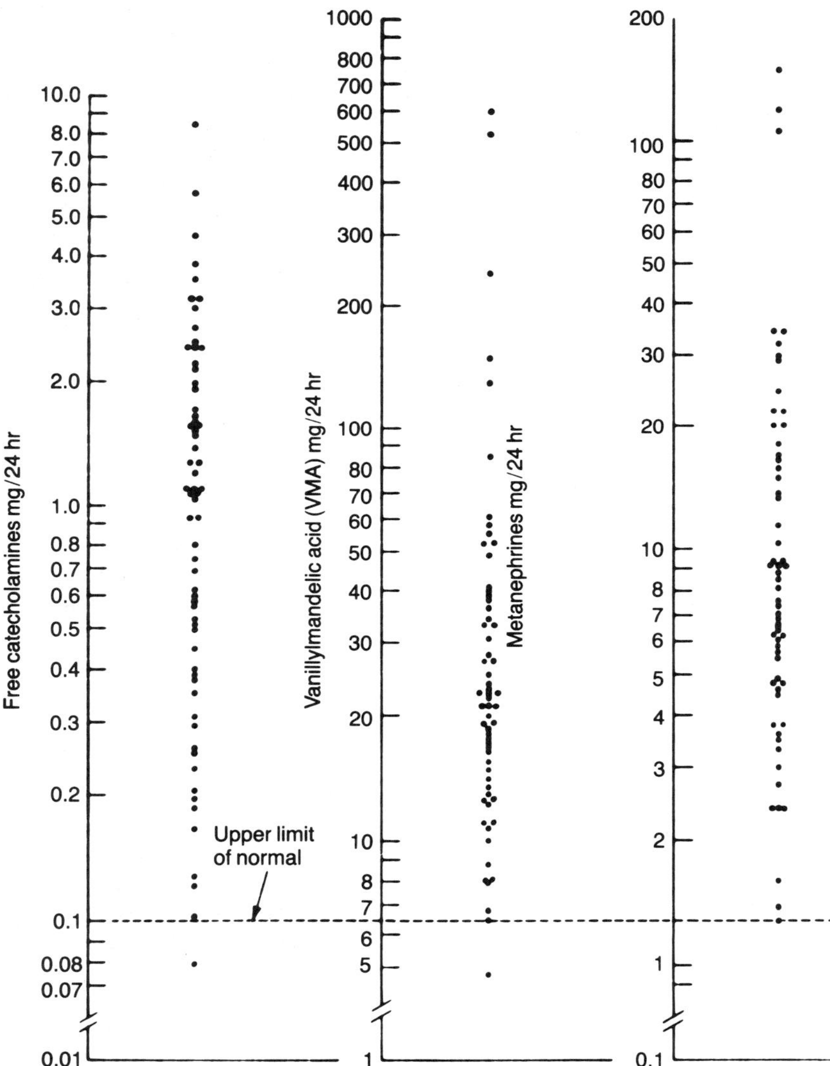

FIGURE 5. Urinary excretion of catecholamines and metabolites in pheochromocytoma. Summary of results of urinary assays on 64 patients with proven pheochromocytoma, representing the experience of the Experimental Therapeutics Branch of the National Institutes of Health up until 1966. The range of values was so great that it required use of differing logarithmic scales. The horizontal broken line designates the upper limits of normal, these being catecholamines = 0.1 mg, vanillylmandelic acid (VMA) = 6.5 mg, and metanephrines = 1.3 mg/day. (Data from Sjoerdsma et. al. [169a].)

0.20–3.5 μg/mg creatinine. Values over 5 μg/mg creatinine are diagnostic of pheochromocytoma. Metanephrines are more consistently elevated in pheochromocytoma patients than VMA or catecholamines and are felt by most authorities to be the best single screening test for pheochromocytoma. The upper limit of normal is 1.3 mg/day using the Pisano method, and if over 2.5 mg/day, it is indicative of pheochromocytoma. However, in Modlin et al.'s series (130) of 72 patients with pheochromocytoma, urinary VMA was elevated in all except one. In van Heerden's review of 106 pheochromocytoma patients operated at the Mayo Clinic, urinary metanephrines were elevated in 95% and VMA in 89% of patients. Only two patients in this series had normal urinary values. Dopamine and its metabolite, homovanillic acid (HVA), are not consistently elevated in pheochromocytoma unless one is dealing with malignant pheochromocytoma or neuroblastoma. Technically speaking, the flurometric methods for determining catecholamines (norepinephrine and epinephrine) are less demanding than those used for measuring metanephrine, and may be elevated following an attack. If completeness of urine collection is questioned, catecholamines or metabolites should be expressed in milligrams of creatinine. This allows short-term collection (2–4 hours) and makes these tests most useful in suspected pheochromocytoma patients with renal insufficiency. Kaplan et al. have shown that urinary metanephrines from single voided urines correlated quite well with 24-hour specimens (97). Table 4 shows normal ranges of urinary catecholamines for children (65). The variability of urinary values with age is readily apparent.

Many drugs, dietary substances, x-ray contrast dyes, and fluorescent substances may interfere with or alter the urinary excretion of catecholamines (15). Methyldopa leads to the highest levels of falsely elevated urinary catecholamines by flurometric methods. Other drugs which could falsely elevate urinary catecholamines include theophylline, ephedrine, levodopa, trifluoperazine, nitroprusside, methyl-glucamine (component of radioopaque contrast media), tricyclic antidepressants, especially desipramine, and clonidine withdrawal. In general, it is wise to ask patients suspected of pheochromocytoma to discontinue all medication at least for

TABLE 4. Excretion of Catecholamine Metabolites by Normal Children[a]

Subjects	Age	VMA Mean	VMA S.D.	HVA Mean	HVA S.D.	M + NM Mean	M + NM S.D.
43	1–12 mo	6.9	± 3.2	12.9	± 9.58	1.64	± 1.32
15	1–2 yr	4.6	± 2.22	12.6	± 6.26	1.68	± 1.13
21	2–5 yr	3.95	± 1.72	7.58	± 3.56	1.25	± 0.77
23	5–10 yr	3.3	± 1.40	4.7	± 2.66	1.13	± 0.78
24	10–15 yr	1.91	± 0.77	2.5	± 2.42	0.60	± 0.48
14	15–18 yr	1.34	± 0.61	1.0	± 0.65	0.24	± 0.23

Source: Data from Gitlow et al. (65).

[a]Excretion in urine expressed as micrograms per milligram of creatinine. VMA=vanillylmandelic acid: HVA=homovanillic acid; M=metanephrine; NM=normetanephrine; S.D.=standard deviation.

1 week before urinary assay. The major drawback with metanephrines is that stress of any kind, i.e., congestive heart failure, shock, sepsis and increased intracranial pressure, will lead to falsely elevated levels. Iron deficiency has also been known to falsely elevate urinary VMA and norepinephrine levels (193). Urinary epinephrine, dopamine, and total metanephrine are normal in iron deficiency.

Pheochromocytoma patients with paroxysmal hypertension usually have elevated 24-hour urinary catecholamines and metabolites. Occasionally, the 24-hour values are normal. In these cases, urine needs to be collected shortly after an attack, spontaneous or provoked.

Fractionated urinary catecholamines may be helpful not only in the localization of pheochromocytoma but also in separating those with essential hypertension from those with pheochromocytoma (8,146). If the urinary content of epinephrine and/or norepinephrine are elevated, the patient's pheochromocytoma is most likely intraadrenal. Although there are epinephrine-producing tumors in the bladder and lung, epinephrine production is primarily confined to the adrenal gland. Moreover, the conversion of norepinephrine to epinephrine requires the presence of cortisol. Hamilton et al. (77) reported that urinary epinephrine over 20 μg/day is characteristic of pheochromocytoma in MEN type II syndrome. Ganguly et al. (59) reported that urinary norepinephrine during sleep was sevenfold higher in patients with pheochromocytoma when compared to those with essential hypertension.

Atuk et al. (7) reported a significant correlation between urinary free catecholamines, blood pressure level, and free catecholamines levels in familial pheochromocytoma. They advanced the concept that the metabolism of catecholamines as well as clinical manifestations may be altered by the aging process.

Plasma Catecholamines

Cryer (35) reviewed the various conditions associated with elevated plasma catecholamines. Hemodynamic effects are first observed when plasma norepinephrine reaches between 1500 to 2000 pg/mL or 10 times the basal levels. Except during heavy exercise, most stressful situations studied such as hypoglycemia, myocardial infarction, surgery failed to elevate plasma norepinephrine over 1500 pg/mL. For epinephrine, hemodynamic effects are seen when level reaches the 50 to 100 pg/mL range. This level of epinephrine is seen in many of the conditions studied, such as during heavy exercise, cigarette smoking, mild hypoglycemia, moderate exercise, myocardial infarction, ketoacidosis and surgery. In this review, 15 patients with pheochromocytomas had mean plasma norepinephrine levels over 2000 pg/mL and epinephrine levels of 280 pg/mL, a value reached by most the aforementioned stressful conditions.

Because of the inherent problems associated with urinary catecholamines determinations such as dietary or drug interference, incomplete urine collection, dependence on intact renal function and catecholomethyltransferase and monoamine oxidase activities, a great deal of effort in recent years has been devoted to the development of sensitive and specific methods to measure plasma catecholamines. Interested readers are directed to the recent reviews on the various techniques for the determination of plasma catecholamines by Raum (151) and Hjemdahl (83). Bravo et al. (19) from the Cleveland Clinic cited several advantages of measuring plasma catecholamines over urinary catecholamines in confirming the diagnosis of pheochromocytoma. First of all, it obviates the need to collect the 24-hour urine. Second, blood is conveniently collected immediately before and after a provocative test and one could correlate catecholamine levels with changes in blood pressure. Third, spontaneous or provoked, changes in catecholamine production could be correlated with the patient's cardiovascular status. In their experience, plasma catecholamines less than 1000 ng/L rules out pheochromocytoma whereas values over 2000 ng/L are almost diagnostic of this disease. In a recent review, the same group reported the superiority of plasma catecholamines over the urinary catecholamines (Figure 6) (19).

There are patients, including those in Bravo's own series, who had

FIGURE 6. Comparison of simultaneously measured indexes of catecholamine production in 43 patients with surgically confirmed pheochromocytoma. The horizontal broken lines represent the the 95% upper confidence limits (i.e., 950 pg/mL) of plasma catecholamine values in 70 subjects with essential hypertension. The broken vertical lines indicate the 95% upper confidence limits of values for urinary vanilmandelic acid (VMA) (i.e., 11 mg/24 hours) and urinary metanephrines (MN) (i.e., 1.8 mg/24 hours) in 30 subjects with essential hypertension. NE + E denotes norepinephrine plus epinephrine. Solid symbols denote false negative tests. All determinations were performed in hospitalized patients. To convert MN and VMA values to micromoles per liter, multiply by 5.265 and 5.046, respectively; to convert NE + E values to nanomoles per liter, convert to micrograms per liter and multiply by 5.911. Data from Bravo and Gifford (19).

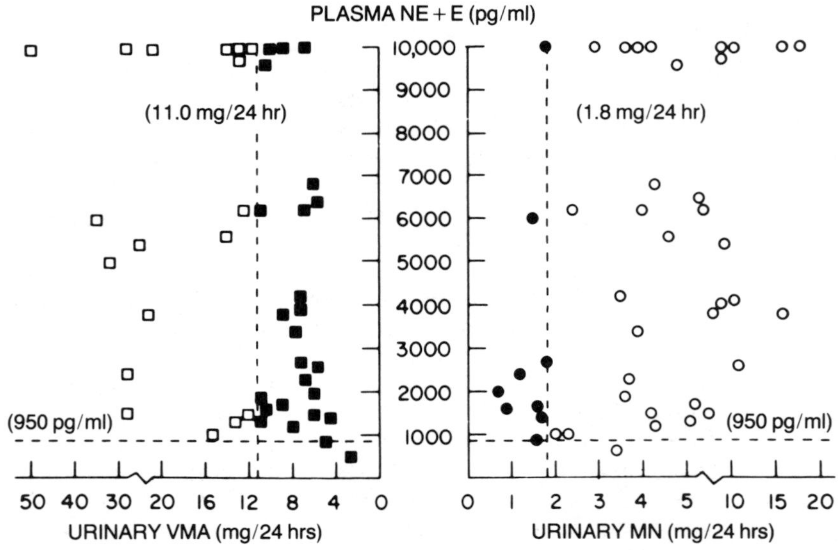

normal plasma catecholamines but abnormal urinary catecholamines. Kaplan (99) pointed out that most published series found a 10 to 30 percent of pheochromocytoma patients who show a falsely negative plasma catecholamine value. Messerli et al. (124) reported patients with pheochromocytoma in the bladder who had repeatedly normal 24-hour urinary catecholamines but well-documented rises in plasma norepinephrine after micturition.

Regardless of which test is superior, certain precautions should be noted when obtaining plasma catecholamines in patients suspected of harboring pheochromocytoma. First, the stress from venipuncture could falsely elevate plasma catecholamines. Therefore, it is important to have the subject in the spine position for 1 hour after placement of an indwelling venous catheter. Second, the red blood cells must be separated from the plasma within 5 minutes because red blood cells and platelets can avidly concentrate catecholamines (8,201). Third, erroneous plasma norepinephrine levels have been reported since radioimmunoassay measures both free and conjugated norepinephrine, whereas the radioenzymatic assay measures only free norepinephrine (6).

Diagnostically, pheochromocytoma could be classified as large or small corresponding to the level of catecholamine secreted. Thus, chronic exposure to a high level of catecholamines leads to down regulation of adrenoreceptors in patients with pheochromocytoma (74). This phenomenon might explain why moderately severe hypertension only occurs in large tumor with plasma norepinephrine many times higher than the smaller ones. It is almost impossible to differentiate patients with small tumors from conditions such as stressful situations, anxiety, or drugs because the rise in plasma catecholamines in these patients is usually less than twofold over basal levels. Brown et al. (21) recently reported the diagnostic utility of plasma norepinephrine and dihydroxyphenylglycol in those patients with borderline elevation of plasma norepinephrine. Kuchel et al. (109) found no correlation between free or conjugated catecholamines and blood pressure or heart rate in 17 patients with pheochromocytoma. However, they did find that conjugated dopamine levels were negatively correlated with both systolic and diastolic blood pressure and that free dopamine level was positively correlated with heart rate.

Provocative Tests: Physical and Chemical

Before the development of sensitive and specific chemical assays for urinary and plasma catecholamines and their metabolites, physicians relied heavily on provocative tests (histamine, tyramine, glucagon) for the diagnosis of pheochromocytoma. At present, there are three reasons why these tests are rarely used: 1) the high prevalence of both false negative and false positive reactions; 2) the possibility of a fatal complication such as shock, cerebral hemorrhage, cerebral vascular accident, or myocardial infarction; 3) the tests are diagnostically inferior to the urinary catecholamines and metabolites measurements.

Glucagon stimulates epinephrine release from the adrenal gland. The glucagon test was felt by many to be the safest and most accurate provocative test form confirming the diagnosis of pheochromocytoma in the past (108). Kaplan (99) states that the only rational use of this test is to identify bilateral medullary hyperplasia in patients with medullary carcinoma of the thyroid in whom the control urine metanephrine values are within the normal range. A positive test requires a threefold rise in plasma catecholamines 1 to 3 minutes after the administration of 1 to 2 mg of glucagon. Concomitant rise of blood pressure, 20/15 mmHg above the pressor response to a cold pressor test is felt by Bravo's group to be desirable (19). For optimal accuracy, this test must be done in a controlled environment, plasma catecholamines determined at the time of peak blood pressure, and plasma values interpreted with regards to responses in normal control subjects. Levinson (112) reported that the plasma norepinephrine response, not epinephrine, predicted the presence or absence of pheochromocytoma in 27 out of 28 patients.

Since 1981 the clonidine suppression test has been shown to be a useful adjunct in the diagnosis of pheochromocytoma by Bravo et al. at the Cleveland Clinic (17). This drug is a centrally acting α-adrenergic agonist which suppresses the release of neurally mediated catecholamine release. The principle behind this suppression test is that the activation of the sympathetic nervous system mediates that normal rise in plasma catecholamines in nonpheochromocytoma subjects whereas in pheochromocytoma patients the rise in plasma catecholamines is the result of diffusion of excess catecholamines into the systemic circulation from the tumor itself. After the administration of an oral dose (0.3 mg), Bravo's group found that the plasma norepinephrine levels in patients with essential hypertension fell to below the normal range but those with pheochromocytoma remained elevated (17). A normal response to clonidine consists of a fall in basal values of norepinephrine and epinephrine to a level below 500 pg/mL in 2–3 hours after drug administration (see Fig. 7). Symptomatic hypotension has been reported to be a serious side effect of this suppression test (22,69). However, Bravo's group argued that this side effect is seen only in patients on concurrent antihypertensive agents. His group made several suggestions when performing this test. First, this should be contraindicated in patients with marked volume depletion. Second, β-adrenergic blocking drugs should be discontinued 48 hours before the test. Third, use only the radioenzymatic assay because it only measures free norepinephrine.

In Europe, Brown et al. (20) have recently popularized another suppression test with pentolinium. This is a preganglionic blocking agent which abolishes the physiologic stimulation of catecholamines secretion but not the autonomous secretion from the tumor. In his series, 18 patients with the tumor failed to show suppression of plasma catecholamines whereas it did suppress the plasma catecholamines in 20 patients with intermittently elevated values. One definite advantage of this suppression test over the clonidine suppression test is that it can be done in the out-patient setting and thus avoid the cost of hospitalization.

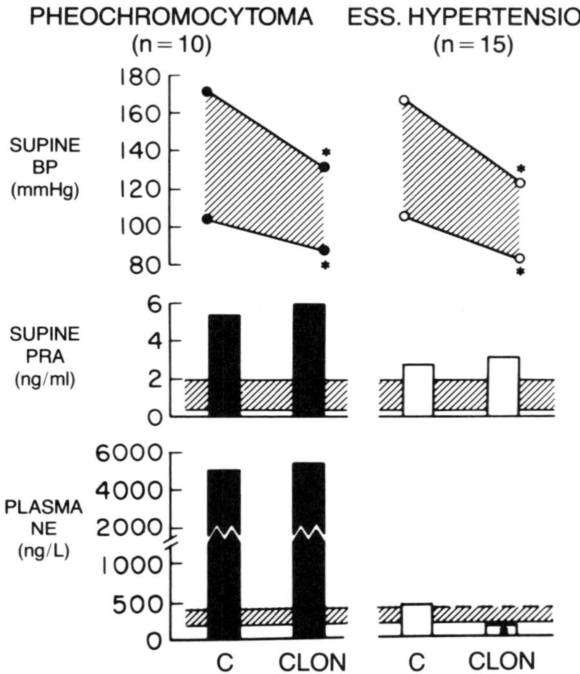

FIGURE 7. Graphic representation of the cardiovascular and humoral responses of 10 patients with proved pheochromocytoma and 15 patients with essential hypertension. For plasma renin activity (PRA) and plasma norepinephrine (NE), the cross-hatched areas indicate the mean (± 2 SD) of values obtained from healthy adult subjects of similar age. (Data from Bravo et al. [18] with permission.)

Other Laboratory Abnormalities

Abnormal laboratory findings associated with pheochromocytoma are listed in Table 5.

Preoperative Localization: Noninvasive vs. Invasive Procedures

Once the diagnosis of pheochromocytoma is confirmed by biochemical and/or provocative tests, it is mandatory to localize the tumor prior to surgical resection. The recent development of sensitive, noninvasive localization procedures such as the computed tomography and adrenal scintigraphy with 131_I-labeled metaiodobenzyl-guanide (MIBG) have revolutionized the approach to tumor localization (56,175,188). These noninvasive procedures have virtually replaced the need for the traditional invasive procedures such as retroperitoneal pneumography, intravenous pyelography, and selective angiography. Abrams et al. (1) compared the

TABLE 5. Abnormal Laboratory Findings in Pheochromocytoma

Abnormal finding	Mechanism(s)	References
1. Carbohydrate intolerance	1. Enhanced glucose production and demand for glucose uptake (α-adrenergic mechanisms) 2. Decreased peripheral sensitivity to insulin-secondary to elevated FFA 3. Direct inhibitory effect of catecholamines on insulin release (α-adrenergic mechanism)	Spergel (172)
2. Elevated plasma free fatty acid	Activation of lipase in adipose tissue	Engelman et al. (51) Rizack (155)
3. Elevated basal metabolic rate	Secondary to elevated FFA	Gifford (64)
4. Polycythemia	1. Increased erythropoietin production (direct) 2. Vasoconstriction of renal vessels leading to renal hypoxia	Bradley (16) Donati (44) Jacob (90)
5. Leukocytosis	Increase mobilization of neutrophils	Samuels (160)
6. Decreased plasma and total blood volume	1. Prolonged vasoconstriction 2. Reduced red cell mass	Johns and Brunges (95) Tarazi (183) Bergman et al. (12)
7. Increased plasma renin and aldosterone	1. Compression of renal artery by tumor 2. Vasoconstriction of renal vessels 3. Direct effect of catecholamines on juxtaglomerular cells and proximal tubular reabsorption of sodium 4. Volume contraction	Maebashi (116) Hiner (82) Van Way and Michelakis (191)
8. Proteinuria (mild to moderate)	Unknown	Howard (85)
9. Uncommon: elevated cholesterol erythrocyte sedimentation rate, BUN, anemia		

Rizza, R. A., et al. (1980) Adrenergic mechanism for the effects of epinephrine in glucose production and clearance in man. J. Clin. Invest 65:682–689.

sensitivity, specificity and accuracy of the computed tomography with ultrasound in 112 patients suspected of adrenal disorder. The sensitivity, specificity, and accuracy of the computed tomography is 84%–98% as compared to 61%–79% for ultrasound. One limitation with the computed tomography is the size of the tumor. In general, a tumor smaller than 1 cm is not easily detected by this procedure. Welch et al. (196) reported the Mayo Clinic experience with the computed tomography from 1976 to 1982 in 60 histologically proved pheochromocytoma and found that this procedure correctly identified 38 out of 41 single intraadrenal tumors, nine out of 10 bilateral adrenal tumors, and eight out of 11 of recurrent tumors. In total, computed tomography correctly localized 51 out of 57 (89%) of the tumors. This procedure only missed two out of five ectopic pheochromocytoma both were found in the organ of Zuckerkandl. From the same institution, van Heerden et al. (189) reported the diagnostic accuracy of computed tomography to be 95% and false negative results in 5%–6%. Stewart et al. (175) from the Cleveland Clinic reported that the diagnostic capacity and false positivity of computed tomography is the same as selective angiography, namely 91% and 9%, respectively. They believe that selective angiography is unnecessary unless the computed tomography fails to localize the tumor. Other utility of the computed tomography includes the identification of metastatic disease, recurrent pheochomocytoma, and tumor localization in patients with MEN syndrome with either normal or equivocal biochemical values (196). Thus, for most hospitals, computed tomography should be the initial localization procedure.

Sission et al. (168) at the University of Michigan popularized the use of 131_I-MIBG as a localization procedure. In their first report, this procedure successfully localized the tumor in four patients who had negative computed tomography. This radiopharmaceutic agent concentrates in adrenal medulla and all adrenergic tissues by competitive inhibition of norepinephrine at catecholamine-storage granules. The uptake of 131_I-MIBG is not inhibited by phenoxybenzamine, propanolol, or a methylparatyrosine but is significantly reduced by tricyclic antidepressant and reserpine (168). Beierwaltes (11) cited five advantages of this localization procedure over computed tomography: 1) a biochemical confirmation of the mass identified by computed tomography; 2) specific diagnosis of pheochromocytoma; 3) detection of extraadrenal pheochromocytoma, especially in the thorax and abdomen; 4) detection of residual pheochromocytoma tissue postoperatively; 5) diagnosis and treatment of malignant pheochromocytoma.

Francis (57) reviewed the advantages and limitations of the 131_I-MIBG scanning technique (Figure 8). Several advantages of this technique over computed tomography include: specificity for pheochromocytoma, ability to image the entire body, and absence of image degradation by surgical clips. The limitations of the MIBG scan include nonavailability of the pharmaceutic tracer, wide range of avidity of both normal and abnormal adrenergic tissues for the tracer, tumor uptake either overlapping with normal adrenal tissue or totally absent. In addition, since this tracer is excreted by the kidney and the bladder, it is difficult to use this technique

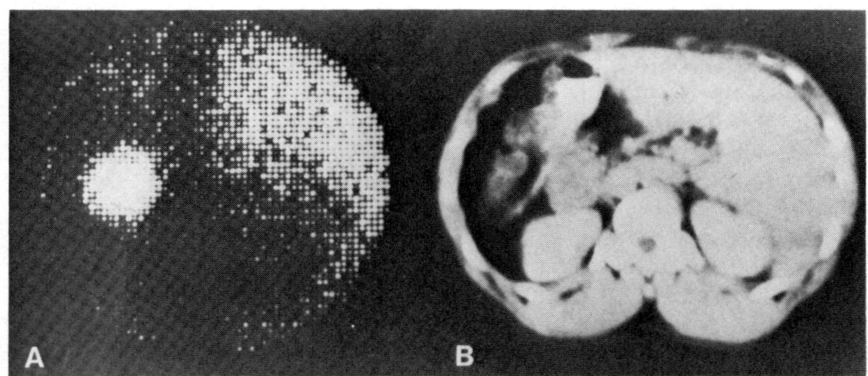

FIGURE 8. **(A)** First pheochromocytoma demonstrated by radionuclide scanning (liver uptake on right but right normal adrenal not imaged). **(B)** CT (reversed to match radionuclide scan) showing "tumor" in front of upper end of left kidney. (Data from Beierwaltes [11] with permission.)

to diagnose pheochromocytoma of the bladder. However, computed tomography may compliment the MIGB scan in several conditions (186). If the MIBG scan is equivocal, computed tomography scan may be helpful. When extraadrenal pheochromocytoma is diagnosed by the MIBG scan, then computed tomography can be used to evaluate local anatomy, especially in the case of suspected intrathoracic tumor. At the University of Michigan, angiography is reserved for the rare patient with negative computed tomography and MIBG scans. As time goes on, this new technique may replace computed tomography as the initial localizing procedure. In short, the recent development of the computed tomography and MIBG scans have not only improved the diagnostic accuracy of tumor localization but also significantly reduce the cost of making the diagnosis since both procedures could be done on the out-patient basis.

Palpation of a neck mass or abdominal mass resulting in reproducing the patient's symptoms with confirmatory elevation of plasma or urinary catecholamines obviously negates the need for any preoperative localization procedure. Likewise, micturition induced attacks of praoxymal hypertension with biochemical confirmation clinches the diagnosis of pheochromocytoma in the bladder without the need for further investigative procedure except cystoscopy. Fluoroscopy plus oblique views of the chest to look at the paravertebral sulcus are at times helpful in detecting small intrathoracic tumor.

TREATMENT: MEDICAL AND SURGICAL

Once the diagnosis of pheochromocytoma is made, with or without localization of the tumor, the patient is usually managed medically with adrenergic antagonists before surgical resection of the tumor. In addition, these adrenergic antagonists are reserved for the long-term use in patients who have metabolic malignant pheochromocytoma or in those who are not surgical candidates because of serious medical complications. The primary objective in the use of these pharmacologic agents is to control the clinical manifestations of catecholamine excess, normalization of blood pressure, pulse rate, electrocardiographic changes, and blood volume.

Norepinephrine is mainly an alpha-stimulator, while epinephrine has mixed alpha-beta-adrenergic effects. Cardiac adrenergic receptors are purely beta in nature. Phenoxybenzamine (Dibenzyline) was first reported by Johns and Brunjes in 1962 to be an effective adrenergic antagonist (95). It inactivates alpha-adrenergic receptors by formation of a stable bond. Orally, it is estimated that only 25% is absorbed; most patients require between 40mg and 60 mg/day. Although its duration is 24 hours and theoretically once-a-day dosage is sufficient, it is recommended that the dose be divided to avoid or minimize any gastrointestinal side effects. If the initial 40 mg/day is not sufficient to achieve therapeutic goal, then an increase of 10–20 mg/day is suggested. Effective adrenergic blockade is usually seen in 5 days to 2 weeks. Blood pressure is controlled in anywhere from 1 to 3 weeks, although complete alpha blockade is usually not obtainable in most patients. The end-point of therapy is a decrease in blood pressure, sweating, weakness and cessation of attack. Roizen set down several criteria for adequate control with phenoxybenzamine prior to surgery: 1) blood pressure less than 165/90 mmHg observed 48 hours before surgery; 2) presence of mild orthostatic hypotension (less than 80/45 mmHg); 3) EKG free of ST or T wave changes for 2 weeks; 4) no more than one premature ventricular contraction every 5 minutes (156). In addition to postural hypotension, nasal stuffiness, inhibition of ejaculation, and tachycardia are other side effects from this drug. Cautious use of phenoxybenzamine is warranted in those patients with severe atherosclerosis or those with significant reduction in renal blood flow. The physician needs to decide whether these preexisting diseases are likely to be improved or worsened when blood pressure is lowered.

Phentolamine (Regitine) is another alpha-adrenergic antagonist used for rapid correction of hypertensive episodes during an attack. The three main side effects are: 1) cardiac stimulation leading to tachycardia, arrhythmia, angina or myocardial infarction; 2) gastrointestinal stimulation leading to abdominal cramps, diarrhea and vomiting; and 3) histamine-like peripheral vasodilation.

Prazosin, a specific α_1-postsynaptic antagonist possesses several unique characteristics which make it a useful adjunct to the α-adrenergic blocking agents (137). In contrast to the nonselective α-adrenergic antagonists, the hypotensive action of this drug is not accompanied by reflex tachycardia. Second, the biologic action of this drug is long enough to allow once a day administration. Third, complete α-blockade is not seen even with chronic therapy. Cubeddu et al. (36) recommend starting with very low doses (0.5 mg) and with patient remaining in bed for 3 hours after the first dose. The same precaution applies to escalating prazosin doses in those patients with coexistent hemoconcentration or recently treated with low sodium diet, diuretic or β blockers. Daily doses should be given in equally divided doses every 6 hours with close monitoring of standing blood pressure. Unlike patients with essential hypertension, patients with pheochromocytoma are exquisitely sensitive to the hypotensive effect after the first dose. In Cubeddu's series, two patients given 1-mg doses of prazosin experienced symptomatic hypotension with fall in systolic blood pressure (74–92 mmHg) and diastolic blood pressure (65–78 mmHg). Most patients with pheochromocytoma require 6–10 mg of this drug. Even though prazosin may be as effective as phenoxybenzamine in terms of blood pressure control, initial experience with this drug shows that the incomplete α-blockade may expose the patient to cardiovascular instability during the induction of anesthesia and surgical resection of the tumor. Thus, additional phenoxybenzamine is often needed.

Beta-adrenergic receptor blockade with propranolol should not be used in the absence of adequate alpha-adrenergic blockade. Prichard and Ross (147) first recommended beta-blockade in pheochromocytoma patients as a useful adjunct to alpha-adrenergic blocking agents. The usual oral dose of propranolol in pheochromocytoma patients is 10 mg three to four times a day although some may require as high as 200 mg/day. Labetalol, a combined α- and β- blocking drug, has been used in Europe with good results in patients with pheochromocytoma (152). However, the predominant β blockade may result in rise in blood pressure.

Tyrosine hydroxylase mediates the rate-limiting step in catecholamine synthesis (tyrosine to dopa). Catecholamine analogues, especially alpha-methylparatyrosine, have been moderately effective in decreasing catecholamine synthesis both in vivo and in vitro (52). In Engelman's study of normal subjects and pheochromocytoma patients, administration of alpha-methylparatyrosine 1–4 g/day orally, resulted in 50%–80% decrease in catecholamine synthesis and normalization of blood pressure in pheochromocytoma patients (52). Atuk recommended starting this drug with 250 mg twice daily and gradually escalating the dose by another 250–500 mg/day and then wait 1 to 2 days to observe clinical response before any further increase in dose. With 2–2.5 g/day, acceptable decrease in catecholamine synthesis is expected. This drug should be started 5–10 days prior to surgery. Addition of other α-blocking agent may be needed in patients with elevated plasma catecholamines. This drug is associated with several unpleasant, dose-dependent side effects such as sleepiness, diarrhea, crystalluria, and extrapyramidal symptoms.

There is a general consensus that α-adrenergic blocking agents should be used preoperatively to control the blood pressure and other unpleasant symptoms of catecholamine excess. However, there is controversy whether or not complete α-blockade is desirable. Reasons cited for α-blockade include the control of unpleasant symptoms from catecholamine excess, reversal of hypovolemia, reduction of hypertensive episode during surgery, reduction of catecholamine-induced myocarditis, better maternal/fetal outcome, protection of myocardial performance, and tissue oxygenation from adverse effects from catecholamines (157). Opponents to complete α-blockade invoke the following reasons. First, it prevents discovery of small tumor during surgery. Second, it prevents the recognition of the second tumor by persistent hypertension after surgical removal of the first tumor. Third, it causes pronounced hypotension after tumor resection, more tachycardia with bleeding, and more oozing of blood during surgery. Last, it increases sensitivity to the hypotensive effects of thiopental and hemorrhage. Desmonts et al. (42) reported no preoperative mortality in 88 patients who did not receive any α-adrenergic blocking agents preoperatively. Even with adequate preoperative α-blocking agents, hypertensive crises can still occur during surgery. Gitlow et al. (65) prefer to switch their patients from oral to parenteral α-adrenergic blocking agents 24 to 48 hours prior to surgery. In van Heerden's series, all but 8 of 106 pheochromocytoma patients received α-adrenergic blocking agents at least 2 weeks plus β-blockers 3 days prior to surgery. They felt that these drugs did not result in total adrenergic blockade but appeared to reduce intraoperative arrhythmias. Manger and Gifford (119) argued that operative morbidity and mortality in highly experienced hands is equally good whether or not preoperative α-and β- blocking agents are used. They recommend that the preoperative therapeutic approach be flexible and individualized.

Surgery of Pheochromocytoma

Nowhere in clinical medicine is the team effort of internist, anesthetist, pharmacologist, and surgeon more needed than in the preoperative, intraoperative, and postoperative management of patients with pheochromocytomas.

Prior to 1950, the mortality from pheochromocytoma in recognized cases ranged from 20% to 25%. In unrecognized cases, the mortality was over 50%. Today, with the advances in our knowledge of adrenolytic agents the pathophysiologies and the many conditions associated with pheochromocytoma, the operative mortality is less than 3% at the Mayo Clinic and at Columbia Presbyterian Medical Center and is zero in 46 cases (40,153) at the Cleveland Clinic. In a 26-year period (1950−1976), Scott et al. (164) reported one fatality out of 32 cases. The unacceptably high operative mortality prior to 1950 was due to 1) hypertensive crisis after induction of anesthesia or surgeon handling the tumor, 2) sudden hypotension immediately after surgical resection of the tumor, and 3) arrhythmias due to the sudden release of catecholamines and/or anesthetic agent sensitizing the myocardium.

The anesthesiologist plays an important role in the surgical management of pheochromocytoma. An excellent review by Desmonts and Marty (43) summarizes various pharmacologic agents used during the induction and maintenance of anesthesia. Induction with thiopental is commonly used. In small doses, thiopental has been shown to reduce plasma catecholamines (96). Halothane, enflurane, and isoflurane have all been used in pheochromocytoma patients. Halothane is to be avoided since it sensitizes the myocardium to catecholamines by reducing the arrhythmogenic threshold for epinephrine (122). On the other hand, enflurane and isoflurane have given good results with low occurrence of arrhythmia (107). Neuroleptanalgesia has been used successfully during surgery, i.e., droperidol, with either fentanyl or phenoperidine. Circulating plasma catecholamines during surgery have been found to be related to the depth of anesthesia (156). This observation is consistent with the clinical experience of van Heerden et al. (189) from the Mayo Clinic who believe that the plane of anesthesia is more important than the specific anesthetic agent used. Vecuronium and pancuronium have been used with few complications. However, gallamine, tubocurare, and sexamethonium are to be avoided because of undesirable side effects.

Regardless of whether or not α-blocking agents are used preoperatively, most patients will experience systolic hypertension (over 200 mmHg) sometime during the intraoperative period. Desmonts and Marty (43) found two distinct origins of elevations of blood pressure. First, noxious stimuli during tracheal intubation, skin incision, and abdominal exploration can cause hypertension which is not consistently related to either an increase in plasma catecholamines or significant hemodynamic changes. Second, palpation of the tumor invariably causes hypertension, marked increase in plasma catecholamines, systemic vascular resistance, and pulmonary wedge pressure. If systolic blood pressure exceed 200 mmHg for over 1 minute, Desmonts and Marty recommend giving one of the following drugs intravenously: Phentolamine, nitroprusside, nitroglycerin, or labetalol (43). Intraoperative arrhythmias, usually premature ventricular contractions, are treated with either intravenous propanolol or lidocaine. Because of lidocaine's short duration of action and lack of negative inotropic effects, many anethesiologists consider it the drug of choice in managing arrhythmia during surgery. Deoreo et al. (40) from the Cleveland Clinic showed that preoperative blood transfusion significantly reduced the incidence of intraoperative hypotension.

A detailed description of the surgical techniques is beyond the scope of this chapter. Interested readers are referred to an excellent monograph by Eddis et al. (48). The anterior transabdominal (transperitoneal) approach is favored by most surgeons; this is because 10% of pheochromocytomas are extraadrenal and, although the tumor is localized preoperatively, up to 8% of adults and 35% of children may harbor multiple tumors. Stewart et al. (175) recommend 1) vertical midline approach in children or when ectopic pheochromocytoma is suspected; and 2) thoracoabdominal nephroadrenalectomy in patients with large tumors, especially on the right side. For patients with MEN type II, total adrenalectomy is indicated because of the high recurrence rate plus accumulating evidence that adrenal hyperplasia precedes the development of pheochromocytoma (89). The general principles of pheochromocytoma surgery are: 1) recognition of the fact that each pheochromocytoma is potentially malignant, and thus it is mandatory for the surgeon to examine all viscera, concentrating on sites where chromaffin tissue is usually found (paraaortic area, lumbar ganglia, perirenal area, organ of Zuckerkandl, pelvis, bladder); 2) recognition of the fact that pheochromocytoma may be bilateral, especially in children and those with MEN syndromes; 3) removal of tumors with capsule intact since fragmentation of the tumor can cause seeding and subsequent recurrence; 4) wide dissection of nearby tissue; 5) palpation of each adrenal and of organs with chromaffin tissue, and noting changes in blood pressure and pulse; 6) removal of any metastases that are found, thus reducing the amount of functioning tissue; 7) after tumor removal if blood pressure failed to decrease a prompt search for a second tumor; 8) right-sided pheochromocytoma usually lies behind the vena cava and dissection may be associated with massive hemorrhage. The four deaths from the Mayo Clinic series of 130 patients were due to uncontrolled hemorrhage. During the immediate postoperative period hypotension and hypertension may be found. Hypotension may be due to one or more mechanisms: 1) alteration of vascular compliance after excision of tumor; 2) residual effect of preoperative medications, i.e., phenoxybenzamine, since it takes 36 hours to dissipate the adrenergic blockade; 3) loss of blood into third space or oozing from incision site (98). On rare occasions, hypotension may be due to myocardial infarction or inadequate steroid replacement in those who underwent bilateral adrenalectomy. Bergman et al. (12) at the National Institutes of Health studied the fluid replacement postoperatively in five patients who underwent surgery and found that they needed anywhere from 3.6 to 8.6 L of fluid during the first day after surgery. Manger and Gifford (119) recommended that the systolic blood pressure be kept at 90–100 mmHg and that intraarterial blood pressure be monitored during the immediate postoperative period in patients with unstable blood pressure. Hypertension during the immediate postoperative period is most likely due to return of normal autonomic reflexes and functional hypervolemic state. This could best be managed by intravenous furosemide. The next most likely cause is residual pheochromocytoma. Response to phentolamine is strong confirmatory evidence that this is indeed the cause. Inadvertent ligation of the renal artery may cause postoperative hypertension.

Mortality rates from the surgical procedure ranges from 17.4% from the Cleveland Clinics to 35% from Vanderbilt, and were higher in the transabdominal approach than in posterior lumbar approach (40,164).

Surgical removal of the tumor usually normalizes the blood pressure. However, the plasma and urinary catecholamines and/or metabolites may remain elevated for several days up to 1 month postoperatively. This may be due to either slow inactivation of circulating catecholamines or excess storage of catecholamines from sympathetic nerves and other tissues.

The 5-year survival in benign tumor is 96%, and for malignant tumor it is 44% (153). In 20%–30% of postoperative patients, blood pressure fails to return to normal. This is especially true in those who had sustained hypertension preoperatively. In the Mayo Clinic series, 28 out of 103 patients remained hypertensive postoperatively. Of these, 10 had sustained hypertension preoperatively, nine had paroxysmal hypertension, and one had MEN syndrome. In the series from Vanderbilt, Scott et al. (164) found that 18 of 27 patients with benign pheochromocytoma remained normotensive 1–20 years postoperatively. The reason for the persistent hypertension is unclear. It could be due to essential hypertension or vascular damage from the hypertension. Postoperative hypertension can be managed with the usual antihypertensive medications.

Surgical treatment of pheochromocytoma during pregnancy deserves consideration. There were 128 cases reported in the literature of pheochromocytoma complicating pregnancy (177). It is important to screen all pregnant females with sustained or paroxysmal hypertension, especially in the presence of typical symptoms and signs of pheochromocytoma. Only 42 of 128 cases were diagnosed prior to delivery. From Schenker and Chowers' series (163), the maternal and fetal mortality were 58% and 55%, respectively, if the diagnosis of pheochromocytoma was not made antepartum. However, if the diagnosis was made, the maternal and fetal mortality were reduced to 18% and 50%, respectively. The general consensus is that an aggressive surgical attempt has to be made whenever pheochromocytoma is diagnosed. Temporary management with alpha- and beta-adrenergic drugs is indicated. If a patient is close to term, it may be technically difficult to remove a pheochromocytoma. In this case, blocking agents are used until term. Fetal maturity shuld be carefully followed. Griffith et al. (75) have successfully managed a pregnant woman with phenoxybenzamine from the 24th to 37th week. Cesarean section followed by adrenalectomy is done with the usual precautions described above.

Malignant pheochromocytoma occurs in 1%–13% of patients and in those patients with extraadrenal pheochromocytoma. The incidence may go up to 30%. In the Mayo Clinic series there were 18 patients with malignant pheochromocytoma (153). The mean survival after surgery was 5.6 years with a range 1 month to 17 years. A few patients did not show evidence of recurrent tumors for many years after surgery. This fact underlines the importance of close follow-up in every postoperative case. Those patients with pulmonary metastases have the worse prognosis. Drasin (45) summarized the cases in the world literature in whom palliative radiotherapy and/or chemotherapy were used. He concluded that chemotherapy with doxorubin hydrochloride and cyclophosphamide in combination with radiation therapy controlled skeletal metastases for about 5 months, when disease progression was again noted. The effects of streptozocin on metastatic pheochromocytoma are mixed (55, 78). A promising agent is 131_I-MIBG which was reported to bring about both subjective and objective benefits in two out of five patients with metastatic pheochromocytoma (11,169).

SUMMARY

Among 35 million Americans with diastolic hypertension, approximately 0.1% have pheochromocytoma. Close to 90% of pheochromocytoma arises from the adrenal gland itself, and the extraadrenal sites include the paraganglia cells of the sympathetic nervous system, the organ of Zuckerkandl, wall of the bladder, paraantic regions, chest, neck, the hilus of the liver, or kidney. Multiple and extraadrenal pheochromocytomas are more common in children. Familial pheochromocytoma is an autosomal dominant disease that is frequently bilateral. About 10% of pheochromocytomas are malignant; histopathologic characteristics fail to distinguish between benign and malignant tumors. The only reliable criteria of malignancy is the presence of metastases or invasion of adjacent tissue. Clinically, pheochromocytoma mimics many diseases. Patients usually have a constellation of symptoms such as severe headache (72%–92%), sweating (60%–70%), palpitations (51%–73%), and hypertension (> 90%). The hypertension could be either sustained (50%–60%) or paroxysmal (about 50%). Symptomatic attacks may be quite variable, anywhere from once every few months to several times daily lasting from less than a minute to a week. Many precipitating factors have been identified, including a variety of drugs. Physical maneuvers, even micturition, can precipitate an attack. Myocarditis, cardiomyopathy, and myocardial infarction have all been associated with pheochromocytoma. Most bladder tumors occur in the adolescent age group between 10 and 19 years. In unsuspected pheochromocytoma in pregnancy, there is a very high maternal and fetal mortality rate.

Symptoms and signs in children with pheochromocytoma differ in several ways from those seen in adults: 90% have sustained hypertension; polydipsia, polyuria, and convulsions are more common. Males predominate and a higher incidence of bilateral and extraadrenal pheochromocytomas exists. Tumors in familial pheochromocytomas are bilateral and frequently associated with the multiple endocrine neuroplasia (MEN) types IIa and IIb or neurocutaneous dysplasias (von Recklinghausen's disease, tuberous sclerosis, Sturge–Weber syndrome, von Hippel-Lindau's disease). It is especially important to screen for pheochromocytoma in MEN Types IIa and IIb since a high percentage of the patients are normotensive and/or asymptomatic.

Urinary metanephrine is the single most reliable screening test for the presence of this tumor since more than 95% of the patients will demonstrate elevated values. Since the list of drugs that are known to interfere with the determination of urinary catecholamines is a large one, it is advisable that all drugs be discontinued for at least 1 week before a urine is collected. Plasma catecholamine is of particular diagnostic importance during a paroxysmal attack. Increased concentration of epinephrine or metanephrine in the urine and/or an elevated plasma epinephrine concentration strongly suggest an adrenal tumor. Preoperative localization of the tumor can be done with various noninvasive, sensitive techniques such as computed tomography and 131_I-MIBG scanning. Computerized tomography appears to be as good as most invasive radiologic procedures. A controversy exists as to whether an alpha-adrenergic blocking agent should be used prior to these invasive procedures. Nonetheless, it is well to remember that any diagnostic procedure that entails minor trauma or stress to the patient could potentially induce an attack. Preoperative beta-blockade is indicated in the presence of tachycardia or angina pectoris only after adequate alpha-blockade. Careful monitoring and prompt control of hypertensive crises (sodium nitroprusside) and arrhythmias (propranolol, lidocaine) are critical to the success of surgery. To prevent postoperative hypotension, correction of blood volume deficit is of paramount importance. In a pregnant patient with pheochromocytoma, it is desirable to remove the tumor especially if it is discovered during the first two trimesters. If the tumor is discovered in the third trimester and the patient can be satisfactorily managed with adrenergic blockade, one could wait until full term and subject the patient to a cesarean section to remove the tumor. In case of malignant tumor with metastases, the therapeutic goal is to remove as much functional tumor tissue as possible. Chemotherapy and/or radiotherapy for this condition have not been too successful. In a few patients, Streptozocin and 131_I-MIBG showed promising results. The 5-year survival of benign tumors is close to 96%, whereas it is only 44% for those with malignant tumors. About 75% of the patients in the successful surgical removal of their tumors become normotensive. Recurrences of pheochromocytoma could appear up to 10 years postoperatively. Those patients with familial pheochromocytoma should be followed for the rest of their life.

Acknowledgement. The author wishes to thank Drs. T. S. Harrison and S. Y. Tan for their helpful comments during the preparation of this chapter.

REFERENCES

1. Abrams, H. L., Siegelman, S. S., Adams, D. F., Sanders, R., Finberg, B. J. Hessell, S. J., and McNeil, B. J. (1982) Computed tomography versus ultrasound of the adrenal gland: A prospective study. Radiology 143, 121–128.
2. Alberts, W. M., McMeekin, J. O., and George, J. M. (1980) Mixed multiple endocrine neoplasia syndromes. JAMA 244, 1236–1237.
3. Allen, J. A., and Raddie, I. C. (1972) The role of circulating catecholamines in sweat production in man. J. Physiol. 227, 801–814.
4. Anderson, R. J. Lufkin, E. G., Sizemore, G. W., Carney, J. A., Sheps, S. G., and Silliman, Y. E. (1981) Acromegaly and pituitary adenoma with phaeochromocytoma: A variant of multiple endocrine neoplasia. Clin. Endocrinol. 14, 605–612.
5. Anton, A. H., Greer, M., Sayre, D. F., and Williams, C. M. (1967) Dihydroxyphenylalanine secretion in a malignant pheochromocytoma. Am. J. Med. 42, 469–475.
6. Aron, D. C., Bravo, E. L., and Kapcala, L. P. (1983) Erroneous plasma norepinephrine levels in radioimmunoassay. Ann. Intern. Med. 98, 1023.
7. Atuk, N. O., McDonald, T., Wood, T., Carpenter, J. T., Walzak, M. P., Donaldson, M., and Gillenwater, J. Y. (1979) Familial pheochromocytoma, hypercalcemia, and von Hippel-Lindau disease. Medicine 58, 209–218.
8. Atuk, N. O. (1983) Pheochromocytoma: Diagnosis, localization and treatment. Hosp. Pract. 18, 187–202.
9. Barnard, P. J., and Jacobson, L. (1965) Malignant phaeochromocytoma associated with argentaffinoma and hypotensive crises: Report of a case. Cent. Afr. J. Med. II, 185–190.
10. Baylin, S. B. (1975) Ectopic production of hormones and other proteins by tumors. Hosp. Pract. 10(10), 117–126.
11. Beierwaltes, W. H. (1983) The localization and treatment of pheochromocytomas with 131_I-MIBG. In: N. W. Thompson and A. I. Vinik (eds.), Endocrine Surgery, Grune and Stratton, New York, pp. 139–150.

12. Bergmann, S. M., Sears, H. F., Jaradpour, N., and Keiser, H. R. (1978) Postoperative management of patients with pheochromocytoma. J. Urol. 120, 109–112.
13. Bertagna, X., Pique, L., Ochoa, C., Luton, J. P., Bricaire, H., Serin, D., Girard, F., Plouin, P. F., Corvol, P., Cesselin, F., and Hamon, M. (1982) Simultaneous measurement of β-endorphin, lipotrophins and metenkephalin in phaeochromocytomas. Acta Endocrinol. 101,72–77.
14. Besterman, E., Bromley, L. L., and Peart, W. S. (1974) An intrapericardial pheochromocytoma. Br. Heart J. 36, 318–320.
15. Blackwell, B., Marley, E., Price, J., and Taylor, D. (1967) Hypertensive interactions between monoamine oxidase inhibitors and foodstuffs. Br. J. Psychiatry 113, 349–365.
16. Bradley, E., Jr., Young, J. D. Jr., and Lentz, G. (1961) Polycythemia secondary to pheochromocytoma. J. Urol. 86, 1–6.
17. Bravo, E. L., Tarazi, R. C., Fouad, F. M., Vidt, D. G., and Gifford, R. W., Jr. (1981) Clonidine suppression test: A useful aid in the diagnosis of pheochromocytoma. N Engl. J. Med. 305, 623–626.
18. Bravo, E. L., Tarazi, R. C., Fouad, F. M., Textor, S. C., Gifford, R. W. Jr. and Vidt, D. G. (1982) Blood pressure regulation in pheochromocytoma. Hypertension 4 (suppl. II), 193–199.
19. Bravo, E. L., and Gifford, R. W. (1984) Pheochromocytoma: Diagnosis, localization and management. N. Engl. J. Med. 311, 1298–1303.
20. Brown, M. J., Allison, D. J., Jenner, D. A., Lewis, P. J., and Dollery, C. T. (1981) Increased sensitivity and accuracy of phaeochromocytoma diagnosis achieved by use of plasma-adrenaline estimations and a pentolinium-suppression test. Lancet 1, 174–177.
21. Brown, M. J. (1984) Simultaneous assay of noradrenaline and its deaminiated metabolites, dihydroxyphenylglycol, in plasma: A simplified approach to the exclusion of phaeochromocytoma in patients with borderline elevation of plasma noradrenaline concentration. Eur. J. Clin. Invest. 14, 67–72.
22. Burris, J. F., D'Angelo, L. J. (1982) Complications of clonidine suppression test for pheochromocytoma. N. Engl. J. Med. 307, 756–757.
23. Calkins, E., and Howard, J. E (1947) Bilateral familial phaeochromocytoma with paroxysmal hypertension: Successful removal of tumors in two cases, with discussion of certain diagnostic procedures and physiological considerations. J. Clin. Endocrinol 7, 475–492.
24. Carmen, C. T., and Brasher, R. E. (1960) Pheochromocytoma as an inherited abnormality. N. Engl. J. Med. 263, 417–423.
25. Carney, J. A., Sizemore, G. W., and Tyce, G. M. (1975) Bilateral adrenal medullary hyperplasia in multiple endocrine neoplasia, type II. The precursor of bilateral pheochromocytoma. Mayo Clinic Proc. 50, 3–10.
26. Carney, J. A., Go, V. L. W., Sizemore, G. W., and Hayles, A. B. (1976) Alimentary-tract ganglioneuromatosis. A major component of the syndrome of multiple neoplasia, type 2b. N. Engl. J. Med. 295, 1287–1291.
27. Carney, J. A., Go, V. L. W., Gordon, H., Northcutt, R. C., Pearse, A. G. E., and Sheps, S. G. (1980) Familial pheochromocytoma and islet cell tumor of the pancreas. Am. J. Med. 68, 515-521.
28. Catalona, W. J., Engleman, K., Ketcham, A. S., and Hammond, W. G. (1971) Familial medullary thyroid carcinoma, pheochromocytoma, and parathyroid adenoma (Sipple's Syndrome). Cancer 28, 1245–1254.
29. Cerny, J. C., Jackson, C. E., Talpos, G. B., Yott, J. B., and Lee, M. W. (1982) Pheochromocytoma in multiple endocrine neoplasia type II: An example of the two-hit theory of neoplasia. Surgery 92, 849–852.
30. Cheng, T. O., and Bashour, T. T. (1976) Striking cardiographic changes associated with pheochromocytoma masquerading as ischemic heart disease. Chest 70, 397–399.
31. Corder, R., Emson, P. C., and Lowry, P. J. (1984) Purification and characterization of human neuropeptide Y from adrenal-medullary phaeochromocytoma tissue. Biochem. J. 219, 699–706.

32. Coupland, R. E. (1965) The Natural History of the Chromaffin Cell. Longmans, Green and Co., London, p. 279.
33. Crout, J. R. (1966) Catecholamine metabolism in pheochromocytoma and essential hypertension. In W. M. Manger (ed.), Hormones and Hypertension, C. C. Thomas, Springfield, IL, pp. 3–40.
34. Cryer, P. E. (1976) Isotope-derivative measurements of plasma norepinephrine and epinephrine in man. Diabetes 25, 1071–1082.
35. Cryer, P. E. (1980) Physiology and pathophysiology of the human sympathoadrenal neuroendocrine system. N. Engl. J. Med. 303, 436–444.
36. Cubeddu, J. X., Zarate, N. A., Rosales, C. B., and Zschaech, D. W. (1982) Prazosin and propranolol in preoperative management of pheochromocytoma. Clin. Pharm. Ther. 32, 156–160.
37. Daggett, P., and Franks, S. (1977) Steroid responsiveness in pheochromocytomas. Br. Med. J. 1, 84.
38. Davis, P., Peart, W. S., and van't Hoff, W. (1955) Malignant phaeochromocytoma with functioning metastases. Lancet 2, 274–275.
39. Dean, R. E. (1958) Pheochromocytoma and pregnancy. Obstet. Gynecol. 11, 35–42.
40. Deoreo, G. A., Jr., Stewart, B. H., Tarazi, R. C., and Gifford, R. W., Jr. (1974) Preoperative blood transfusion in the safe surgical management of pheochromocytoma: a review of 46 cases. J. Urol. 111, 715–721.
41. Desai, P. B. (1959) Microscopic phaeochromocytoma of the adrenal. Indian J. Surg. 21, 1–7.
42. Desmonts, J. M., LeHouelleur, J., Remond, P., and Duvaledestin, P. (1977) Anaesthetic management of patients with phaeochromocytoma. A review of 102 cases. Br. J. Anaesth. 49, 991–998.
43. Desmonts, J. M., and Marty, J. (1984) Anaesthetic management of patients with phaeochromocytoma. Br. J. Anaesth. 56, 781–788.
44. Donati, R. M., McCarthy, J. M., Lange, R. D., and Gallagher, N. I. (1963) Erythrocythemia and neoplastic tumors. Ann. Intern. Med. 58, 47–55.
45. Drasin, H. (1978) Treatment of malignant pheochromocytoma. West. J. Med. 128, 106–111.
46. Ducatman, B. S., Scheithauer, B. W., van Heerden, J. A., and Sheedy, P. F. (1983) Simultaneous phaeochromocytoma and renal cell carcinoma: Report of a case and review of the literature. Br. J. Surg. 70, 415–418.
47. Dunn, F. G., de Carvalho, J. G. R., Kem, D. C., Higgins, J. R., and Frohlich, E. D. (1976) Pheochromocytoma crisis induced by saralasin. New Eng. J. Med. 295, 605–607.
48. Eddis, J. A., Ayala, L. A., and Egdahl, R. H. (1975) Manual of Endocrine Surgery. New York, Heidelberg, Berlin, Springer–Verlag.
49. Eisenberg, A. A., and Wallerstein, H. (1932) Pheochromocytoma of the suprarenal medulla (paraganglioma). Arch. Pathol. 14, 818–836.
50. Engel, A., and von Euler, U. S. (1950) Diagnostic value of increased urinary output of noradrenaline in pheochromocytoma. Lancet 2, 387.
51. Engelman, K., Mueller, P. S., and Sjoerdsma, A. (1964) Elevated plasma free fatty acid concentrations in patients with pheochromocytoma. Changes with therapy and correlations with the basal metabolic rate. N. Eng. J. Med. 270, 865–870.
52. Engelman, K., Horwitz, D., Jequier, E., and Sjoerdsma, A. (1968) Biochemical and pharmacologic effects of α-methyltyrosine in man. J. Clin. Invest. 47, 577–594.
53. Engleman, K., and Portnoy, B. (1970) A sensitive double-isotope derivative assay for norepinephrine and epinephrine. Cir. Res. 26, 53–57.
54. Feldman, J. M., Blalock, J. A., Zern, R. T., and Wells, S. A. (1979) The relationship between enzyme activity and the catecholamine content and secretion of pheochromocytomas. J. Clin. Endo. Meta. 49, 445–451.
55. Feldman, J. M., (1983) Treatment of metastatic pheochromocytoma with streptozocin. Arch. Intern. Med. 143:1799–1800.

56. Fisher, M., Vetter, W., Winterberg, B., Hengstmann, J., Zidek, W., Friemann, J. and Vetter, H. (1984) Scintigraphic localization of phaeochromocytomas. Clin. Endocrinol. 20, 1–7.
57. Francis, I. R., Glazer, G. M., Shapiro, B., Sisson, J. C., and Gross, B. H. (1983) Complementary roles of CT and 131I MIBG scintigraphy in diagnosing pheochromocytoma. Am. J. Rad. 141, 719–725.
58. Frankel, F. (1886) Ein Fall von doppelseitigem, völlig latent verlaufenen Nebennierentumor und gleichzeitiger Nephritis mit Veranderungen am Circulationsapparat und Retinitis. Virchows Arch. Pathol. Anat. Physiol. 103, 244–263.
59. Ganguly, A., Henry, D. P., Yune, H. Y., Pratt, J. H., Grim, C. E., Donohue, J. P., and Weinberger, M. H. (1979) Diagnosis and localization of pheochromocytoma: Detection by measurement of urinary norepinephrine excretion during sleep, plasma norepinephrine concentration and computerized axial tomography (CT-scan). Am. J. Med. 67, 21–26.
60. Ganguly, A., Grim, C. E., Weinberger, M. H., and Henry, D. P. (1984) Rapid cyclic fluctuations of blood pressure associated with an adrenal pheochromocytoma. Hypertension 6, 281–284.
61. Geffen, L. B., Rush, R. A., Louis, W. J., and Doyle, A. E. (1973) Plasma catecholamine and dopamine-β-hydroxylase amounts in phaeochromocytoma. Clin. Sci. 44, 421–424.
62. Gemmell, A. A. (1955) Phaeochromocytoma and the obstetrician. J. Obstet. Gynaecol. Br. Commonw. 62, 195–202.
63. Gifford, R. W., Jr., Kvale, W. F., Maher, F. T., Roth, G. M., and Priestley, J. T. (1964) Clinical features, diagnosis and treatment of pheochromocytoma: A review of 76 cases. Mayo Clin. Proc. 39, 281–302.
64. Gifford, R. W., Jr. (1961) Hypertensive emergencies and their treatment. Med. Clin. North Am. 45, 441–452.
65. Gitlow, S. E., Mendlowitz, M., Wilk, E. K., Wilk, S., Wolf, R. L., and Bertani, L. M. (1968) Excretion of catecholamine metabolites by normal children. J. Lab. Clin. Med. 72, 612–620.
66. Gitlow, S. E., Mendlowitz, M., and Bertani, L. M. (1970) The biochemical techniques for detecting and establishing the presence of a pheochromocytoma. A review of ten years' experience. Am. J. Cardiol. 26, 270–279.
67. Gitlow, S. E., Pertsemlidis, D., and Dziedzic, S. W. (1983) Pheochromocytoma. In: D. T. Krieger and C. W. Bardin (eds.), Current Therapy in Endocrinology, C. V. Mosby Co., St. Louis, pp. 110–117.
68. Gittes, R. F. and Mahoney, E. M. (1977) Pheochromocytoma. Urologic Clinics of North America 4(2), 239–256.
69. Given, B. G., Taylor, T., Lilly, L. S., and Dzau, V. J. (1983) Symptomatic hypotension following the clinidine suppression test for pheochromocytoma. Arch. Intern. Med. 143, 2195–2196.
70. Goodall, McC., and Stone, C. (1960) Adrenaline and noradrenaline producing tumors of the adrenal medulla and sympathetic nerves. Ann. Surg. 151, 391–398.
71. Gorlin, R. J., Sedano, H. O., Vickers, R. A., and Cervenka, J. (1968) Multiple mucosal neuromas, pheochromocytoma and medullary carcinoma of the thyroid—a syndrome. Cancer 22, 293–299.
72. Graham, J. B. (1951) Pheochromocytoma and hypertension. An analysis of 207 cases. Int. Abst. Surg. 92, 105–121.
73. Gravier, M., Bernheim, M. (1924) Cancer bilateral des glandes surrenales avec generalisation mediastinale et syphilis pulmonaire concomitant. Lyon Med. 134, 223.
74. Greenacre, J. K., Conally, M. E. (1978) Desensitization of the beta-adrenoceptor of lymphocytes from normal subjects and patients with pheochromocytoma: Studies in vivo. Br. J. Clin. Pharmacol. 5, 191–197.
75. Griffith, M. I., Felts, J. H., James, F. M., Meyers, R. T., Shealy, G. M., and Woodruff, L. F., Jr. (1974) Successful control of pheochromocytoma in pregnancy. J. Am. Med. Assoc. 229, 437–439.

76. Gupta, K. K. (1975) Pheochromocytoma and myocardial infarction. Lancet 1, 281–282.

77. Hamilton, B. P., Landsberg, L., and Levine, R. J. (1978) Measurement of urinary epinephrine in screening for pheochromocytoma in multiple endocrine neoplasia type II. Am. J. Med. 65, 1027–1032.

78. Hamilton, B. P. M., Cheikh, I. E., and Rivera, L. E. (1977) Attempted treatment of inoperable pheochromocytoma with streptozotocin. Arch. Intern. Med. 137, 762–765.

79. Hassoun, J., Monges, G., Giraud, P., Henry, J. F., Charpin, C., Payan, H., and Toga, M. (1984) Immunohistochemical study of pheochromocytomas: An investigation of methionine-enkaphalin, vasoactive intestinal peptide, somatostatin, corticotropin, β-endorphin and calcitonin in 16 tumors. Am. J. Pathol. 114, 56–63.

80. Hermann, H., and Mornex, R. (1964) Human tumours secreting catecholamines: Clinical and physiopathological study of the pheochromocytomas. Pergamon, Oxford, New York, pp. 207.

81. Hill, C. S., Ibanez, M. L., Samaan, N. A., Ahern, M. J., and Clark, R. L. (1973) Medullary (solid) carcinoma of the thyroid gland: An analysis of the M.D. Anderson Hospital experience with patients with the tumor, its special features and its histogenesis. Medicine 52, 141–171.

82. Hiner, L. B., Gruskin, A. B., Baluarte, H. J., Cote, M. L., Sapire, D. W., and Levitsky, D. (1976) Plasma renin activity and intrarenal blood flow distribution in a child with a pheochromocytoma. J. Pediatr. 89, 950–952.

83. Hjemdahl, P. (1984) Catecholamine measurements by high-performance liquid chromatography. Am. J. Physiol. 247, E 13–20.

84. Hollenhorst, R. W. (1948) The ocular changes associated with pheochromocytoma. Am. J. Med. Sci. 216, 226–233.

85. Howard, J. E., and Barker, W. H. (1937) Paroxysmal hypertension and other clinical manifestations associated with benign chromaffin cell tumors (phaeochromocytoma). Bull. Johns Hopkins Hosp. 61, 371–410.

86. Huang, S. K., Rosenberg, M. J., and Denes, P. (1984) Short PR interval and narrow QRS complex associated with pheochromocytoma electrophysiologic observations. J. Am. Coll. Cardiol. 3, 872–875.

87. Hume, D. M. (1960) Pheochromocytoma in the adult and in the child. Am. J. Surg. 99, 458–496.

88. Imura, H., Kato, Y., Masaki, I., Masachika, M., and Mikio, Y. (1971) Effect of adrenergic blocking or stimulating agents on plasma GH, IRI and blood FFA levels in man. J. Clin. Invest. 50, 1069–1079.

89. Irvin, G. L., Fishman, L. M., and Sher, J. A. (1983) Familial pheochromocytoma. Surgery 93, 938–941.

90. Jacob, H. S. (1974) The polycythemias and their relationship to erythropoietin. In: Dowling, H. F., ed., Disease-a-Month, Chicago, Year Book Medical Publishers, August.

91. Jaffe, B. M. (1978) The diarrheagenic syndrome: Verner-Morrison WDHA syndrome in: S. R. Friesen and R. E. Bolinger (eds.), Surgical Endocrinology: Clinical Syndromes, J. B. Lippincott Co., Philadelphia, pp. 215–235.

92. James, R. E., Baker, H. L., Jr., and Scanlon, P. W. (1972) The roentgenologic aspects of metastatic pheochromocytoma. Am. J. Roentgenol. Radium Ther. Nucl. Med. 115, 783–793.

93. Jelliffe, R. S. (1952) Phaeochromocytoma presenting as a cardiac and abdominal catastrophe. Br. Med. J. 2, 76–77.

94. Jiang, N.-S., Stoffer, S. S., Pikler, G. M., Wadel, O., and Sheps, S. G. (1973) Laboratory and clinical observations with a two-column plasma catecholamine assay. Mayo Clin. Proc. 48, 47–49.

95. Johns, V. J., Jr., and Brunjes, S. (1962) Pheochromocytoma. Am. J. Cardiol. 9, 120–125.

96. Joyce, J. T., Roizen, M. F., and Eger, E. I. (1983) Effects of thiopental induction on sympathetic activity. Anesthesiology 59, 19–22.

97. Kaplan, N. M., Kramer, N. J., Holland, O. B., Sheps, S. G., and Gromez-Sanchez, C. (1977) Single-voided urine metanephrine assays in screening for pheochromocytoma. Arch.Int. Med. 137, 190–193.

98. Kaplan, N. A. (1978) Clinical Hypertension. Medcom Press, New York.

99. Kaplan, N. M. (1982) Pheochromocytoma. In: Clinical Hypertension, 3 ed. Williams and Wilkins, Baltimore, ch. 10.

100. Kaufman, B. H., Telander, R. L., van Heerden, J. A., Zimmerman, D., Sheps, S. G., and Dawson, B. (1983) Pheochromocytoma in the pediatric age groups: Current status. J. Ped. Surg. 18, 879–884.

101. Kaufmann, J. F. (1974) Pheochromocytoma and tricyclic antidepressants. JAMA 229, 1282.

102. Kawashima, K. (1911) Uber einen Fall von maltiplen Hautfibromen met Nebennierengeschwulst. Virchows. Arch. 203, 66–74.

103. Khairi, M. R. A., Dexter, R. N., Burzynski, N. J., and Johnston, C. C., Jr. (1975) Mucosal neuroma, pheochromocytoma and medullary thyroid carcinoma: Multiple endocrine neophasia type 3. Medicine 54, 89–112.

104. Kirkendahl, W. M., Liechty, R. D., and Culp, D. A. (1965) Diagnosis and treatment of patients with pheochromocytoma. Arch. Intern. Med. 115, 529–536.

105. Kline, I. K. (1961) Myocardial alterations associated with pheochromocytomas. Am. J. Pathol. 38, 539–552.

106. Kohn, A. (1902) Das chromaffine Gewebe. Z. Anat. Entwicklungsgesch. 12, 253.

107. Kreul, J. F., Dauchot, P. J. and Anton, A. M. (1976) Hemodynamic and catecholamine studies during pheochromocytoma. Anesthesiology 44, 265–268.

108. Kuchel, O., Hamet, P., Buu, N. T., et al. (1981) Basis of false-positive glucagon tests for pheochromocytoma. Clin. Pharmacol. Ther. 29, 687–694.

109. Kuchel, O., Buu, N. T., Bourque, M., Hamet, P., and Larochelle, P. (1982) The hemodynamic relevance of free and conjugated dopamine in pheochromocytoma. J. Clini. Endo. Metab. 54, 1268–1270.

110. Kukreja, S. C., Hargis, G. K., Rosenthal, I. M., and Williams, G. A. (1973) Pheochromocytoma causing excessive parathyroid hormone production and hypercalcemia. Ann. Intern. Med. 79, 838–840.

111. L'abbé, M., Tinel, J., and Doumer, E. (1922) Crises solaires et hypertension paroxystique en rapport avec une tumeur surrénale. Bull. Soc. Méd. Hôp. 46, 982–990.

112. Levinson, P. D., Hamilton, B. P., Mersey, J. H., and Kowarski, A. A. (1983) Plasma norepinephrine and epinephrine responses to glucagon in patients with suspected pheochromocytomas. Metabolism 32, 998–1001.

113. Ljungberg, O., Cederquist, E., and von Studnitz, W. (1967) Medullary thyroid carcinomas and pheochromocytoma: A familial chromaffinomatosis. Br. Med. J. 1, 279–281.

114. Lloyd, R. V., Shapiro, B., Sisson, J. C., Kalff, V., Thompson, N. W., and Beierwalter, W. A. (1984) An immunohistochemical study of pheochromocytomas. Arch Pathol. Lab. Med 108, 541–544.

115. Louis, W. J., Doyle, A. E., Heath, W. C., and Robinson, M. J. (1972) Secretion of dopa in phaeochromocytoma. Br. Med. J. 4, 325–327.

116. Maebashi, M., Miura, Y., Yoshinaga, K., and Sato, K. (1968) Plasma renin activity in pheochromocytoma. Jpn. Circ. J. 32, 1427–1432.

117. Maloney, J. M. (1955) Pheochromocytoma in pregnancy. N. Engl. J. Med. 253, 242–243.

118. Manasse, P. (1896) Zur histologie and histogenese der primären nierengeschwülste. Virchows. Arch. Pathol. Anat. 145, 113–157.

119. Manger, W. M., and Gifford, R. W. (1977) Pheochromocytoma. Springer-Verlag, New York.

120. Manger, W. M., Wakim, K. G., and Bollman, L. J. (1959) Chemical Quantitation of Epinephrine and Norepinephrine in Plasma. C. C. Thomas, Springfield, IL, p. 398.

121. Manley, E., and Blackwell, B. (1970) Interactions of monoamine oxidase inhibitors, amines, and foodstuffs. Adv. Pharmacol. Chemother. 8, 185–239.
122. Maze, M., and Mason, D. M. (1983) Aetiology and treatment of halothane-induced arrhythmias. In: R. I. Mazze (ed.), Inhalation Anaesthesiology, W. B. Saunders, Philadelphia, p. 301.
123. Melicow, M. M., Uson, A. C., and Veenema, R. J. (1973) Malignant non-functioning pheochromocytoma of the organ of Zuckerkandl masquerading as a primary carcinoma of the prostate with metastases. J. Urol. 110, 97–103.
124. Messerli, F. H., Finn, M., and MacPhee, A. A. (1982) Pheochromocytoma of the urinary bladder: Systemic hemodynamics and circulating catecholamine levels. JAMA 247, 1863–1864.
125. Miller, G. L., and Wynn, J. (1971) Acromegaly, pheochromocytoma, toxic goiter, diabetes mellitus and endometriosis. Arch. Intern. Med. 127, 299–303.
126. Miller, S. S., Sizemore, G. W., Sheps, S. G., and Tyce, G. M. (1975) Parathyroid function in patients with pheochromocytoma. Ann. Intern. Med. 82, 372–375.
127. Minno, A. M., Bennett, W. A., and Kvale, W. F. (1954) Pheochromocytoma. A study of 15 cases diagnosed at autopsy. N. Engl. J. Med. 251, 959–965.
128. Minopoli, M. and Bordi, C. (1983) Changing patterns of sex distribution in familial medullary carcinoma of the thyroid and associated phaeochromocytoma. Clin. Endo. 18, 645–648.
129. Misugi, K., Misugi, N., and Newton, W. A. (1968) Fine structural study of neuroblastoma, ganglioneuroblastoma, and pheochromocytoma. Arch. Pathol. 86, 160–170.
130. Modlin, I. M., Farndon, J. R., Sheperd, A., Johnston, I. D. A., Kennedy, T. L., Montgomery, D. A. D., and Welbourn, R. B. (1979) Phaeochromocytomas in 72 patients: clinical and diagnostic features, treatment and long term results. Br. J. Surg. 66, 456–465.
131. Moertel, C. G., Beahrs, O. H., Wooner, L. B., and Tyce, G. M. (1965) "Malignant carcinoid syndrome" associated with non-carcinoid tumors. N. Engl. J. Med. 273, 244–248.
132. Moon, H. D., Koneff, A. A., Li, C. C., and Simpson, M. E. (1956) Pheochromocytomas of adrenals in male rats chronically injected with pituitary growth hormone. Proc. Soc. Exp. Biol. Med. 93, 74–77.
133. Moorhead, E. L. II, Caldwell, J. R., Kelly, A. R. and Morales, A. R. (1966) The diagnosis of pheochromocytoma. Analysis of 26 cases. JAMA 196, 1107–1113.
134. Mulrow, P. J., Cohn, G. L., and Yesner, R. R. (1959) Isolation of cortisol from a pheochromocytoma. Yale J. Biol. Med. 31, 363–372.
135. Nakano, Y., Imura, H., Yawata, M., Shinpo, S., Ikeda, M., Morimoto, M., Manabe, S., Kato, Y., and Fukase, M. (1968) In: D. G. Mexico (ed.), 3rd International Congress of Endocrinology. Abstracts of brief communications, Excerpta Medica Foundation, Amsterdam, New York, p. 63.
136. Neff, F. C., Tice, G. M., Walker, G. A., and Ockerblad, N. (1942) Adrenal tumor in female infant with hypertrichosis, hypertension, overdevelopment of external genitalia, obesity, but absence of breast enlargement. J. Clin. Endocrinol. 2, 125–127.
137. Nicholson, J. P. Jr., Vaughn, D., Jr., Pickering, T. G., et al. (1983) Pheochromocytoma and prazosin Ann. Intern. Med. 99, 477–479.
138. Ochi, K., Yoshioka, S., Morita, M., Takeuchi, M. (1981) Pheochromocytoma of bladder. Urology 17, 228–230.
139. O'Connor, D. T., Frigon, R. P., and Deftos, L. J. (1983) Immunoreactive calcitonin in catecholamine storage vesicles of human pheochromocytoma. J. Clin. Endocrinol. Metab. 56, 582–585.
140. Page, L. R., and Copeland, R. B. (1968) Pheochromocytoma. In: H. F. Dowling (ed.), Disease-a-Month, Chicago Year Book Medical Publishers, Chicago, January.
141. Pearse, A. G. E. (1968) Common cytochemical and ultrastructural characteristics of cells producing polypeptide hormones (the APUD series) and their relevance to

thyroid and ultimobranchial C cells and calcitonin. Proc. R. Soc. London, Ser. B 170, 71–80.

142. Pearse, A. G. E. (1978) The APUD Concept: Embryology, cytochemistry and ultrastructure of the diffuse neuroendocrine system. In: S. R. Frisen and R. E. Bolinger (eds.), Surgical Endocrinology: Clinical Syndromes, J. B. Lippincott, Philadelphia, pp. 18–34.
143. Peelen, J. W., and DeGroat, A. (1955) Pheochromocytoma complicated by pregnancy: Case report. Am. J. Obstet. Gynec. 69, 1054–1061.
144. Pick, L. (1912) Das Ganglioma embryonale sympathicum (Sympathoma embryonale), eine typische bösartige geschwuestform des sympathischen nervensystems. Ber. Klin. Wochenschr. 49, 16–22.
145. Pisano, J. J. (1960) A simple analysis for normetanephrine and metanephrine in urine. Clin. Chim. Acta 5, 406–414.
146. Plouin, P. F., Duclos, J. M., Menard J., Comoy, E., Bohuon, C., and Alexandre, J. M. (1981) Biochemical tests for diagnosis of phaeochromocytoma: Urinary versus plasma determinations. Br. Med J. 282, 853–854.
147. Prichard, B. N. C., and Ross, E. J. (1966) Use of propranolol in conjunction with alpha receptor blocking drugs in pheochromocytoma. Am. J. Cardiol. 18, 394–398.
148. Pugh, R. C. B., Gresham, G. A., and Mullaney, J. (1960) Pheochromocytoma of the urinary bladder. J. Path. Bact. 79, 89–107.
149. Radtke, W. E., Kazmier, F. J., Rutherford, B. D., and Sheps, S. G. (1975) Cardiovascular complications of pheochromocytoma crisis. Am. J. Cardiol. 35, 701–705.
150. Ramsay, I. D., and Langlands, J. H. M. (1962) Phaeochromocytoma with hypotension and polycythaemia. Lancet 2, 126–128.
151. Raum, W. J. (1984) Methods of plasma catecholamine measurement including radioimmunoassay. Am. J. Physiol. 247, E4–12.
152. Reach, G., Thibonnier, M., Chevillard, C., Corvol, P., and Milliez, P. (1980) Effect of labetalol on blood pressure and plasma catecholamine concentrations in patients with phaeochromocytoma. Br. Med. J. 3, 1300–1301.
153. Remine, W. H., Chong, G. C., van Heerden, J. A., Sheps, S. G., and Harrison, E. G., Jr. (1974) Current management of pheochromocytoma. Ann. Surg. 179, 740–748.
154. Reimer, R. (1927) Sobre um caso de syndrome de Addison produzida por "paraganglioma da capsula suprarenal." Folha Med. 8, 3.
155. Rizack, M. A. (1966) An epinephrine-sensitive lipolytic activity in adipose tissue. J. Biol. Chem. 236, 657-662.
155a. Rizza, R. A., Cryer, P. E., Haymond, M. W., and Gerich, J. E. (1980) Adrenergic mechanism for the effects of epiphrine in glucose production and clearance in man. J. Clin. Invest. 65, 682–689.
156. Roizen, M. F., Horigan, R. W., Frazer, B. M. (1981) Anesthetic doses blocking adrenergic (stress) and cardiovascular responses to incision. Anesthesiology 54, 390–398.
157. Roizen, M. F., Hunt, T. K., Beaupre, P. N., et al. (1983) The effect of alpha-adrenergic blockade on cardiac performance and tissue oxygen delivery during excision of pheochromocytoma. Surgery 82, 941–945.
158. Russell, D. S., and Rubenstein, L. J. (1971) In: C. E. Lumsden (ed.), Pathology of Tumours of the Nervous System, 3rd edition, Williams and Wilkins, Baltimore, p. 344.
159. Saint-Pierre, A., Lejosne, Ch., and Perrin, A. (1974) Aspects electrocardiographiques des pheochromocytomes. Coeur Med. Interne 13, 59–73.
160. Samuels, A. J. (1951) Primary and secondary leucocyte changes following the intramuscular injection of epinephrine hydrochloride. J. Clin. Invest. 30, 941–947.
161. Sano, T., Saito, H., Inaba, H. et al. (1983) Immunoreactive somatostatin and vasoactive intestinal polypeptide in adrenal pheochromocytoma: An immunochemical and ultrastructural study. Cancer 52, 282–289.
162. Sayer, W. J., Moser, M., and Mattingly, T. W. (1954) Pheochromocytoma and the abnormal electrocardiogram. Am. Heart J. 48, 42–53.

163. Schenker, J. G., and Chowers, I. (1971) Pheochromocytoma and pregnancy. Obstet. and Gynecol. Surg. 26, 739–747.
163a. Schonebeck, J. (1969) Malignant pheochromocytoma. Scand. J. Urol. Nephrol. 3, 64–68.
164. Scott, H. W., Jr., Oates, J. A., Nies, A. S., Burko, H., Page, D. L., and Rhamy, R. K. (1976) Pheochromocytoma: Present diagnosis and management. Ann. Surg. 183, 587–593.
165. Shapiro, B., Sisson, J. C., Lloyd, R., Nakajo, M., Satterlee, W., and Beierwaltes, W. H. (1984) Malignant phaeochromocytoma: Clinical, biochemical and scintigraphic characterization. Clin. Endocrinol. 20, 289–203.
166. Sherwin, R. P. (1968) The adrenal medulla, paraganglia and related tissues. In: J. M. B. Bloodworth, Jr. (ed.), Endocrine Pathology. Williams and Wilkins, Baltimore, pp. 256–315.
167. Sipple, J. H. (1961) The association of pheochromocytoma with carcinoma of the thyroid gland. Am. J. Med. 31, 163–166.
168. Sission, J. C., Frager, M. S., Valk, T. W., et al. (1981) Scintigraphic localization of pheochromocytoma. N. Engl. J. Med. 305, 12–17.
169. Sission, J. C., Shapiro, B., Beierwaltes, W. H., et al. (1984) Radiopharmaceutical treatment of malignant pheochromocytoma. J. Nucl. Med. 25, 197–207.
169a. Sjoerdoma, A., Engman, A., Waldman, K. et al. (1966) Pheochromocytoma: Current concepts of diagnosis and treatment. Ann. Int. Med. 65, 1302–1305.
170. Sloand, C. M., and Thompson, B. T. (1984) Propranolol-induced pulmonary edema and shock in a patient with pheochromocytoma. Arch. Intern. Med. 144, 173–174.
171. Smithwick, R. H., Greer, W. E. R., Robertson, C. W., and Wilkins, R. W. (1950). Pheochromocytoma: A discussion of symptoms, signs and procedures of diagnostic value. N. Engl. J. Med. 242, 252–257.
172. Spergel, G., Bleicher, S. J., and Ertel, N. H. (1968). Carbohydrate and fat metabolism in patients with pheochromocytoma. N. Engl. J. Med. 278, 803–809.
173. Stackpole, R. H., Melicow, M. M., and Uson, A. C. (1963) Pheochromocytoma in children. Pediatrics 63, 315–330.
174. Steiner, A. L., Goodman, A. D., and Powers, S. R. (1968). Study of a kindred with pheochromocytoma, medullary thyroid carcinoma, hyperparathyroidism and Cushing's disease: Multiple endocrine neoplasia, type 2. Medicine 47, 371–409.
175. Stewart, B. H., Bravo, E. L., Haaga, J., Meaney, T. F., and Tarazi, R. (1978). Localization of pheochromocytoma by computed tomography. N. Engl. J. Med. 299, 460–461.
176. Stewart, B. H. (1983) Adrenal surgery-current state of the art. J. Urol. 129, 1-7.
177. Stonham, J., and Wakefield, C. (1983) Pheochromocytoma in pregnancy. Anesthesia 38, 654–658.
178. Suda, T., Tomori, N., Tozawa, F., et al. (1984) Immunoreactive corticotropin and corticotropin-releasing factor in human hypothalamus, adrenal, lung cancer, and pheochromocytoma. J. Clin. Endocrinol. Metab. 58, 919–923.
179. Suda, T., Tozawa, F., Tachibana, S., et al. (1983) Multiple forms of immunoreactive dynorphin in human pituitary and pheochromocytoma. Life Sci. 32, 865–870.
180. Sutton, St. J. M. G., Sheps, S. G., and Lie, J. T. (1981) Prevalence of clinically unsuspected pheochromocytoma: Review of 50-year autopsy series. Mayo Clin. Proc. 56, 354–360.
181. Symington, T., and Goodall, A. L. (1953) Studies in phaeochromocytoma: I. Pathological aspects. Glasgow Med. J. 34, 75–96.
182. Tannenbaum, M. (1970) Ultrastructural pathology of adrenal medullary tumors. In: S. C. Sommers (ed.), Pathology Annual. Appleton-Century-Croft, New York, pp. 145–171.
183. Tarazi, R. C., Frohlich, E. D., and Dustan, H. P. (1971) Plasma volume changes with long-term beta-adrenergic blockade. Am. Heart J. 82, 770–776.

184. Taub, M. A., Osburne, R. C., Georges, L. P., and Sode, J. (1982) Malignant pheochromoctyoma: Severe clinical exacerbation and release of stored catecholamines during lymphoma chemotherapy. Cancer 50, 1739–1741.

185. Thomas, J. E., Rooke, E. D., and Kvale, W. F. (1966) The neurologist's experience with pheochromocytoma. A review of 100 cases. J. Am. Med. Assoc. 197, 754–758.

186. Thomas, J. L., Bernardino, M. E., Samaan, N. A., and Hickey, R. C. (1980) CT of pheochromocytoma. Am. J. Radio. 135, 477–482.

187. Trump, D. L., Livingston, J. N., Baylin, S. B. (1977) Watery diarrhea syndrome in an adult with ganglioneuroma pheochromocytoma. Cancer 40, 1526–1532.

188. Valk, T. W., Frager, M. S., Gross, M. D., et al. (1981) Spectrum of pheochromocytoma in multiple endocrine neoplasia. Ann. Intern. Med. 94, 762–767.

189. Van Heerden, J. A., Sheps, S. G., Hamberger, B., et al. (1982) Pheochromocytoma: Current status and changing trends. Surgery 91, 367–373.

190. Van Vliet, P. D., Burchell, H. B., and Titus, J. L. (1966) Focal myocarditis associated with pheochromocytoma. N. Engl. J. Med. 274, 1102–1108.

191. Van Way, C. W., III, Michelakie, A. M., Alper, B. J.,Hutcheson, J. K., Rhamy, R. K., Scott, H. W., Jr. (1970) Renal vein renin studies in a patient with renal hilar pheochromocytoma and renal artery stenosis. Ann Surg 172, 212–217.

192. Velasquez, G., D'Souzam, V. J., Hackshaw, B. T., et al. (1984) Phaeochromocytoma and cardiomyopathy. Br. J. Radio. 57, 89–92.

193. Voorhess, M. L., Stuart, M. J., Stockman, J. A., and Oski, F. A. (1975) Iron deficiency anemia and increased urinary norepinephrine excretion. J. Pediatr. 86, 542–547.

194. Voute, P. A., Jr., Wadman, S. K., and van Putten, W. J. (1970) Congenital neuroblastoma. Symptoms in the mother during pregnancy. Clin. Pediatr. J. 9, 206–207.

195. Warren, S., Grozdev, L., Gates, O., and Chute, R. N. (1966) Radiation-induced adrenal medullary tumors in the rat. Arch. Path. 82, 115–118.

196. Welch, T. J., Sheedy, P. F., van Heerden, J. A., Sheps, S. G. et al. (1983) Pheochromocytoma: value of computed tomography. Radiology 48, 501–503.

197. Wilk, E. K., Gitlow, S. E., and Bertani, L. M. (1968) A modification of the Taniguchi method for the determination of normetanephrine and metanephrine. Clin. Chim. Acta 20, 147–148.

198. Yoshimasa, T., Nakao, K., Li, S., et al. (1983) Plasma methionine-enkephalin and leucine-enkephalin in normal subjects and patients with pheochromocytoma. J. Clin. Endocrinol. Metab. 57, 706–712.

199. Zelch, J. V., Meaney, T. F., and Belhobek, G. H. (1974) Radiologic approach to the patient with suspected pheochromocytoma. Radiology 111, 279–284.

200. Zimmerman, I. J., Biron, R. E., and McMahon, H. E. (1953) Pheochromocytomas of the urinary bladder. N. Engl. J. Med. 249, 25–26.

201. Zweifler, A. J., and Julius, S. (1982) Increased platelet catecholamine content in pheochromocytoma: A diagnostic test in patients with elevated plasma catecholamines. N. Engl. J. Med. 306, 890–894.

INDEX

A

Acetylcholine, 23, 24, 25–26
ACTH (adrenocorticotropic hormone), 46, 106, 123–125, 132–133, 140, 141–142, 143–144, 153, 159–160
  familial unresponsiveness to, 291
  plasma levels, in Cushing's syndrome, 266–267
  precursor, 124
  radioimmunoassay, 267–268
  reactions stimulated by, 139–142
  release, 119–123
  secretion, 105–106
  stimulation, 56–57, 58
ACTH receptor, 125, 126–128
ACTH stimulation test, 269
  prolonged, 296
  rapid, 296
ACTH syndrome, ectopic, *See* Ectopic Cushing's syndrome
Actin, 28
Actinomycin D, 90–91, 92, 96, 98
Activation, 178–181
Activity-structure relationships, 189–190
Acute adrenocortical insufficiency, *See* Adrenal crisis
Addison's disease, 284, 301, 403
  autoimmune or idiopathic, 285–288
  clinical manifestations and pathophysiology, 292–294
  definition and historical perspective, 284
  diagnosis, 295–296
  familial types, 291
  incidence, 285
  infection and, 289
  laboratory findings, 294–295
  pathogenesis, 285
  therapy, 299–300
Adenoma, 254–255
  aldosterone-producing, 325
Adenyl cyclase, 135
Adenylate cyclase, 26, 92
Adipose tissue, 174–175
  lipid mobilization and glucose metabolism in, effect of glucocorticoids on, 90–93
Adrenal cortex, 45
  hormone receptors of, 169–191
  hypofunction, *See* Addison's

Adrenal cortex [cont.]
disease, Adrenal insufficiency, Adrenocortical insufficiency
Adrenal crisis, 285, 302–303
Adrenal Cushing's syndrome, 254–255
treatment, 278–279
Adrenal hyperplasia
bilateral, 248, 249–254
congenital, 349–350, 363–376
Adrenal insufficiency, 87, 341, 346
from adrenal hemorrhage, 289
classification, 284–285
differential diagnosis, 297–298
iatrogenic, 289–291
primary, *See* Addison's disease
therapy, 298–300
tuberculosis and other infections and, 289
See also Adrenaocortical insufficiency
Adrenal medulla, 1, 46
Adrenal steroids, *See* Steroids
Adrenalectomy
for Cushing's disease, 275
effects, 86–87, 98, 100, 101, 102, 103
Adrenergic blocking, 416–417, 418
β-Adrenergic receptor, *See* Beta adrenergic receptor
Adrenocortical hypoplasia, 292
Adrenocortical insufficiency
acute, *See* Adrenal crisis
chronic, 292–294
effects, 86–87
primary, *See* Addison's disease
secondary, 300–302
Adrenocortical membrane, 128–132
Adrenocorticoid(s)
abnormalities, 230–237
action, 214–237
colon and, 227–230
water balance and, 224–227
Adrenocorticotropic hormone, *See* ACTH
Adrenogenital syndrome, 363
Adrenoleukodystrophy, 291–292
Adrenoxin, 66, 67
ALD, *See* Adrenoleukodystrophy
Aldactone, 333–334
Aldosterone, 45, 153, 201–202, 227
binding, 176, 202–203
deficiency, 234–235
effect
on energy generation, 211–213
on RNA synthesis, 206
formation, 73–74
-induced proteins, 207–211
induction of protein synthesis, 206–207
metabolism, 77–78
secretion, 162
Aldosterone-producing adenoma, 325
Aldosterone receptor, 204–206
Aldosterone stimulating factor, 153–162
Aldosteronism, 236–237
primary, 325–334
secondary, 336–346
Aldosteronoma, 349
Alkaline phosphatase, 98
Alpha-adrenergic antagonist, 415
Amino acid, uptake, 101
L-Amino acid decarboxylase, aromatic, 6
Aminoglutethimide, *See* Cytadren
cAMP, *See* Cyclic AMP
Amphotericin B, 227
Anatomic-physiologic correlations, 56–59
Androgen(s), 363
formation, 74
Androgen receptors, 190
Androgenital syndrome, *See* Congenital adrenal hyperplasia
Anesthesiology, 417–418
Angiography, for Cushing's syndrome, 271–273
Angiotensin
pressor response to, 102
II, 45–46, 153
III, 157
Anterior pituitary gland, 144
Antiinflammatory agent, glucocorticoids as, 103–105
Apudomas, 386–387
Aromatic-L-amino acid decarboxylase, 6
Arterial supply, 47, 52–53
Ascorbic acid, 142, 143
ATP, 18, 19, 20–21, 22, 185
ATPase, 18, 19, 20, 21
Autoimmune Addison's disease, 285–286

B

Bartter's syndrome, 331t, 332, 344–345
Beta-adrenergic receptor, 416
Bilateral adrenal hyperplasia, 248, 249–250
Bilateral nodular hyperplasia, 325
Binding, nuclear, 181–182
Bladder, *See* Urinary bladder
Blood pressure, in pheochromocytoma, 391
Brain, 173–174, 183–184, 188
Bromocriptine, 277

C

Calcium (CA^{+2}), 25, 97
ions, 132–134
release, 26–27
Calmodulin, 30
Carcinoma, 254–255
Cardiac failure, 341–342

Cardiomyopathy, catecholamine, 394–395
Catecholamine(s), 390, 417
plasma levels, pheochromocytoma and, 407–409
release, 23–32
storage, 13–23
storage complex, 21–23
synthesis, 1, 2–13
urinary free, 404, 405, 406, 407
Catecholamine cardiomyopathy, 394–395
Cell response, to mineralocorticoids, 202–213
Cellular action, 202–213
Central nervous system, 160–161
Children, pheochromocytoma in, 385–386, 396–397
Cholesterol, 139, 140
side chain cleavage, 68–69
Cholesterol demolase, deficiency, 371
Chromaffin, 418
cells, 386
granule, 13–21, 27, 28, 30–31
"Chromaffin system," 384
Chromaffinoma, 386
Chromogranin A, 16
Chromomembrin B, 14
Cirrhosis, *See* Liver, cirrhosis
Citrate, 90
Citric acid cycle, 212
Colon, 201, 227–230
Congenital adrenal hyperplasia (CAH), 349–350, 363–376
Cortex, *See* Adrenal cortex
Cortexolone-receptor complex, 172–173
Cortical collecting tubule, 214–218
Corticosterone, 45
aldosterone formation from, 73–74
Corticotropin-releasing factor (CRF), 121–122, 252–253
Corticotropin-releasing factor stimulation test, 268–269
Cortisol, 45, 87, 89, 91, 94, 96, 104, 105, 202
metabolism, 75–77
plasma levels, in Cushing's syndrome, 263
urinary free, 263
Cortisone, metabolism, 104
CRF, *See* Corticotropin-releasing factor
Cushing's disease, 248, 249–254
treatment, 274–278
Cushing's syndrome, 300, 403
classification and pathogenesis, 248–256
clinical manifestations, 257–261
course and prognosis, 279–280
definition and historical perspective, 247–248
diagnosis, 261
differential, 265–273
tests, 264–265
screening tests, 261–264
treatment, 274–279
complications, 280–281
Cyclic AMP, 26, 88, 92, 100, 134, 135, 136
Cycloheximide, 91, 96–97, 98
Cyproheptadine, 276–277
Cytadren (Aminoglutethimide), 227, 334–335
Cytochrome P-450, 66–68, 71–72, 72–73
Cytosol, 173

D

Deoxycorticosterone (DOC), 87, 103, 156–157
Developmental anatomy, 59–62
Dexamethasone, 91, 92, 93, 98, 103
Dexamethasone-suppressible hyperaldosteronism, 372
Dexamethasone suppression test, 282
high-dose, 265–266
low-dose, 264–265
overnight, 261, 262
Dibenzyline (phenoxybenzamine), 415
Disease states, receptors and, 190
Distal tubule, 214–218
DNA
binding to, 182
synthesis, 94, 98
DOCA, 214, 215, 216–218, 222
Dopamine, 161
Dopamine antagonist, 161
Dopamine-β-hydroxylase, 6–8
Drug-induced hypertensive crisis, 403–404

E

Ectopic ACTH syndrome, *See* Ectopic Cushing's syndrome
Ectopic Cushing's syndrome, 255–256
treatment, 279
Edema
secondary aldosteronism with, 340, 342–343
secondary aldosteronism without, 344–346
Electrocardiographic changes, in pheochromocytoma, 394–395
Electrolyte metabolism, 201–237
disorders, 230–237
Electron, transport, 66–68
Endocrine diseases, associated with pheochromocytoma, 402
β-Endorphins, 106
Energy, generation, 211–213

Enflurane, 417–418
Epinephrine, 1, 87, 390, 392, 417
  synthesis, 8–9
Estrogens, formation, 74
Exocytosis, 23, 25, 32

F

Familial cytomegalic adrenocortical hypoplasia, 292
Fatty acids, release, 91–92
Feedback, 143–144
Feminizing tumor, 283
Fetal zone, 61–62
Fibroblast, 177, 178, 185
Flavin-adenine dinucleotide (FAD), 212
Flavin mononucleotide (FMN), 212
Flavoprotein, 66
Fucose, uptake, 91

G

Gallstones, 403
Gamma amino butyric acid (GABA), 277
Gastronemius muscle, 100
Genetics, related to congenital adrenal hyperplasia, 364–365
Glomerular filtration rate, 224
Glucagon, 92
Glucocorticoid(s), 87, 223–224, 363
  biochemical changes, in target tissues, 94–107
  effects
    on glucose metabolism and uptake, 87–89, 90–93
    on lipid metabolism, 90–93
    on protein metabolism, 93–94
  for congenital adrenal hyperplasia, 373–374
  excess, 235–236
  glomerular filtration rate and, 224
Glucocorticoid receptors
  activation or transformation, 178–181
  distribution, 170–175
  properties, 176–178
Gluconeogenesis, 86
Glucose, 96
  blood levels, 86
  metabolism, 87–89, 90–93, 97
  uptake, 89, 96
Glucose-6-phosphatase, 88
Glucosuria, 87
Glycogen, synthesis, 89
Glycogen phosphorylase, 88
Glycogen synthase, 98
Gross anatomy, 46–49
Growth hormone, 90, 161
  elevation, 402–403
  production, 106–107

H

Halothane, 417
Heart, 90, 184
  effect of glucocorticoids on, 102–103
  murmurs, 393–394
Hemorrhage, adrenal, 289
Hexose monophosphate (HMP) shunt, 212–213
HLA genotyping, 365
Hormonal treatment, for congenital adrenal hyperplasia, 373
Hormone receptors, of adrenal cortex, 169–191
Histamines, 105
Hydrogen (H^+) secretion, 222–223
  renal, 219–223
17-Hydroxycorticosteroids (17-OHCS), urinary levels, in Cushing's syndrome, 263–264
18-Hydroxy-deoxycorticosterone (18-OH DOC), 156, 157, 332, 335
11-Hydroxylase, deficiency, 373
11β-Hydroxylase, deficiency, 369–370
17α-Hydroxylase, deficiency, 370–371
18-Hydroxylase, deficiency, 364, 371–372
21-Hydroxylase, deficiency, 365, 366, 367–369, 373
Hydroxylase system, 11, 18, 72–73
17α-Hydroxylation, 71
21-Hydroxylation, 71–72
3β-Hydroxysteroid, deficiency, 370
3β-Hydroxysteroid dehydrogenase, 69–70
18-Hydroxy-tetrahydro-deoxycortisone (18-OH TH-DOC), 335–336
Hyperaldosteronism, 372
Hypercortisolism, 248
Hyperkalemia, 346
Hypermineralocorticoidism, 325–334, 346–350
Hypertension, 326, 330, 332
  low renin, 334–336
  malignant, 346
  paroxysmal, 390
  in pheochromocytoma, 391, 392
  renovascular, 346
Hypertensive crisis, 403–404, 417
Hypoaldosteronism
  pseudohypoaldosteronism, 350
  selective, 346–350
Hypokalemia, 326, 330, 332
Hypomineralocorticoidism, 346–350
Hyponatremia, 294
Hyporeninemic hypoaldosteronism, 347–349
Hypothalamo-pituitary-adrenocortical system, 145
Hypothalamus, 120, 144, 173
  dysfunction, 253–254

I

Iatrogenic adrenal insufficiency, 289–290
Idiopathic Addison's disease, *See* Autoimmune Addison's disease
Idiopathic edema, 342–343
Immunosuppressive agent, glucocorticosteroids as, 103–105
Indomethacin, 155–156
Insulin, 91
  effects, 90
Insulin hypoglycemia, 297–298
Insulin sensitivity, 98
Insulin tolerance test, 269

J

Juxtaglomerular cells, 154

K

17-Ketosteroid(s), 264
Δ^5-3-Ketosteroid isomerase, 70–71
Kidney, 184

L

L-amino acid decarboxylase, aromatic, 6
"Labile protein," 136–139
Lipid
  mobilization, 90–93
  synthesis, 213
Lipolysis, 92
Lipolytic hormones, 91
β-Lipoprotein, 106
Liver, 86–87, 93–94, 171, 177, 178, 181–182
  cirrhosis, 340–341
  effect of glucocorticoids on, 97–100
  glucocorticoids, 89
  glycogen content, 88
Low renin hypertension, 334–336
Lung, 174, 188
  effect of glucocorticoids on, 101
Lymphocytolysis, 97
Lymphoid tissue, effect of glucocorticoids on, 94–97, 104
Lysosomes, 104

M

Macrophages, 104
Macula densa, 155
Magnesium 161–162
Malignant hypertension, 346
Malignant pheochromocytoma, 400–402
Mammary tissue, 174
Medulla, *See* Adrenal medulla
Medullary collecting duct, 218
α-Melanocyte stimulating hormone (αMSH), 124
β-Melanocyte stimulating hormone (βMSH), 124
Membrane receptors, 184–185
Menstrual cycle, aldosterone during, 337, 338
Messenger RNA, synthesis, 98
Metabolic acidosis, 233
Metanephrines, total, 404, 406, 407
Metastatic destruction of adrenal glands, 290–291
Metergoline, 276, 277
Methyl prednisolone, 93
Metoclopramide, 161
Metopyrone, *See* Metyrapone
Metyrapone (Metopyrone), 277–278
Metyrapone test, 268, 297
MIBG scan, 413–414
Microscopic anatomy, 49–56
Migration inhibiting factor (MIF), 105
Mineralocorticoid(s), 100–101, 101–102, 160–162, 201, 363
  ACTH, 159–160
    See also ACTH
  cellular action, 202–213
  for congenital adrenal hyperplasia, 375
  excess, 236–237
  exogenous, 221–223
  potassium, 158–159
  renin-angiotensin system, 153–157
  resistance to, 234–235
Mineralocorticoid receptors, 175–176, 204–206
Mitochondria, 66–68
Mitotane (o,p'-DDD), 277–278
Molybdate, 180–181
MSH, *See* Melanocyte stimulating hormone
Multiple endocrine neoplasia (MEN)
  type II, 400, 418
  type IIa, 398
  type III, 398, 400
Murmers, 393–394
Muscle, 174
  effect of glucocorticoids on, 100–101
Myosin, 28

N

Nelson's syndrome, 252, 253, 267, 277
Nephrotic syndrome, 342
Neural events, 118–119
Neuroectodermal dysplasias, 402–403
Neurohormones, 119–123
Neutrophils, 105
Nodular hyperplasia, 325
Norepinephrine, 1, 92, 390, 391, 394
Nuclear binding, 181–182
Nuclei, 173

O

Oral contraceptives, 345–346
Organ of Zuckerkandl, 413
Overnight dexamethasone suppression test, 261, 262

P

Paraganglioma, 386
Paroxysmal hypertension, 390
Phenoxybenzamine (Dibenzyline), 415
Phentolamine (Regitine), 415
Phenylethanolamine-N-methyltransferase (PNMT), 8–10
Pheochromocytoma, 383, 420–421
  clinical manifestations, 390–403
  diagnosis, 404–414
  drug-induced hypertensive crisis, 403–404
  etiology, 385–386
  history, 384
  incidence, 384
  malignant, 400–402
  pathology, 386–390
  treatment, 414–420
Phosphatidic acid phosphatase (PAPase), 101
Phosphodiesterase, activity, 92
Phosphoenolpyruvate, 88–89
Phosphoenolpyruvate carboxylase, 99
Phospholipids, 1291–132
Physiologic-anatomic correlations, 56–59
Pituitary-Cushing's syndrome, 248
  treatment, 274–278
Pituitary gland, 173
  anterior, 144
  effect of glucocorticoids on, 105–107
  irradiation, 275–276
  tumors, 252, 253
Pituitary system, control mechanisms in, 117–145
"Polyglandular syndrome," 247
Potassium (K^+), 102, 158–159
  depletion, 219–221
  excretion, 213
  transport, 214
Prazosin, 415–416
Prednisone, 103
  See also Cortisone
Pregnancy
  aldosterone secretion during, 337–339
  pheochromocytoma in, 395–396
  toxemia of, 339–340
Pregnenolone, 68, 69, 139, 140
  conversions from, 69–73
Preoperative localization, of pheochromocytoma, 411–414
Primary adrenocortical insufficiency, *See* Addison's disease
Primary aldosteronism, 325–334
Prolactin, 161
Prolonged ACTH stimulation test, 296
Proopiomelanicortin, 124
Prostacyclin (PGI), 93
Prostaglandin(s), 132, 155, 156
  PGE_1, 93
  prostacyclin, 93
  synthesis, 93
Protein(s)
  aldosterone-induced, 207–211
  binding, 205
  fraction, 162
  labile, 136–139
  metabolism, 93–94
  synthesis, 95–96, 206–207
Provocative tests, for pheochromocytoma, 409–410
Proximal tubule, 214
Pseudohypoaldosteronism, 234, 350
Psychological treatment, for congenital adrenal hyperplasia, 376
Pyridoxal phosphate, 181

R

Radiologic examination, for Cushing's syndrome, 270–271
Rapid ACTH stimulation test, 296
Rapid metyrapone test, 297
Receptor
  concentrations, regulation, 185–187
  correlation of physiologic activity with, 187
  disease states and, 190
  forms, 183–184
  ontogeny of, 187–188
  See also specific receptor
Regitine (phentolamine), 415
Renal H^+ secretion, 219–223
Renal tubule, 201
Renin
  low renin hypertension, 334–336
  plasma levels
    during pregnancy, 338
    in primary aldosteronism, 326
  pressor reponse to, 102
Renin-angiotensin system, 153–157, 293
Renin hypertension, 334–336
Renin-secreting tumor, 331t, 332–333, 346
Renovascular hypertension, 346
RNA, synthesis, 95, 98, 206

S

Salivary ducts, 201
Salt-wasting, 332, 367–368

Secondary adrenal insufficiency, 284, 300–302
Secondary aldosteronism, 335–336
Serotinin, 276
Short-circuit current (SCC), 208, 219
Sipple's syndrome, 399–400
Sodium (Na^2), 102, 160
  absorption, 227–228
  -calcium exchange, 25
  deficiency, 228–229
  effect on tyrosine uptake, 4
  excretion, 213
  transport, 214
Sodium chloride, 102
  loading, 222
Sodium-potassium (Na-K) ATPase, 208, 209–211
Sodium pump, 208
Sodium-wasting, *See* Salt-wasting
Steroid(s)
  biosynthesis, 65–74, 139–142
    inhibitors, 277–278
  hydroxylation, 66–68
  metabolism, 74–78
Steroid-diabetes, 87
Steroidogenesis, 363–364
Stress, 87, 118–119, 119–120
Structure-activity relationships, 189–190
Sugar, uptake, 96
Suprarenal glands, 45–46
  anatomic-physiologic correlations, 56–59
  developmental anatomy, 59–62
  gross anatomy, 46–49
  microscopic anatomy, 49–56
Surficants, 101
Surgical treatment
  for congenital adrenal hyperplasia, 375
  for pheochromocytoma, 417–420
  for primary aldosteronism, 333
Sweat ducts, 201
Synexin, 29, 30

T

T lymphocytes, 104
Target tissues, biochemical changes in, 94–107
Tetrahydro aldosterone, 78
"Tetrahydro" compounds, 75, 76
Thiopental, 417
Thymidine, 95
Thymocytes, 177–178, 185
Thymus cell, 95
Thymus gland, 97
Thyroid carcinoma, 398, 399
Triamcinolone, 223–224
Tryptophan oxygenase activity, 100
Tuberculosis, 289
Tyrosine, transport, 4–5
Tyrosine aminotransferase, 99
Tyrosine hydroxylase, 5–6, 11
  activation, 11–12
  inhibition, 10
  synthesis, 12

U

Urinary bladder, 218–219
  pheochromocytoma of, 397–398

V

^{V}max, 41, 98–99
Vanillylmandelic acid (VMA), 404, 406
Vascular tissue, effect of glucocorticoids on, 101–102
Vasopressin stimulation test, 298
Virilizing tumors, 281–283
VMA, *See* Vanillylmandelic acid
von Hippel-Landau disease, 402
Von Recklinghausen's disease, 402

W

Water
  balance, 224–227
  metabolism, 201–237
    disorders, 230–237

Z

Zona fasciculata, 51, 53, 55, 56, 169
Zona glomerulosa, 49, 51, 53, 57, 157, 169
Zona reticularis, 51, 53, 55, 56, 169